Chronobiotechnology and Chronobiological Engineering

NATO ASI Series

Advanced Science Institutes Series

A Series presenting the results of activities sponsored by the NATO Science Committee, which aims at the dissemination of advanced scientific and technological knowledge, with a view to strengthening links between scientific communities.

The Series is published by an international board of publishers in conjunction with the NATO Scientific Affairs Division

A	Life Sciences	Plenum Publishing Corporation
B	Physics	London and New York
C	Mathematical and Physical Sciences	D. Reidel Publishing Company Dordrecht, Boston, Lancaster and Tokyo
D	Behavioural and Social Sciences	Martinus Nijhoff Publishers Boston, Dordrecht and Lancaster
E	Applied Sciences	
F	Computer and Systems Sciences	Springer-Verlag Berlin, Heidelberg, New York
G	Ecological Sciences	London, Paris, Tokyo
H	Cell Biology	

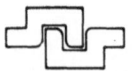

Series E: Applied Sciences – No. 120

Chronobiotechnology and Chronobiological Engineering

Editors:

Lawrence E. Scheving, Ph.D.
Rebsamen Professor Anatomical Sciences
University of Arkansas for Medical Sciences
Little Rock, Arkansas, USA

Franz Halberg, M.D.
Head of Chronobiology Laboratories
Professor of Laboratory Medicine and Pathology
University of Minnesota School of Medicine
Minneapolis, Minnesota, USA

Charles F. Ehret, Ph.D.
Senior Scientist
Argonne National Laboratories
Argonne, Illinois, USA

1987 **Martinus Nijhoff Publishers**
Dordrecht / Boston / Lancaster
Published in cooperation with NATO Scientific Affairs Division

Proceedings of the NATO Advanced Research Workshop on "Chronobiotechnology and Chronobiological Engineering", Cardiff, Wales, UK, April 21–25, 1985

ISBN-13: 978-94-010-8086-6   e-ISBN-13: 978-94-009-3547-1
DOI: 10.1007/978-94-009-3547-1

Distributors for the United States and Canada: Kluwer Academic Publishers, P.O. Box 358, Accord-Station, Hingham, MA 02018-0358, USA

Distributors for the UK and Ireland: Kluwer Academic Publishers, MTP Press Ltd, Falcon House, Queen Square, Lancaster LA1 1RN, UK

Distributors for all other countries: Kluwer Academic Publishers Group, Distribution Center, P.O. Box 322, 3300 AH Dordrecht, The Netherlands

PREFACE

High blood pressure (BP) (with fats and smoking) is one of the three
roots of cardio-cerebro-renovascular disease affecting up to 25% of the
adult population. Hence, high blood pressure should be recognized and
treated, to reduce any complications and prolong life, as noted by Michael
Weber of the Veterans Administration Hospital in Long Beach, California.
He further emphasizes the need for monitoring before one starts the
treatment of high blood pressure. Indeed, he refers to the results of the
Australian study on mild hypertension with a large percentage of placebo-
responders and rightly suggests that many people are treated who should
not be because of 'white-coat-associated high blood pressure'. He also
points to the lack of standardization of techniques for data analysis and
of methods of BP measurement. Ambulatory monitoring under usual conditions without concomitant recording of events does not allow even a
qualitative assessment of the impact of varying stimuli, in Weber's
opinion.

Paolo Scarpelli of the University of Florence proposes several
clinical applications of automatic monitoring, namely in patients with
malignant hypertension and in iatrogenous and hence reversible MESOR-
hypertension. That automatic instrumentation is highly desirable for
young children is another point of the presentation by Scarpelli. He
documents the difficulty in obtaining reliable measurements on 9-year-
olds. Such lack of reliability notwithstanding, he can, by the use of
rhythmometric methods, find differences in the dynamics of BP variability
between groups of 9-year-olds who have or do not have a family history of
high blood pressure. Scarpelli presents such evidence to advocate that
instrumentation yet to be engineered should eventually allow every child
to be reliably and automatically monitored, with event recorders and
soft-ware for rhythm analysis.

The contribution to this volume of the perinatologist Paul Meis is a
logical next step in extending the need for monitoring instrumentation to
the neonatal unit, as well as to pregnancy. Automatic neonatal blood
pressure monitoring instrumentation is provided by Nippon Colin Ltd.
(Komaki, Japan). With its use, inter-cardiovascular risk group differences are detected, but hardware for any chronobioengineering is not
enough in itself. Additional ingredients are needed: the realization
that we are dealing with dynamic functions that have predictable since
rhythmic elements, Table 1, and that concepts that result in data reduction to the mean and a standard deviation are not invariably sufficient to
exploit the information from chronobioengineering. Figure 1 shows the
dynamic indices that have already proved of some value, as a first step in
dealing with the dynamics of body function.

That one must pay attention to the waveform, be it by signal averaging or by harmonic analysis, is a point made by the over-viewer of the sessions on blood pressure, Germaine Cornelissen of the University of Minnesota Chronobiology Laboratories. She has fitted 95 harmonics to each of 80 24-h series sampled at 7.5-minute intervals and has found prominent harmonics among the first 10. She suggests that the 11th to 95th harmonics represent mostly noise. She then documents that the amplitudes of the first 10 harmonics exceed those from the extrapolated noise characteristics, and suggests that these contribute most markedly to the circadian waveform. She empha-sizes the availability of software for extracting information on dynamic endpoints. Her contribution strengthens Michael Weber's conclusion that although unsuccessful monitoring procedures still can occur, investigators and

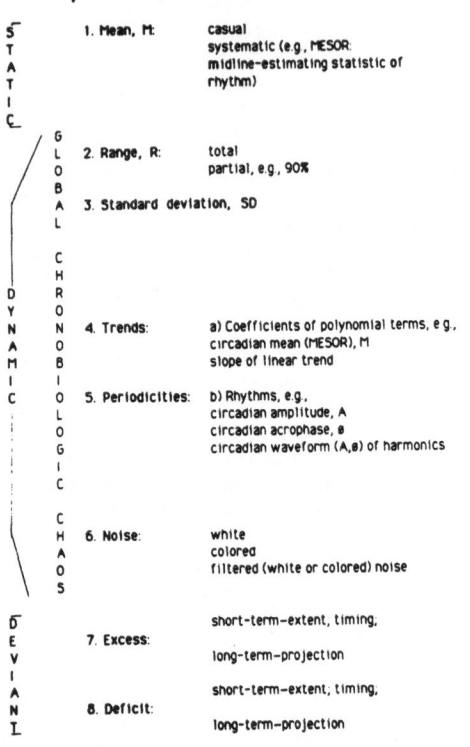

Table 1

Dynamic endpoints complement static ones

STATIC (GLOBAL CHRONOBIOLOGIC CHAOS)	1. Mean, M:	casual systematic (e.g., MESOR: midline-estimating statistic of rhythm)
	2. Range, R:	total partial, e.g., 90%
	3. Standard deviation, SD	
DYNAMIC	4. Trends:	a) Coefficients of polynomial terms, e.g., circadian mean (MESOR), M slope of linear trend
	5. Periodicities:	b) Rhythms, e.g., circadian amplitude, A circadian acrophase, ø circadian waveform (A,ø) of harmonics
	6. Noise:	white colored filtered (white or colored) noise
DEVIANT	7. Excess:	short-term—extent, timing; long-term—projection
	8. Deficit:	short-term—extent; timing; long-term—projection

clinicians can now use the technique of ambulatory blood pressure monitoring with such a high level of confidence that they will generate usable data. That such non-invasive instrumentation is now available is a contribution of another of the authors in this volume, Verlin McCall of Irvine, California. He introduced the Pressurometer III, an important research tool, and tested it, with his brother Willifred McCall, a physician in everyday practice, where ambulatroy blood pressure monitoring belongs. Because of its weight and the need to put on electrodes, however, the Pressurometer is not the ideal instrument for long-term monitoring in the home.

The machine produced by Instruments for Cardiac Research (Liverpool, New York; a subsidiary of Squibb) has the unquestionable merit that it requires no electrodes. It does not have a rechargable battery and is by no means light in weight. It replicates the human observer in that it exhibits digit preference, an imperfection that will eventually be remedied.

DEFINITION OF RHYTHM PARAMETERS

MESOR

MESOR, M rhythm-adjusted mean (midline-estimating statistic of rhythm), defined as average value of rhythmic function (e.g., cosine curve) fitted to data; expressed in same units as original data. Note that MESOR will differ from arithmetic mean if data unequidistant (e.g., concentrated near crest of rhythm) and/or cover non-integral number of cycles.

period

rhythmic function

Period, τ duration of one complete cycle in rhythmic function; expressed in time units, such as seconds, hours, days or years, or in physiologic units such as complete cardiac, respiratory or menstrual cycle; equated to 360° for angular expression of acrophase.

amplitude

MESOR

total predictable change (double amplitude)

Amplitude, A half of total predictable change in rhythm, defined by rhythmic function fitted to data; expressed in original or "relative" units, e.g., as percentage of series mean or MESOR.

reference time   acrophase

rhythmic function

time

Acrophase, ø lag from reference time of rhythm's crest-time, defined by rhythmic function fitted to data; usually expressed in (negative) degrees, with 360° ≅ period, 0° = reference time; customary time units (e.g., clock-hours and minutes, days, weeks, months or years) or physiologic units (e.g., number of heart beats, respiratory or menstrual cycles) also appropriate for rhythm synchronized with corresponding period.

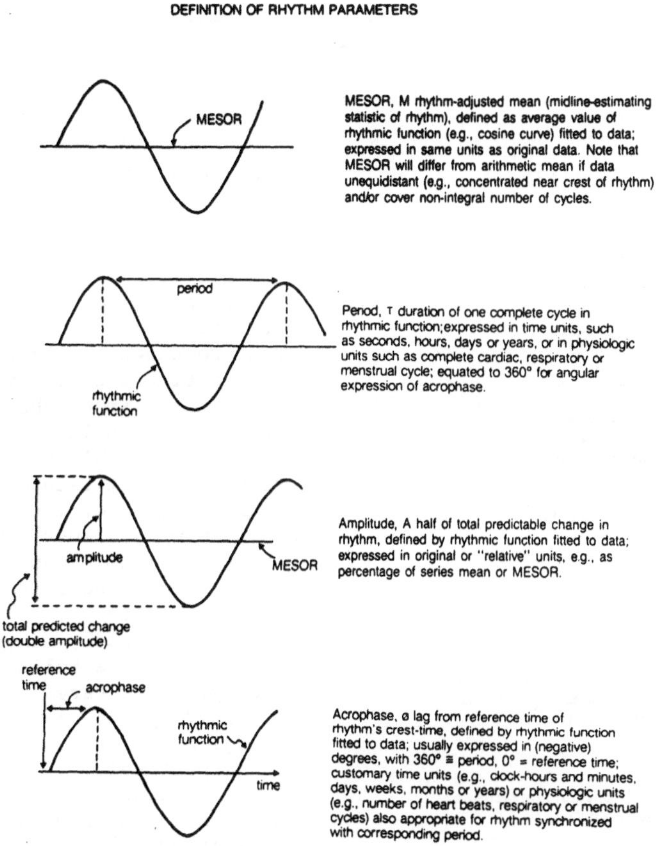

Figure 1: Definitions (for more detail, see Glossary of chronobiology, Chronobiologia 4, Suppl. 1: 189 pp.).

Lighter instruments are needed, and they are being produced. Room-restricted instrumentation, which can be carried with a handle but is too heavy to be worn, constitutes another need; the front-runner in this field is a machine manufactured by Nippon Colin (Komaki, Japan). This machine is used extensively in research by a number of chronobiologists in conjunction with software for rhythmometry that has to complement this machine and the fully ambulatory ones. Such progress notwithstanding, however, and with exceptions as noted above, in the view of most participants, the chronoengineering for software in dealing with the variability of blood pressure is the most urgently needed item.

For the pessimists among us, instrumentation available today provides no more than a choice between the proverbial devil and the deep blue sea. As to devils, first study Table 2. At first it appears that machines qualifying for this label are those encountered in public places that compute 'good days' and 'bad days' once one's birthday is indicated and some money inserted. Everybody knows (we hope!) that these machines are a put-on and have no basis in published scientific fact. All in all, the birthday-determined biorhythm machines are innocuous; of course, it has nothing to do with hardware and software engineering for rhythm assessment.

There are, however, also machines in public places that are clearly dangerous; they measure a single blood pressure or heart rate, as do individuals at health fairs (conventions of buyers and sellers of health information), often with a 'free' blood pressure included. Any single measurement may unduly alarm a person who is in the best of health. For instance, one may have been running to catch a plane. The plane's departure delayed, one finds time, at the airport, to take his blood pressure. This reading will be unduly high, if for no other reason than apprehension.

Another person may be lulled into a false sense of safety by a single acceptable reading. Indeed, the danger of both false positive and false negative diagnoses looms large, in view of the variability of blood pressure shown in Figure 2. The time has come to do something about the fact that a single measurement of blood pressure, heart rate or a single value of many other functions must not serve as the sole basis for decisions regarding health when, in clinically healthy men, systolic and diastolic blood pressure vary within 24 hours, on the average by 69 and 56 mm Hg, respectively.

The presentations at the session on electro-cardiographic monitoring emphasize the need for instruments that record for durations longer than 24 hours. This need can be shown in two ways. A first pertinent fact, from the viewpoint of classical cardiology, is that of 12 monitoring days, one day may be devoid of any and all ECG-recorded ischemia, whereas on subsequent days, there is consistently ECG evidence for ischemic attacks (Biagini et al., 1981). What is even more interesting, a pattern of ischemia can be the expression of several rhythms with different frequencies. In the case of Biagini et al. (1981), two components are actually phase-drifting circadians, each with a

Table 2

**PUT-ONS:
ONE OF THEM DANGEROUS**

Machines:

Sell you information on:
1) Birthday biorhythms:
Your "good" and "bad" days

2) Health measures:
Your blood pressure and pulse

Results:

1) Your "good" or "bad" days may
not be true at all

2) Your physiologic measures are true only for a moment
(whether or not influenced by your arm size or the
machine's operating condition)

Action

If you judge your health by single physiologic measures,
this is the dangerous put-on

Alternative:
Chronobiology

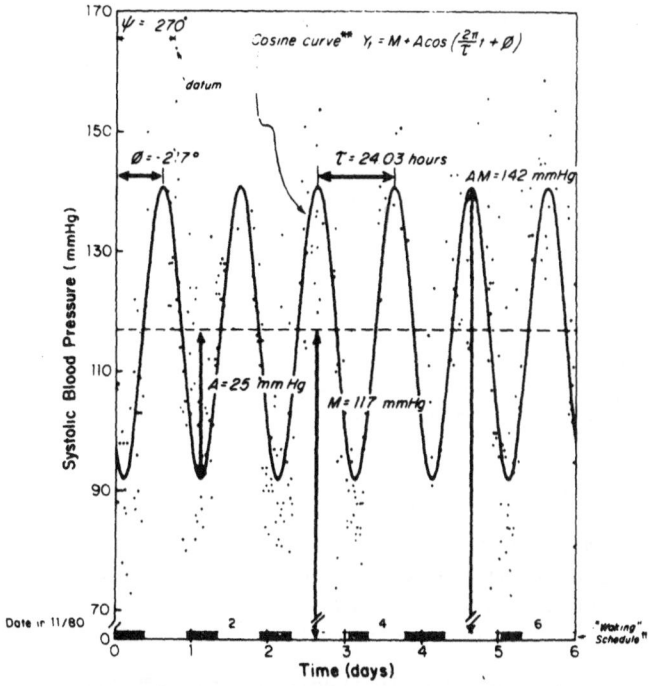

Parameters of Circadian Rhythm
in Systolic Blood Pressure
Estimated by Non-Linear Least Squares Procedure*

$\psi = 270°$

Cosine curve** $Y_t = M + A\cos\left(\frac{2\pi}{\tau}t + \emptyset\right)$

datum

$\emptyset = -2I7°$

$\tau = 24.03$ hours

AM = 142 mmHg

$A = 25$ mm Hg

$M = 117$ mmHg

Systolic Blood Pressure (mmHg)

Date in 11/80

"Waking"
Schedule"

Time (days)

*Applied to automatically recorded data from healthy woman 60 years of age

Fitted to data by non-linear least squares, with Y_t = value of curve at time t, M = mesor = average value of curve over integral number of cycles, A = amplitude = half of difference between highest and lowest value of curve; AM = acrometron = highest predicted value, τ = period = duration of one complete cycle; $\emptyset$ = acrophase = timing of highest value in curve (here in relation to 00 on first day of data collection), with 360° = τ. = macrophase = timing of highest value Procedure also provides confidence interval for parameter. (M, A, τ, and $\emptyset$)

"From automatic octometry, rest-span shaded

Figure 2: Physiologic variability can be rendered predictable and such predictability can be exploited when other approaches fail (Chronobiologia 8: 351-366, 1981; Postgrad. Med. 79: 44-46, 1986).

confidence interval for the period that does not cover precisely 24 hours (Halberg, this volume). It then becomes a rhetorical questions whether a 24-h ECG sufficies as a representative record. An analogy might be considered to further emphasize the limitations of 24-hour records for circadian and infra-dian studies. One-day monitoring of a circadian rhythm (in any variable) is equivalent to taking the pulse by monitoring for a duration correspond-ing to the average time of a single heartbeat. During, say, a second of monitoring, one may not pick up a single beat. To drive this analogy to the absurd, one may have to conclude that the patient has no heartbeat.

Figure 3, a summary of data collected by Charles Leach, another symposium participant, provides yet another reason for the need to construct recorders that monitor for spans exceeding one day. The periodicity observed by him is an infradian one; just as one wouldn't wish to monitor a circadian rhythm during an 8-hour span, one shouldn't limit monitoring to a single day to characterize a rhythm with a period of several days.

Ivan Bourgeois of Medtronic BV in Kerkrade, Holland, the chairperson of the cardiology session, considered the indications and specifications for a chronobiologic pacing of the human heart. His firm, Medtronic, has already introduced pacemakers guided by instantaneous motor or respiratory activity. With him, one can emphasize the need for pacing not only in the light of instantaneous demands, but anticipatory changes in pacing may have value. A programmable pacemaker with a built-in recorder and physiologic laboratory could take into account the rhythm structure of pathology.

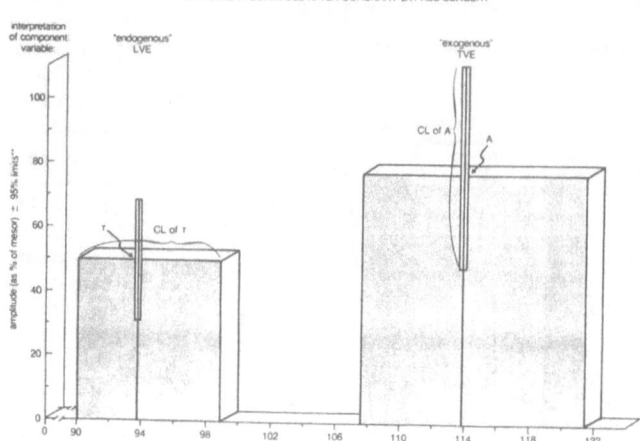

INFRADIAN COMPONENTS OF DIFFERING PERIOD (τ) CHARACTERIZE HOURLY
TOTAL VENTRICULAR ECTOPIES (TVE) AND LONGEST RUNS OF VE (LVE)
IN A PATIENT COMATOSE AFTER CORONARY BYPASS SURGERY'

Figure 3: The presence of rhythms with periods of 3.5 days or even longer
periods makes it mandatory at the outset to monitor the electrocardiogram
for spans exceeding 24 hours (Chronobiologia 10: 138, 1983).

What applies for electrical treatment in theory has already been
applied to drug administration devices. The most advanced system was
presented by Robert E. Fischell of the Johns Hopkins University Applied
Physics Laboratory. He has devised a microprocessor-controlled
implantable, externally programmable medication system aimed particulary
at the release of insulin into the human body. The system equals a fully
implantable, programmable infusion pump consisting of a patient's
programming unit, a medication programming unit, and a medication
injection unit. The infusion pump is refilled at intervals of several
months; it serves as an artificial pancreas.

This latter topic is succinctly discussed, on the basis of extensive
experience, by the president of the University of Montpellier and chairperson of the session on pumps, Jacques Mirouze. Pumps used by him
already assure a minimal uninterrupted insulin supply (around 1 unit/hr)
and are adjustable so that more insulin is delivered with meals and
physical exercise. As noted for the pacemaker and as applies to the pump
as well, a proper program will anticipate spontaneous rhythmic changes in
demand and will provide for rhythm-stage-dependent responses to meals. A
contribution to this volume by Yves Lazorthes and Jean-Claude Verdier of
the University of Toulouse, France, considers automatic drug administration devices and their mechanisms, as well as their application in
treating cancer pain, spasticity or malignant brain tumors themselves.
Anthony F. Yapel and Felix Theeuwes, of 3M and Alza Corps., respectively,
introduce their technologies applicable to chronotherapy. 3M already
offers a product line of volumetric external infusion pumps and Alza's

mini-osmotic pump is extensively used in experimental research. With the Medtronic implantable externally programmable pump, Marco Cavallini, now of the University of Rome, documents, for the first time in a middle-sized animal (beagle), a clear gain from the use of sinusoidal schedules originally introduced in Minnesota for treatment with ara-C, and now extended by him for treatment with cyclosporine.

Another highlight of the meeting was the session on data acquisition and analysis sytems. Its chairperson, Martin Knapp of the University of Nottingham, England, was responsible for introducing a clinical system involving computers for bedside monitoring, e.g., after a transplantation. In this session, Ramon C. Hermida of the University of Madrid made the point that indices such as the rhythm parameters defined in Figure 1 may well be used as such, but that chronobiologic methodology includes, in addition, a wealth of other methods. From the viewpoint of chronobioengineering, sooner or later, the software of today should become the hardware of tomorrow. For the storage of chronobiologic data, Robert M. Goodman of the Franklin Institute (Philadelphia, Pennsylvania) presents a device that allows large scale data acquisition and storage. Salvatore Romano of the University of Florence shows the need for using multiple methods to check on results. In this context, he provides an independent confirmation of the finding on 9-year-olds that the dynamics (rather than the static mean) separate groups of children with or without a family history of high blood pressure.

Jean De Prins of the Free University of Brussels reviews the problems associated with actual data collection and shows that "noise" originates in different ways. He distinguishes different noise types, including fluctuations of the biological system itself, flutucations external to the organism monitored yet measured by the transducer and noise originating from both the transducer and the sampling device. This noise may be redistributed over the frequency range investigated (aliasing). De Prins reemphasizes that mathematical theories rely on simplifying assumptions (such as normality, independence of errors, stationarity and erogodicity) that are not necessarily verified in practice. Accordingly, he concludes that in view of different experimental conditions, an array of methods of analysis has to be considered, each with its own domain of applicability.

The Table of Contents lists many internationally known contributors to this volume. The major point may well be that the challenge of chronobiologic engineering should take us, in everyday medical practice and in self-help for health care, to wedding chronobiologic software to the hardware. This critical step would allow a fuller exploitation of data collected with classical tools, such as thermometers and sphygmomanoneters, and of those obtained with automatic recorders, which should sooner or later be provided not only with solid-state memories but also with proper analyzers. The Cardiff symposium volume, if it did no more, assembles hard data to document the need for both software and hardware engineering, so that the predictable and rhythmic dynamics, that are the web of all life, can be properly assessed.

References
1. Biagini A., C. Carpeggiani, M.G. Mazzei, R. Testa, C. Michelassi, R.
    Antonelli, A. L'Abbate, A. Naseri 1981: Distribuzione ora ria degli
    episodi di angiana a riposo. Effetto della terapia medica. G. Ital.
    Cardiol. 11:4-11.

2. Halberg F. In press: Perspectives of chronobiologic engineering. In:
    Proc. NATO Advances Research Workshop, Chronobiotechnology and
    Chronobiological Engineering, Cardiff, Wales, April 21-25, 1985.

Franz Halberg

ACKNOWLEDGEMENTS

Several organizations and their officers were instrumental in making the Advanced Study Workshop and this volume possible. Foremost among those were Drs. M. di Lullo, of the Scientific Affairs Division of NATO and Frederick Hegge of the Department of Behavioral Biology - Division of Neuropsychiatry of Walter Reed Army Institute of Research, Washington, D.C. whose organizations provided the primary funding of the workshop. Both individuals gave much encouragement and advice to the Director.

Our hosts in Cardiff, Wales, Drs. Keith Griffiths and Douglas W. Wilson and their staffs from the Tenovus Institute for Cancer Research left no stone unturned to make sure that we were subjected to hospitality of the highest quality and at the lowest possible cost. Douglas Wilson was attentive to every detail before, during and after the meeting. The following companies also made significant and much appreciated contributions to the development and support of this program:

MEDTRONICS Europe
SPACELABS, INC., U.S.A.
3M, Minneapolis, U.S.A.
NOVO RESEARCH INSTITUTE, Copenhagen
ICELANDIC AIRLINES, Reykjavik, Iceland

Opening Remarks: RATIONALE AND GOALS OF THIS WORKSHOP

Lawrence E. Scheving,
Dept. of Anatomy, University of Arkansas for Medical Sciences,
Little Rock, AR, 72205, U.S.A.

A well-attended NATO-sponsored Advanced Study Institute was held in
Hannover, Federal Republic of Germany, from 13-25 July 1979. The
subject title of that school was "Chronobiology: Principles and
Applications to Shifts in Schedules". The proceedings, edited by L.E.
Scheving and F. Halberg were published by Sijthoff and Noordhoff in
1980. It was a two-week course which dealt with the broad subject of
chronobiology, but it tended to focus on the practical problems of
shiftwork and of transmeridian travel (jet-lag). We believe that this
tutorial course had impact. A number of the faculty and students who
attended are now among the leaders working on, or heading up projects
on, shiftwork and jet-lag throughout the world. Thus, the institute
helped to intensify worldwide lay interest in problems of shiftwork and
the associated changes in internal time structure.
  An emergent consensus from the 1979 NATO school was that although
the state-of-the-art of laboratory-based measurements of circadian
function had reached a high level of sophistication and practicality,
this clearly was not the case for our capacity to measure rhythms with
several frequencies on vital human functions in the field.
  In everyday life, many rhythms are extremely noisy. Although such
rhythms have been measured and certain components of them became clearly
evident, measurements done by the subjects themselves or by staff are
cumbersome and time consuming, and they interfere with the work itself.
Thus there arises an uncertainty as to how much self-measurement is
tolerable and when automatic-measurement becomes mandatory.
Self-measurements are useful and indispensible for certain purposes and
conditions. They cannot readily serve, however, for the assessment of
certain ultradian rhythms with very high frequencies which we now know
interact with circadian rhythms. Moreover, in a variety of conditions,
the rhythms in self-measured or automatically obtained data are still
covert and are revealed only by special methods of analysis.
  A major task for the chronobiologist of the future is to resolve
better the temporal structure of man as well as the experimental animal.
To do this he will need reliable, socially acceptable instrumentation
that is comfortable to use over long spans of time. But this is not
enough. There is also an urgent need to be able to analyze in a
meaningful, understandable way, the data collected as one goes; thus
rapid reduction of data is essential.
  With the above as a background, the organizers saw the need for a
workshop that would deal specifically with what kinds of continuous
monitoring devices are available, how they can be improved, and how are
the data handled once they are collected? Our overall objective in
planning was to bring together, from industry, government and the
university, some of the world's leadership in this area. We decided
that the fields to be covered would include the monitoring of body core
and surface temperatures, gross body movement, psychophysiological
performance (with special emphasis on the nervous system), circulation

and respiration, as well as vigilance, visual acuity, cognitive functions, reaction time and well being. Also of great concern was how to improve chronobiologically patient monitoring; treatment devices, such as cardiac pacemakers; and drug-administration systems, such as pumps and oral and transdermal systems. Further within the scope of the meeting was the collection of biophysical, biochemical, and numerical analyses of blood, urine, sweat, and saliva in both the human and experimental animal.

A major fundamental rhythmic variable measured in the past has been body temperature, and this will be the subject of the first panel. From this panel of 11 top experts from around the world we should learn first, from the reviewer the historical development of instrumentation, why is body temperature an important variable to monitor, the problems encountered, and the state-of-the-art of the instrumentation used to measure temperature. What are the problems for the subject who must wear such instruments over long spans of time in contrast to wearing them over short spans of time.

Most important there should emerge from this panel, as from every other panel, recommendations as to how technology might be improved to resolve better the whole spectrum of rhythmic frequencies characterizing this fundamental rhythmic variable. I am pleased to say that a new technology for monitoring deep body temperature through microwave sensors has emerged; and the developer of that technology D. V. Land of Glasgow is on hand to explain what I believe will become the "wave-of-the-future" for obtaining clinically valuable information about internal temperature variation. The technique is passive, non-invasive, and completely safe. The publication that follows this workshop should serve as an up-to-date reference for anyone interested in this particular subject.

The second panel will deal first with the monitoring of motor activity and the electromyogram: Of what practical use are the data obtained from the actograph? The reviewer should tell us why it is important to monitor motor activity, the historical development of such monitoring equipment, and the state-of-the-art of the present equipment; he has played a major role in bringing about the latest technology. Most important we want to know its limitations as well as how such monitoring can be improved and how one handles the large amount of data obtained? Following this, we will hear about the more up-to-date ways now available for monitoring vigilance and psychological endpoints. We know that in the past many of these measurements depended on pencil and paper tests; but now more sophisicated techniques have been developed, and we would expect to learn from this group what is desirable for advancement in the future.

The final afternoon panel will deal with monitoring of eye movements, respiration, and electroencephalogram recordings, and their importance and reliability in health as well as sleep. We should learn whether the instrumentation available today is adequate for long term measurement or monitoring of the EMG, EOG, and the EEG directly and simultaneously. Do the instruments available reliably differentiate dream (REM) sleep from non-dream sleep? For example, are the instruments that give an analog recording of the parameters of sleep as good as those that give us direct recordings of EMG activity, eye movements or EEG activity? Can the instruments at hand differentiate a true from an artifact signal and can the intrepreter distinguish one from the other or does he have no idea as to which is which? Can you believe summary data?

Tomorrow morning we deal with monitoring of blood pressure, a subject that has been a great interest to me. It has been widely documented for blood pressure that self-measurement can complement measurements by medical or paramedical staff. We now know that developments in instrumentation, the use of automatic blood-pressure monitors, complements (rather than replaces) the conventional sphygmomanometer. What the automatic instrument does is to provide more refined cardiovascular profiles which are necessary to better resolve and therefore to better understand changes in blood pressure. We have arrived at a stage where most clinicians accept the fact that blood pressure, especially in the hypertensive, shows a remarkably circadian rhythm. But, it also is a variable that is characterized by many other frequencies including weekly or circaseptan rhythms.

The blood-pressure panel will be followed by a group dealing with chronobiological electrocardiographic monitoring; and from this panel we should learn what are the chronobiological implications of screening, diagnosis, and, most important, treatment. What is the state-of-the-art of instrumentation; what is needed for advancement?

Since the biological time structure is continually changing, we know that any response to a drug or any other agent will vary. The experimental evidence is overwhelming that the timing of drugs according to the body rhythms can bring about a therapeutic advantage. This is especially important in the timing of cancer chemotherapeutic agents, but it also is important to a diabetic patient receiving insulin as well as in the regulation of blood coagulation. Can the physician afford to ignore this variation in susceptibility to various types of medication? This indeed is a very important panel and those involved are pioneers in this endeavor. The current practice of medicine largely disregards timing of drug administration. The development of extra- corporal programmable drug-delivery systems will make clinical "chronotherapy" both possible and economical. Science and technology must come to grips with the best way to administer drugs chronobiologically. There is a great potential in this field, both for industry, and, more importantly, for the health of man.

There are problems associated with clinical laboratory instrumentation; this is a difficult area because it usually involves the monitoring of biochemical variables, but it is an area that we must address in the future. Overviewing this session is a very competent clinician and laboratory specialist. The same problems pertain to laboratory monitoring of the temporal structure of animals and plants, and again we are fortunate in having an exceptional panel of experts.

Finally the panel on data acquisition and analysis systems on the morning of the last day has an important task before it. It is essential to continue to develop better tools for automatic data collection and transfer, as well as for transient and definitive data-base storage. Any information gained from a given subject should be analyzed as it is collected, for the purposes of monitoring, yet it should also be accumulated for the derivation of individualized reference values for that subject to assist in decision-making. It is extremely important that data obtained are meaningful to the referring physician and also compatible with a computerized medicine information system. The stored data can also form part of a data base for the construction of peer-group reference values and for even broader research purposes.

Since storage and analytical capabilities are limited, it becomes essential that the variables that we do select to study are important in performance as well as systemic functions such as core temperature, cardiovascular indices, performance vigilance, and automatically monitored body chemistry; such variables will have to be compared for their relative merits. Only then will it be possible to investigate and eventually optimize those factors that underlie a given worker's ability to perform mentally and physically.

We should also develop answers for those who continually ask the questions: How do we measure? How do we schedule? Or more generally, how do we use chronobiology in industrial hygiene as well as in preventive medicine. Of central importance is the question of relevant functions and sample design. If we can record only a limited number of variables from a subject: 1) Which ones are essential and which are non-essential, redundant, or of less importance? There is already general agreement that core temperature and motor activity measurements are high on the list of essentials, 2) What rank is given to respiratory, circulatory, and neural-system parameters? 3) When do we wish to extract simultaneously from our subjects some measures of vigilance, visual acuity, cognitive functions, and sense of well-being? 4) What priorty do we give the collection of blood, urine, breath, sweat, and saliva samples? 5) What are the practical limitations in terms of sampling frequency and duration? (6) What kinds of sensors and collecting devices are presently available, and are they sufficient to the task? 7) What kinds of interpretive techniques are presently available (inferential statistical graphic, beyond doubly plotting, etc.), are they sufficient to the task, and what changes are needed? and 8) What kinds of interventions, strategies to effect mitigation, are available, are they sufficient to the task, and what changes do we need?

Each of the above questions represents a problem for which we already have available some fairly reasonable, although not entirely satisfactory, answers. For each question, we ask our panels of experts to come up with some answers and to make suggestions for the future.

XIX

Perspectives of chronobiologic engineering

Franz Halberg, Professor of Laboratory Medicine, Pathology, Physiology and Biology; Director, Chronobiology Laboratories, University of Minnesota, 5-187 Lyon Laboratories, University of Minnesota, Minneapolis, MN 55455, USA

Dedicated to George W. Thorn, Emeritus Hersey Professor of Medicine at Harvard University, where the work leading to this field started.

Introduction

The precise periodicity of a metronome is not a characteristic of health or disease. A *roughly* recurrent pattern, in turn, is described in many forms of life, including human beings. Bioperiodic patterns can be recognized in most processes or events from womb to tomb, but they are not readily quantified by the unaided eye. Up to the late 40s, statistical aspects of the reproducibility of changing patterns of recurrence were not usually measured. Long time series were not economically measurable. Few had the patience of Santorio (1657), who in the 17th century had accumulated a time series of 30-year length. On the basis of usually only a few measurements, it was attractive for the classical physiologist to postulate a regulation for constancy as the major homeostatic feature of life. Along this line of thinking and acting, bioperiodicities were second-order phenomena, buried in mostly unpublished laboratory records or in the noise term of mathematical models.

In the past several decades, various designs, methods of data collection and statistical analyses have been developed into a new technologic endeavor. This is the study of chronobiology, of predictable since rhythmic biologic changes. Briefly, chronobiology resolves a dynamic time structure. Evidence has accumulated on the ubiquity and critical importance of rhythms. The stage of about 24-h (circadian) rhythms tips the scale between death and survival, in the organism's response to the identical physical, bacteriologic or pharmacologic stimulus, Figure 1a-c (Halberg, 1962). Such data have been analyzed by classical statistical methods, e.g., by analyses of variance. Indeed, a significant effect of time is then found (P<.05).

One should be able to say more than that there is a rhythm; it is rewarding to resolve certain characteristics of rhythmic change. At this point, the computer is helpful. With its aid, dense and long data series on most of one's vital functions are easily collected and analyzed. Chronobiologically-analyzed ambulatory electrocardiographic, electroencephalographic, core and surface temperature, motor activity and blood pressure records, usher in a new era (Halberg E. et al., 1978, 1979, 1981a and b).

No longer are data series interrupted as they had to be when conventional tools such as the thermometer or sphygmomanometer only were available for self-measurements. Automatically, one now monitors during sleep and during waking activities, under both usual and unusual conditions, for some variables during weeks rather than merely days. Such extensive series need not be used merely for the computation of a mean. These series can yield dynamic characteristics, along with a more reliable mean, when used as input for a chronobiologic algorithm. The algorithm provides a specific output from the given input; it has to be so precisely defined that it can be implemented on a computer (Knuth, 1977). By algorithms in the form of special programs applied to biologic time series, a computer resolves rhythms. These are rigorously defined as recurrent patterns, validated and quantified with error estimates by inferential statistical means (Halberg, 1969). By computer, several characteristics such as those in Figure 2a-e, describing the extent and timing of change, are readily resolved.

An alternative is the mistaken identification of rhythms as unqualified effects of time of day or season. This view is subjective, can be misleading and can become a source of harm. Figures 3a and b show the consequences of a difference in period or amplitude, respectively, for two rhythms being compared at one or the other time of day. The investigator who finds a decrease may advocate

Circadian-stage-dependent pathologic response of central nervous system to fixed physical stimulus*

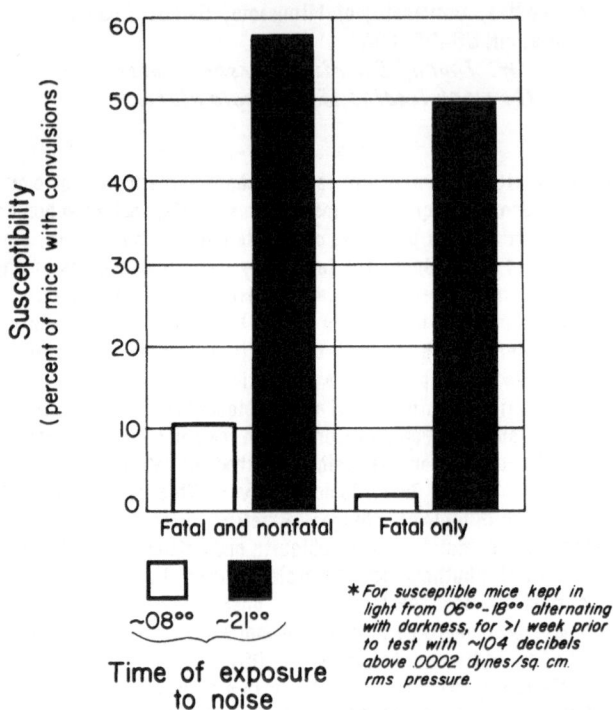

Fig. 1a: Within-day change in susceptibility to audiogenic convulsions. Two groups of mice were picked at random for tests at 08^{00} (day) or 21^{00} (night). The animals had been kept in light from 06^{00} to 18^{00}, alternating with darkness, with food freely available. Separate groups of mice were placed for 60 seconds into a tub and were exposed to auditory stimulation by bells, roughly to 104 decibels above 0.002 dynes/sq cm rms pressure. Note in the figure on the left that the same stimulus, namely exposure to the noise of bells in a tub, will bring about convulsions in over 50% of the mice at one test time, but in hardly more than 10% of the animals at another test time ($P<.05$). Note further from the right of the same figure that nearly 50% of the animals die from these convulsions at one time and only very few at another time ($P<.05$). © 1958 by Halberg.

substitution treatment; a colleague who finds an increase may advocate the opposite, yet in either case there is *no* change in overall mean. Differences in phase or waveform (not shown) can be equally confusing. The dangers of such misinterpretations would be limited if rhythms were the exception. Figure 4a,b, showing drastic within-day differences in the count of certain blood cells, was interpreted as an exception in the early fifties; bioperiodicities continue to be described as unusual phenomena, yet by the 80s, painstaking work with a combination of biophysical,

Manipulability of timing of an extreme physiologic (dashing) and several pathologic responses (audiogenic convulsion and death) explored by 2-timepoint spot checks.*

Note also apparent increase in overall susceptibility at 8 days after shift of synchronizing lighting regimen.

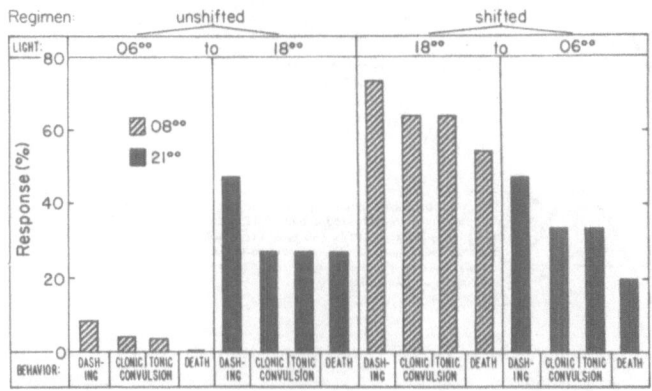

*Total of 102 D₉ mice of both sexes, ~5 weeks of age, tested by exposure to ~104 decibels above .0002 dynes/sq cm rms pressure on 2 regimens, each with light for 12 hours alternating with darkness for 12 hours but with the regimen shifted in one case (right) in its temporal placement along 24-hour scale. Response sequence: Dashing, clonic convulsion, tonic convulsion and death, not initiated in some animals and not completed in others.

Fig. 1b: Unfavorable responses to the exposure of mice susceptible to convulsions and death from convulsions, and to dashing in response to noise, can be shifted in their time location. If animals are maintained in light from 06⁰⁰ to 18⁰⁰, many more die from exposure to noise at 21⁰⁰ rather than 08⁰⁰. The reverse holds true after the animals have been kept for several weeks in light from 18⁰⁰ to 06⁰⁰. The unshifted animals had been standardized on the given regimen from birth; the shifted animals have been on the changing schedule for 8 days. The increase in overall susceptibility at 8 days after the synchronizer shift (P<.05) occurs during the time of a decrease in susceptibility with age and is ascertained by a comparison with unshifted controls. In this particular case, a transient desynchronization among those circadian rhythms developed at this age may be harmful, leading to an increased susceptibility to convulsions. This result, however, has to be checked by denser sampling, e.g., at 4-hour intervals, around the clock, to rule out changes in waveform and/or an incomplete adjustment to the new synchronizer schedule as factors contributing to the result. © 1958 by Halberg.

Fig. 1c: Different timing of susceptibility rhythms to different agents. Subgroups of comparable mice kept in LD12:12, exposed to the same potentially noxious stimulus at different times, 4 hrs apart, in order to test for changes in susceptibility during 24 hrs, show drastically different outcomes in mortality. Life or death from the cardiac drug ouabain, from a bacterial poison, *E. coli* endotoxin, from noise and from other agents including anti-cancer drugs (not shown) are a function of an organism's time structure. Results are expressed as % of the mean ≡ 100%. Within-day differences are all statistically significant. © 1962 by Halberg.

biochemical and behavioral methods has documented rhythms as *the dynamics of all life*. As a developing

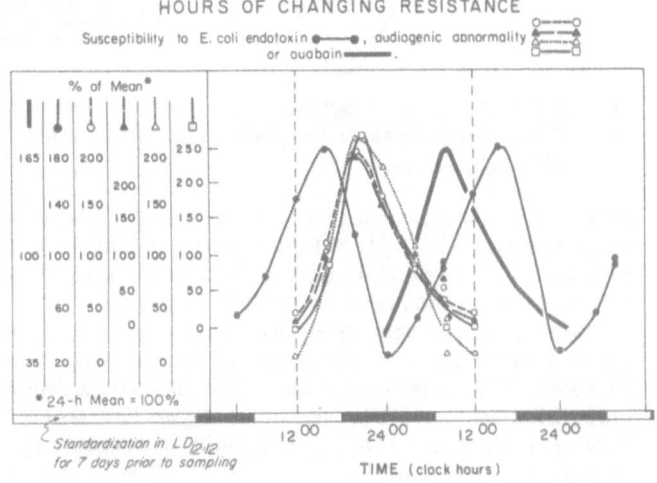

4

DEFINITION OF RHYTHM PARAMETERS

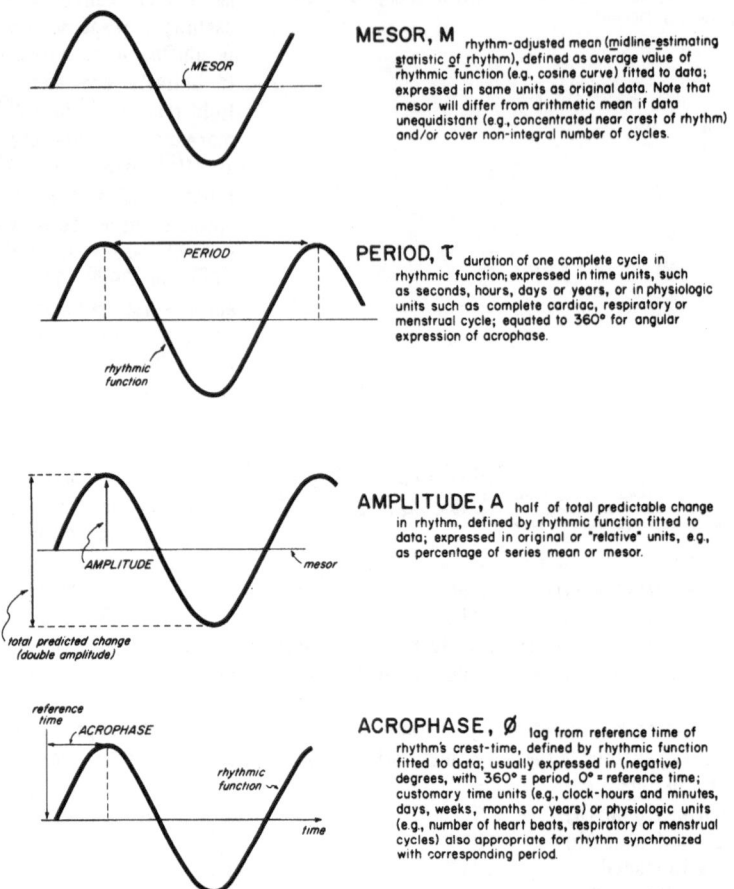

MESOR, M rhythm-adjusted mean (<u>m</u>idline-<u>e</u>stimating <u>s</u>tatistic <u>o</u>f <u>r</u>hythm), defined as average value of rhythmic function (e.g., cosine curve) fitted to data; expressed in same units as original data. Note that mesor will differ from arithmetic mean if data unequidistant (e.g., concentrated near crest of rhythm) and/or cover non-integral number of cycles.

PERIOD, τ duration of one complete cycle in rhythmic function; expressed in time units, such as seconds, hours, days or years, or in physiologic units such as complete cardiac, respiratory or menstrual cycle; equated to 360° for angular expression of acrophase.

AMPLITUDE, A half of total predictable change in rhythm, defined by rhythmic function fitted to data; expressed in original or "relative" units, e.g., as percentage of series mean or mesor.

ACROPHASE, Ø lag from reference time of rhythm's crest-time, defined by rhythmic function fitted to data; usually expressed in (negative) degrees, with 360° ≡ period, 0° = reference time; customary time units (e.g., clock-hours and minutes, days, weeks, months or years) or physiologic units (e.g., number of heart beats, respiratory or menstrual cycles) also appropriate for rhythm synchronized with corresponding period.

<u>Fig. 2a</u>: Characteristics of rhythms. The period, amplitude or acrophase, may change with the risk of developing a disease or in disease, in the absence of any increase in mean (cf. Figure 2e left). ©1985 by Halberg.

science, chronobiology is concerned with the objective quantification of ubiquitous rhythms with many frequencies, Table 1, as biologic structures in time (Halberg, 1969, 1983). Time structure characterizes all levels of biologic organization, whether it is a population, a person or the interaction of molecules in a cell or test tube, Figure 4c.

Many biologic processes are already documented to exhibit computer-validated rhythms in the stricter sense of the word defined above. They are found in bacteria and unicells (Rogers and Greenbank, 1929; Halberg and Conner, 1961; Edmunds and Halberg, 1981; Schweiger and Halberg, 1982; Halberg et al., 1985), along with mammals (Halberg and Visscher, 1952; Halberg, 1959; Scheving, 1976; Brown et al., 1982), including human beings (Halberg, 1959, 1960, 1982; Halberg et al., 1973; Smolensky et al., 1972). Rhythms in time complement cells in space. Many rhythms are shown to persist and free-run, with periods differing from precise environmental

Table 1: Period ranges for terms describing components in a spectrum of biologic rhythms[a]

Rhythms with different frequencies (or reciprocals of frequency, i.e., periods) usually characterize the same variable, if it is measured with sufficient density and for a long span. Here, different variables are listed to allude to the ubiquity of rhythms.

Domain Region	Range				Illustrative example	Validated free-running from reference period (lit.)	
ultradian	$\tau <$	20		h			
circacentuminutan	$\tau =$	1.7 ±	1	"	EEG-sleep-wakefulness of narcoleptics[1,2]		
" semidian	$\tau =$	12 ±	1	"			
circadian	$\tau <$	24 ±	4	"	Human adrenal cortical cycle	yes[3]	24 h
dian	$\tau <$	24 ±	0.2	h	Murine core temperature synchronized by 12 h light alternating with 12 h darkness[4-6]	yes[4-6]	24 h
infradian	$\tau >$	28		"			
circadidian	$\tau =$	2 ±	0.5	d			
" semiseptan	$\tau =$	3.5 ±	1	"	Sudden human death[7]		
" septan	$\tau =$	7 ±	2.5	"	Human 17-ketosteroid excretion[8]	yes	7 d
					Egg-laying of *Folsomia candida*[9]		
					Luminescence of *Gonyaulax*[10]		
					Response of *Acetabularia*[11]		
" diseptan	$\tau =$	14 ±	3	"			
" vigintan	$\tau =$	21 ±	3	"			
" trigintan	$\tau =$	30 ±	5	"	Human gonadal cycle[8,12]		
circannual	$\tau =$	1 y ±	2	m	Gonadal index of catfish[13,14]	yes	1 y
circaseptennian*	$\tau =$	7 y ±	2	y	Gonadal index of marine invertebrates[15,16]		
" duodecennian*	$\tau =$	12 y ±	4	"	Human blood pressure[17]	yes*	¶

[a] τ = period; h = hour; d = day; m = month; y = year. Terms coined to roughly approximate validated rhythms. By analogy to usage in physics, where frequencies higher than those audible or visible are called **ultra**sonic and **ultra**violet, frequencies higher than one cycle per 20 h are designated as **ultra**dian. By the same token, as frequencies lower than audible or visible are called **infra**sonic and **infra**red, rhythms with a frequency lower than one cycle per 28 h are designated as **infra**dian. The suffix *-ennian* instead of *-annual* for periods longer than 1 year serves to avoid the connotation of "annual" as a suffix after numbers larger than 1 to denote events that repeat themselves within the year, as in *biannual* or *triannual,* meaning twice or thrice a year. The change from *duo-* (used earlier in *circaduodian,)* to *di-* is prompted by the desire for consistency (e.g., with *circadiseptan)* and by the need to use an infix that denotes a doubling (rather than the addition of two, as done advisedly in *circaduodecennian,)*. A term such as *circasemidian* (and, perhaps, others if left unqualified) describes only a spectral component, without any implication as to whether the component represents a rhythm in its own right, rather than merely the waveform of a rhythm with a different (e.g., lower) frequency. Physiologic tests are required to distinguish these possibilities. Prominent rhythms in various speciies are cited above to emphasize the ubiquity of spectral organization. Most frequencies here cited are also likely to characterize a single human variable such as heart rate.

William MacDonald, John W. Clark, Michael V. Molitor and, for the past decade, Robert P. Sonkowsky, all at one time professors in the Classics Department, University of Minnesota, kindly participated in the coining and/or updating of these terms. While originally proposed as adjectives, their use as nouns also seems acceptable, for the sake of brevity.

*Tentative and awaiting analysis of as-yet unavailable longer series. ¶Sunspot cycle during same span.

References to Table 1

1. Passouant P., Halberg F., Genicot R., Popoviciu L., Baldy-Moulinier M.: La périodicité des accès narcoleptiques et le rythme ultradien du sommeil rapide. Rev. neurol. (Paris) 121: 155-164, 1969.

2. Halberg F.: More on educative chronobiology, health and the computer. Int. J. Chronobiol. 2: 87-105, 1974.

3. Halberg F.: Physiologic considerations underlying rhythmometry, with special reference to emotional illness. Symposium on Biological Cycles and Psychiatry. In: Symposium Bel-Air III, Geneva, Masson et Cie., 1968, pp. 73-126.

4. Halberg F.: Beobachtungen über 24 Stunden-Periodik in standardisierter Versuchsanordnung vor und nach Epinephrektomie und bilateraler optischer Enukleation. 20th meeting of the German Physiologic Society, Homburg/Saar, September 1953. Ber. ges. Physiol. 162: 354-355, 1954.

5. Halberg F.: Physiologic 24-hour periodicity: general and procedural considerations with reference to the adrenal cycle. Z. Vitamin-, Hormon- u. Fermentforsch. 10: 225-296, 1959.

6. Halberg F., Nelson W., Runge W.J., Schmitt O.H., Pitts G.C., Tremor J., Reynolds O.E.: Plans for orbital study of rat biorhythms. Results of interest beyond the Biosatellite program. Space Life Sci. 2: 437-471, 1971.

7. Halberg F.: Preface. In: Chronobiology 1982-1983, E. Haus, H. Kabat, eds., S. Karger, Basel, 1984, pp. v-viii.

8. Halberg F., Engeli M., Hamburger C., Hillman D.: Spectral resolution of low-frequency, small-amplitude rhythms in excreted 17-ketosteroid; probable androgen-induced circaseptan desynchronization. Acta endocr. (Kbh.) Suppl. 103: 5-54, 1965.

9. Chiba Y., Cutkomp L.K., Halberg F.: Circaseptan (7-day) oviposition rhythm and growth of spring tail, *Folsomia candida (Collembola: Isotomidae)*. Int. J. Cycle Res. 4: 59-66, 1973.

10. Halberg F., Hastings W., Cornélissen G., Broda H.: *Gonyaulax polyedra* 'talks' both 'circadian' and 'circaseptan'. Chronobiologia 12: 185, 1985.

11. Schweiger H-G., Halberg F.: Can a unicell measure the week and an isolated cytoplasm measure half a week? Notiziario SIBioC 6: 525-526, 1982.

12. Ferin M., Halberg F., Richart R.M., Vande Wiele R. (eds.): Biorhythms and Human Reproduction. Int. Inst. for the Study of Human Reproduction Conference Proceedings, John Wiley and Sons Inc., New York, 1974.

13. Sundararaj B.I., Vasal S., Halberg F.: Circannual rhythmic ovarian recrudescence in the catfish, *Heteropneustes fossilis*. Int. J. Chronobiol. 1: 362-373, 1973.

14. Sundararaj B.I., Vasal S., Halberg F.: Circannual rhythmic ovarian recrudescence in the catfish, *Heteropneustes fossilis* (Bloch). In: Toward Chronopharmacology, Proc. 8th IUPHAR Cong. and Sat. Symposia, Nagasaki, July 27-28, 1981, R. Takahashi, F. Halberg and C. Walker, eds., Pergamon Press, Oxford/New York, 1982, pp. 319-337.

15. Halberg F., Shankaraiah K., Halberg Francine, Giese A.C.: The chronobiology of murine invertebrates: methods of analysis. In press.

16. Pearse J.S., Pearse V.B., Giese A., Sothern R.B., Halberg F.: Circannual rhythm with similar timing characterizes gonadal index of a marine invertebrate (ochre star) studied 30 years apart. Proc. Int. Soc. Chronobiol., Little Rock, Ark., Nov. 3-6, 1985, in press.

17. Sothern R.B., Halberg F.: Circadian and infradian blood pressure rhythms of a man 20-37 years of age. Proc. 2nd Int. Conf. Medico-Social Aspects of Chronobiology, Florence, October 2, 1984, in press.

ADVANTAGES OF RHYTHMOMETRY

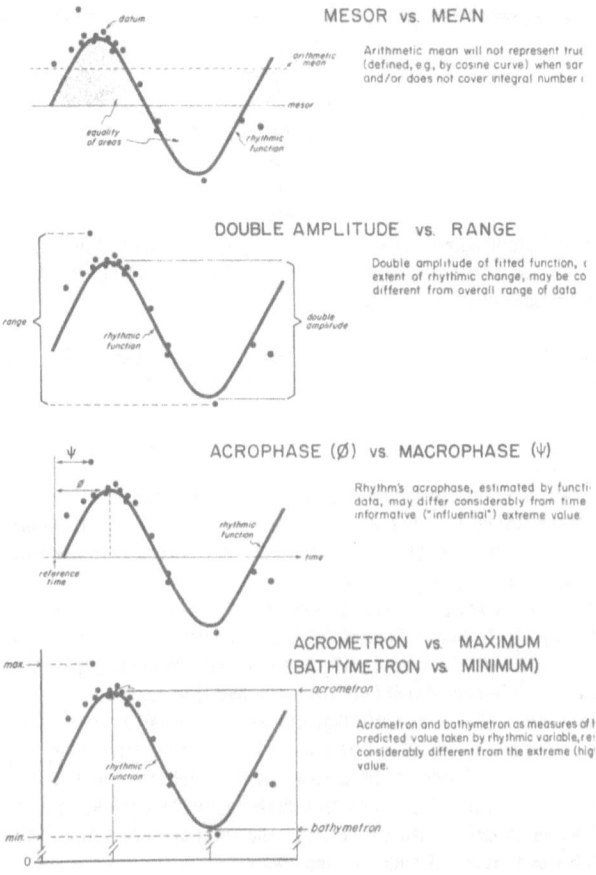

MESOR vs. MEAN

Arithmetic mean will not represent true
(defined, e.g., by cosine curve) when sar
and/or does not cover integral number of

DOUBLE AMPLITUDE vs. RANGE

Double amplitude of fitted function, o
extent of rhythmic change, may be co
different from overall range of data

ACROPHASE (∅) vs. MACROPHASE (Ψ)

Rhythm's acrophase, estimated by functio
data, may differ considerably from time
informative ("influential") extreme value

ACROMETRON vs. MAXIMUM
(BATHYMETRON vs. MINIMUM)

Acrometron and bathymetron as measures of h
predicted value taken by rhythmic variable, rei
considerably different from the extreme (hig
value.

Fig. 2b: Advantages of rhythmometry. ©1985 by Halberg.

counterparts such as 24 hours, 7 days or a year. These slight, yet statistically significant differences are interpreted as supporting a partly genetic basis for rhythms (Halberg, 1959, 1969). Recently, such suggestions have been further supported by results on twins reared apart, Table 2. The variability within twin pairs, even though they were reared far apart, was much smaller than that among twin pairs. The heritability of dynamic characteristics of human circadian rhythms (Table 2) is thus demonstrated (Halberg, 1983; Hanson et al., 1984). Accordingly, rhythms should come into the mainstream of all biology and medicine. As ubiquitous phenomena, almost certainly many more rhythms with widely differing frequencies will continue to be recorded and quantified by modern computer-associated hardware and software. The view of rhythms merely as the expression of some timekeeping mechanism is also an important focus, but one of much more limited scope. Birthday-determined biorhythms, in turn, are beyond the scope of currently legitimate science.

We here introduce the importance of rhythms by their relevance to major biomedical problems of our age (Halberg et al., 1959, 1979; Halberg, 1960, 1983; Menzel, 1962; Reinberg & Halberg,

8

Table 2
Certain features of our make-up in time are inherited
Genetic aspects of circadian heart rate characteristics[1]

Variability of rhythm characteristics *within* twin pairs reared apart is smaller than that among pairs

Rhythm characteristics	Intraclass correlation	95% confidence interval
MESOR	.679	.32-.87
Amplitude	.609	.21-.84
Acrophase	.658	.28-.56
Mean correlation	.649	

[1] Results based on hourly averages of heart rate from about 24-hour monitoring of 8 pairs of women, 8 pairs of men and one set of male triplets. Results in keeping with those obtained in the interim in a larger number of pairs of twins.

1971; Scheving et al., 1974; Haus et al., 1980, 1981a and b; Walker et al., 1981; Hermida et al., 1982; Takahashi et al., 1982; Halberg and Wetterberg, 1983; Haus & Kabat, 1984; Reinberg et al., 1984; Reale et al., 1985).

I. Monitoring the heart

The electrocardiographic assessment of the risk of sudden death is a prime concern of current medicine. In this context, there are two ways to look at the status quo in cardiac monitoring. The optimist takes pride in progress. In 1985, we have indeed acquired both hardware and software for automatically recording an ambulatory 24-hour ECG.

The realist may wonder whether current versions of 24-hour ECG monitoring should not be more fully exploited. By 1610, Santorio Santorio's Pulsilogium quantitatively assessed heart rate, as cited by Wesseling et al. (1982). By 1657, Santorio had made observations on his body weight for 30 years. He found a 30-day bioperiodicity in a healthy man, that likely characterizes the cardiovascular system as well. The Pulsilogium was eventually superseded by ECGs. Early electrocardiographers recorded quite a few cardiac cycles before interpreting them. Once it will be realized that circadian characteristics of the ECG can also be valuable, as will be documented below, a 24-hour record, i.e., the record of a single circadian cycle (by analogy to a single cardiac cycle) will also be recognized as an extremely short one. The interpretation of a 24-h record only then becomes as unacceptable as that of only one cardiac cycle.

Apart from the record's brevity, the usually descriptive analysis of 24-h ECG records is complicated by the large variability in the rate of a given abnormality examined that may not be properly resolved by conventional analyses. This variability appears to be unpredictable, only until it is being analyzed for rhythms. Some ECG instrumentation is programmed to reduce data to hourly values (Biagini et al., 1981; Orth-Gomér et al., 1982; Berry and Fox, 1983). Others go to further steps of data reduction seeking a single number (Lown et al., 1971). A linear regression, to approach relations between counts of abnormality in a reference span and after treatment, does not assess any time pattern (Sami et al., 1980). The classical analysis of variance of the ECG, a useful procedure indeed, does not in itself estimate the rhythmic characteristics of within-patient variability (Morganroth et al., 1978). The record of a patient with 1 abnormal event every hour for 240 hours may not be equivalent to that of another patient, exhibiting 240 ectopies during a single clock-hour and none during the ensuing 239 hours. Actually, a patient may not show a single cardiac ischemia on a first day of monitoring, but may exhibit a reasonable number of such abnormalities on each of 11 following days (Biagini et al., 1981). A seemingly random pattern may first appear as clock-hour-dependent but may reveal added predictable features on time series analyses, Table 3. Indeed in this case, two phase-drifting circadian and an infradian period are demonstrated.

Table 3

There is more to a time series than meets the unaided eye. The isolation of rhythms in time series can be compared to the isolation of chemical compounds. Several rhythmic components can be found in a given data set, just as several compounds may be isolated from materials in a test tube.

Multiple rhythmic components of ECG-ischemic episodes of a patient monitored for 12 days*

Data¶	Period (τ) (95% interval) (hours)			Amplitude (95% interval) (N/hour)		
hourly totals	τ_1= 4.2	(	-)	0.26	(0.08,	0.44)
" "	τ_2=11.80	(11.65,	11.95)	0.49	(0.30,	0.60)
" "	τ_3=22.90	(22.23,	23.25)	1.06	(0.49,	1.62)
" "	τ_4=23.35	(22.40,	23.69)	1.09	(0.52,	1.65)
24-h totals	τ_5=79.12	(72.37,	88.50)	0.23	(~0.00,	0.50)
	[3.30	(3.02,	3.69)]			

*The two clearly phase-drifting (if not free-running) circadian rhythms are validated by linear-nonlinear least-squares rhythmometry. The 11.8-hour component is probably descriptive of the waveform of the contributing two circadian rhythms. The tentatively presented ultradian and infradian components await further study in longer and denser data.
¶Hourly and 24-hourly totals are actually fitted with a trend (results on trend [P<.001] not shown). The period of τ_5 (in days) is given in brackets.

Original data: Biagini A., Carpeggiani C., Mazzei M.G., Testa R., Michelassi C., Antonelli R., L'Abbate A., Naseri A.: Distribuzione ora ria degli episodi di angiana a riposo. Effetto della terapia medica. G. Ital. Cardiol. 11: 4-11, 1981.

Time-specified treatment certainly will have to take such rhythms into account.

For a comparison of clinically defined groups in research, the 24-hour ECG record has considerable value, notably when it is analyzed in the light of advanced methods for time series analysis. Chronobiologic computer techniques can be applied to the 24-h ECGs of men with coronary heart disease (CHD) who die or survive within a 5-year follow-up. As compared to those of survivors, hourly ventricular ectopic beats (VEB) of men who die from CHD within a 5-year follow-up have a higher mean (called by chronobiologists a midline-estimating statistic of rhythm [MESOR, M]), Figure 2. Moreover, two other circadian characteristics of the hourly incidence of VEBs differ in the two groups. These are the amplitude (A), a measure of the extent of reproducible change, and the acrophase ($\emptyset$), a measure of reproducible timing. VEBs in those who die show more than twice the circadian A and a later timing of $\emptyset$, Figure 5a,b (Orth-Gomér et al., in press). A comparison of all 3 rhythm characteristics (M, A and $\emptyset$) separates the survivors from those who died of CHD (P=0.002). The usual reliance on total VEB incidence does not separate these two groups (P=.084) at the 5-year follow-up.

By evaluating three circadian characteristics (M, A & $\emptyset$) describing the predictable since rhythmic variation in VEB incidence, rather than relying only on abnormality per unit time, the possibility of recognizing candidates for sudden, presumably coronary death at the 5-year follow-up is increased. This is a practical group result at a given test time. Once the observation span is lengthened, both the classical approach and the time series analysis achieve a separation of the patients who die or live. The fact that the chronobiologic method achieves this separation earlier suggests that it is more sensitive. This point matters when the results of the group study are to be transferred to an individual. As noted, a single day's electrocardiographic monitoring is not representative, if it can show zero abnormality, yet is followed by considerable ischemia on each of

Parameters of Circadian Rhythm in Systolic Blood Pressure Estimated by Non-Linear Least Squares Procedure*

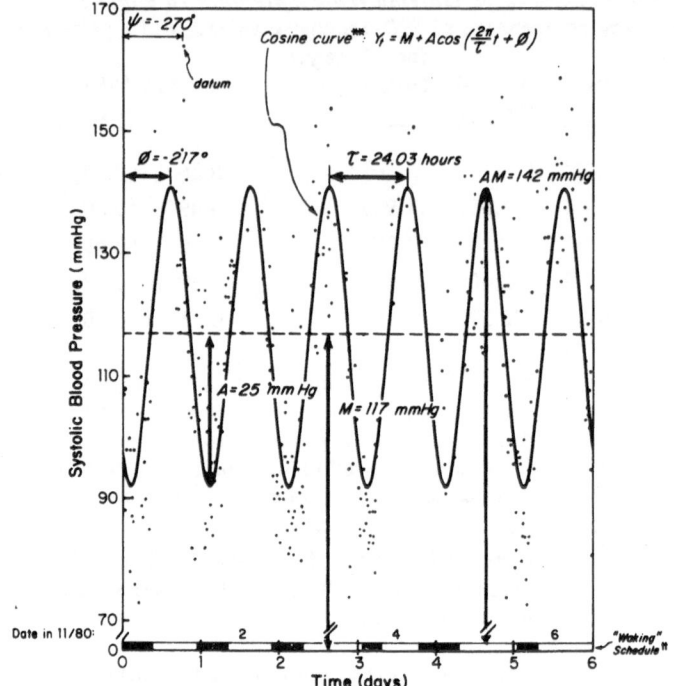

*Applied to automatically recorded data from healthy woman 60 years of age.

**Fitted to data by non-linear least squares, with Y_t = value of curve at time t; M = mesor = average value of curve over integral number of cycles; A = amplitude = half of difference between highest and lowest value of curve; AM = acrometron = highest predicted value; τ = period = duration of one complete cycle; $\emptyset$ = acrophase = timing of highest value in curve (here in relation to 00^{00} on first day of data collection), with $360° \approx \tau$. ψ = macrophase = timing of highest value. Procedure also provides confidence interval for parameters ($M, A, \tau,$ and $\emptyset$).

††From automatic actometry; rest-span shaded.

Fig. 2c: Original systolic blood pressures in Torr (approximated by mm Hg) obtained over 6 consecutive days, each value shown as a dot. The fit by nonlinear least squares of a 24-h cosine curve results in a period deviating only slightly from 24 hours. This period is compatible with a 24-hour synchronization of the circadian rhythm, since its confidence interval overlaps the 24.00-hour value (Fig. 2d). Around the MESOR of 117 mm Hg, the double-amplitude of 50 mm Hg is hardly negligible. The data are denser by night than by day; hence, the correct MESOR seems too high to the naked eye. The MESOR of a curve fitted by hand would be lower, but would constitute an optical illusion. Curves should not be fitted by hand; a computer is more reliable. ©1981 by Halberg.

11 successive days (Biagini et al., 1981). Hence, in the case of suspicion of certain diseases, it may be necessary to cover by ECG, for any one individual, more than a single 24-hour span.

One may ask whether the group result as a whole, based on 24-h records from 41 different individuals (namely from 34 patients who live for 5 years after

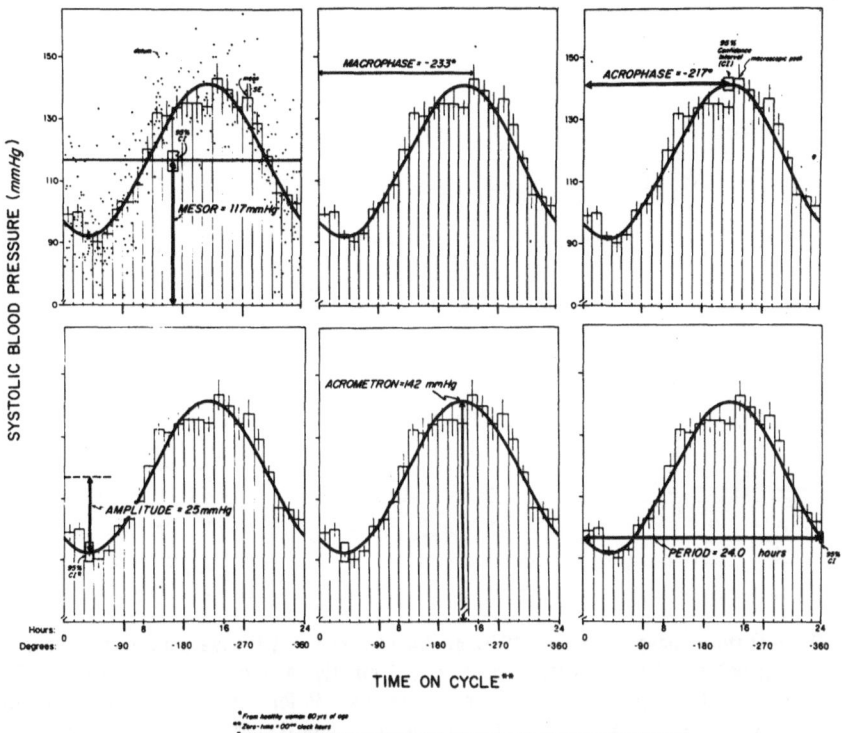

HYPOTHESIS TESTING* AND ESTIMATION OF
CIRCADIAN PARAMETERS OF SYSTOLIC BLOOD PRESSURE
ESTIMATED BY NON-LINEAR LEAST-SQUARES FIT
OF COSINE CURVE TO 7 DAYS OF DATA' (summarized by plexogram)

Fig. 2d: Summary of the Figure 2c data in a plexogram, i.e., with individual values stacked along the scale of a single idealized day, as shown with the MESOR in the top section on the left. The uncertainty of the MESOR is also shown as a 95% confidence interval (95% CI). Interval estimates are also given for three other parameters: the acrophase, amplitude and period. In addition, the figure demonstrates the so-called macrophase and the acrometron. What matters is not what these endpoints are called, but rather what they *mean*. The macrophase, i.e., the macroscopic peak, is not the acrophase (Fig. 2b); it has been shown that the acrophase is the more stable endpoint. The acrometron, the sum of MESOR and amplitude, is a fixed if arbitrary upper limit and should be replaced by time-varying limits as soon as they can be specified from work under properly defined reference conditions. ©1981 by Halberg.

their myocardial infarction and from 7 patients who die within the same span) can be used for a consideration of the sampling needed to draw an inferential statistical inference for the given individual's prospects for the ensuing 5 years. Along this line of thought, 41 days of monitoring may be too much, if day-to-day variability, in any one subject, is smaller than the variability among subjects. These variabilities remain to be compared. The duration of ECG monitoring needed to assess the 'personalized' chances of sudden death may be determined in a given individual on the basis of as-one-goes sequential analyses for circadian rhythm

DIFFERENCES IN CIRCADIAN AMPLITUDE IN THE FACE OF SIMILAR MESORS OF SYSTOLIC BLOOD PRESSURE
IN 2 CLINICALLY-HEALTHY MEN*

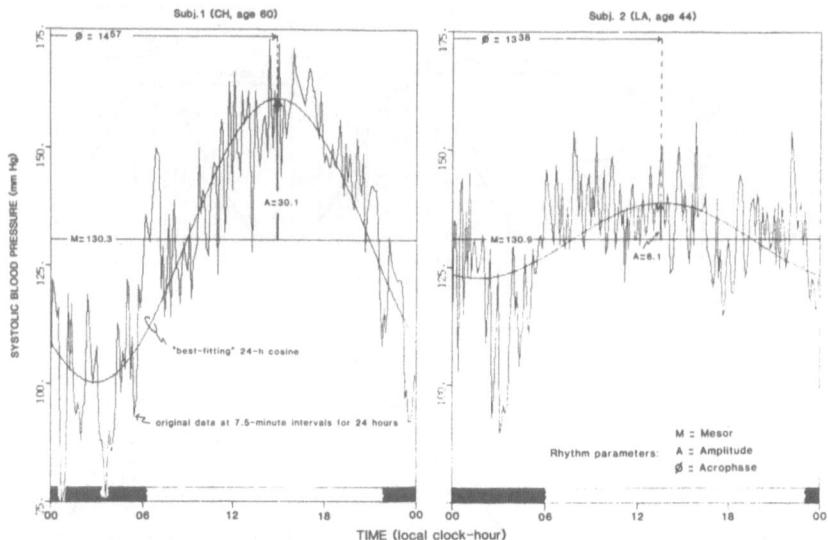

*Each wearing Pressurometer III from Delmar Avionics ,(Irvine,CA) for 24 hrs

<u>Fig. 2e</u>: 24-h systolic blood pressure (SBP) profile of 2 men, with widely differing circadian amplitudes, one being of 30.1 mm Hg, the other of 8.1 mm Hg. As a first approximation, in the case on the left, the fit of a single 24-h cosine curve accounts for a predictable change in SBP equivalent to the double amplitude, i.e., for a change of 60 mm Hg per day. The SBP MESOR is within the usual range of MESOR-variation; actually, it is the same as that of the man providing the profile on the right of the same figure. ©1984 by Halberg.

characteristics. The input into such software remains to be specified. Candidate endpoints remain to be sought among the variables yielded by Holter monitoring, to be tested for each given purpose such as diagnosis, prognosis, the timing of therapy and the assessment of its effects. The promise of the chronobiologically interpreted ECG applies to both drug administration and electrical pacing. Whatever the application, Figure 5a,b suggests that cardiac monitoring in 1985 can exploit information on circadian and other dynamics of the human heart. With respect to the assessment of a group difference, at least at a particular (5-year) post-infarction timepoint, chronobiologic criteria for the interpretation of no more than hourly VEBs succeeded where conventional ones failed.

II. Treating cancer

The war against cancer is hardly won, even if some progress in a few conditions by radiotherapy and/or chemotherapy is encouraging. In view of the realistically reviewed status quo (Kolata, 1985), any additional improvement deserves serious consideration, notably when it already has led to the gains in Figure 6a,b (Halberg, 1977, 1982; Halberg and Halberg, 1984).

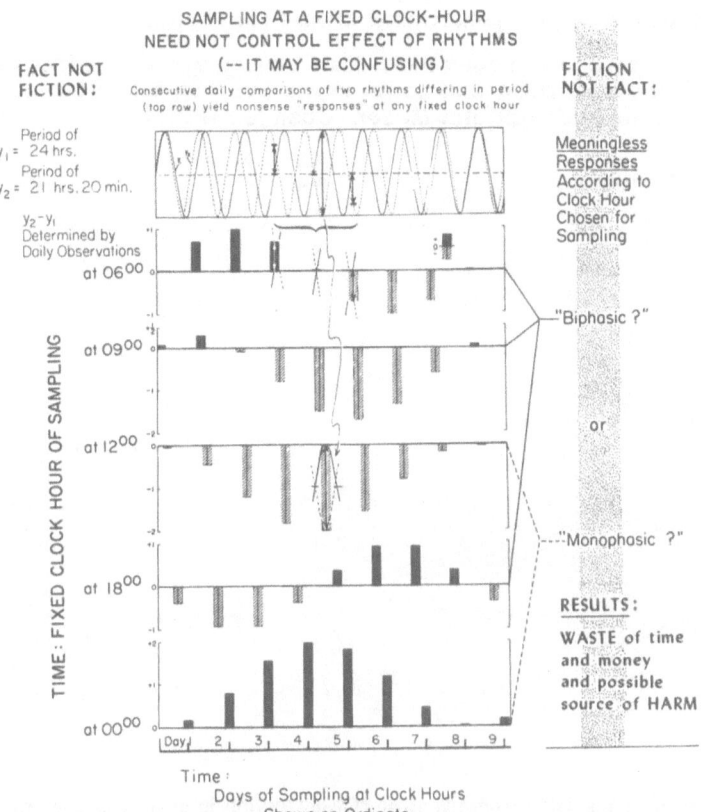

SAMPLING AT A FIXED CLOCK-HOUR
NEED NOT CONTROL EFFECT OF RHYTHMS
(--IT MAY BE CONFUSING)

FACT NOT
FICTION:

Consecutive daily comparisons of two rhythms differing in period
(top row) yield nonsense "responses" at any fixed clock hour

FICTION
NOT FACT:

Period of
y_1 = 24 hrs.

Period of
y_2 = 21 hrs. 20 min.

y_2-y_1
Determined by
Daily Observations

at 06:00

Meaningless
Responses
According to
Clock Hour
Chosen for
Sampling

at 09:00

"Biphasic ?"

TIME: FIXED CLOCK HOUR OF SAMPLING

at 12:00

or

at 18:00

"Monophasic ?"

RESULTS:

WASTE of time
and money
and possible
source of HARM

at 00:00

Day 2 3 4 5 6 7 8 9

Time:
Days of Sampling at Clock Hours
Shown on Ordinate

Fig. 3a: Confusion arising from a difference in period of the rhythms of two individuals or groups, compared at a fixed convenient time of day. This difference between the two groups being compared will undergo drastically different changes with time, simply as a function of the particular clock-hour chosen for observation. More specifically, the figure shows the time-course of an inter-group difference between synchronized controls and desynchronized experimentals, when comparisons are made 24 hours apart, at one or the other clock-hour. A given physiologic function, y, is assumed to be circadian periodic in both groups compared. y_1 could represent the very common 24-hour synchronized case, while y_2 could differ in period from y_1 by 160 minutes in time. On the plot, y_1 and y_2 start out in phase at 06, in each case.

The figure models a control, being compared with a subject exhibiting a circadian desynchronization. A similar finding may also occur in a comparison of a 24-h synchronized subject with a subject undergoing a schedule shift. Such patterns may be found in a plethora of publications on functions previously demonstrated as circadian periodic. The value of such responses is questioned, even if everybody samples at the same clock-hour. Thus, if a student working daily at noon records a drop, e.g., in the biochemical value of a patient, a replacement therapy will be advocated. This would be disputed (and should be) by a colleague working at midnight who records a rise and recommends the opposite treatment. Were it not that the more prominent investigators of circadian systems are themselves synchronized by rather similar

14

social schedules, such disputes would be much more frequent. Whether or not a response is contested, however, matters little. Actually, the undisputed 'result' is the more dangerous one, since it can be the basis of unwarranted clinical action. ©1960 by Halberg.

Plasma Aldosterone in Young Individuals as Compared to Older Ones is *Higher* in the Morning and *Lower* in the Evening, Since Circadian Amplitude, but not Mesor, Changes with Age*

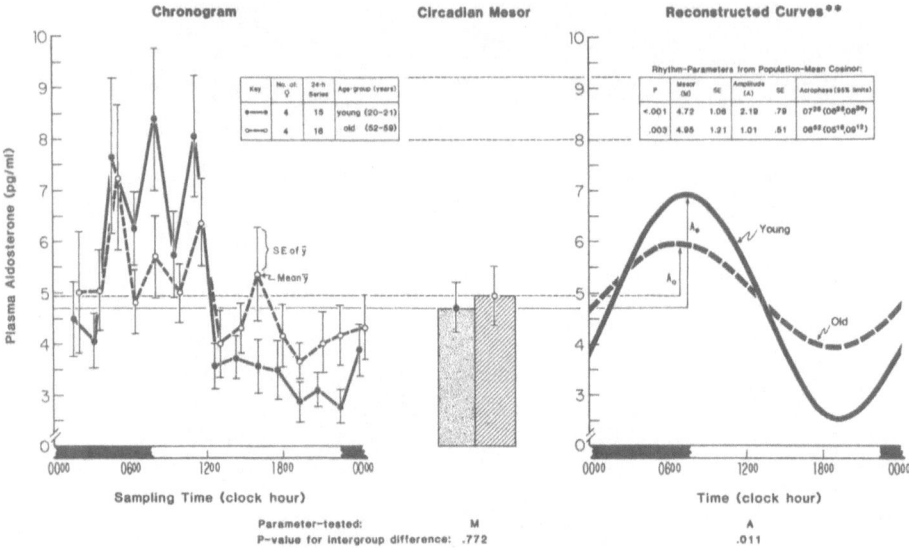

*Diurnally active, nocturnally resting Japanese women sampled every 100 minutes throughout 24-hour spans in each of the 4 seasons.
** Each cosine curve (representing rhythm) drawn on basis of parameter estimates from population-mean cosinor (see box).

Fig. 3b: The confusion arising from the study of two individuals or groups when the rhythms' amplitudes differ. Depending on the time of day when the two groups are being compared, e.g., with sampling at peak or trough time, young individuals will have the higher or the lower circulating aldosterone concentration, respectively. Opposing interpretations of the data will lead to a dispute; a third colleague who will sample, e.g., at the midline crossing, will claim that both of the other investigators are wrong and that there is no age effect. The heuristic value of conclusions drawn from work at a fixed time of day is limited. ©1983 by Halberg.

II.1. *Chronoradiobiology.* The importance of timing radiation is demonstrated under controlled conditions in the laboratory. The dose of whole-body irradiation that kills about 50% of exposed mice within 30 days varies drastically as a function of the circadian rhythm stage at irradiation time, Figure 7, mostly as a function of documented changes in the susceptibility of the bone marrow (Halberg, 1960, 1982; Haus et al., 1974). As Figure 7 also shows, these results are not a time-of-day effect. The timing of these rhythmic changes in bone marrow susceptibility and mortality can be shifted by manipulating the regimen of lighting. Whereas highest resistance to radiation exposure occurs in the early afternoon, on one lighting regimen, it occurs about 12 hours later on a long-maintained different regimen. In addition to the mammalian host, certain tumors also exhibit circadian rhythms. A technology transfer to the clinic of this basic information is documented in Figure 8.

II.2. *Chronoradiotherapy.* Nearly 50 patients in India with large tumors in or near the mouth received radiotherapy (Rx) in Chandigarh, India, at different times related to when the tumor (or the region close to the tumor) was warmest. After taking temperature readings of each patient's

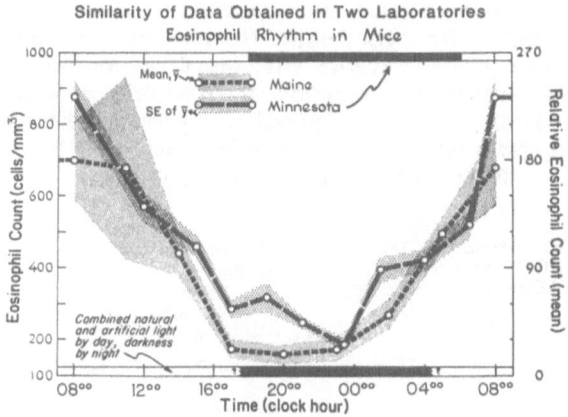

Similarity of Data Obtained in Two Laboratories
Eosinophil Rhythm in Mice

Fig. 4a: Chronogram displays data obtained under only slightly different conditions of illumination in two different laboratories, a year and many miles apart. Mice of different sex from different stocks were studied. The design of one study provided for sampling at intervals of several days on the same animals in Minnesota. In the other study, in Maine, separate, presumably comparable groups were sampled at intervals during a 24-h span. Actual counts are shown for the confirmatory data from Maine (vertical scale on left), whereas data from Minnesota are expressed as relative change, i.e., as percentage of the mean equated to 100%, in relation to the vertical scale on the right. Use of the latter procedure renders comparable data on rhythms occurring around different means. Some similarity of the rather large changes is recognized by the naked eye. ©1959 by Halberg.

Fig. 4b: Reproducibility is a key word for rhythm assessment. It is, however, a relative matter, depending on conditions, not all of them reproduced in "replications" of a given study. The impressive similarity in Figure 4a is reproduced to a considerable yet more limited extent in Fig. 4b. Data from Utah and Arkansas and another profile from Minnesota are added to those in Fig. 4a. Three new strains are explored; again, animals of the two sexes are added. It becomes clear that some procedure other than a description of the peak time or the trough time is needed to assess the extent of reproducibility of rhythm characteristics. This is the purpose of the display on the right.

Replication of Circadian Rhythm in Circulating Eosinophils of Mice of Different Stock and Sex
Studied in Different Laboratories over a 27-year Span

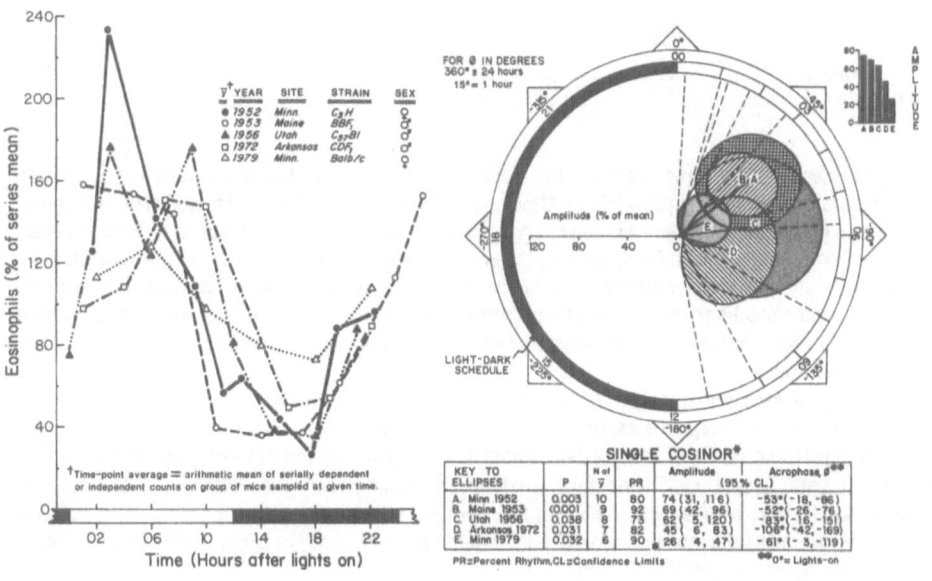

16

This display, the so-called single cosinor, provides a measure of the timing of high values by the angle of a vector and of the extent of change by the vector length. The uncertainties of these estimates are described by confidence regions. While the rhythm is reproduced, as a non-random event, with statistical significance, the point estimates can vary drastically, if for instance the two studies in Minnesota are compared (see also Figs. 14d-14g). In any event, the rhythm as such is not an exception. A *somewhat* reproducible change not only in circulating blood eosinophils but in many other variables as well is actually the rule in biology (see Fig. 4c). ©1982 by Halberg.

FROM CLOCK—CALENDAR OVER RHYTHM—RESTRICTED—PROGRAM (top middle and right)
TO BIOLOGIC—TIME—STRUCTURE* (bottom middle and right).
MOLECULAR TO SOCIETAL

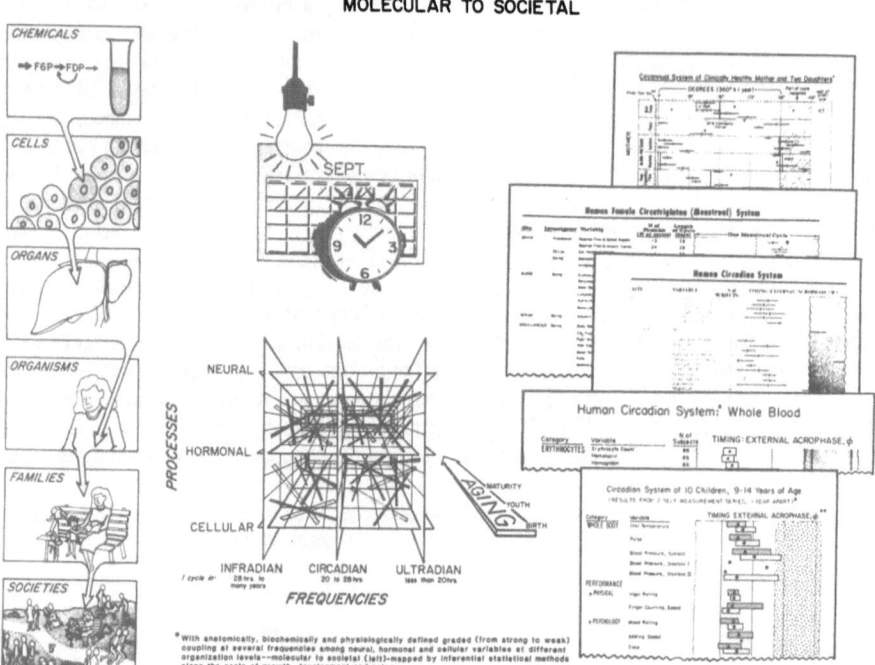

Fig. 4c: Abstract timekeeping mechanisms such as 'biologic' clocks and calendars constitute interesting analogies. Focus upon biologic timekeeping mechanisms such as the adrenal, pituitary, hypothalamus or pineal is preferred. Sharper focus upon specific loci pertinent to a given problem such as the fasciculata of the adrenal cortex, the anterior lobe of the pituitary, the suprachiasmatic nuclei of the hypothalamus or specific cells of the pineal is warranted and is best complemented by reference to biochemical entities. Such a focus, while important, is of much more limited scope than the recognition that rhythms, as the dynamics of all life, must come into the mainstream of all biology and medicine.

Rhythms are now assessed in solutions of chemicals, in unicells as well as in cell cultures, in organs, organisms, families and societies. In mammals in particular, they are found at the neural, hormonal and cellular levels of integration. Apart from any discussion of clocks and calendars that may prompt (but cannot substitute for) anatomical, biophysical, biochemical, physiologic or behavioral work, it is necessary to map rhythms as they take place, with infradian, circadian and ultradian frequencies intermodulating with each other and with superimposed trends in the context of growth, development and aging. ©1980 by Halberg.

Table 4
Different approaches to the estimation of benefit from the radiotherapy of human perioral cancers all reveal that timing is important in determining outcomes.

Perioral tumor regression rates (in %/week) as a function of circadian stage (in relation to tumor temperature macrophase, γ_T) of radiotherapy

Data summary[1]

Approach[2]	N	Data limits low	Data limits high	Range of change original	%	Mean ± SE (SD)
IA	5	7.9	16.6	8.7	110.3	12.1 ± 1.5 (3.4)
IB	39	3.5	21.5	18.0	514.3	12.2 ± 0.8 (4.7)
II	39	3.0	17.5	14.5	481.8	8.8 ± 0.6 (3.7)

Rhythmometric summary

Approach	% rhythm	P (H_0: A=0)	MESOR ± SE (%/week)	Amplitude (95% CI)	Acrophase[3]
IA	96	0.042	11.2 ± 0.5	4.9 (1.8, 8.0)	-354° (-320, -25)
IB	32	0.001	11.6 ± 0.7	4.1 (2.1; 6.2)	-332° (-304,-356)
II	48	<0.001	8.0 ± 0.5	4.2 (2.7; 5.6)	-353° (-336, -9)

Diagnostic tests[4]

Approach	Sinus	Norm	Hom. var.
IA	NA	>.050	0.828
IB	0.252	>.050	0.871
II	0.262	>.050	0.231

1) N = number of data; SE = standard error; SD = standard deviation; CI = confidence interval.
2) Approach differs in the estimation of tumor regression rate. In approach I, a usual linear regression model is fitted to means of data from all patients treated at a given circadian stage (A) or using all individual data (B). In approach II, the regression line is constrained to pass through the origin and all individual data are used; 8 patients per treatment time; tumor regression estimated weekly over 5 weeks; tumor regression not evaluated on 5th week for one patient.
3) $360° \equiv 24$ h; $0° = \gamma_T$; radiotherapy administered at γ_T, ± 4 h from γ_T or ± 8 h from γ_T.
4) P-values from test of assumptions underlying the use of the single cosinor method. P>0.05 validates the cosinor results, whereas P<0.05 provides information concerning data departure from underlying assumptions; NA indicates that the test could not be performed (no replicate); 'sinus' relates to the sinusoidality test, i.e., a test of goodness of fit for the cosine model; 'normal' checks the normality of residuals (Shapiro-Wilk test); 'hom var' tests the homogeneity of variance; since none of these tests yields P-values < 0.05, transformations or alternate models need not be considered.
Original data: Deka A., Chatterjee B., Gupta B.D., Balakrishnan C., Dutta T.K.: Temperature rhythm—an index of tumour regression and mucositis during the radiation treatment of oral cancers. Ind. J. Cancer 13: 44-50, 1976.

18

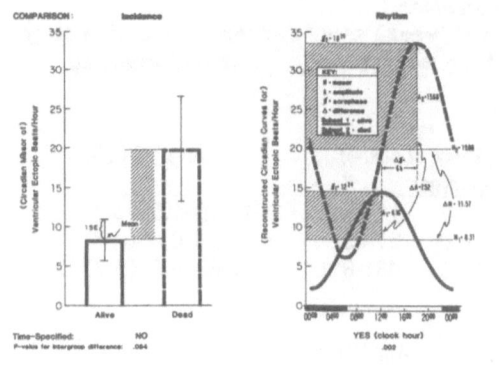

Ventricular Ectopic Beats (VEBs) in Patients with Ischemic Heart Disease Who Survived (——) or Died (←——→) within 5 Years of 24-Hour ECG Recording

Homeostatic Approach (left) and Chronobiologic Approach (right) to the Prediction of Sudden Death

Fig. 5a: Classical physiology and medicine assess the incidence of abnormality (left of figure), e.g., ventricular ectopies (with the implied viewpoint of homeostasis, i.e., an imaginary regulation for constancy, with random variability around a set-point). In so doing, one ignores the very dynamics of life at all levels of organization, including the heart. A chronobiologic approach that relies on the recognition and quantification of a spectrum of rhythms is now possible with time series of appropriate density and length, collected with modern hardware and software. Note that the P-value for the intergroup difference in the incidence of VEBs is .084 if one follows a homeostatic approach. This P-value improves considerably when circadian rhythm characteristics are assessed (Figure 4b, right). The approach to an entire spectrum of rhythms in more detailed records over longer spans should be even more useful. From Orth-Gomér et al., in press.

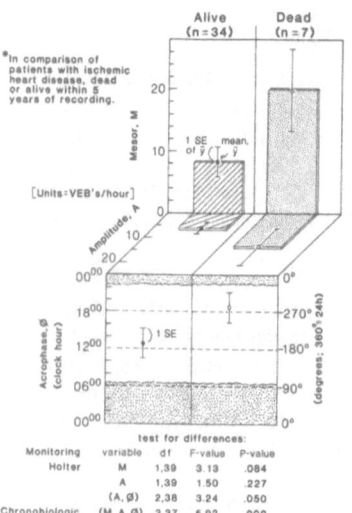

Chronobiologic Monitoring Succeeds (P=.002) to Predict Life or Death When Traditional Holter Monitoring Fails (P = .084)*

Fig. 5b: A group approach to assessing chances of sudden death in this figure, elaborating on Figure 5a, is no substitute for an individualized approach. Note nonetheless that the amplitude-acrophase pair in itself resolves the inter-group difference at the 5% level, while a chronobiologic approach taking three rhythm characteristics into account yields a P of .002. It should be realized that these analyses deal with only a single frequency, the circadian, and ignore even the circadian waveform, as well as ultradians and infradians. For qualification, see text. From Orth-Gomér et al., in press.

continued from page 14

tumor every 2 hours for several days, the average time of peak tumor temperature was determined in each case. The patients were then assigned to different groups with differently timed Rx to find the best Rx time. Eight patients received Rx at the temperature peak. Four other groups, each consisting of 8 patients, received Rx either 4 or 8 hours before or after their tumors' temperature peak. After 5 weeks of Rx, 5 days a week, tumors had shrunk the fastest and were about 30% of their original size in patients who received Rx at the peak tumor temperature time. The tumors in patients who received the same Rx 8 hours after their tumor's peak temperature time had shrunk to only slightly less than 70% of their original size, as seen on the left of Figure 8. Details of various approaches, all validating the merits of chronotherapy, are given in Table 4. Thus, the beneficial therapeutic effect (tumor shrinkage) of radiotherapy was enhanced more than 100% by timing Rx according to a circadian variation in tumor temperature (Deka, 1975; Deka et al., 1976; Halberg et al., 1977).

More importantly, a follow-up 2 years after completion of Rx showed that more than 60% of those treated at the time of peak of their tumor temperature were still alive and disease-free,

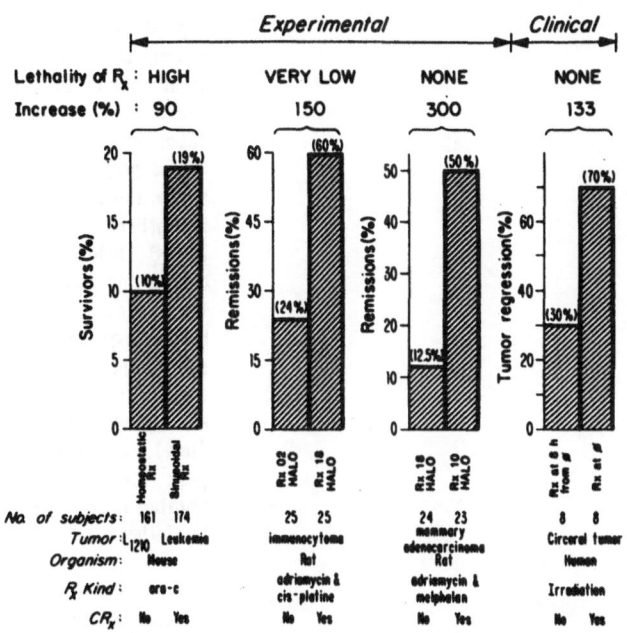

Fig. 6a: Chronotherapy in the laboratory (first 3 studies) and clinical details of time course in Fig. 8. ©1980 by Halberg.

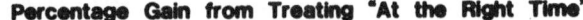

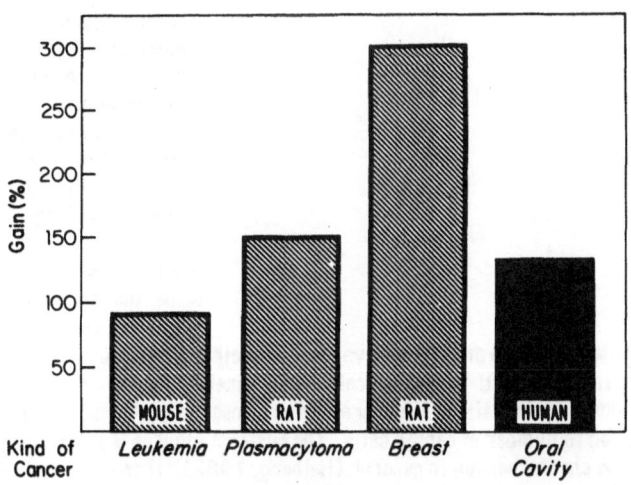

Fig. 6b: Percentage gain in treating several malignant tumors at the right time (23). ©1980 by Halberg.

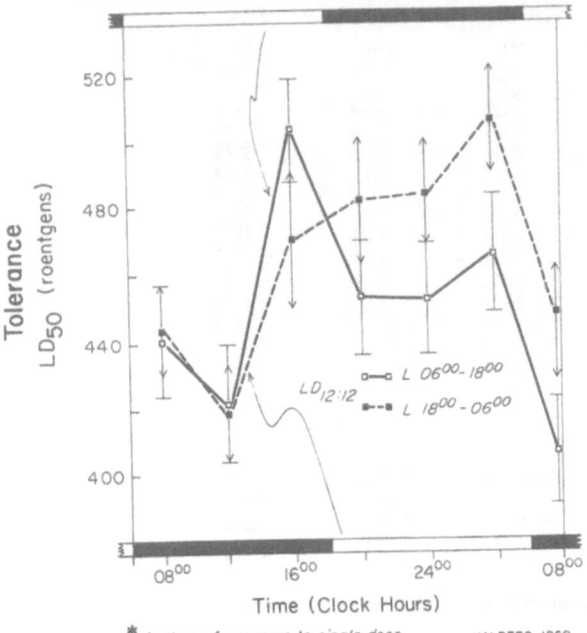

CHRONOTOLERANCE
Gauged by
LD_{50} From Whole Body X-Irradiation of C-Mice In Relation To Circadian System Stage *

Tolerance
LD_{50} (roentgens)

520

480

440

$LD_{12:12}$ o—o $L\ 06^{00}-18^{00}$
●--● $L\ 18^{00}-06^{00}$

400

08^{00} 16^{00} 24^{00} 08^{00}
Time (Clock Hours)

At time of exposure to single dose   HALBERG, 1960

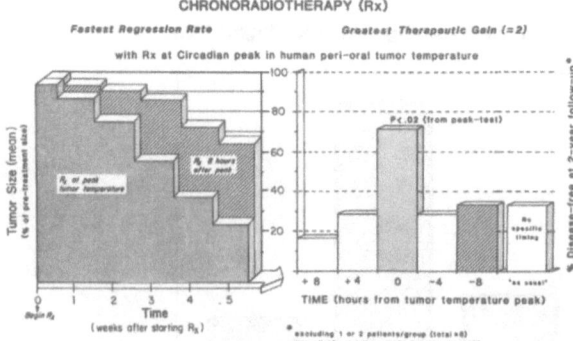

CHRONORADIOTHERAPY (Rx)

Fastest Regression Rate   Greatest Therapeutic Gain (=2)

with Rx at Circadian peak in human peri-oral tumor temperature

Tumor Size (mean)
(% of pre-treatment size)

% Disease-free at 2-year follow-up*

100
80
60
40
20

R_x at peak
tumor temperature

R_x 8 hours
after peak

P<.03 (from peak-test)

R_x
specific
timing

0   1   2   3   4   .5
Begin R_x Time
(weeks after starting R_x)

+8   +4   0   -4   -8   "as usual"
TIME (hours from tumor temperature peak)

* excluding 1 or 2 patients/group (total =8)
unavailable at follow-up (Halberg et al., 1977)

Fig. 7: The dose of whole-body x-irradiation which kills 50% of the animals within 30 days (LD50/30) depends on the stage of the circadian system at the time of exposure. The single dose, LD50/30 (obtained in 1958 in the Chronobiology Laboratories, University of Minnesota), varies by nearly 100 r as a function of circadian timing. ©1960 by Halberg.

Fig. 8 (below): Timing complements dosing for gain in treating cancer. Tumor regression is of about 70% on the average when treatment is given at peak tumor temperature, whereas it may only be of about 30% on the average with treatment at other times (left). A gain of 2 from treatment at peak tumor temperature as marker rhythm is shown on the right. ©1970 by Halberg.

compared with only 35% or less of the patients treated 4 or 8 hours before or after tumor peak temperature or in the control group "treated as usual", as shown on the right of Figure 8. Statistical analyses in Table 4 of these two-year follow-up data of the chronobiologic treatment of oral cancers in India support the use of the circadian tumor if not peritumoral temperature peak as a circadian rhythmic marker for timing radiotherapy.

II.3. *Chronochemotherapy.* One method for testing anti-cancer treatments in the laboratory is to administer a drug (for chemotherapy) every 3 hours over a 24-hour span in order to frequently if not continually bathe the body with the anti-cancer substance, and thus to catch any cancer cells that might enter a certain drug-sensitive stage of their cell division cycles. The drug then has the best chance to inhibit or kill the cancer cell. Unfortunately, healthy tissue is also destroyed by the drug. This results in undesired, life-threatening damage, e.g., to the bone marrow, along with the desired reduction in number of cancer cells. The abstract Figures 9 and 10 portray the available evidence underlying chronotherapy in general (Halberg, 1982). It is well-known for many agents, including drugs, that a given dose of a potentially harmful agent can be tolerated better at one time than at another time (Figure 9, left). It seems reasonable, therefore, to vary dosing with timing (Figure 9, right). To emphasize these points, Figure 10 left combines the foregoing rationale: a

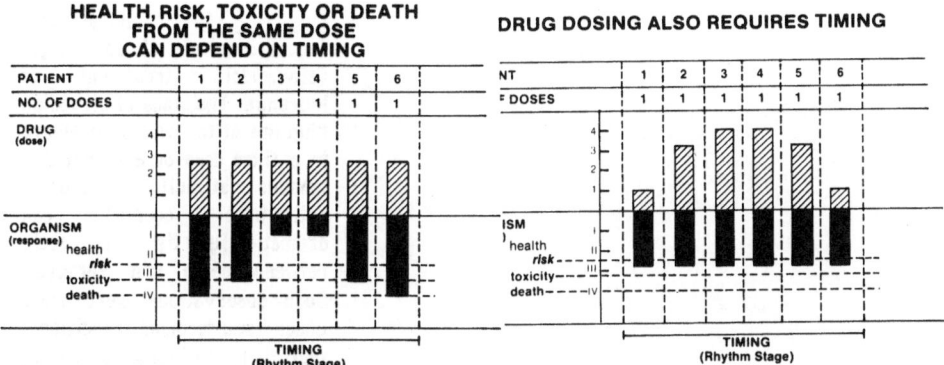

Fig. 9: Abstract schemes representing a wealth of information on the importance of rhythm stage in the outcome of a desired or undesired response, including death. © 1973 by Halberg.

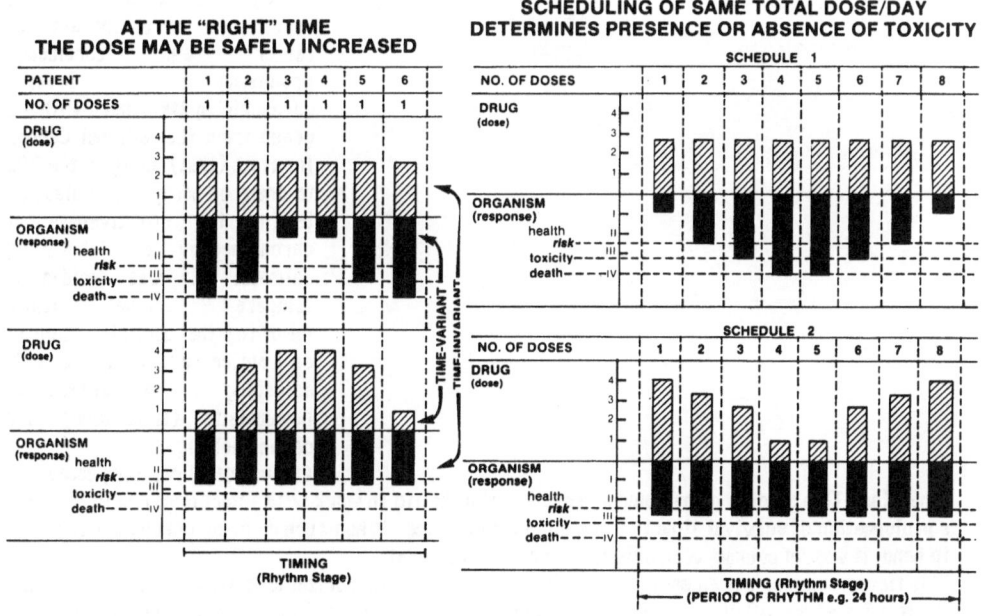

Fig. 10: Further abstract summaries of decades of work from many laboratories documenting the rational basis of chronotherapy. © 1973 by Halberg.

time-variant response characterizes a time-invariant dosing of different patients and *vice versa*, a time-variant dosing is required for a desired time-invariant response in different patients (Figure 10, left) (Halberg, 1962; Halberg et al., 1973, 1977).

The same rationale applies to multiple dosing as well, as shown at the right of Figure 10. Figures 11 and 12 carry this same rationale to a critical laboratory experiment on the model of L1210 mouse leukemia. As background to Figures 9-12, in a series of studies (not shown here [Halberg et al., 1973; Scheving et al., 1976]), the toxicity of a drug called arabinosyl cytosine

22

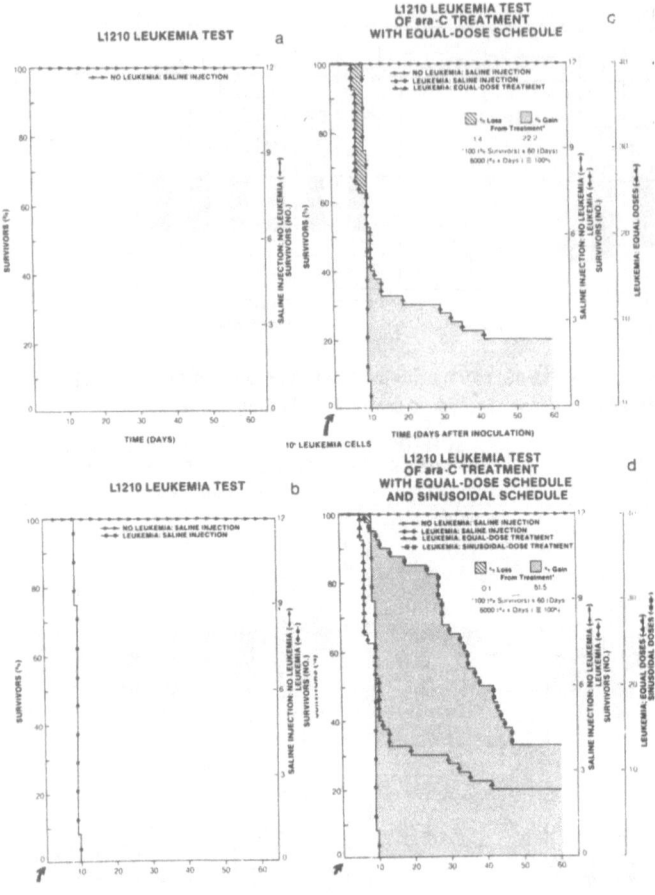

Fig. 11: Homeostatic (equal-dose) vs. chronobiologic (sinusoidal) treatment of leukemia. The stage of circadian rhythms at the time of exposure to a fixed dose of a potentially noxious stimulus (including antimitotic agents) can dramatically tip the scale between death and survival. Such observations were made under standardized conditions, including continuous darkness, to document that rhythms were not simply a function of the lighting regimen or of the time of day. On the basis of such results, a chronotherapy of cancer was considered promising. Several chronobiologists met with a group from the National Cancer Institute (USA) early in the 70s to draw up acceptable rules for testing the effectiveness of chronotherapy on laboratory animals. It was decided to compare survival times following the administration of an anticancer drug, ara-C, according to 4 courses of homeostatic (fixed-dose) and chronobiologic (sinusoidally-varying dose) schedules. This study demonstrated a reduction of lethality in work with intact mice and in terms of a prolongation of survival time in work on leukemic mice. When such gains by chronotherapy were in hand, it was, of course, desirable to improve the cure rate.

This figure summarizes an early study of cure rate. In a, the horizontal bottom scale indicates that the test lasted for 60 days; the vertical scales show that 12 animals were used to test the effect of saline injection in the absence of leukemia and that 12 is equated to 100% in this case. It can also be seen from the line with arrows on top of the graph that all 12 mice survived the saline injection. To complete the drawing of the 'tennis court', leukemia cells are given to another 12 animals on day 0, as shown in b. They survive for only a few days; by day 10 they are all dead. In c, a major homeostatic contribution to the treatment by ara-C made in non-chronobiologic terms is shown. A new scale on the right shows that we are now dealing with a larger group consisting of 40 animals. First, it can be seen that some animals die slightly earlier; this is simply a reminder of the calculated risk that one takes in deciding for chemotherapy. The loss is very small when compared with the drastic gain. Indeed, some animals live for 60 days and are probably cured. Others have a prolonged survival time. Any prolongation of survival and some cures when previously there were none is remarkable. The question remains, however, whether there can be improvement; indeed there can, as shown in d. The premature deaths are reduced to a truly negligible value; the survival time of most animals is prolonged and cure rate raised. The final summary in Fig. 12 shows that, by

23

sinusoidal chronotherapy as compared to homeostatic equal-dose treatment, the cure rate has been
nearly doubled. If the now-minimal loss is subtracted, the therapeutic benefit is still substantial
and can be further improved in other, much less toxic models. For statistical considerations,
follow-up work by others and ourselves, and references, see Halberg et al.[7]. © 1973 by Halberg.

**L1210 LEUKEMIA TEST OF ara-C TREATMENT
WITH EQUAL-DOSE OR SINUSOIDAL SCHEDULE,
AS COMPARED TO SALINE INJECTION (≡0)**

<u>Fig. 12</u>: Gain from sinusoidal chronotherapy as
compared to homeostatic equal-dose treatment.
© 1973 by Halberg.

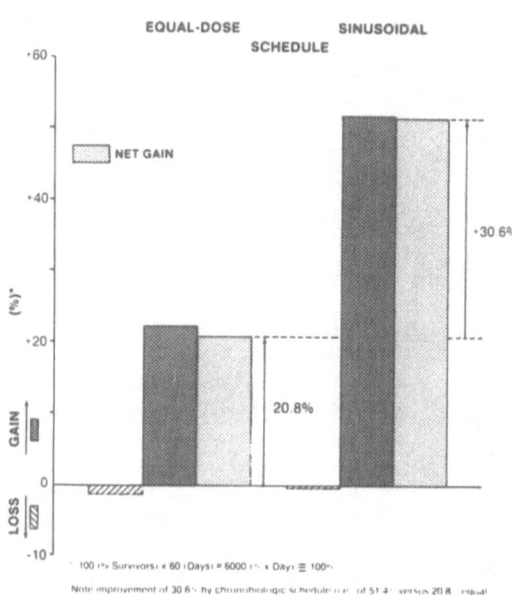

(briefly ara-C) was reduced by varying the
drug administration mode in keeping with the
principle shown at the bottom of Figure 10. In
one study, over 70% of intact mice die from
damage caused by ara-C when 8 equal 3-hourly
doses are given over a 24-hour span, followed
by 2 days of no treatment and then this entire
3-day cycle is repeated 3 more times. Instead
of 8 equal doses, 8 sinusoidal doses (that rise
and fall throughout the 24 hours) can be given,
so as to yield a total dose of drug/day
corresponding to that given in equal doses. With
the rightly timed "peak and valley" of these
gradually increasing and then decreasing doses,
up to 70% of the mice survive the treatment.
This increase in survival--higher drug
tolerance--is dependent on when the highest and
lowest doses are given (see abstract Figure 10).

In this case, most mice survive the drug
when large doses are given during their usual
resting span (in mid- to late light on a 24-h
cycle of light and darkness), when the bone

marrow is most resistant (as can also be seen from Figure 7, in response to radiation rather than
ara-C). Most mice die when largest doses are given 12 hours later, that is late in the activity
(dark) span. Thus, properly timed sinusoidal dosing reduces toxicity. A follow-up study carried
out concomitantly in laboratories at Arkansas and Minnesota on benefit from the superior tolerance
associated with the proper timing of sinusoidal ara-C treatment yielded nearly identical results
(Scheving et al., 1976).

Once data on cyclic changes in drug tolerance were in hand, it was reasonable to extend their
scope to the actual treatment of disease. In another series of experiments, instead of using intact
animals, mice were first given leukemia and were later treated with ara-C: nearly twice as many
were cured when, instead of equal doses, varying doses were given in such a way that the highest
doses were given in the middle of the resting (light) span (Halberg et al., 1973; Haus et al., 1972).
An early illustrative experiment is shown in Figures 11 and 12.

Anti-leukemic drugs are only one category among many for which it has been shown that by
treating at the 'right' time with the 'right' schedule of doses, tolerance can be increased under
controlled laboratory conditions. Cases in point are drugs acting upon a breast cancer and a
plasmacytoma of the rat; gains of up to several hundred per cent were obtained by the timing of
single or multiple-agent chemotherapy (Halberg and Delbarre, 1977; Halberg and Halberg, 1984).
These experimental gains complement the clinical gain of two—a doubling of therapeutic
benefit—from chronoradiotherapy, shown in Figure 6.

II.4. *Immunotherapy*. Treating rats carrying a transplantable plasmacytoma with properly
timed injections of an immunomodulating drug, lentinan, the malignant growth can be slowed with a
schedule simulating certain rhythmic patterns and speeded up with another pattern, both patterns

24

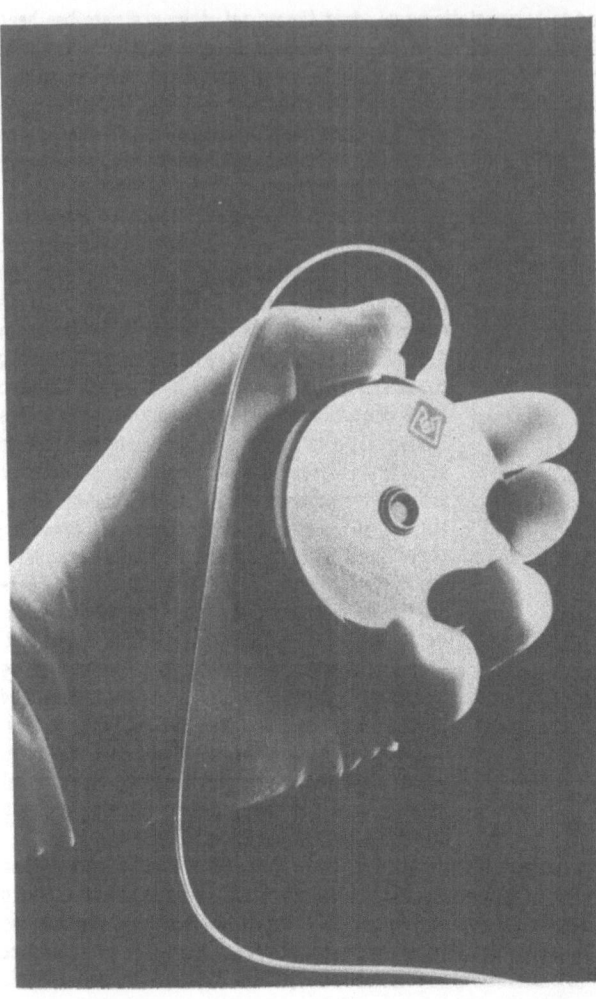

Fig. 13a: Hand-held implantable externally programmable Medtronic pump. Courtesy of Medtronic Inc., Minneapolis, MN.

totalling the same dose/day. It is important to note, for this case and several others, that optimization by drug patterning has to take into account rhythmic changes with several frequencies. Once several frequencies are involved, however, as is the case for cyclosporine (Halberg, Sanchez and Fernandez, 1983), special drug administration devices can be particularly helpful, as will be discussed next.

III. Chronotherapy via the drug pump

A Medtronic implantable and externally programmable pump (Figure 13a,b) was used on 21 outbred beagle dogs to administer cyclosporine with one of several circadian sinusoidal schedules or at a constant rate. The dogs were kept in 12 h of light alternating with 12 h of darkness. This experiment is described in a series of steps visualized in Figure 14 (Cavallini et al., in press a). Fig. 14a presents results on 9 dogs. When they are untreated, they live 5-7 days. This average of about 6 days can be improved by treatment with cyclosporine, as shown in Fig. 14b. Four animals suffice to document the point of a statistically significant improvement from cyclosporine. This improvement is kept to a modest prolongation so as not to unduly prolong the suffering of the animals and the cost. Against these two reference standards, the results obtained with the sinusoidal schedules given via the drug pump can be compared. With the pump and programmer described in Figure 13, one can indeed implement the several sinusoidal schedules shown in the top half of Fig. 14c. The sinusoidal timing of cyclosporine consisted of gradually increasing and then decreasing doses. Different dogs received the peak daily dose at a preselected circadian stage. Daily treatment with a sinusoid peaking at the right time, shortly after the middle of the daily dark span, greatly increased the effect obtained as compared to the effect of the same daily dose injected at a constant rate or injected with the sinusoidal schedule peaking at the wrong time (during the light span in the laboratory).

Figure 14 introduces, with the results, the cosinor method of data analysis. The data for each dog are shown as such in the bottom half of Fig. 14c. Connecting the data at each timepoint with a line (using the mean, when there are 2 dogs at one timepoint) does not help clarify whether the differences represent random variability. The fit of a 24-h cosine curve in Fig. 14d in turn serves

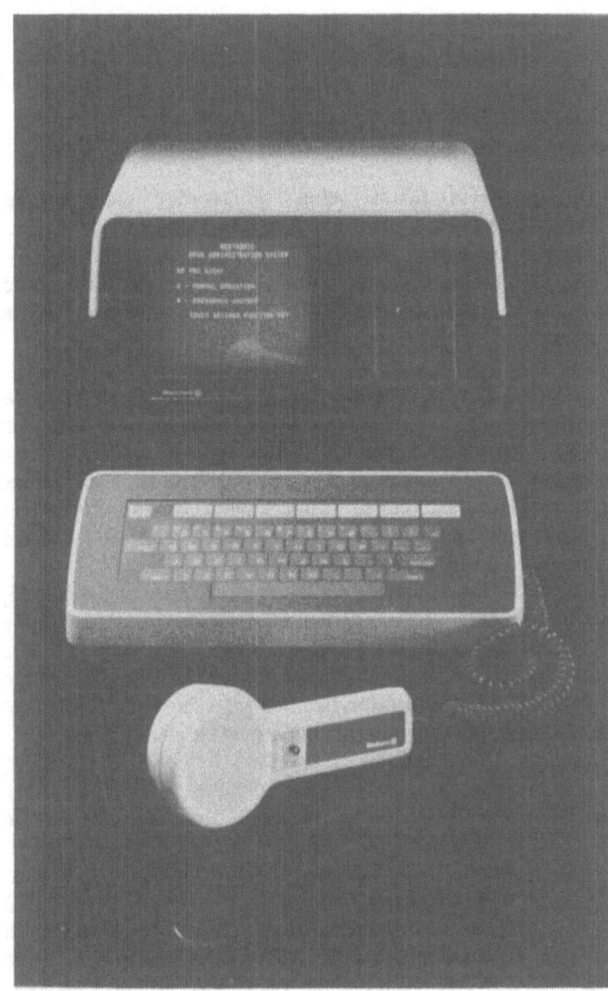

Fig. 13b: External programmer of implantable Medtronic pump, used to vary rate of cyclosporine (or any other) infusion according, e.g., to circadian sinusoidal schedules (see Figure 14c). Courtesy of Medtronic Inc., Minneapolis, MN.

this purpose of asking about the likelihood that the results are a matter of chance. With the fit shown in Figure 14d, one can test whether the amplitude of the fitted cosine curve is likely to be zero. In rejecting the zero-amplitude assumption (result not shown), the rhythm can indeed be validated, as is the case for the results on cyclosporine in this figure. One can then proceed to an estimation of rhythm characteristics, shown in Fig. 14e; it can be seen that the amplitude is at 5.23 days. This amplitude is one-half of the total predictable change due to the organism's rhythmic response, i.e., to drug timing. The double amplitude or the total predictable change (not the range of variability) is 10 days. The best treatment time is also given by the acrophase, an indication of the lag from some arbitrary zero-time (in this case midnight) of the peak in the curve best-approximating all data. It does appear that this best time is 2h 24 min after the reference (i.e., after midnight).

Figure 14f shows the Figure 14e results in a different way, along polar coordinates, as a step toward the estimation of the uncertainty of the rhythm characteristics. These characteristics are displayed on a clock-face. Midnight is shown on top, noon at the bottom, and 6 a.m. and 6 p.m. are shown on the left and right, respectively. Negative degrees are shown in a clockwise fashion so that midnight corresponds to 0°, 06^{00} to -90°, noon to -180°; other times are readily computed if it is realized that 360° are equated to 24 hours, 15° to 1 hour and hence 1° to 4 minutes. A confidence region for the uncertainty of the best time for highest concentrations of the sinusoidal cyclosporine schedule is also given, in Figure 14g, as the elliptical region around the tip of the vector representing the amplitude-acrophase pair.

Once the cyclosporine sinusoid peaking at night was known to be associated with best results, whereas a sinusoid peaking around noon yielded the worst results, two different treatment times were used for follow-up work with oral doses. These were so chosen that one led to blood concentrations that peaked at the anticipated best circadian stage (around 02^{30}), the second, about

PROLONGATION OF CANINE RENAL ALLOGRAFT FUNCTION OPTIMIZED BY CIRCADIAN SINUSOIDAL CYCLOSPORINE TREATMENT VIA IMPLANTED (MEDTRONIC) PUMP.

FIRST UNTREATED OR UNDERTREATED CONTROL GROUP: TIME TO REJECTION IN THE ABSENCE OF TREATMENT OR WHEN LESS THAN 50% OF INTENDED CYCLOSPORINE DOSE IS ACTUALLY ADMINISTERED

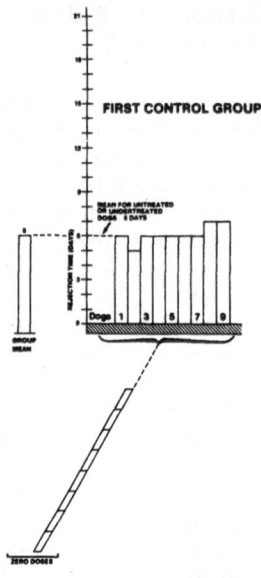

Fig. 14a: The canine animal preparation used for the chronotherapy-test with the pump described in Figure 13a. From Cavallini et al., in press.

Fig. 14b: (below) Treatment with equal doses (the homeostatic approach) prolongs life (P<.05). From Cavallini et al., in press.

12 hours later, at the anticipated worst circadian stage. By the choice of these oral treatment times, allowance was made for differences in route of administration, for reproducing the time courses of the desired and the undesired cyclosporine concentrations in blood. Pharmacokinetic studies indicated that the intended timing of changing blood concentrations was indeed achieved (Cavallini et al., in press a-c).

This follow-up study on kidney-allografted dogs validated, with the oral administration of cyclosporine, the results obtained earlier by the use of the pump. As a start, 10 dogs were paired; each had one kidney removed and discarded, while the other kidney was removed and transplanted into its partner in the pair. Within each pair, one dog was assigned to one treatment time while the other was assigned to the other treatment time. This was done to compensate for inter-dog differences by keeping the immunologic barrier similar within a pair of dogs. The two groups treated at 2 different times were thus rendered comparable. In order to prevent the transplanted kidney from being rejected, cyclosporine was given orally once each day for as long as the kidney functioned. One dog in each pair received the drug at 08^{30} every day, while the second dog received the drug at 20^{30}.

Treatment notwithstanding, all dogs receiving cyclosporine in the morning had rejected their grafted kidney by 10 days after surgery. Rejections in this group started as early as 6 days after surgery and were roughly comparable to those of the earlier series, Figure 15. Of the 5 dogs treated in the evening, the predicted right time, only one dog had rejected the transplanted kidney at 15 days after surgery. Even in this case, there is a 50% increase over the longest graft survival time for dogs receiving the drug in the same dose in the morning (at the wrong time). The grafts in the other 4 dogs treated in the evening (at the right time) were still functioning at

SECOND "HOMEOSTATICALLY"-TREATED CONTROL GROUP: EFFECT OF EQUAL CYCLOSPORINE DOSES: UNAMBIGUOUS PROLONGATION OF GRAFT FUNCTION GAIN KEPT SMALL IN ORDER TO REDUCE STUDY DURATION AND COST

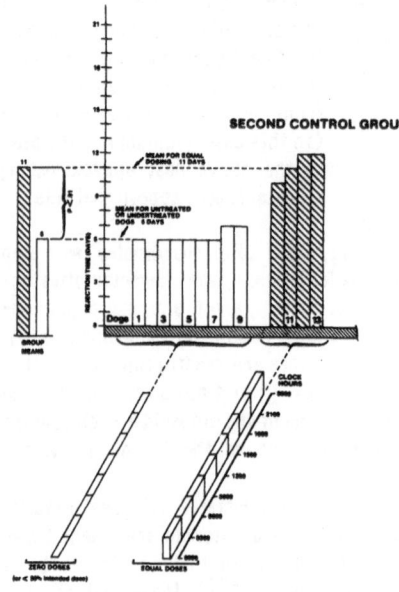

MACROSCOPIC VIEW OF CHANGES IN REJECTION TIME AS A FUNCTION OF CIRCADIAN TIMING OF PEAK CYCLOSPORINE ADMINISTRATION.

Fig. 14c: Treatment with sinusoidally varying doses, with different time location of high and low doses, has different effects. From Cavallini et al., in press.

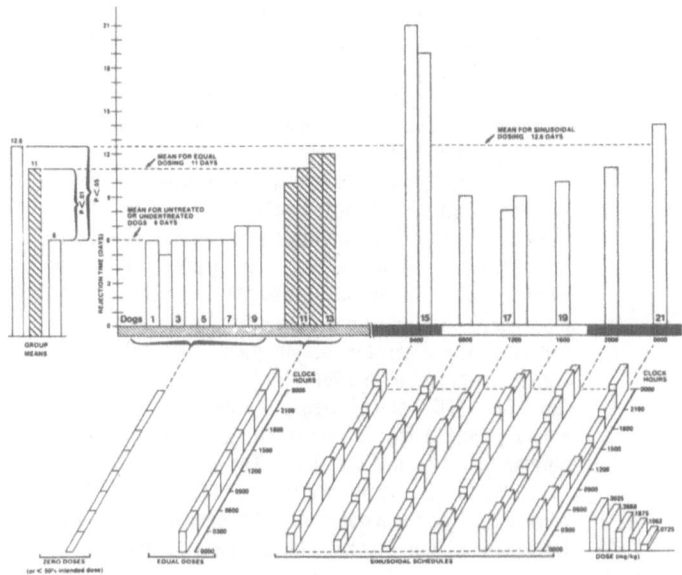

the time of the first summary. One of these dogs had lived for more than a month after surgery, while its partner, treated at the wrong time, had rejected within 1 week after surgery, Figure 15. These statistically highly significant results on the first 5 pairs were confirmed by follow-up work on other pairs of dogs (Cavallini et al., in press c).

A high-technology product, the drug pump, served in this case as a tool for therapy research leading the way toward a conventional (oral) therapy mode optimized according to circadian rhythms. It has been shown in the interim, however, that much added gain can be derived from a therapy with

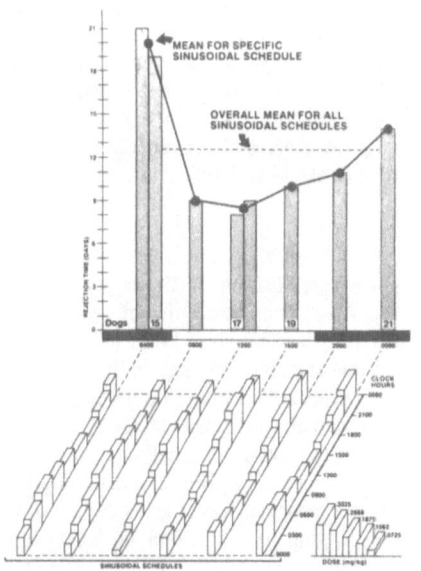

cyclosporine also optimized according to built-in about-7-day circaseptan rhythms. When multiple circadian and circaseptan patterns, Figure 16, are to be administered, drug pumps become an indispensable tool. In combination with the use of marker rhythms, they can provide the properly timed "peaks and valleys" in drug concentration, as these are needed for an optimal therapeutic effect.

For some of the work with ara-C in Figures 11 and 12, a former laboratory staff member, an Olympic runner (he had to be one!), administered the sinusoidal drug patterns. His effort was considerable: he injected 270 mice within 180 minutes; that is, he injected each mouse within less than 60 seconds. At this feverish pace, he continued reinjecting large groups of mice every 3 hours, for 48 hours. He repeated this 48-hour marathon after a rest day for 3 more cycles. The addition of a second about-7-day (circaseptan) pattern to the circadian one is unrealistic if a pump is unavailable. The same demanding patterns, however, are now easily and automatically implemented in the patient by an implantable externally programmable pump, Figure 13. Indeed, more complex schedules than a single set of increasing and decreasing doses during 24 hours can

FIT OF A COSINE CURVE PROVIDES MEANS FOR RHYTHM DETECTION AND FOR PARAMETER ESTIMATION (WITH CONFIDENCE LIMITS): THE FIT REVEALS MARKED DIFFERENCES IN REJECTION TIME AS A FUNCTION OF THE TIMING OF HIGHEST CYCLOSPORINE DOSE.

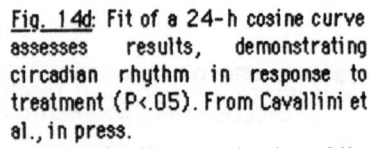

Fig. 14d: Fit of a 24-h cosine curve assesses results, demonstrating circadian rhythm in response to treatment (P<.05). From Cavallini et al., in press.

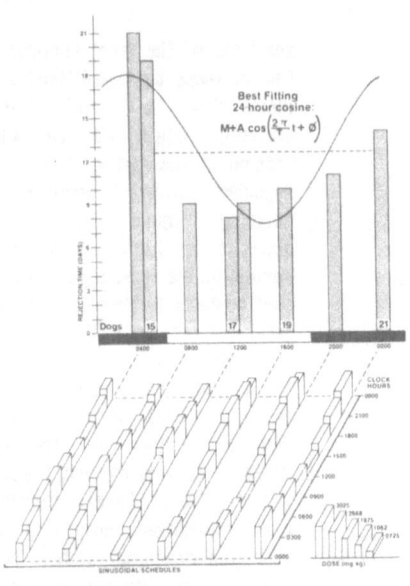

and should be given with the pump in view of the exhaustive evidence documenting the clinical importance of circadian-circaseptan intermodulation. The possiblity must also be kept in mind that a fixed-rate drug administration is likely to result in complex response patterns, such as those shown in Figure 16.

The next task is to administer drugs according to marker rhythms monitored automatically. Monitored information should be analyzed as one goes and results of analyses should govern the pattern of drug administration. This "closing of the loop" between the dispenser (the pump) and the sensor (of the organism) constitutes a desirable development. As yet only a limited number of marker rhythms, such as those of the ECG, EEG, blood pressure, respiration, motor activity and body temperature, can be monitored automatically around the clock. The need to collect data manually is now eliminated in these instances, but the need to analyze them automatically remains. Even with this qualification, marker rhythmometry is particularly useful when the period of a patient's rhythms is different from precisely 24 hours. The data from ambulatory monitoring devices already available for implementing marker rhythm assessment in the fields of potential chronotherapy, including that of cancer, have to be properly analyzed to test the possible merits of various applications in fields including, among others, cardiology and immunology. Eventually, there may be many pacemaker-pump combinations for properly scheduled electrical and pharmacologic combination treatment. Until such aims are realized, however, it seems reasonable to suggest, on the basis of available evidence, that all treatment should be timed. This suggestion is supported beyond the Figure 15 data by the finding that even the action of a placebo, in human beings (Günther et al., 1980) as well as rats (Cavallini et al., in press b), depends upon drug administration time.

IV. How many pacemakers?

Chronobiology pertains by the benefits derived from a specification of timing to all drug delivery, as a complement to dosing, Figures 9, 10 and 16. Apart from the timing of conventional treatment modes, an understanding of the body's dynamics may lead to novel kinds of treatment. Eventually, the malfunction of neuro-endocrine pacemakers that complement those in the heart may also be treated. By virtue of the hormones it rhythmically secretes, the ovary is a pacemaker in a sex-related cycle. The different zones of the adrenal cortex contain still another set of chemical pacemakers. Cortisol, an adrenal cortical hormone influencing sugar metabolism, undergoing rhythms in its own right, Figure 17a,b, coordinates several (but not all) about 24-hour rhythms (Halberg, 1983). Aldosterone, another adrenal cortical hormone influencing salt and water handling, changes the characteristics of its about-yearly rhythm as a function of the risk of developing a high blood pressure, Figure 18 (Halberg et al., 1981; Hermida and Halberg, 1984a,b; Hermida et al., 1984, 1985a). These compounds are parts of neuroendocrine networks that coordinate the changes associated with the risk of developing major diseases of our civilization. Even some aspects of personality depend upon the third hormone from the adrenal cortex,

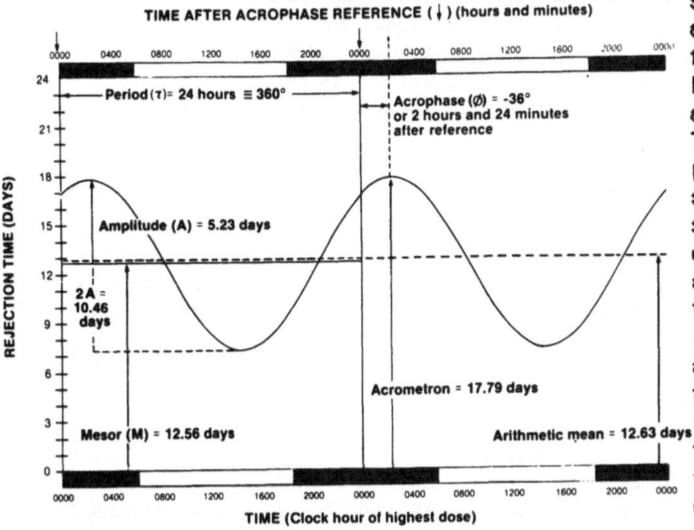

PARAMETER ESTIMATION:
MESOR: (CIRCADIAN) RHYTHM-ADJUSTED AVERAGE
REJECTION TIME WITH DIFFERENTLY TIMED
SINUSOIDAL SCHEDULES;
AMPLITUDE: MEASURE OF MAXIMAL
PREDICTABLE GAIN
ACROPHASE: MEASURE OF OPTIMAL SINUSOIDAL
SCHEDULE OF CYCLOSPORINE ADMINISTRATION.
ACROMETRON = MESOR + AMPLITUDE:
MEASURE OF LONGEST PREDICTABLE
GRAFT FUNCTION

Fig. 14e: A presentation of rhythm parameters, estimated by the 24-h cosine curve fit, approximates the extent and timing of gain. From Cavallini et al., in press.

dehydroepiandrosterone sulfate, Figure 19a-c (Hermida et al., 1985b). These steroids, which are also apparently produced periodically in the brain (Synguelakis et al., 1985), interact with several systems to which they are coupled by so-called feed-sidewards (Halberg, 1983; Halberg et al., 1983; Sánchez et al., 1983a and b), Figure 20. The organism's pacemakers and paceresetters intermodulate at several frequencies, providing spontaneously paced yet environmentally responsive and adjustive schedules for all tissues (Halberg, 1983).

TIME AFTER ACROPHASE REFERENCE (↓) (hours and minutes)

Period (τ)= 24 hours ≡ 360°
Acrophase (Ø) = -36° or 2 hours and 24 minutes after reference
Amplitude (A) = 5.23 days
2A = 10.46 days
Acrometron = 17.79 days
Mesor (M) = 12.56 days
Arithmetic mean = 12.63 days
REJECTION TIME (DAYS)
TIME (Clock hour of highest dose)

For the smooth function of an organism, various intermodulating schedules need not be rigidly maintained if the individual is to function in a fashion integrated with the environment for an optimal quality of life. Schedules can be shifted in keeping with the demands of modern life. Transient desynchronization can be an asset rather than necessarily a detriment; it can delay a genetically-determined rise in blood pressure mean (J. Halberg et al., 1980). Schedule shifts can be beneficial even in the model of an isolated cytoplasm, Figure 21a-c (Schweiger and Halberg, 1982). The frequency at which schedule shifts are implemented is critical in this context (Hayes et al., 1981; Halberg, 1983).

Artificial pacing may be required, however, when the internal circadian-infradian schedule adjustments fail, i.e., when there is a neuroendocrine block. The drug pump represents a potential chemical pacemaker, pacing with the ultradian, circadian and infradian frequencies characterizing the organism in health. Today, drug administration devices can aim to take into account the cellular rhythms of a cancer, e.g., in the human breast, by timing the delivery of anti-cancer drugs so as to reduce if not avoid their toxicity and preferably also to improve the desired effect. Figure 22a shows the goal and Figure 22b the results of work in our laboratory toward that goal (cf. also Figure 6a; Halberg et al., 1980). Tomorrow, drug administration devices may serve to correct "failing" circadian and other rhythms at several levels of rhythmic organization, Figure 4c. Such timing devices may then become as important in medicine as is the now-conventional electrical pacemaker for a failing heart.

The cardiac pacemaker itself will have to become chronobiologic beyond sensing *instantaneous* demands from within the heart, from respiration or overall muscular activity, to cite only a few of its current capabilities. Should cardiac pacing also anticipate what may be described as a long-term automatically sensed, analyzed and thus identified chronobiologic demand of the organism as a whole? An artificial cardiac pacemaker may well be taught, by software, the 'languages' of the many rhythms with different frequencies that are all preparatory for optimal function. Accumulating (if indirect) evidence for the desirability of implementing changes that are *anticipatory of*

Table 5

The same dose of the same molecule given at different times can influence cancer development in opposite ways. A polysaccharide, lentinan, given in the same total dose for a week prior to the transplantation of a plasmacytoma into the LOU rat, can accelerate tumor development and shorten lifespan when given with one pattern, yet delay carcinogenesis and prolong life when given with another pattern (Halberg et al., 1983). In the following tabulation, a spontaneous cancer appearance is delayed by the hormone melatonin at the "right time" in a dose ineffective when given at the "wrong time"

Melatonin modulates cancer appearance in mouse breast

Rx kind:	Rx time (hours after lights-on)					
	03	07	11	15	19	23
Saline	26.7±2.1	27.2±1.3	24.2±1.8	22.9±1.8	24.1±2.7	27.4±1.6
Melatonin	25.9±2.1	28.4±2.5	26.7±1.2	28.3±1.5	29.6±1.5	24.9±1.8

Mean difference (in weeks): melatonin minus saline

-0.7	+1.2	+2.5	+5.4	+5.5	-2.5

*Difference in time to tumor appearance (in weeks) for 180 $C3CF_1$ female mice (30/timepoint) treated daily with melatonin as compared to 180 mice treated with saline alone, with treatment started before the appearance of any tumors. Results summarized 38 weeks after start of treatment when 50% of mice, including 30 untreated mice, had developed a tumor. Melatonin given daily at two circadian times *delays* breast cancer appearance by more than 5 weeks, whereas the same dose given at another circadian time *accelerates* mammary carcinogenesis by 2.5 weeks, on the average. *This change in kind of melatonin effect is significant at the 0.002 level* (Table 2).

Table 6

The Table 5 results could be a matter of chance. This is highly unlikely, however, in view of the following analyses. An inferential statistical procedure supports the inference that the response to melatonin depends upon the state of the circadian rhythmic system of the host prone to develop breast cancer.

Cosinor summary of Table 5 data*

P	MESOR ± SE weeks	Amplitude (95% confidence limits)	Acrophase**
.002	1.6 ± 0.7	3.6 (1.1, 6.1)	14^{56} (11^{24}, 17^{24})

*Result of least-squares fit of 24-h cosine function to the difference, at 6 circadian times, of a total of 87 individual values for tumor appearance in melatonin-treated mice and the mean-value at each corresponding timepoint for saline-treated mice. Results summarized 38 weeks after onset of treatment when 50% of mice (including 30 untreated mice) had developed a tumor (Table 1).

The MESOR represents a 1.6-week *average* delay by melatonin of breast cancer appearance, irrespective of treatment time and as compared to mean time of tumor appearance in saline-injected controls. The average extent of *predictable* change around this MESOR, the double amplitude, averages 7.2 weeks. As a function of timing, the melatonin effect changes from an inhibition to an enhancement of mammary carcinogenesis.

**In hours and minutes after reference = light-onset in LD12:12.

Original data: Wrba H., Halberg F., Dutter A.: Placebo-accelerated murine mammary carcinogenesis possibly partly reversed by melatonin. Proc. Int. Soc. Chronobiol., Little Rock, Ark., Nov. 3-6, 1985, in press.

AMPLITUDE/ACROPHASE PAIR, SHOWN ON POLAR COORDINATES, ILLUSTRATES EXTENT OF GAIN DERIVED FROM TIMING WITH OPTIMAL SINUSOIDAL ADMINISTRATION SCHEDULE.

CIRCADIAN OPTIMIZATION OF PROLONGATION BY CYCLOSPORINE OF CANINE KIDNEY ALLOGRAFT FUNCTION

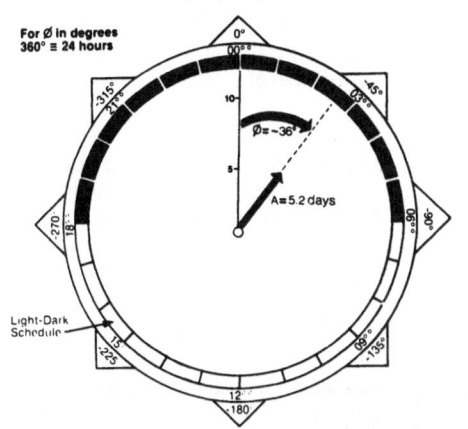

POINT AND INTERVAL ESTIMATES SHOULD BE ROUTINELY GIVEN IN GAUGING BENEFIT. ARE THESE RESULTS SIGNIFICANT IN THEMSELVES? WE ARE DEALING ONLY WITH 8 DOGS.

<u>Fig. 14f</u>: Rhythm parameters are given in polar plot as length and angle of a vector. From Cavallini et al., in press.

increased need as well as responsive to demand stems from this fledgling science of chronobiology, the computer-aided study of biologic time structure, notably of rhythms.

Timing pertains even to biotechnology, as is apparent from Figure 23. The effect of the same dose of the same molecule upon the same basic endpoint can be inhibitory for the ensuing 24 hours when given at one stage of the circadian rhythm and stimulatory for 24 hours when given at another. When this molecule is given at still other circadian stages, it can be inhibitory first and stimulatory thereafter, or vice versa (Walker et al., 1985). It follows that in molecular biology, timing is also likely to be useful if not critical. It was shown much earlier that pituitary growth hormone stimulates mitotic activity in mouse liver when given at one time, but does not do so when given at another time (Littman et al., 1958) and that this effect is detected at one time, but not at another (Halberg et al., 1973). The circumstance that an effect is detected at one time but not at another was noteworthy; the finding that with one administration time, the effect is obtained, whereas at another time it is not and that these times are predictably rhythmic, was remarkable. The observation that the effect might be actually opposite at different predictable times should prompt action.

In the latter case, timing should take precedence over dosing. This is particularly important when timing can make the difference between an inhibition and a stimulation not only of DNA-labeling in health, Fig. 23, but also of carcinogenesis (Tables 5 and 6). The mechanisms underlying such changes, including reversals of response, may be viewed as so-called feed-sidewards, Figure 24. It can be shown that depending upon the circadian stage of murine adrenal cells or of the bisected adrenals, their *in vitro* production of corticosterone, stimulated by a pituitary preincubation fluid, is attenuated, amplified or left unaffected by the addition of an aqueous pineal homogenate (APH). The pineal, the pituitary and the adrenals are characterized by variables that are rhythmic with several frequencies (Halberg, 1983).

Once it was clear that in several *ex vivo* systems, the addition of APH results in an attenuation, amplification or no effect, depending on the circadian stages of the pineal and the pituitary, follow-up work then sought to gain insight into biochemically specifiable mechanisms of this 'chronomodulation', by keeping one of the constituents constant as a first step, i.e., by replacing the pituitary preincubation medium with a synthetic short-chain ACTH 1-17 (and thereafter replacing APH with melatonin) (Sánchez et al., 1983a and b). Figure 25 shows the feed-sideward thus demonstrated: a circadian rhythmic pineal interaction with the ACTH 1-17 effect upon the bisected adrenal. In this interaction of Figure 25, the hypothalamus, as an integrator, has been removed; the pituitary is replaced by a molecule which is the same at all test times and is added in a fixed dose to the incubation medium; only the pineal and the adrenal thus interact in their varying stages. The chemical detective work and the search for its biophysical basis thus begun can now continue. There

**MEASURE OF UNCERTAINTY ON AMPLITUDE
AND ACROPHASE PAIR ESTIMATES RELIABILITY
OF BENEFIT DERIVED FROM OPTIMAL SCHEDULE
OF CYCLOSPORINE ADMINISTRATION.**

CIRCADIAN OPTIMIZATION OF PROLONGATION
BY CYCLOSPORINE OF
CANINE KIDNEY ALLOGRAFT FUNCTION

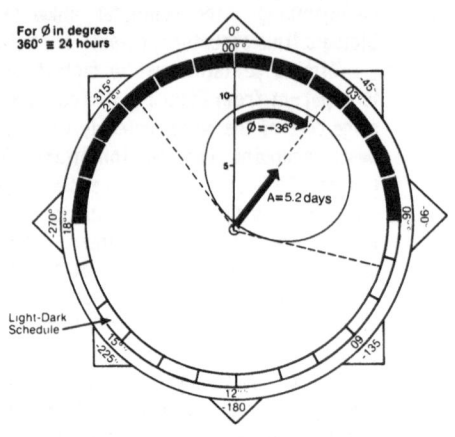

P	No. Obs.	PR	Mesor SE (Days to Rejection)	Amplitude(A) (95% CL)	Acrophase (Ø)
0.041	8	72	12.6 1.1	5.2 (.3,10.2)	-36° (-321,-108)

P = Probability of hypothesis: Amplitude = 0; No. obs. = Number of observations
PR = Percent Rhythm (percentage of variability accounted for by cosine curve)
95% CL = Conservative 95% confidence limits derived from cosinor ellipse

**CANINE RENAL ALLOGRAFT FUNCTION OPTIMIZED BY STUDY OF 6
DIFFERENTLY TIMED CIRCADIAN-SINUSOIDAL CYCLOSPORINE INFUSIONS
VIA IMPLANTED (MEDTRONIC) PUMP
RESULTS USED FOR OPTIMAL TIMING OF SINGLE DAILY
ORAL CYCLOSPORINE DOSE**

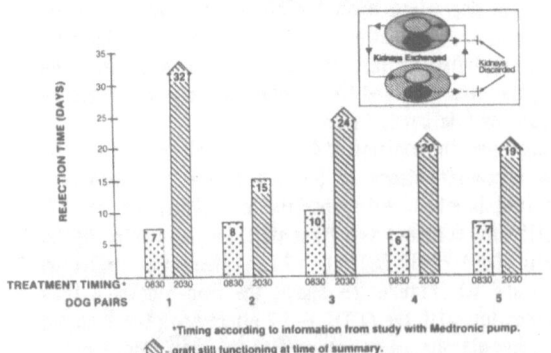

**SINGLE ORAL CYCLOSPORINE DOSE TIMED TO ACHIEVE
BEST OR WORST EFFECTS;
TIMING PREDICTED FROM RESULTS OF PUMP-DELIVERED, SYSTEMATICALLY
PROGRAMMED, DIFFERENTLY-TIMED SINUSOIDAL PATTERNS**

Fig. 14g: Uncertainty of parameters is shown by 95% confidence region. From Cavallini et al., in press.

Fig. 15 (below): In dogs kept in light from 06:00 to 18:00, treated either at 08:30 or at 20:30 with a single daily oral dose of 12.5 mg/kg cyclosporine, the evening dose is over twice as effective as the morning dose in prolonging kidney allograft function. A pharmacokinetic difference is not detected at these particular treatment times. From Cavallini et al., in press.

are likely to be many such intermodulations, as suggested by the results in Figure 23. The mechanisms of the organism's time structure, including feed-sideward in networks, are the more interesting since they may also serve as a model for better engineering.

To the extent that the data and concepts conveyed in the figures of this introductory paper constitute fact, the current concepts of physiologic homeostasis are fancy and the basic fabric of biomedical thought and action must be reconsidered. Concepts that regard rhythmic variation as random variability draw a curtain of ignorance over the very range of the dynamics of health, Figure 26. Chronobiology in turn provides a challenge for engineering in assessing physiologic changes that are hardly trivial if they can tip the scale between death and survival and that can now be resolved by available software, provided that it can be wedded to proper hardware for the collection of the data bases necessary as reference standards.

Conclusions

Christopher William Hufeland (1797), private physician and friend of Goethe, Schiller and Herder, refers to what we now call the circadian period as the unit of our natural chronology, also pertinent to *The Art of Prolonging Life,*

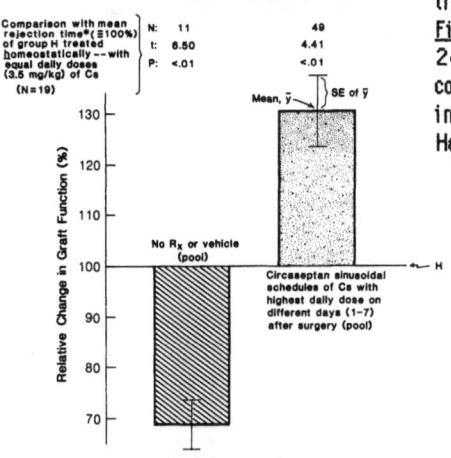

Circaseptan Optimization of Cyclosporine (Cs)
Transplant-Immunotherapy
15–27-Week-Old Diabetic Male Ma Lewis (RT-1^L)
Recipient Rats Bearing Segmental Pancreatic Allografts
from Donor ACI Rats (RT-1^a)

Comparison with mean rejection time*(≡100%) of group H treated homeostatically — with equal daily doses (3.5 mg/kg) of Cs (N=19)			
N:	11	49	
t:	6.50	4.41	
P:	<.01	<.01	

Mean, ȳ   SE of ȳ

No R$_x$ or vehicle (pool)

Circaseptan sinusoidal schedules of Cs with highest daily dose on different days (1–7) after surgery (pool)

H

Relative Change in Graft Function (%)

*Time to rejection determined by onset-time of hyperglycemia (>200 mg% lasting ≥ 3 days)

Fig. 16: As compared to treatment with equal daily doses, circaseptan dosing schedules (that vary quasi-sinusoidally with a 7-day cycle, irrespective of the timing of the highest dose) prolong graft function.

Fig. 17a: Individualized range specified along the 24-h scale for acceptable variability in plasma cortisol of a clinically healthy adult woman for the interpretation of single samples. © 1981 by Halberg.

Individual Circadian Merodesm

Tolerance intervals determined separately for 3-hour spans, indicate limits within which 90% of measurements would be expected to fall with 90% confidence.

N=72

Cortisol (plasma, μg/dl)

TIME (CLOCK HOURS)

←dark span→

*Note that a value of 5 (μg/dl) is suspiciously high for a blood sample taken at 23⁰⁰, but suspiciously low for one taken during the morning or at noon (between 06⁰⁰ and 13⁰⁰). The same value of 5 is "usual" (or "unusual") at certain other times.

the subtitle of his book, *Makrobiotik*. Indeed, the human body, as well as all other living systems, represents a network of interacting rhythms. Nearly two centuries ago, Autenrieth (1801a,b,c) described the physiologic variations of body temperature and pulse by the naked eye. Menzel (1962) was one of the first to study body temperature variations by means of an automatic temperature recorder and to use his results as a marker rhythm and also to initiate curve-fitting. Nonetheless, until the computer and the use of inferential statistics become ubiquitous, the clinical significance of physiologic changes cannot be exploited systematically in the clinic. Rhythms don't work like old-fashioned deterministic clocks, with wheels that make each other move in unison. They represent more than the feed-forward or feedback of classical endocrinology, regulating for constancy with deviations from constancy representing noise. Multiple interactions among rhythmic structures result in feed-sidewards and in rhythms of several orders, some more or less spontaneous, others reactive and still others modulatory. In a thus-chronomodulated system, the same molecule or its byproducts can at one time be a stimulator, at another time be an inhibitor and at still another time be inactive. A given molecule can function as a hormone at one time and as a neurotransmitter at another time. An understanding of this well-integrated time structure is a prerequisite for modern preventive and curative medicine. Chronobiology can explain many of the contradictions found in today's bioscience, but this is not the

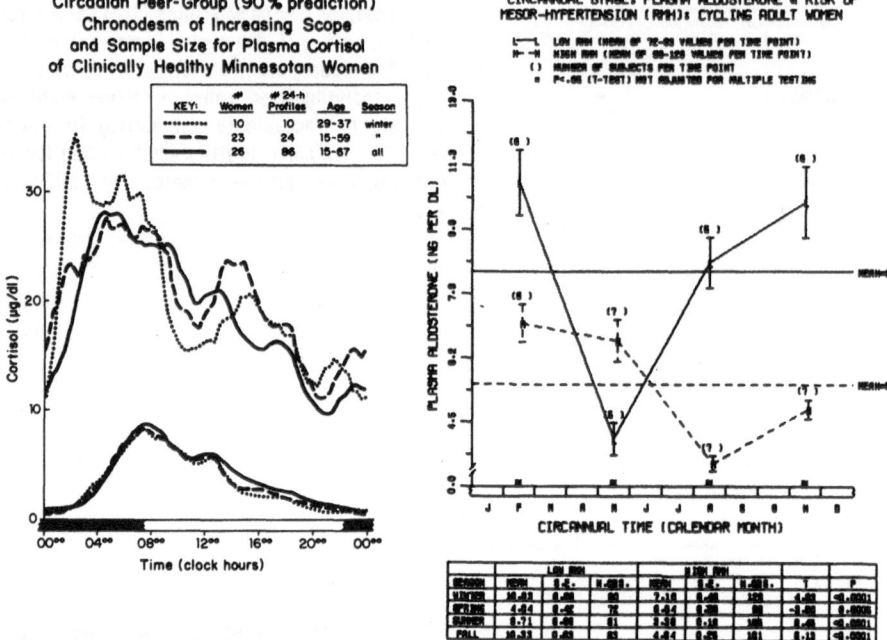

Fig. 17b: Circadian peer-group reference ranges constructed as 95% prediction intervals for the interpretation of single samples from adult women, in winter or in all seasons. These ranges serve only to illustrate the application of procedures for obtaining reference standards for endocrine determinations specified by clock-hour and the subject's living routine. Data from many more subjects are required for reliable chronodesms. Short-term fluctuations in the limits should be interpreted with special caution. The greater extent of irregularity in the upper limit, as compared to the lower, is attributable to the back-transformation of limits computed from log-transformed data. The exact pattern of irregularities depends in part on the particular data span and increment selected for the computations. The construction of chronodesms based on a model that allows for variation not only in the mean but also in the standard deviation avoids such irregularities, but requires more elaborate calculations. For the purpose of this introduction, the point may be made that there are drastic changes in hormone concentration, even when data are averaged for a group. As compared to Figure 17a, the limits in Figure 17b are broader. Individualized reference standards are indeed preferred, but are costly. From Nelson et al., 1983.

Fig. 18: Changes along the scale of a year in circulating plasma aldosterone in two groups of women at high (dashed line) or low (continuous line) risk of developing a high blood pressure. From Hermida and Halberg, 1984a.

primary aim of this field.

Chronobiology, the study of a biologic time structure, resolves the dynamics of organisms; it has its own computer-assisted methods of data collection and data analysis. By the use of such methods with special designs, this science has unearthed a wide-ranging body of biologic facts. These facts, rhythms with different frequencies at different organization levels, are of critical importance; they tip the scale between life and death in response to many stimuli. A physical stimulus such as noise, to which susceptible mice are exposed, or a bacterial endotoxin, and a long list of drugs can be

Biogenesis of:

ADRENAL CORTICOIDS　　ANDROGEN&ESTROGEN

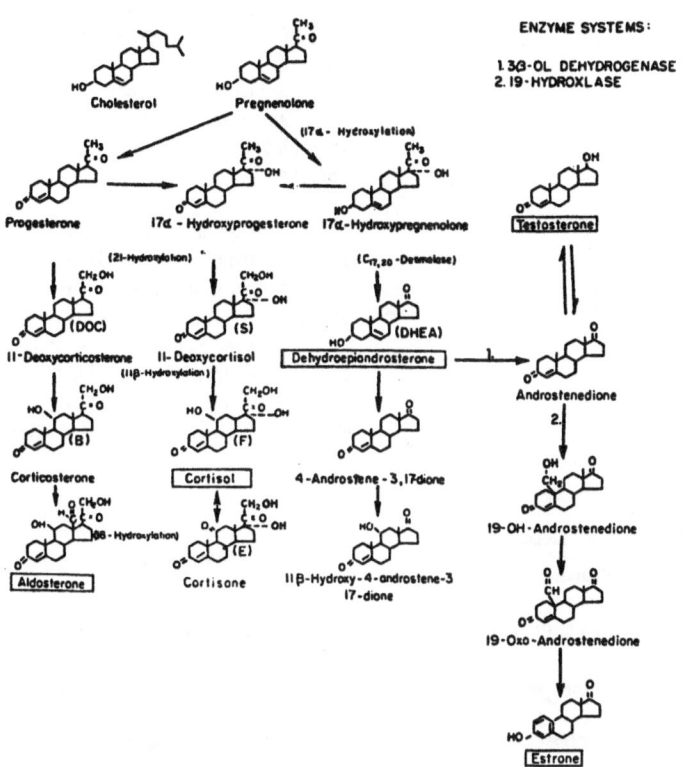

Fig. 19a: Metabolic scheme of steroid synthesis showing sites of switching mechanisms. Along the 24-hour scale, the production and/or release of aldosterone increases first during rest and coordinates salt and water metabolism. An increase in circulating cortisol follows promptly, during rest, and coordinates carbohydrate metabolism. The production of dehydroepiandrosterone sulfate, a step toward sexogens (androgen and estrogen), follows in the afternoon. The rhythms of these compounds (in rectangles) are indicators, if not determinants, of the risk of developing certain civilization diseases (Halberg, 1983). After F. Ungar, from Halberg, 1983.

well-tolerated without any obvious side effect at one time, but 12 hours earlier or later a stimulus of the same intensity and kind, including the same dose of a given drug, can kill most animals exposed to it.

With respect to a biotechnology, the fact is pertinent that the same dose of the same molecule given just 12 hours apart can have dramatically different effects. An inhibition of DNA synthesis or a stimulation, is a function of the timing of the drug's administration. Far-reaching consequences beyond improving yield, to opening new approaches, are reasonable to expect.

With respect to physiologic monitoring, the assessment of the risk of sudden death has been improved by a dynamically, i.e., chronobiologically evaluated electrocardiography. More generally, biophysical and biochemical modes of disease risk assessment can exploit changes in the characteristics of rhythms with several frequencies that are associated with risk. Here is a challenge for future chronobioengineering. New perspectives are also opened by chronobiology for

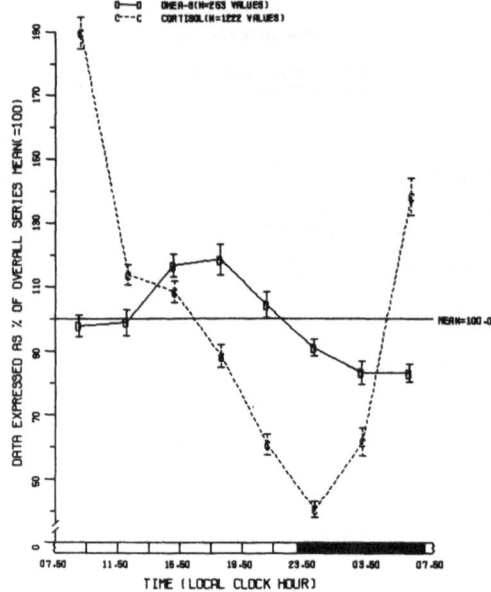

COMPARISON OF DHEA-S AND CORTISOL IN PLASMA SAMPLED IN WINTER IN 17 SERIES FROM 16 JAPANESE+MINNESOTAN WOMEN (29-36 YEARS-OF-AGE) (MEAN & STANDARD ERROR OVER 3-H SPANS)

Fig. 19b: Difference in circadian extent of change and timing of circulating cortisol and DHEA-S in clinically healthy women, shown as time plots for a single season. © 1985 by Halberg.

Fig. 19c (below): Cosinor summary of a map in Fig. 19b, extended in scope to all seasons, yet separated by geographic area. © 1985 by Halberg.

those concerned with pacing and drug administration. Timing is an already-tested dimension of drug administration devices. Use of the Medtronic pump has doubled the benefit from cyclosporine treatment. Modern hardware can now be wedded to chronobiologic software for physiologic monitoring in the service of disease prevention as well as treatment.

Circadian Rhythm in Plasma Cortisol and Dehydroepiandrosterone-sulfate (DHEA-S) in Women in Japan and Minnesota*

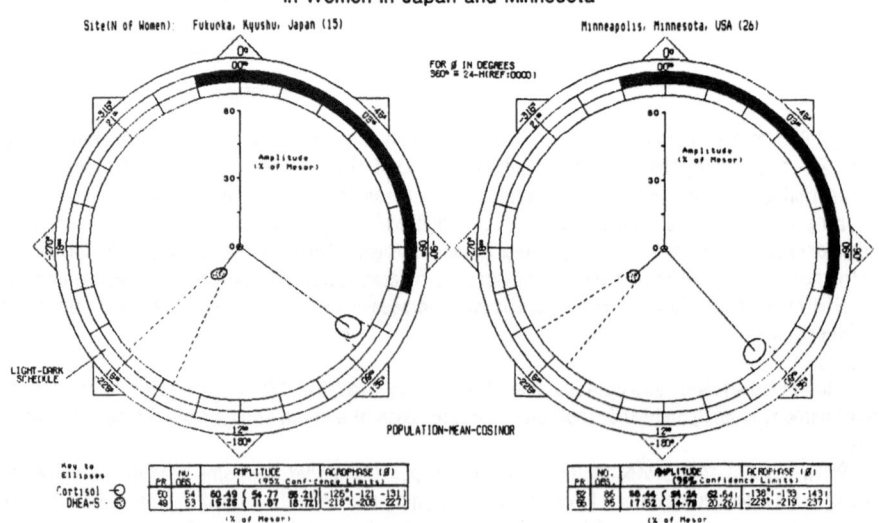

*Sampled around-the-clock in each of 4 seasons at 20-minute intervals for Cortisol and 100-minute intervals for DHEA-S via i.v catheter. Women in 3 age categories (15-21, 29-36 and 44-59 years) pooled for summary.

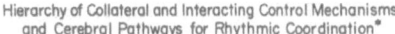

Hierarchy of Collateral and Interacting Control Mechanisms and Cerebral Pathways for Rhythmic Coordination*

Mortality of Musca Autumnalis Pupae in Response to Repeated Synchronizer-Shifts Depends on Interval between Shifts, Possibly Interacting with Circaseptan Rhythm

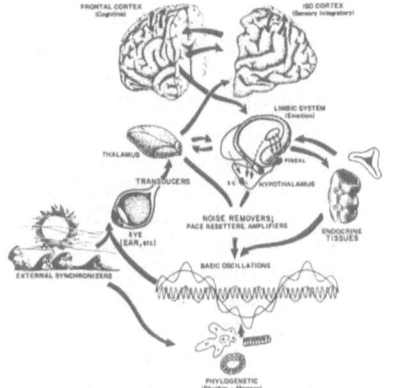

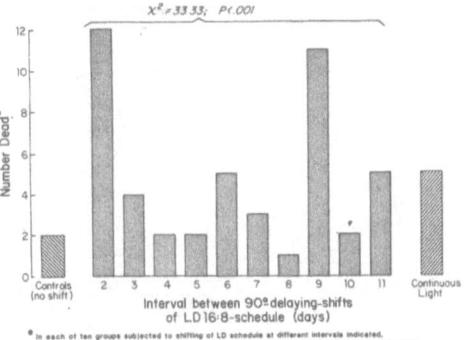

*INTEGRATION AND ADAPTATION AT SEVERAL FREQUENCIES

Fig. 20 (left): Hierarchy of collateral and interacting coordinating mechanisms and cerebral pathways for rhythmic integration and adaptation in the form of rhythms at several frequencies. In other words, the figure represents the abstract spectrum of multiple frequencies and anatomic sites involved in ecchronisms, providing harbingers of risk or disease and representing potential chronopathologies. On the one hand, ecchronisms are manifested and quantifiable (and perhaps correctable) as simple (or complex) changes of one (or several) rhythm characteristics (Figure 2) occurring under specified conditions. Cases in point are changes of MESOR, amplitude, acrophase, waveform (all at one or several periods, or their reciprocals, the frequencies) and changes of the period itself. The consequences, if any, of an internal or external desynchronization under conditions, when the period is usually synchronized are now amenable to ambulatory study.

On the other hand, rhythm alterations may involve so-called spectral compromises in which one spectral component is frequency-multiplied or -demultiplied in relation to the rhythm with a particular frequency under consideration. Thus, a circadian frequency, desynchronized from the exact 24-h periodicity, may tend toward a frequency-multiplied circaseptan period, each period involving one or several underlying (e.g., biochemical) mechanism(s). Such spectral changes are possible at single and/or multiple sites and/or frequencies, within the time structure of the organism as a whole. Spectral compromises may constitute even more general and particularly critical phenomena when they occur between 1. the set of frequencies characteristic of the organism and 2. the set of frequencies characterizing the individual's socio-ecologic setting. The aim to achieve (by drugs if not otherwise) a 'normalization' of the spectrum of rhythms includes a focus upon organismic mechanisms of timing. These consist of a set of neural, hormonal and cellular networks with a prominent adrenal cycle as pacemaker for some variables and with a suprachiasmatic pace- and amplitude-modulator for overall metabolism as gauged by body core temperature. Quantification of health by checks at specified times of certain organ systems may reveal some ecchronism as a harbinger of chronopathology, before the need for a biopsy. In other cases, ecchronism itself may be part of a disease; e.g., an amplitude change in blood pressure may constitute actual chronopathology. The extent to which the model here proposed (the animal with suprachiasmatic nuclear lesions) involves complex ecchronism at levels other than the overall metabolism is now objectively measurable and thus amenable to rigorous study. From this broader viewpoint, rats with bilateral suprachiasmatic lesions offer themselves as useful models to experimental physiologists, pathologists and pharmacologists. Graph drawn by Prof. Erwin W. Powell, from Halberg et al., 1979.

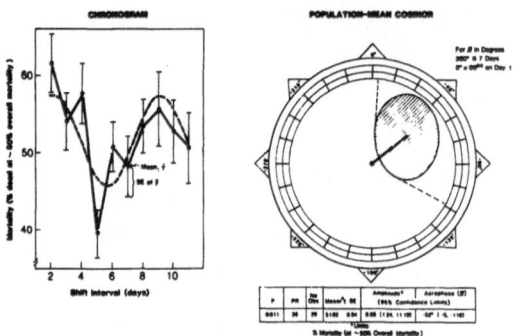

About 7-Day (Circaseptan) Frequency Response of Insect to Circadian Manipulation

Increased Mortality of Intact *Musca autumnalis* Exposed to Repeated 90°-Shift of LD16:8 Lighting Schedule (6-hr lengthening of single dark span) for a Lifetime Exhibits Circaseptan Rhythm as A Function of Shift Interval*

Fig. 21a (top right, preceding page): A study of the mortality of face flies exposed to 6-hour shifts of a regimen of 16 hours of light alternating with 8 hours of darkness, implemented at intervals of 2-11 days. Note the very high mortality in the case of shifts at 2-day intervals, and again with shifts at 9-day intervals. The data suggest a circadian-circaseptan interaction that may underlie the susceptibility of an organism to schedule shifts. The data suggest further that by manipulating the frequency of schedule shifts, undesired effects, such as an increased mortality, can be reduced. Such lifespan-shortening or -lengthening by lighting schedules representing routines of living is of broad interest, whether one's goal is fighting insect pests or improving the quality and duration of human shift-workers. From Hayes et al., 1981.

Fig. 21b: Summary of studies by Hayes et al. (1981) revealing a circaseptan rhythm in mortality in response to lighting schedule shifts at different intervals. The population-mean cosinor summary of the percentage of deaths/group (at 50% overall mortality) from 29 experiments involving adult flies demonstrates that mortality was highest for shift intervals of ~2 or ~9 days. Thick dashed line (left) is best-fitting 7-day cosine, represented by corresponding thick dashed vector (right). Dashed thin tangents (right) indicate 95% confidence intervals of acrophase. Analysis of data by Hayes et al., 1981; cf. Halberg, 1983.

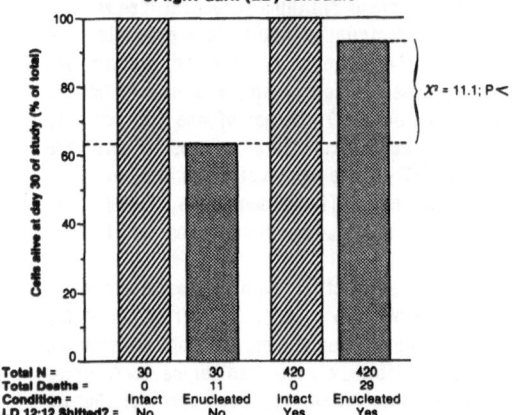

Adverse effect of enucleation upon survival of *Acetabularia mediterranea* counter-acted by shifts of light-dark (LD) schedule*

$X^2 = 11.1; P < .001$

Total N =	30	30	420	420
Total Deaths =	0	11	0	29
Condition =	Intact	Enucleated	Intact	Enucleated
LD 12:12 Shifted? =	No	No	Yes	Yes

* For 30 days, 30 intact and 30 enucleated cells were monitored in unshifted LD 12:12 schedule. Comparable groups were subjected to 12-hour shifts of light-dark schedule every 2, 3, 4, 5, 6, 7, 8, 9, 10, 11, 12, 13, 14 or 15 days.

Fig. 21c: Lighting regimen shifts may prolong (rather than shorten) the lifespan of an isolated (if debilitated) cytoplasm (Schweiger and Halberg, 1981). From Schweiger and Halberg, 1982.

References

1. Am. J. Anat. 168: 363-594 (1983).
2. Autenrieth J.H.F. (1801a): Handbuch der empirischen, menschlichen Physiologie, Vol. 1, Tübingen, pp. 106-111.
3. Autenrieth J.H.F. (1801b): Handbuch der empirischen, menschlichen Physiologie, Vol. 1, Tübingen, pp. 208-209.
4. Autenrieth J.H.F. (1801c): Handbuch der empirischen, menschlichen Physiologie, Vol. 1, Tübingen, pp. 342-343.
5. Berry D.A., Fox T.L. (1983): Regression analysis applied to PVC histories: a statistical procedure for evaluating antiarrhythmic drug efficacy. Statistics in Medicine 2: 331-343.

TREATMENT AS USUAL (WITHOUT CONSIDERATION OF RHYTHMS): TREATMENT MAY FAIL BEFORE SUCCESS IS ACHIEVED

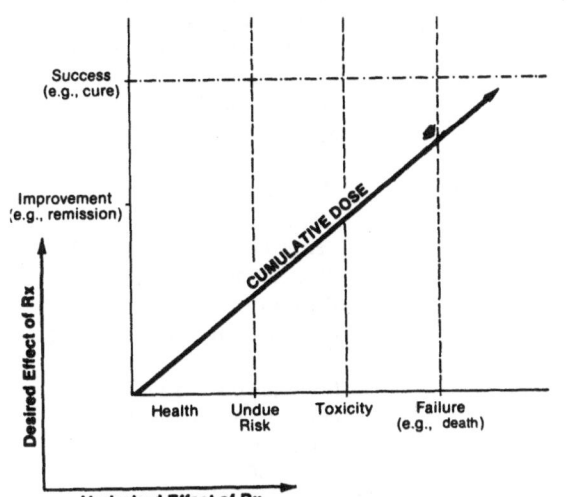

BY IDENTIFYING THE OPTIMAL CIRCADIAN STAGE, THE 'USUAL' CUMULATIVE DOSE MAY NOT LEAD TO FAILURE BUT WITH TOXICITY, TO SUCCESS

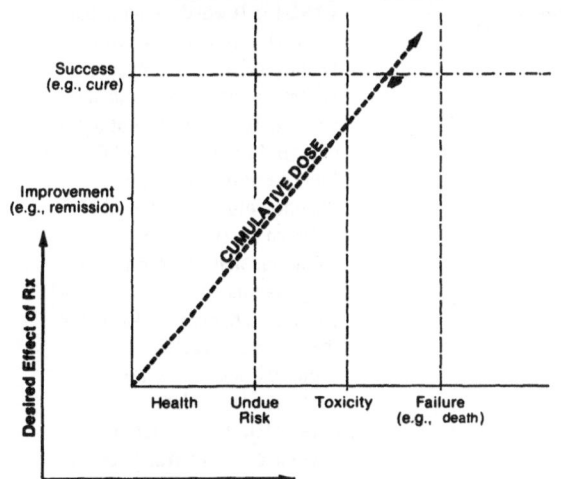

Fig. 22a (parts 1 & 2 this page, parts 3 & 4 next): Abstract aim of curing human breast cancer with or without toxicity by timing according to several rhythmic patterns that can now be administered by a pump. © 1985 by Halberg.

6. Biagini A., Carpeggiani C., Mazzei M.G., Testa R., Michelassi C., Antonelli R., L'Abbate A., Naseri A. (1981): Distribuzione oraria degli episodi di angina a riposo. Effetto della terapia medica. G. Ital. Cardiol. 11: 4-11.

7. Biological Laboratory, Cold Spring Harbor, LI, NY (1960): Vol. XXV: *Biological Clocks*. Cold Spr. Harb. Symp. quant. Biol. 25, 524 pp.

8. Brown H.E., Halberg F., Scheving L.E., Pauly J.E. (1982): Reproducibility of murine circadian eosinophil rhythms (with differences in geographic locations, method, strain, age and sex) over several decades. In: *Toward Chronopharmacology*, Takahashi R., Halberg F. and Walker C., eds., pp. 349-356, Pergamon Press, Oxford/New York.

9. Cavallini M., Halberg F., Cornélissen G., Enrichens F., Margarit C. (in press a): Organ transplantation and broader chronotherapy with implantable pump and computer programs for marker rhythm assessment. J. Controlled Release.

10. Cavallini M., Halberg F., Liu T., Magnus G. (in press b): Coordinated optimization of device, administration pattern, route and time scale for (e.g., cyclosporine) chronotherapy. Proc. 2nd Int. Conf. Medico-Social Aspects of Chronobiology, Florence, Oct. 2, 1984.

11. Cavallini M., Halberg F., Sutherland D.E.R., Cornélissen G., Heil J., Najarian J.S. (in press c): Optimization by timing of oral cyclosporine to prevent acute kidney allograft rejection in dogs. Transplantation.

12. Deka A.C. (1975): Application of chronobiology to radiotherapy of tumours of the oral cavity. M.D. Thesis, Post-Graduate Institute of Medical Education and Research, Chandigarh, India.

13. Deka A.C., Chatterjee B., Gupta B.D., Balakrishnan C., Dutta T.K. (1976): Temperature rhythm—an index of tumour regression and mucositis during the radiation treatment of oral

40

**CIRCADIAN TIMING CAN THUS MAKE THE DIFFERENCE
BETWEEN SUCCESS AT THE COST OF TOXICITY (·--)
AND FAILURE (—)**

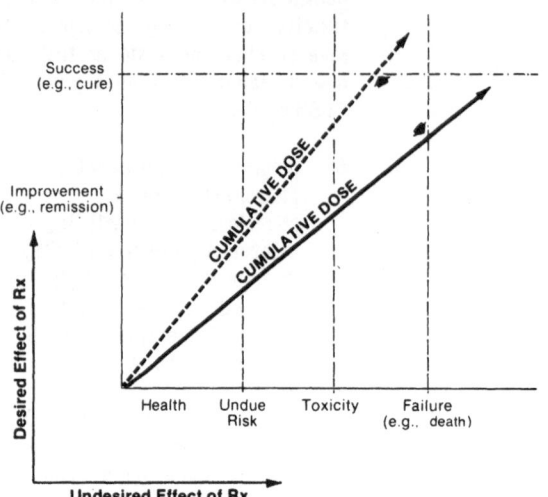

**TIMING ACCOUNTING FOR RHYTHMS WITH SEVERAL FREQUENCIES
MAY ACHIEVE THE ULTIMATE GOAL:
SUCCESS WITHOUT UNDUE RISK OR TOXICITY**

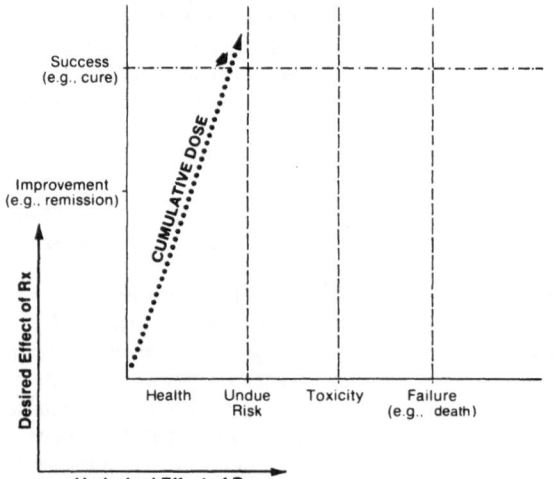

cancers. Ind. J. Cancer 13: 44-50, 1976.

14. Edmunds L.N., Halberg F. (1981): Circadian time structure of *Euglena:* a model system amenable to quantification. In: *Neoplasms—Comparative Pathology of Growth in Animals, Plants and Man,* Kaiser H., ed., pp. 105-133, Williams and Wilkins, Baltimore.

15. Günther R., Herold M., Halberg E., Halberg F. (1980): Circadian placebo and ACTH effects on urinary cortisol in arthritics. Peptides 1: 387-390.

16. Halberg E., Fanning R., Halberg F., Cornélissen G., Wilson D., Griffiths K., Simpson H. (1981): Toward a chronopsy: Part III. Automatic monitoring of rectal, axillary and breast surface temperature and of wrist activity; effects of age and of ambulatory surgery followed by nosocomial infection. Chronobiologia 8: 253-271.

17. Halberg E., Halberg F., Cornélissen G., Simpson H.W., Taggett-Anderson M.A. (1979): Toward a chronopsy: Part II. A thermopsy revealing asymmetrical circadian variation in surface temperature of human female breasts and literature review. Chronobiologia 6: 231-257.

18. Halberg E., Halberg F., Haus E., Cornélissen G., Wallach L.A., Smolensky M., Garcia Sainz M., Simpson H.W., Shons A.R. (1978): Toward a chronopsy: Part I. A chronobiologic case report and a thermopsy complementing the biopsy. Chronobiologia 5: 241-250.

19. Halberg E., Halberg F., Shankaraiah K. (1981): Plexo-serial linear-nonlinear rhythmometry of blood pressure, pulse and motor activity by a couple in their sixties. Chronobiologia 8: 351-366.

20. Halberg F. (1959): Physiologic 24-hour periodicity; general and procedural considerations with reference to the adrenal cycle. Z. Vitamin-, Hormon- u. Fermentforsch. 10: 225-296.

21. Halberg F. (1960): Temporal coordination of physiologic function. Cold Spr. Harb. Symp. quant. Biol. 25: 289-310.

Chronopolychemotherapy of 13762 Mammary Adenocarcinoma
in ♀ Fischer Rats

Treatment with 0.8mg/kg of Adriamycin i.p. in 7 Doses during 9-Day Span
(5 Days/Week) Beginning 11 Days after Tumor Inoculation
Followed by 1.6 mg/kg of Phenylalanine Mustard p.o. in 7 Doses
during 17-Day Span (3 Days/Week)

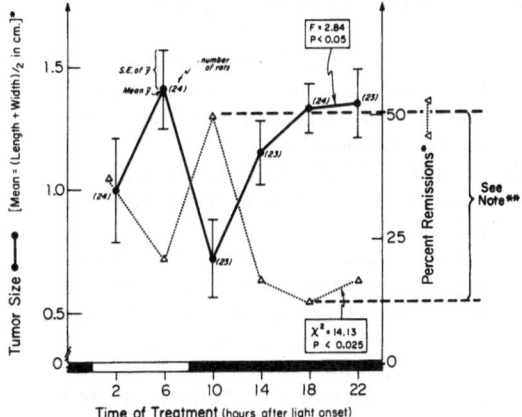

*Data summarized at 50% reduction of mean tumor size
irrespective of treatment time (36 days after tumor
inoculation).

**Note large difference in observed % remission between
animals treated at 10 and 18 hours.

Fig. 22b: A step toward the aim in Figure 22a in work on the therapy of a mammary adenocarcinoma in the rat, taking at least circadian timing into account. From Halberg et al., 1980.

Fig. 23: Depending upon the circadian system's stage encountered by the agent tested at administration time, results can be drastically different; the same dose of a given molecule may stimulate or inhibit DNA labelling in bone for the ensuing 24 hrs. At other test times, within 24 hrs, inhibition may be seen first, followed by stimulation or vice versa. These results reveal the importance of a chronobiologic approach to biotechnology (Walker et al., 1985). From Walker et al., 1985.

22. Halberg F. (1962): Physiologic 24-hour rhythms: A determinant of response to environmental agents. In: *Man's Dependence on the Earthly Atmosphere*, K.E. Schaffer ed., pp. 48-98, Macmillan, New York.

Chronomodulatory ACTH 1-17 Effects Upon Metaphyseal Bone DNA Labelling[†]

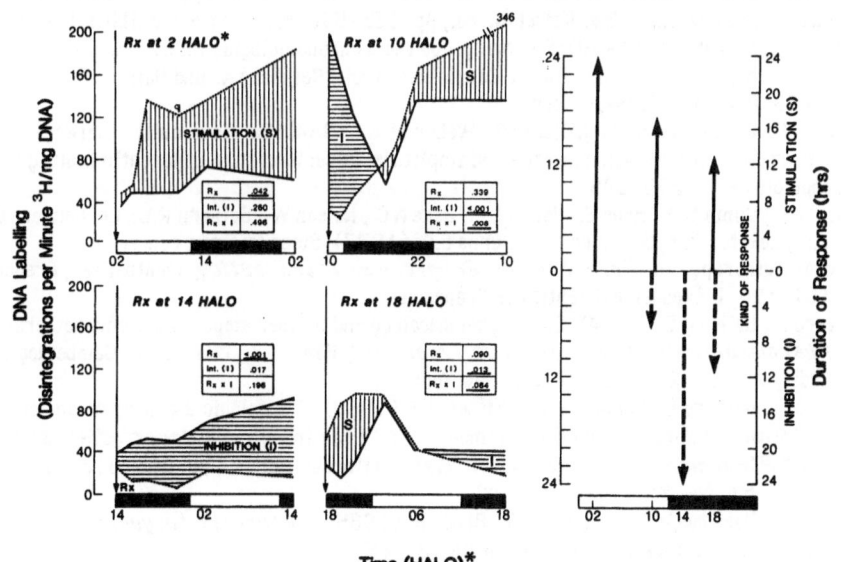

Key: —— Placebo
        ---- 20 IU/kg ACTH 1-17
        * Hours After Light Onset for mice (♀CD2F₁)
          on

† Results of 2-way analysis of variance at each circadian stage
  in boxes: main effects are kind of Rx (placebo vs. ACTH 1-17)
  & Rx-to-kill interval (2, 4, 8, 12, & 24 hrs)

¶ Outlier (that would raise mean to 338) removed

23. Halberg F. (1969): Chronobiology. Ann. Rev. Physiol. 31: 675-725.
24. Halberg F. (1977): Zusammenfassung der Tagung. Nova Acta leopoldina 46: 754-755.

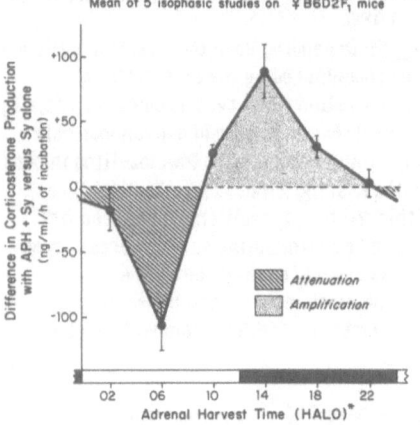

Lack of Effect, Attenuation or Amplification by Aqueous Pineal Homogenate (APH) of Corticosterone Production by Bisected Adrenals in Response to ACTH 1-17 (Sy)

Mean of 5 isophasic studies on ♀ B6D2F₁ mice

Attenuation
Amplification

02 06 10 14 18 22
Adrenal Harvest Time (HALO)*

*_Hours After Light On_

Fig. 24: Chronomodulation leading to effects such as those in Fig. 25, namely rhythmic sequences of attenuation, amplification and/or no effect, in the interaction of three entities, usually periodic in themselves. From Sánchez et al., 1983b.

25. Halberg F. (1982): Chronopharmacology and chronotherapy. In: *Cellular Pacemakers,* D.O. Carpenter ed., pp. 261-297, John Wiley and Sons Inc., New York.

26. Halberg F. (1983): Quo vadis basic and clinical chronobiology: promise for health maintenance. Am. J. Anat. 168: 543-594.

27. Halberg F., Conner R.L. (1961): Circadian organization and microbiology: variance spectra and a periodogram on behavior of *Escherichia coli* growing in fluid culture. Proc. Minn. Acad. Sci. 29: 227-239.

28. Halberg F., Cornélissen G., Sothern R.B., Wallach L.A., Halberg E., Ahlgren A., Kuzel M., Radke A., Barbosa J., Goetz F., Buckley J., Mandel J., Schuman L., Haus E., Lakatua D., Sackett L., Berg H., Wendt H.W., Kawasaki T., Ueno M., Uezono K., Matsuoka M., Omae T., Tarquini B., Cagnoni M., Garcia Sainz M., Perez Vega E., Wilson D., Griffiths K., Donati L., Tatti P., Vasta M., Locatelli I., Camagna A., Lauro R., Tritsch G., Wetterberg L. (1981): International geographic studies of oncological interest on chronobiological variables. In: *Neoplasms—Comparative Pathology of Growth in Animals, Plants and Man,* Kaiser H., ed., pp. 553-596, Williams and Wilkins, Baltimore.

29. Halberg F., Delbarre F. (1979): Summary: quo vadis chronobiologia. In: *Chronopharmacology,* Proc. Satellite Symp. 7th Int. Cong. Pharmacol., Reinberg A. and Halberg F., eds., pp. 403-426, Pergamon Press, Oxford.

30. Halberg F., Drayer J.I.M, Cornélissen G., Weber M.A. (1984): Cardiovascular reference data base for recognizing circadian mesor- and amplitude-hypertension in apparently healthy men. Chronobiologia 11: 275-298.

31. Halberg F., Gupta B.D., Haus E., Halberg E., Deka A.C., Nelson W., Sothern R.B., Cornélissen G., Lee J.K., Lakatua D.J., Scheving L.E., Burns E.R. (1977): Steps toward a cancer chronopolytherapy. In: *Proc. XIV Int. Congress of Therapeutics,* Montpellier, France, pp. 151-196, L'Expansion Scientifique Française.

32. Halberg F., Halberg E. (1984): Chronopharmacology and further steps toward chronotherapy. In: *Pharmacokinetic Basis for Drug Treatment,* Benet L.Z., Massoud N., Gambertoglio J.G., eds., pp. 221-248, Raven Press, New York.

33. Halberg F., Halberg E., Barnum C.P., Bittner J.J. (1959): Physiologic 24-hour periodicity in human beings and mice, the lighting regimen and daily routine. In: *Photoperiodism and Related Phenomena in Plants and Animals,* Withrow R.B., ed., pp. 803-878, Ed. Publ. #55, Am. Assn. Adv. Sci., Washington, DC.

34. Halberg F., Hastings W., Cornélissen G., Broda H. (1985): *Gonyaulax polyedra* 'talks' both 'circadian' and 'circaseptan'. Chronobiologia 12: 185.

35. Halberg F., Haus E., Cardoso S.S., Scheving L.E., Kühl J.F.W., Shiotsuka R., Rosene G., Pauly J.E., Runge W., Spalding J.F., Lee J.K., Good R.A. (1973): Toward a chronotherapy of neoplasia: Tolerance of treatment depends upon host rhythms. Experientia (Basel) 29: 909-934.

36. Halberg F., Lubanovic W.A., Sothern R.B., Brockway B., Powell E.W., Pasley J.N., Scheving L.E. (1979): Nomifensine chronopharmacology, schedule shifts and circadian temperature rhythms in di-suprachiasmatically lesioned rats—modeling emotional chronopathology and

FEEDSIDEWARDS:

**MULTIPLE RHYTHMIC INTERACTIONS AMONG SEVERAL
BIOPERIODIC ENTITIES RESULTING IN PREDICTABLE**
RHYTHMIC SEQUENCES OF ATTENUATION, AMPLIFICATION AND NO-EFFECT
**BY MODULATOR UPON THE INTERACTION OF
ACTOR AND REACTOR**

As can be seen from the two diagrams below, the roles of modulator, actor and reactor may vary among interacting units

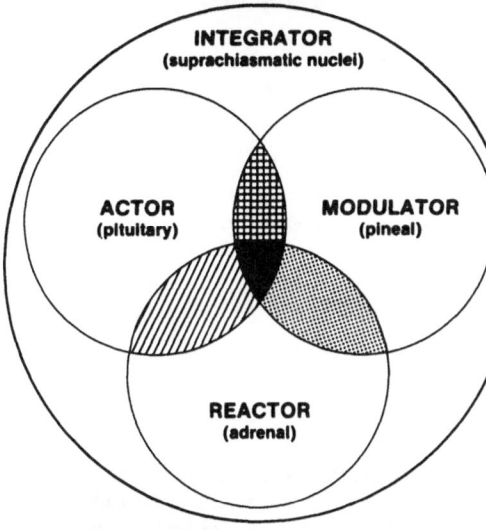

1. ▨ ACTOR ◄──► REACTOR

2. ▦ MODULATOR ◄──► ACTOR

3. ▨ MODULATOR ◄──► REACTOR

4. ■ FEEDSIDEWARD

Fig. 25: Chronomodulation by the pineal of the adrenal response to ACTH (see Figure 24). © 1985 by Halberg.

chronotherapy. Chronobiologia 6: 405-424.

37. Halberg F., Nelson W., Levi F., Culley D., Bogden A., Taylor D.J. (1980): Chronotherapy of mammary cancer in rats. Int. J. Chronobiol. 7: 85-99.

38. Halberg F., Powell E.W., Lubanovic W., Sothern R.B., Brockway B., Pasley J.N., Scheving L.E. (1977): The chronopathology and experimental as well as clinical therapy of emotional disorders. In: Halberg F., Carandente F., Cornelissen G., Katinas G.S.: Glossary of chronobiology (see insert). Chronobiologia 4, Suppl. 1, 189 pp.

39. Halberg F., Sánchez de la Peña S., Fernandes G. (1983): Immunochronopharmacology. In: *Advances in Immunopharmacology,* Hadden J., Chedid L., Dukor P., Spreafico F., Willoughby D., eds., pp. 463-478, Pergamon Press, Oxford.

40. Halberg F., Scheving L.E., Lucas E., Cornélissen G., Sothern R.B., Halberg E., Halberg J., Halberg Francine, Carter J., Straub K.D., Redmond D.P. (1984): Chronobiology of human blood pressure in the light of static (room-restricted) automatic monitoring. Chronobiologia 11: 217-247.

41. Halberg F., Scheving L.E., Powell E.W., Hayes D.K. (eds.) (1981): *Chronobiology,* Proc. XIII Int. Conf. Int. Soc. Chronobiol., Pavia, Italy, Sept. 4-7, 1977, Il Ponte, Milan.

42. Halberg F., Visscher M.B. (1952): A difference between the effects of dietary calorie restriction on the estrous cycle and on the 24-hour adrenal cortical cycle in rodents. Endocrinology 51: 329-335.

43. Halberg F., Wetterberg L. (1983): Chronobiology of plasma and urinary melatonin in breast cancer. Chronobiologia 10: 130.

44. Halberg J., Halberg E., Hayes D.K., Smith R.D., Halberg E., Delea C.S., Danielson R.S., Bartter F.C. (1980): Schedule shifts, life quality and quantity—modeled by murine blood pressure elevation and arthropod lifespan. Int. J. Chronobiol. 7: 17-64.

45. Halberg J., Halberg E., Regal P., Halberg F. (1981): Changes with age characterize circadian rhythms in telemetered core temperature of stroke-prone rats. J. Gerontol. 36: 28-30.

46. Hanson B.R., Halberg F., Tuna N., Bouchard T.J. Jr, Lykken D.T., Cornélissen G., Heston L.L. (1984): Rhythmometry reveals heritability of circadian characteristics of heart rate of human twins reared apart. Cardiologia 29: 267-282.

47. Haus E., Halberg F., Loken M.K. (1974): Circadian susceptibility-resistance cycle of bone

44

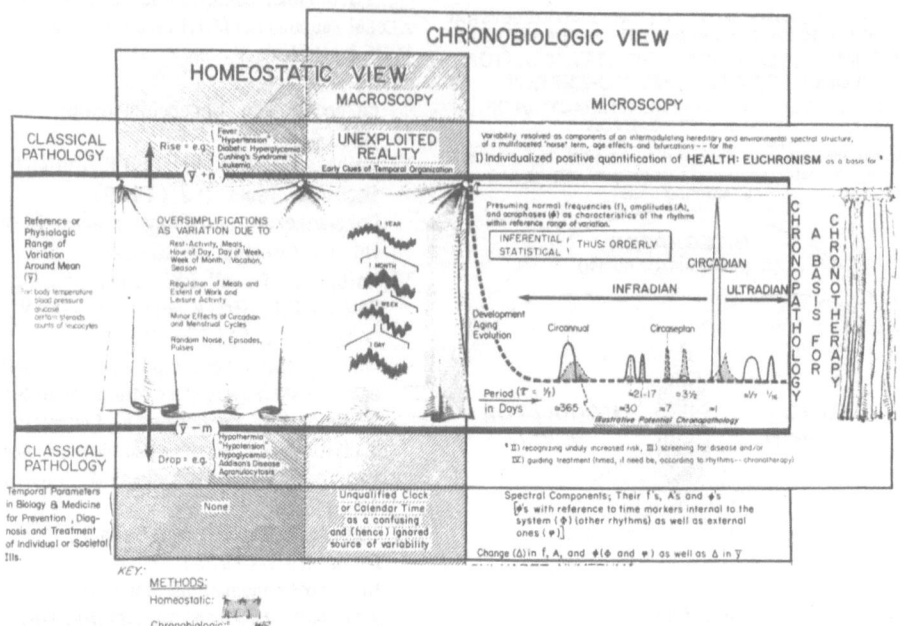

Fig. 26: Two views of body function. Homeostatically, one seeks increases or decreases, under the assumption that the body is regulated for constancy. In this case, one admits of some changes as a function of the clock-hour, the time of week or the time of year, and at best attempts to "control" for such effects by fixing sampling times by convenience. This approach is not always appropriate and can be extremely misleading (see Figure 3). The chronobiologic view, in turn, removes the curtain of ignorance drawn over the range of physiologic variation, and provides dynamic endpoints, as rhythm characteristics. Information on rhythm alteration serves for detection of the risk of developing cardiovascular disease (Figure 18), for an early diagnosis of possible abnormality (Figure 2e left), and for improving benefit from treatment by timing non-drug or drug therapy (Figures 6 and 14). © 1980 by Halberg.

marrow cells to whole-body X-irradiation in BALB/c mice. In: *Chronobiology*, Proc. Int. Soc. for the Study of Biological Rhythms, Little Rock, Ark., Scheving L.E., Halberg F. and Pauly J.E., eds., pp. 115-122, Georg Thieme Publishers, Stuttgart/Igaku Shoin Ltd., Tokyo.

48. Haus E., Halberg F., Scheving L., Cardoso S., Kühl J.F.W., Sothern R., Shiotsuka R.N., Hwang D.S., Pauly J.E. (1972): Increased tolerance of leukemic mice to arabinosyl cytosine given on schedule adjusted to circadian system. Science 177: 80-82.

49. Haus E., Kabat H. (eds.) (1984): Chronobiology 1982-1983. 574 pp. S. Karger, Basel.

50. Haus E., Lakatua D.J., Halberg F., Halberg E., Cornélissen G., Sackett L.L., Berg H.G., Kawasaki T., Ueno M., Uezono K., Matsuoka M., Omae T. (1980): Chronobiologic studies of plasma prolactin in women in Kyushu, Japan, and Minnesota, USA. J. Clin. Endocr. Metab. 51: 632-640.

51. Hayes D.K., Halberg F., Cornélissen G., Stebbings J.H. (1981): Chronobiologic concepts and biomathematical methods applicable to design and analyses of time series studies of human health. Proc. Environmetrics 81, Summaries of Conference Presentations, SIAM, pp. 318-319.

52. Hermida R.C., Halberg F. (1984a): Assessment of the risk of mesor-hypertension. Chronobiologia 11: 249-262.
53. Hermida R.C., Halberg F., Bingham C. (1985a): Bootstrapping and added data support plasma aldosterone as a time-dependent discriminant of cardiovascular risk (CR). Chronobiologia 12: 186.
54. Hermida R.C., Halberg F., Del Pozo F. (1985b): Chronobiologic pattern discrimination of plasma hormones, notably DHEA-S and TSH, classifies an expansive personality. Chronobiologia 12: 105-136.
55. Hermida Dominguez R.C., Halberg F., del Pozo F., Haus E. (1982): Toward chronobiologic pattern discrimination of the risk of developing breast cancer and other diseases. Rev. Esp. Oncol. 29: 199-267.
56. Hermida Dominguez R., Halberg F., Halberg E., Haus E., Lakatua D., Uezono K., Kawasaki T., Mandel J.S., Del Pozo Guerrero F. (1984b): Endocrine chronorisk of mesor-hypertension in clinically healthy women sought by circadian and circannual pattern discrimination. In: SIRMCE Congress 1982, Influence of Environment on Man, November 17-20, 1982, Vienna, pp. 74-162.
57. Hufeland C.W. (1797): *Makrobiotik, The Art of Prolonging Life*. 2nd English trans., printed for J. Bell, London, p. 201.
58. Knuth D.E. (1977): Algorithms. Scientific American 236: 63-80.
59. Kolata G. (1985): Is the war on cancer being won? Science 229: 543-544.
60. Litman T., Halberg F., Ellis S., Bittner J.J. (1958): Pituitary growth hormone and mitoses in immature mouse liver. Endocrinology 62: 361-364.
61. Lown B., Wolf M. (1971): Approaches to sudden death from coronary heart disease. Circulation 44: 130-142.
62. Menzel W. (1962): Menschliche Tag-Nacht-Rhythmik und Schichtarbeit. Benno Schwabe & Co. Verlag, Basel/Stuttgart, 189 pp.
63. Morganroth J., Michelson E.L., Horowitz L.N., Josephson M.E., Pearlman A.S., Dunkman W.B.: Limitations of routine long-term electrocardiographic monitoring to assess ventricular ectopic frequency. Circulation 58: 408-414, 1978.
64. Nelson W., Cornélissen G., Hinkley D., Bingham C., Halberg F.: Construction of rhythm-specified reference intervals and regions, with emphasis on 'hybrid' data, illustrated for plasma cortisol. Chronobiologia 10: 179-183, 1983.
65. Orth-Gomér K., Halberg F., Sothern R., Åkerstedt T., Theorell T., Cornélissen G. (1982): The circadian rhythm of ventricular arrhythmias. In: Toward Chronopharmacology, R. Takahashi, F. Halberg and C. Walker, eds., pp. 191-202, Pergamon Press, Oxford/New York.
66. Orth-Gomér K., Cornélissen G., Halberg F., Sothern R., Åkerstedt T. (in press): Relative merits of chronobiologic vs. conventional Holter monitoring. Proc. 2nd Int. Conf. Medico-Social Aspects of Chronobiology, Florence, Oct. 2, 1984.
67. Reinberg A., Halberg F. (1971): Circadian chronopharmacology. Ann. Rev. Pharmacol. 2: 455-492.
68. Reinberg A., Smolensky M., Labrecque G. (eds.) (1984): *Annual Review of Chronopharmacology*, Proc. 1st Int. Montreux Conf. of Biological Rhythms and Medications, Montreux, Switzerland, March 26-30, 1984, Pergamon Press, Oxford.
69. Reale L., Tarquini B., Halberg F. (eds.) (1985, in press): *Proc. 2nd Int. Conf. Medico-Social Aspects of Chronobiology,* Florence, October 2, 1984.
70. Rogers L.A., Greenbank G.R. (1929): The intermittent growth of bacterial cultures. J. Bacteriol. 19: 181-190.
71. Sami M., Kraemer H., Harrison D.C., Houston N., Shimasaki C., DeBusk R.F. (1980): A new method for evaluating antiarrhythmic drug efficacy. Circulation 62: 1172-1179.
72. Sánchez de la Peña S., Halberg F., Halberg E., Ungar F., Cornélissen G., Sánchez E., Brown G., Scheving L.E., Yunis E.G., Vecsei P. (1983a): Pineal modulation of ACTH 1-17 effect upon murine corticosterone production. Brain Res. Bull. 11: 117-125.

73. Sánchez de la Peña S., Halberg F., Ungar F., Haus E., Lakatua D., Scheving L.E., Sánchez E., Yecsei P. (1983b): Circadian pineal modulation of pituitary effect on murine corticosterone *in vitro*. Brain Res. Bull. 10: 559–565.

74. Santorio S. (1657): De Statica Medicina. Hagæ–Comitis, ex typographia A. Ylaco.

75. Scheving L.E. (1976): The dimension of time in biology and medicine: chronobiology. Endeavour 35: 66–72.

76. Scheving L.E., Halberg F., Pauly J.E. (eds.) (1974): *Chronobiology*. Proc. Int. Soc. for the Study of Biological Rhythms, Little Rock, Ark., Georg Thieme Publishers, Stuttgart/Igaku Shoin Ltd., Tokyo.

77. Scheving L.E., Haus E., Kühl J.F.W., Pauly J.E, Halberg F., Cardoso S. (1976): Close reproduction by different laboratories of characteristics of circadian rhythm in 1-β-D-arabinofuranosylcytosine tolerance by mice. Cancer Res. 36: 1133–1137.

78. Schweiger H-G., Halberg F. (1982): Can a unicell measure the week and an isolated cytoplasm measure half a week? Notiziario SIBioC 6: 525–526.

79. Smolensky M., Halberg F., Sargent F. II (1972): Chronobiology of the life sequence. In: *Advances in Climatic Physiology*, Itoh S., Ogata K. and Yoshimura H., eds., pp. 281–318, Igaku Shoin Ltd., Tokyo.

80. Synguelakis M., Robel P., Baulieu E-E., Halberg F. (in press): Circadian rhythms of pregnenolone (P), dehydroepiandrosterone (D) and corticosterone (B) in rat plasma and brain in a comparative physiologic context. Proc. Int. Soc. Chronobiol, Little Rock, Ark., Nov. 3–6, 1985.

81. Takahashi R., Halberg F., Walker C. (eds.) (1982): *Toward Chronopharmacology*, Proc. 8th IUPHAR Cong. and Sat. Symposia, Nagasaki, July 27–28, 1981, Pergamon Press, Oxford/New York.

82. Walker C.M., Winget C.M., Soliman K.F.A. (eds.) (1981): *Chronopharmacology and Chronotherapeutics*. Florida A & M University Foundation, Tallahassee, Florida.

83. Walker W.Y., Russell J.E., Simmons D.J., Scheving L.E., Cornélissen G., Halberg F. (1985): Effect of an adrenocorticotropin analogue, ACTH 1-17, on DNA synthesis in murine metaphyseal bone. Biochem. Pharmacol. 34: 1191–1196.

84. Wesseling K.H., de Wit B., Settels J.J., Klawer W.H., Arntzenius A.C. (1982): On the indirect registration of finger blood pressure after Peñáz. Funkt. Biol. Med. 1: 245–250.

85. Wrba H., Halberg F., Dutter A. (in press): Melatonin circadian-stage-dependently delays breast cancer development in mice injected daily for several months. In: Proc. 1st Int. Workshop on Neuroimmunomodulation, Bethesda, MD, Nov. 27–30, 1984.

86. Wrba H., Halberg F., Dutter A. (in press): Placebo-accelerated murine mammary carcinogenesis possibly partly reversed by melatonin. Proc. Int. Soc. Chronobiol., Little Rock, Ark., Nov. 3–6, 1985.

Support: U.S. Public Health Service (GM-13981); Medtronic Inc. (Minneapolis, MN 55455, USA). This paper was originally prepared for a Medtronom and for Chronobiologia. The author is indebted to Medtronic Inc. (Minneapolis, MN, USA) and to the journal Chronobiologia (Milan, Italy) for permission to use the figures in this presentation.

Modern drug administration devices for the chronobiologic optimization of conventional treatment modes

M. Cavallini*, F. Halberg**, G. Cornélissen**, D.E.R. Sutherland**
*Department of Surgery, University of Rome, Rome, Italy
**Departments of Laboratory Medicine and Pathology and Surgery, University of Minnesota, Minneapolis, MN, USA

Introduction

In specifying new drug administration modes, one must keep in mind the merits of conventional routes. Indeed, we shall show herein that a modern administration device aids the scheduling of cyclosporine (Cs) according to a conventional treatment mode. Cs is a hydrophobic 11-amino-acid cyclic polypeptide (1), produced by two soil fungi, soluble in lipids or organic solvents, that was found to have immunosuppressive properties by Borel et al. (2,3) at Sandoz Ltd. (Basel, Switzerland). Studies in experimental animals by Calne et al. (4) and other investigators (5) showed that Cs could prevent or greatly delay the onset of organ allograft rejection. The mechanism of action of Cs is not well understood. The drug depresses humoral and cellular immunity, with a preferential and reversible action against T lymphocytes (6,7). These effects are not accompanied by the bone marrow depression that is frequent during treatment with azathioprine. Among its side effects, recent clinical trials have shown nephrotoxicity and hepatotoxicity at the usual therapeutic doses in transplanted patients (8-10). Our studies on the rat and the dog underline the importance of chronopharmacology and chronotherapy and how modern instrumentation can optimize the schedule of Cs administration.

Results in the rat

Male inbred Lewis rats kept in light (L) and darkness (D) alternating at 12-h intervals (LD12:12) were studied for both toxicity and immunosuppression by Cs. Treatment during the dark span (the rat's habitual active span) was associated with a statistically significant increase in the immunosuppression effect of Cs (11,12). The allograft studies, male inbred Lewis rats, were recipients of a heterotopic intra-abdominal heart allograft from ACI rats. A circadian and a circannual variation in the immunosuppressive effect, manifested by a prolongation of graft function, were noted (12). A subsequent study with segmental pancreas allograft from ACI rats into diabetic male Lewis inbred rats extended the scope of the previous results. The circadian stage at treatment time with Cs again determined the extent of prolongation of graft function (13,14).

Results in the dog

The effects of timing Cs administration were tested on nephrectomized dogs bearing an allografted kidney. 1.5 mg/kg of Cs per day were given via an externally programmable implanted Medtronic pump at a continuous injection rate or with one of 6 changing rates, each involving 8 different doses, increasing and then decreasing sinusoidally every day, with the total dose per day equal to that in dogs infused at a constant rate. With both the constant and the sinusoidal rate, Cs prolonged graft function with statistical significance. Moreover, some sinusoidal infusion schedules were better than others. The assumption that the differences among dogs treated with different sinusoidal schedules varied randomly was rejected by the fit of a 24-hour cosine function. This approach demonstrated a statistically significant circadian rhythm in response to sinusoidal Cs treatment. A circadian sinusoidal schedule of Cs peaking in the middle of the dark span was associated with a gain factor of nearly 2 (100% increase) in graft survival (when the duration of graft function associated with Cs delivery peaking in the middle of the light span was equated to

100%) (15). Accordingly, we tested and validated, in the experimental model of kidney-allografted dogs, the possibility that the results obtained with a pump could be exploited for the more conventional oral administration of the drug (16).

In dogs kept in light from 06^{00} to 18^{00}, treated at 08^{30} or at 20^{30} with a single daily oral dose of 12.5 mg/kg Cs, a similar peak Cs concentration in blood was reached approximately at the times documented as the best ($3^{22}\pm1^{13}$) or the worst ($15^{42}\pm0^{41}$) in prior studies with multiple sinusoidal drug schedules via an implanted, externally programmable pump. In the absence of a pharmacokinetic difference, the evening dose was more effective than the morning dose in prolonging kidney allograft function, as shown by life table statistics (P=0.01). The prior results from a modern drug administration device, a drug pump, by specifying circadian timing, thus served to optimize the conventional treatment mode: the oral administration of cyclosporine.

Discussion and conclusion

Modern technology such as an implantable externally programmable pump allows the administration of drugs according to factors that can be optimized for the individual patient. The importance of drug administration devices allowing the optimization of patterned schedules on an individualized basis is perhaps more generally recognized for applications in the treatment of diabetes.

A microprocessor-controlled Programmable Implantable Medication System (PIMS) for the release of insulin and other medications into the human body is described by Fischell (17). The system includes a fully implantable programmable infusion pump, a patient's programming unit, a medication programming unit, and a medication injection unit. A command link allows the infusion pump to be programmed after implantation. Using the programming unit, the physician tailors the basal and post-prandial insulin infusion profiles to the patient's needs. The patient can also manually request appropriate amounts of post-prandial insulin. The infusion pump can be refilled at several-month intervals.

Against the background of chronobiologic studies, it becomes apparent that optimization of drug administration via treatment timing is possible for an array of other medications, as illustrated herein for the case of Cs. Administration by the pump is not only more convenient, and not only allows the administration of patterns that cannot be readily achieved orally or by infusion into ambulatory subjects for long spans, but it can also serve for extrapolation concerning the best conventional (e.g., oral) treatment time.

References

1. Dreyfus M., Hyerri E., Hotman H., et al.: Cyclosporin A and C new metabolites from trichoderma polysporum. Eur. J. Appl. Microbiol. 3: 125, 1976.
2. Borel, J.F., C. Feurer, C. Magnee et al.: Effects of the new anti-lymphocytic polypeptide cyclosporin A in animals. Immunol. 32: 1017, 1977.
3. Borel, J.F., C. Feurer, H.Y. Gubler, et al.: Biological effects of the new anti-lymphocytic agent Cyclosporin A. Agents and Actions 6: 468, 1976.
4. Calne R.Y., D.J.G. White: Cyclosporin A--a powerful immunosuppressant in dogs with renal allografts. IRCS J. Med. Sci. 5: 595, 1977.
5. Morris, P.J.: Cyclosporin A overview. Transplantation 32: 349, 1981.
6. Kunkl A., Klaus G.G.B.: Selective effects of Cyclosporin A on functional B-cell subsets in the mouse. J. Immunol. 125: 1562, 1980.
7. Hess A.D., Tutschka P.J.: Effect of cyclosporin A on human lymphocyte responses in vitro. I) Cs-A allows for the expression of alloantigen-activated suppressor cells while preferentially inhibiting the induction of cytolitic effector lymphocytes in MLR. J. Immunol. 124: 2601, 1980.
8. Ferguson R.M., Rynasiewicz J.J., Sutherland D.E.R., et al.: Cyclosporin A in renal transplantation preliminary reports of 100 patients in a prospective randomized trial. Surgery 92: 175, 1982.

9. Powles R.J., Clink H.M., Spence D.: Cyclosporin A to prevent graft vs. host disease in man after allogeneic bone marrow transplantation. Lancet i: 327, 1980.
10. Klintmalm G.B.C., Iwatsuki S., Starzl T.E.: Nephrotoxicity of cyclosporin A in liver and kidney transplant patients. Lancet 1: 470, 1981.
11. Cavallini M., Magnus G., Halberg F., Florack G., Sutherland D.E.R.: Murine model for a chronoimmunotherapy of allotransplantation: Circadian and circannual variation in cyclosporine effects. Eur. Surg. Res. 15 (Suppl. 1): 19-20, 1983.
12. Cavallini M., Magnus G., Halberg F., Liu T., Sibley R., Najarian J.S., Sutherland D.E.R.: Benefit from circadian timing of cyclosporine revealed by delay of rejection of murine heart allograft. Transpl. Proc. 15 (Suppl. 1): 2960-2966, 1983.
13. Liu T., Cavallini M., Halberg F., Cornélissen G., Field J., Sutherland D.E.R: Multifrequency chronotherapy with circaseptan and eventually circannual optimization may follow early circadian-sinusoidal pump-implemented infusions of cyclosporine – In: Annual Review of Chronopharmacology, Proc. 1st Int. Montreux Conf. of Biological Rhythms and Medications, Montreux, Switzerland, March 26-30, 1984, A. Reinberg, M. Smolensky, G. Labrecque, eds., Pergamon Press, Oxford, 1984, pp. 133-136.
14. Sutherland D., Cavallini M., Halberg F., Liu T., Magnus G., Carandente O.: Chronobiology of transplantation and cyclosporine timing with special reference to segmental pancreas transplantation. Chronobiologia 10: 163-164, 1983.
15. Cavallini M., Halberg F., Cornélissen G., Enrichens F., Margarit C.: Organ transplantation and broader chronotherapy with implantable pump and computer programs for marker rhythm assessment. J. Controlled Release, in press.
16. Cavallini M., Halberg F., Sutherland D.E.R., Cornélissen G., Heil J., Najarian J.S.: Optimization by timing of oral cyclosporine to prevent acute kidney allograft rejection in dogs. Transplantation, in press.
17. Fischell R.E.: Microprocessor application to an artificial pancreas. Preprint, 11 pp., 1980.

Implantable and programmable drug administration system for chronopharmacological applications

P. Guiot and I. Bourgeois

Research and Support Center, Medtronic, Kerkrade, The Netherlands

Some drugs given by continuous infusion do not present constant therapeutic indices. Drug activity and/or toxicity are dependent upon when in the circadian cycle the drug is administered. An implantable device sensitive to non-invasive telemetry dealing with various administration parameters was developed by Medtronic. A 20 ml collapsible reservoir, roller pump, stepper motor, microprocessor, lithium-thionyl chloride battery, antenna and acoustic transducer are hermetically housed in the Drug Administration Device (DAD). The device is cylindrical, 7 cm in diameter and 2.7 cm thick, and weighs 175 g empty. Access to the reservoir is possible through a percutaneously palpable septum sealed filling port. Septum, internal pump tubing and catheter connected to the DAD are made of silicon rubber. All metallic components are made of titanium. A programmer consisting of computer screen console, keyboard, programming wand and printer allows non-invasive examination and instruction of the DAD. The patient's initials, drug name and concentration, as well as the metrology used, define the pump profile. Audible alarms within the pump warn the patient when the reservoir volume or the battery voltage are low. A *bolus* occurs once at the pump's maximum dispensing rate (0.9 ml/hr). The time during which the bolus occurs and the drug concentration determine the dose. A *multi-step bolus* occurs once, in a series of 1-10 doses at specified rates. A *bolus-delay* occurs intermittently, at prescribed dose and at specified intervals. A *continuous* mode of infusion occurs at a specified hourly rate. A *continuous-complex* mode of infusion consists of a series of 1-10 doses at specified intervals. This maximum 10 blocks histogram is continuously repeated. Experiments performed with the DAD have already shown that sinusoidal timing for cyclosporine administration highly increase time before kidney allograft rejection in dogs (Cavallini et al., in press). Since adriamycin cardiotoxicity is reduced when administered in the morning, it should be possible to construct an administration pattern devoid of major toxicity.

Cavallini M., Halberg F., Cornélissen G., Enrichens F., Margarit C.: Organ transplantation and broader chronotherapy with implantable pump and computer programs for marker rhythm assessment. J. Controlled Release, in press.

Pumps for providing insulin

J. Mirouze, J.L. Selam and C. Saeidi
University of Montpellier, France

Pumps with insulin are utilized to assure a supply of this hormone which is continuous but is adjusted to the varying needs of those patients with diabetes mellitus who are insulin-dependent and difficult to treat by conventional or so-called optimal injections of insulin. Such insulin infusions constitute the most recent therapeutic acquisition of diabetology; they assure a minimal insulin supply, around 1 unit per hour, without interruption throughout the night and are adaptable as a function of the fluctuations in blood sugar associated with meals, physical exercise, and also the unpredictabilities of the unstable forms of the disease. Adjustments for fast or slow delivery are made by the patient.

Our experience in Montpellier dates back to July 1, 1980. We have followed a total of 60 patients, two-thirds of them with unstable diabetes and one-third with 'difficult' diabetes with explosive complications or pregnancies. The tools used varied; they include a) syringe-type, b) peristaltic and/or c) electromagnetic pumps, from the a) Lilly, Miles, Nordisk, Travenol, etc., b) Siemens and c) Pacesetter companies.

Three ways of providing insulin are theoretically possible. The venous route is chosen for the artificial pancreas and for the macropumps used on patients while they are in the hospital. The subcutaneous route is used most often with portable pumps; all varieties of ordinary conventional insulin are utilizable, but the manipulations of the material have to be frequent, since the pump has to be filled every 1-3 days and the entry site of the catheter has to be changed every 1-6 days. The peritoneal route should logically not be utilized, except for pumps with large reservoirs, lasting 2-4 weeks. This route requires insulin preparations that are stable for such long spans, which are currently not commercially available. The catheter is manipulated only in the case of malfunction, notably in the case of partial or total obstruction. The peritoneal route, as compared to the subcutaneous and in particular the intravenous routes, has the advantage of reducing the number of manipulations, of assuring a more acceptable glycemia, and of providing for greatest comfort. This is the only logical route for implantable pumps that as yet are utilized only exceptionally in our clinic. Complications are rare and sometimes relate to the mechanical frailties of the pump or to the malfunctioning of the catheter; these complications lead to metabolic problems in the diabetic patient as well as to occasional infections of the subcutaneous path of the catheter.

At this time, treatment by pump can be visualized only for properly educated diabetics who know their diabetes and their insulin requirements and accept the iterative practice of the self-monitoring of their glycemia, having learned how to manipulate the pump from a medical staff which is alert and available for 24 hours each day. A specific autonomous organization in support of pump treatment is indispensable as soon as the number of thus chronically treated patients increases and until provisions are made in a future chronobiologic pump to overcome all of the above-mentioned shortcomings.

References

1. Mirouze J., Selam J.L.: Clinical experience in human diabetics with portable implantable insulin minipumps. Life Support System 1: 39-50, 1983.

2. Mirouze J., Selam J.L., Rodier M., Lapinski H., Saeidi C., Richard J.L.: Traitement du diabète sucre par infusion insulinique. Bul. Acad. Nat. Med. 168: 80-90, 1984.
3. Richard J.L., Mirouze J., Cavaille G.: Le pancréas artificiel. Description et application. Rev. Europ. Technol. Biomed. 2: 92-100, 1983.
4. Selam J.L., Mirouze J.: Actualités sur les indications et l'utilisation des pompes à insuline chez les diabétiques. Encyclopédie Médico-Chirurgicale. Nutrition 9: 10508-5, 1983.
5. Selam J.L., Mirouze J.: Quel est l'avenir de l'infusion continue d'insuline par voie péritonéale? Diabète et Métabolisme 10: 221-223, 1984.

DRUG DELIVERY TECHNOLOGIES AT 3M

ANTHONY F. YAPEL, JR.
BIOSCIENCES LABORATORY
3M
ST. PAUL, MINNESOTA, USA

INTRODUCTION

I would like to thank Professor Franz Halberg for recently introducing me to the areas of chronobiology and chronopharmacology and for inviting me to participate in this International Workshop on Chronobiology. I have personally been involved in various aspects of drug delivery over the past decade, but much of my research has pertained to controlled release and sustained release drug delivery systems. More often than not, my personal research objectives and those of my colleagues have focused on trying to develop sustained release systems with "zero order" drug diffusion characteristics rather than dosage forms with "pulsed" drug release characteristics. Although it is my personal belief that sustained release drug delivery systems definitely have their place in today's health care environment, I have learned both from Professor Halberg and from discussions with various participants in this workshop that pulsed drug dosing given at appropriate times in the circadian cycle may not only be more efficacious but much safer than most current methods of drug administration to patients.

Today I'd like to describe for you several types of patented technologies which have been developed at 3M over the past several years. Some have been designed specifically for sustained release drug delivery applications. Others have been developed for non-drug related applications which, with appropriate modification, might have applicability in chronotherapy.

INFUSION PUMPS

Probably the 3M technology most directly applicable to chronotherapy is a product line of precision volumetric infusion pumps. AVI, Inc., a 3M subsidiary, manufactures a series of three different, quite versatile, non-implantable pumps (Models AVI 100, AVI 400 and AVI Micro 110) which can be used in a variety of drug delivery applications. These include venous infusions, arterial infusions, all types of nutritional support needs, chemotherapy applications, neonatal applications and special procedures such as streptokinase administration. One of the unique features of the AVI pumps is their ability to intravenously infuse medication into a patient in a very steady, continuous, nonpulsating fashion. They also provide the user with programmable control over the dose volume infused and the rate at which the fluid is delivered.

The key component of the AVI disposable administration set used with the pumps is a three-chambered, flexible polyvinyl chloride cassette which is interchangeable between infusion pump models. Due to its valveless design, it may be used for gravity infusion of fluids as well. Mechanical manipulation of this flexible cassette in each of the three AVI pumps takes place by a piston and valve arrangement which gives precise control over both the delivery rate and the volume infused.

Each of the AVI pumps provides for patient safety by monitoring a number of potential alarm conditions, any one which will halt delivery of the infusate and activate both audible and visual indicators on the pump. Some of these alarm conditions include an "empty infusate bag" signal, excessive back pressure in the infusion line, air bubbles in the infusion line, etc.

Some of the key infusion characteristics of the AVI pumps are as follows. Both the AVI 400 and AVI 100 are programmable from 1 - 999 ml/hr in 1 ml/hr increments. When small infusion rates are required, as in neonatal applications, the AVI Micro 110 is programmable at one-tenth that rate. Infusion volumes are likewise programmable, ranging from 1 - 9,999 ml in 1 ml increments for the AVI 400 and AVI 100 to one-tenth that volume range for the AVI Micro 110. The volumetric accuracy of all pumps is +/- 2%. In case of occlusion in the infusion line, this is immediately detected by the pump and pressure is immediately removed. Occlusion pressures can be adjusted at either 4 or 9 psi. The pumps are able to achieve their smooth, continuous delivery of fluid by dividing each ml into 960 parts for the AVI 400 and 2400 parts for the AVI 110.

Both the AVI 100 and AVI Micro 110 can be programmed to deliver infusate at a constant, selected rate as a function of time. The AVI 400 can do this also, but offers an additional advantage in that it is capable of delivering so-called "piggyback" drug administrations automatically. In the piggyback mode, two different fluids can be delivered with independent infusion rates and volumes, or alternatively, a single infusate can be delivered in this stepwise fashion. Only one container and one set of infusion tubing is needed each day with no resetting or reprogramming of the pump being necessary. It is also possible to have the programming algorithm in the AVI 400 factory-modified to produce essentially any desired infusion rate profile as a function of time. This capability would obviously be of considerable value in chronotherapy applications.

AEROSOL DRUG DELIVERY

Another 3M technology which could be useful in selected chronopharmacological applications is the delivery of drugs to the lungs by aerosol. 3M's Riker Laboratories is one of the world's leading producers of aerosols for administration of drugs to the lung, particularly for bronchial emergencies like asthma attacks. Riker, in fact, developed and marketed the first metered dose aerosols for inhalation therapy in 1956, forming the foundation of today's medicinal aerosol technology.

At the heart of aerosol drug delivery systems is a unique, metered aerosol valve which can be made to deliver a precise dose of drug ranging from 25 microliters to 100 microliters. These valves are designed to deliver the final dose as accurately as the first. The aerosol cannisters themselves are generally made from either aluminum or poly-vinylchloride-coated glass, the choice being dependent on the corrosive characteristics of the drug or solvent being loaded into the cannister. The cannisters can be cold filled with drug by gravity at dry ice temperatures; alter-natively, they can be pressure filled with drug at room temperature. The choice often depends on drug stability and/or economic considerations. Either solid, micronized particulate drugs or drugs in solution can be delivered from the aerosol cannisters which are pressurized by selected Freon propellants used alone or in various combinations to provide optimum propellant characteristics for each drug candidate.

Precise control of drug particle size (or droplet size in the case of drugs in solution) in the range from 1 to 5 microns as well as control of propellant characteristics are necessary to insure that the aerosolized drug is deposited in the airways and alveoli of the lung rather than impacting in the back of the throat which will occur if the drug par-ticle size is too large. Drug impacting in the throat is ultimately swallowed and much reduced in efficacy, particu-larly if the purpose of its administration is to treat a lung disease like asthma. Particulate or droplet drug size and shape reaching the lung can be regulated to some degree through use of "adapters" which are attached to the orifice of the aerosol cannister. Adapters are available in various sizes and shapes and aid in controlling the region of depo-sition of the aerosolized drug particles/droplets in the lung.

Although many of us probably consider inhalation aero-sols primarily for use only in bronchial emergencies, they may also be a very effective method for delivering other drugs to the systemic circulation to treat a variety of ail-ments. For example, next to intravenous injection, inhala-tion has the potential of being one of the faster acting noninvasive methods for administering a drug to the body. In the alveoli of the lung, a drug molecule has the opportu-nity to pass rapidly through a membrane that averages only 1.5 microns in thickness directly into the bloodstream. Potentially, lower drug doses would be needed because the drug is targeted directly to the bloodstream and experiences no "first pass effect" in the liver. Aerosol drug delivery to the systemic circulation thus offers the advantage of relatively low drug degradation (compared to oral delivery) and a uniform, precise dose of drug which can approximate an injection.

The aerosol method of drug delivery could thus have important implications in the chronotherapy of both diseases of the lung and other illnesses of the body. Once the optimum time and frequency of drug dosing has been established for a patient by the chronopharmacologist, aerosol delivery of the appropriate medication via the lung should be painless and relatively convenient since both the timing and dose of the drug can be easily adjusted by either the physician or the patient.

MICROSPHERE DRUG DELIVERY SYSTEMS

For clarification, I will define a microsphere intended for use as a drug delivery device as a solid, spherical matrix containing dissolved or entrapped biologically active material. At 3M, we have been able to prepare both protein and polysaccharide microspheres from a variety of starting materials including albumin, various enzymes, dextran and starch (1,2). We have also developed methods to make them magnetically responsive (2).

Our objective in developing these microspheres was to utilize them to deliver drugs directly to diseased target organs. These carriers were designed to have certain required properties, including the ability to bind drugs and release them in a controlled manner. They were also designed to be body degradable and directable to specific internal or external sites by various routes including intravenous, intramuscular, inhalation, topical and oral methods of administration.

Protein microspheres, in particular, are relatively easy to prepare. Using serum albumin of any animal species as an example, one simply injects an aqueous solution of the protein into rapidly stirred vegetable oil (e.g., cottonseed oil), heats at an elevated temperature (e.g., 150 degrees C) for an appropriate time period (e.g., 1 hour) to drive water from and insolubilize the protein, and then filters the resulting spheres from the bath (3). The size of the spheres is controlled in large part by the rate of stirring and can generally be adjusted relatively easily in the range from 5 - 100 microns.

There are several methods which can be used to load the microspheres with drugs. In the "equilibration" method, one simply allows a dissolved drug of choice to equilibrate with the preformed microspheres prepared as described above. Drug interactions will take place with various hydrophobic and/or hydrophilic binding sites on the spheres to ultimately produce a microsphere carrier containing bound drug. We have been successful in loading a number of drug classes into albumin microspheres using this technique including narcotics, antiseptics, antituberculars, antibacterials, anti-inflammatories, barbiturates and analgesics (1). However, sphere loadings are rather low using the equilibration method, ranging from 1% - 5% by weight of drug.

A preferred method of microsphere loading is termed "entrapment". In this method, the free drug is dissolved in solution with the native albumin prior to sphere formation. In the case of water insoluble drugs, they can be micronized and dispersed in the albumin solution. The drug-containing solution or dispersion is then injected as described above into hot, stirred vegetable oil to form microspheres containing both chemically bound and physically entrapped drug. The advantages offered include much higher microsphere drug loadings (up to 60% loadings by weight possible) and no restriction to solvent soluble drugs (as is the case with the equilibration method). In cases where heating would inactivate or otherwise alter a specific drug, it is possible to alternatively chemically crosslink the microspheres at room temperature in the vegetable oil bath by using such common protein crosslinking agents as glutaraldehyde or formaldehyde (1,2,3).

Drug release from the microspheres can be controlled by several methods which adjust the porosity, insolubility and biodegradability of the carrier spheres. These include varying the time and temperature of heat crosslinking, varying the time of chemical crosslinking at room temperature (or any other chosen temperature), and varying the concentrations of drug and carrier within the spheres. Generally speaking, the higher the ratio of carrier to drug concentration, the slower will be the release of drug from the microspheres. In vivo biodegradability of the spheres can be adjusted from hours to many months by controlling the microsphere crosslinking conditions (1,2,3).

Appropriately sized microspheres can be conveniently utilized to target drugs of choice to specific organs of the body. For example, intravenously injecting microspheres in the 10 - 80 micron particle size range will result in their depositing very quickly in the capillary bed of the lungs where they are filtered out with 99% efficiency, releasing entrapped drug to this target tissue. Smaller microspheres less than 5 microns in diameter will pass through the capillary bed of the lungs, enter the reticuloendothelial system and ultimately deposit in the liver and spleen with relatively high efficiency (>90%), releasing appropriate drug to those target tissues. Inhalation, intramuscular and oral routes of microsphere delivery are also reasonable, although with inhalation the microspheres must be small (1- 5 micron range) to permit passage into the deep airways without undesirable impaction in the back of the throat as discussed previously.

In summary, using the methods described above (see also references (1), (2), (3)), it is possible to incorporate water soluble drugs, water insoluble dispersions of drugs, mixtures of water soluble and insoluble drugs, and heat sensitive drugs into albumin and other microsphere carriers. By carefully adjusting the size of the microspheres, precise targeting of the carriers to the lungs, liver and spleen is readily achievable.

Although the use of microsphere drug delivery systems

in chronotherapy is not as straightforward as the use of infusion pumps or possibly even aerosols, they do offer the
advantage of specific organ targeting. In this regard, by
appropriately adjusting the time and temperature of sphere
crosslinking, it may be possible to produce several classes
of microspheres containing the same drug but releasing it at
different rates, some quickly but others gradually more
slowly. By appropriately mixing these microspheres and administering them in a single dose, it is conceivable that
one could generate a drug release profile that produced
pulses of drug as a function of time as spheres of different
crosslink density released their contents.

MAGNETICALLY RESPONSIVE MICROSPHERES

Using either heat or chemical crosslinking methods
identical to those described above, it is possible to incorporate magnetically responsive materials in albumin or other
protein microspheres by dispersing them in the native protein solution just prior to forming the spheres in the vegetable oil bath (2,3). Magnetic iron oxide as well as a
number of other metallic magnetic complexes can be used.
Widder, Senyei and coworkers (4,5,6,7) have demonstrated
that at least in smaller test animals, such magnetic microspheres loaded with drugs can be targeted to specific sites
within the animal's body with externally placed magnets.
They have specifically used this approach to target albumin
microspheres containing the antitumor agent Adriamycin to
tumors in rats and have observed significant regression of
such tumors following microsphere treatment.

In separate but related studies, Langer (8) has also
demonstrated enhanced drug delivery from magnetically
responsive polymer carriers in the presence of oscillating
magnetic fields. When the oscillating magnetic field is
turned on, the amount of drug released from the carriers is
significantly higher than when the magnetic field is off.
The oscillatory magnetic fields apparently cause microscopic
movements of the magnetic particles within the carrier,
opening up diffusion pathways which allow more drug to be
released from the carrier.

The type of approach being pioneered by Langer could
have definite bearing on chronotherapy applications. By
applying an oscillating external magnetic field to a magnetically responsive drug delivery system like albumin microspheres or a drug-containing polymer implant, for example,
one could potentially increase the diffusional output of
drug from the carriers in a regulated, pulsatile fashion at
times most suitable for a patient's chronotherapeutic treatment. If, in addition, this drug could be targeted to a
specific site or organ of interest in the body either by
virtue of the size of the spheres or via external magnetic
fields, certainly some interesting chronotherapeutic applications could result.

TRANSDERMAL DRUG DELIVERY

Transdermal drug delivery systems have received a considerable amount of attention from the pharmaceutical industry during the past several years, particularly since the introduction of the nitroglycerin transdermal patches for treating angina by G.D. Searle, Key Pharmaceuticals and Alza/Ciba-Geigy in the United States and more recently by Pharma Schwartz in Germany.

There are three basic approaches being utilized today in the development of transdermal drug delivery devices. In the first approach, a polymer matrix containing the drug is simply taped down to the skin. The drug passes from the matrix directly to the skin. Examples of this type of device include Key Pharmaceutical's "Nitro Dur" and G.D. Searle's "Nitro Disc" products. In the second approach, a solution or ointment of drug is provided between a backing and rate controlling membrane. The drug passes through the rate controlling membrane and an adhesive before contacting the skin. An example of this type of system is Alza/Ciba-Geigy's "Transderm Nitro" nitroglycerin patch. In the third approach, the drug is simply incorporated into the adhesive itself. Pharma Schwartz's "Deponit" transdermal nitroglycerin product is an example of this type of system. All of these transdermal products contain relatively impermeable backings which help direct the drug to the skin. They also contain adhesives and release liners as essential components of construction.

Although today's transdermal systems are designed to provide a constant, zero order release of drug to the systemic circulation, the potential exists for chronotherapy applications. The most obvious application is to simply apply a transdermal patch containing a drug of choice to the skin and then remove it at an optimum time dictated by the chronopharmacologist. Pulsed dosing of drug to the systemic circulation would be achieved by continually applying and removing the patch at specific time intervals dictated by chronotherapy. This presumes, of course, that the drug (or a combination of drug and penetration enhancer) is able to penetrate the skin with relative ease.

SUMMARY

In summary, I've presented to you a selected number of drug delivery techniques, one of which, the infusion pumps, is directly applicable to chronotherapy. Most of the others, however, have been developed specifically for sustained release drug delivery applications. I've suggested some possible modifications of these sustained release technologies which, with additional development, might have potential application in chronopharmacology or chronotherapy. As someone personally untrained in chronobiology, I hope that I have been able to provide you with some basis for further thought and discussion of these concepts and their possible use in chronotherapy.

REFERENCES

1. Yapel, AF: U.S. Patent 4,147,767, to 3M Company, 1979.
2. Yapel, AF: U.S. Patent 4,169,804, to 3M Company, 1979.
3. Yapel, AF: in Methods in Enzymology, Vol. 112, pg. 3, 1985.
4. Widder, KJ and Senyei, AE: U.S. Patent 4,247,406, 1981.
5. Senyei, AE and Widder, KJ: U.S. Patent 4,357,259, to Northwestern University, 1982.
6. Senyei, AE, Driscoll, CF and Widder, KJ: in Methods in Enzymology, Vol. 112, pg. 56, 1985.
7. Widder, KJ, Senyei AE and Scarpelli, DG: Proc. Soc. Exp. Biol. Med., Vol. 158, 141, 1978.
8. Langer R, Brown L and Edelman, E: in Methods in Enzymology, Vol. 112, pg. 399, 1985.

THE MINI-OSMOTIC PUMP AS A TOOL IN CHRONOBIOLOGY

F. THEEUWES   Alza Corporation, 950 Page Mill Road, Palo Alto CA

1. INTRODUCTION

The majority of drugs are usually administered in impulse or bolus form as a consequence of release mechanisms of conventional dosage forms (e.g., pills, tablets, capsules, injections). Both drug administration regimen and drug discovery processes have been dependent on these input functions in the past.

The ideal drug administration regimen should result from a basic understanding of the concentration-effect relationships, and the tools that will allow study of these relationships should be flexible. Various reports in the literature indicate that concentration-effect relationships are not invariant, but dependent on other events: exogenous, as induced by drug-drug interactions; or endogenous, as indicated by chronobiological processes.

In the last 15 years, a variety of infusion pumps have become available that allow different administration regimens. The mini-osmotic pump is such a system (Ref. 1). It is designed to deliver at constant volumetric delivery rate dV/dt, however, the mass delivery rate dm/dt can be programmed to be any function of time by suitably programming the concentration in an added displacement unit.

2. SYSTEM DESCRIPTION

The pump is shown in Figure 1 in cross section indication from inside to outside the drug reservoir, osmotically active sleeve, and semipermeable membrane.

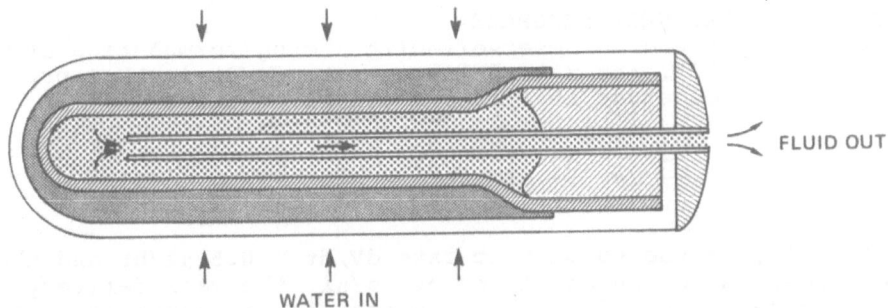

FIGURE 1.   Cross section of mini-osmotic pump in use.

62

The membrane forms the external housing and binds to the drug reservoir, thereby enclosing the osmotic sleeve between reservoir and membrane. The system is fabricated with empty reservoir which can be filled with experimental drug formulations. Two size systems (Ref. 2) are presently available with reservoir capacity respectively of 200 μl and 2 ml, as shown in Figure 2. The release rate in vivo is equal to the rate in vitro as shown in Figure 3.

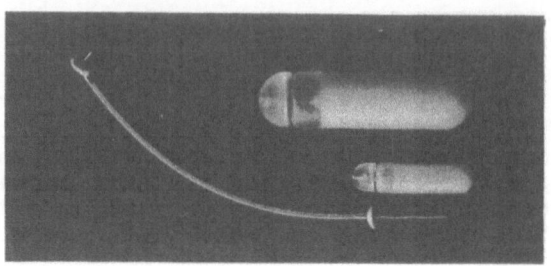

FIGURE 2. Photograph of the two sizes of mini-osmotic pumps.

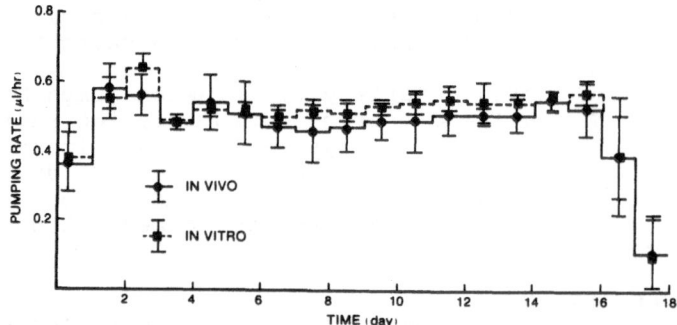

FIGURE 3. In vivo release rate compared to in vivo rate

3. DRUG MASS DELIVERY PROGRAMS

By filling the drug reservoir with a drug formulation at concentration "C", the mass delivery rate dm/dt is thus programmed to be constant at a rate shown in equation (1)

$$\frac{dm}{dt} = \frac{dV}{dt} \times C \qquad (1)$$

For example, if the volumetric rate dV/dt = 0.5 μl/hr and the drug concentration 50 mg/ml, or 50 μg/μl, the mass delivery rate will be dm/dt = 25 μg/hr. In addition to constant mass delivery rates, a variety of drug programmed rates that are predetermined as a function of time can be achieved. Such rates can be accomplished by coupling a volume displacement

unit containing the drug program to the pump, which is now
filled with an inert fluid, such as isotonic saline. An example of such a program is shown in Figure 4 where a catheter
tube containing a drug program C (t) that is alternating by
formed regions of drug spaced by an immissible fluid containing no drug.

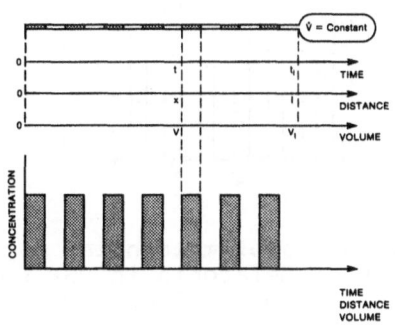

FIGURE 4. Catheter displacement tube filled with a drug
program of on-off type.

A program of the on-off type was for the first time achieved
by H.J. Lynch, R.W. Rivest, and R.J. Wurtman (Ref. 3) producing
artificial induction of melatonin rhythms in pinealectomized
rats. The apparatus used to program the tubing to separate the
aqueous drug solution by blank mineral oil spacers is shown in
Figure 5(A). The tubing was coiled around the pump, as shown
in Figure 5(B). The resultant urinary recovery profile is
shown in Figure 6.

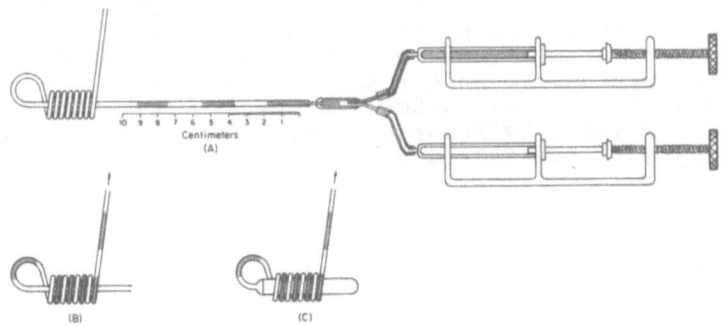

FIGURE 5. Programmed microinfusion apparatus. (A) Individual
components of the infusate program are forced from microsyrin-
ges, via a manifold, into the straight feeder portion of a
thermoformed capillary tubing forming the linearly arrayed
program. (B) The program is then driven, with additional vehicle, into the coiled portion of the tubing. (C) The feeder
portion of the tubing is cut off, a saline-filled osmotic mini-
pump is attached, and the assembly is ready for implantation.

64

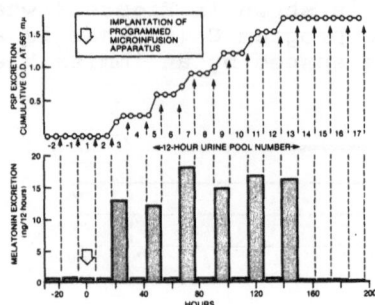

FIGURE 6. Rhythmic infusion of melatonin. A programmed infusate, consisting of 10 µg melatonin in PSP solution alternating with melatonin-free mineral oil, was implanted in a
pinealectomized rat (rat C). 6-hour urine samples were collected and pooled according to the cyclic appearance of PSP,
and the melatonin content of the urine samples was measured.

4. CONCLUSIONS
    There is a considerable and growing body of evidence indi-
cating that the pharmacodynamics of some drugs depends on the
time of administration during a relevant biological cycle. It
is expected that the pace of such chronobiological research
will accelerate in the near future and that the mini-osmotic
pump will prove to be a valuable tool in such research.

REFERENCES

1. Theeuwes F, Yum SI: Principles of the Design and Operation
   of Generic Osmotic Pumps for the Delivery of Semisolid or
   Liquid Drug Formulations. Ann. Biomed. Eng. 4, 343, 1977.
2. ALZA Corporation "Technical Applications File."
3. Lynch JL, Rivest RW, Wurtman RJ: Artificial Induction of
   Melatonin Rhythms by Programmed Microinfusion. Neuroendo-
   crinology 31: 106-111, 1980.

IMPLANTABLE SYSTEMS FOR LOCAL CHRONIC ADMINISTRATION OF DRUG APPLICATION
IN NEUROPHARMACOLOGY

YVES LAZORTHES and JEAN-CLAUDE VERDIE-Neurosurgical University Clinic, CHU
Rangueil, Toulouse

Recent neurobiological data concerning the existence of multiple receptor sites and the individualization of specific neurotransmitters have
forced us to step back and take another look at some of our preconceived
ideas about the central nervous system. The concept of a chemical neuro-
transmission, complementary and specific to a given transmission, has
progressively been associated with the electric model.

A better knowledge of the action mechanisms of the endogenous and exogenous ligands has allowed us to dispose of numerous active compounds.
The systemic approach to drug administration requires large doses that
eventually reach the action site, but only after having selectively crossed the bloodbrain barrier. In addition, the quantity of drugs administered causes a variety of undesirable side effects. The difference between
the dosage which is administered systemically and the dosage which is actually therapeutically effective is the basis of development of a new
therapeutical approach: locoregional neuropharmacology. This method has
progressively developed for several sites of administration (epidural, intrathecal, intraventricular, intravascular, intraparenchymally, etc.) for
numerous drugs (opiates, antimitotics, antispastics, neuromediators, etc.)
and for a variety of indications.

The need for chronic administration of drugs either through continuous perfusion or by repeated injections led to the development of implantable systems, permitting us to:

a. Increase the comfort and quality of life of those treated on an
out-patient basis.

b. Develop the concept of "pharmacological neurosurgery" which
appears to be a method of the future as it is not only effective, conservative, and selective, but also completely reversible.

c. To optimize the therapeutic effects of chronotherapy.

1. MATERIAL
The implantable systems are connected to supple silicone catheters
whose distal ends are positioned near the particular action site. There
are two types of systems.

1.1. Reservoirs
These consist of small-volume injection sites which are shunted to
the area to be perfused. The goal of these "access sites" is to transform
a lumbar or an intraventricular puncture or an intra-arterial injection
into a simple transcutaneous injection. There are two models:

a. 1) Silicone, dome-shaped capsules originating from the Ommaya
reservoir but with a flat bottom and side outlet. The CORDIS "unidose"
reservoir is the most widely known; it consist of a stainless steel rein-
forced bottom to prevent perforation while injecting. These small-volume
injector-reservoirs (1-2 ml volume) correspond to a single-dose injection.

Their dome is self-sealing to resist subcutaneous leakage during and after needle penetration and to permit multiple injections (using a 25 G or smaller needle).

b. 2) Stainless steel injection sites with a self-sealing chamber. This is the PORT-A-CATH system manufactured by PHARMACIA ; it can be connected to an intravenous or intra-arterial catheter as well as to a catheter to be placed epidurally or in the subarachnoid space.

These implantable reservoirs allow drugs to be administered either by repeated injections or by slow continuous perfusion (maximum rate 1 is liter/hour). They provide no autonomy to the patient who must depend on a prescription "on demand". It is difficult to be sure you are injecting the entire contents of the reservoir, and unfortunately, none of these systems includes an integral anti-bacterial filter.

In order to provide his patients with a certain autonomy, Poletti (36) devised a system whereby a lumbar catheter was connected in the lining of the abdomen. He incorporated a high-pressure Hakim valve and on-off valve, permitting the transcutaneous injection of a 0.1 bolus. This combination of pre-existing parts represents an original, economical solution; however, it is bulky and not very functional.

1.2. Implantable micro-pumps

These pumps have a large enough reservoir capacity to allow patient autonomy and they can easily be refilled through simple percutaneous injection. The different systems currently available vary in their working mechanisms and in their capability to insure safety and provide accurate, variable prescriptions.

1) If we consider the working mechanisms, we can differentiate between the following:

a. Pumps whose means of propulsion is chemical, in the form of Fluorocarbon gaseous pressure (Freon). In 1969, B. J. Blackshear (3,4) invented the system which is manufactured by INFUSAID . The disc-shaped pump is 3 cm high and has a diameter of 9 cm; its empty weight is 200 grams and it has a reservoir capacity of 50 ml. The pump is separated into two chambers by titanium bellows. The inner drug chamber contains the solution to be infused and the outer charging chamber contains a fluorocarbon liquid in equilibrium with its vapor phase. At 37°C, the vapor pressure exerted by this substance is approximately 300 mm Hg greater than atmospheric pressure. This vapor pressure provides the power source, exerting pressure on the bellows and forcing the infusate through a 0.22 micron bacterial filter and flow-regulating resistance element. The pump is placed beneath the skin, and the inner drug chamber is refilled by percutaneous injection. The pressure of this injection condenses the driving vapor, thus simultaneously filling the pump and recharging the power source.

b. The electro-mechanical peristaltic pumps are the most well-known. The peristaltic pump consists of a flexible tube placed in a metallic U-shaped chamber. Rollers squeeze the tubing walls at variable speeds which propels the drug at a variable flow-rate. The most sophisticated model is the one manufactured by MEDTRONIC, INC.: the Drug Administration Device or DAD 8600 model. The reservoir, drug pathways and exterior of the DAD are constructed of titanium elastomers; it measures 2.75 cm high and has a diameter of 7 cm. Its empty weights is 175 grams with a reservoir capacity of 20 ml. The 8601 model includes a bacterial retentive filter of 22 microns. Energy is provided by a lithium thionyl-chloride battery with a life expectancy of approximately 10 years. The programable infusion parameters are controlled by a microprocessor which is

hermetically sealed in the leakproof DAD case (10,14). The pump made by
SIEMENS[++] (IDE Model) is similar (Table I).

TABLE 1. . IMPLANTABLE DRUG DELIVERY DEVICES

Systems	Mechanisms	Dimensions (cm)	EW	Infusion modes	R V	A	P	S
INFUSAID Mod. 400	Vapor Pressure	3 X 9	208	Continuous 2-6 ml/24h	47	No	No	Yes
MEDTRONIC Mod. 8600	Peristaltic	2.7 X 7	175	Variable 0-0.9 ml/h	20	Yes	Yes	No
SIEMENS Mod. IDI	Peristaltic	8.5 X 6 X 2.2	170	Variable (24 steps)	10	Yes	Yes	No
PACE-SETTER Johns Hopkins	Solenoid pulsatlie	8.1 X 2	170	Variable (2 µl steps)	7.5	Yes	Yes	No
CORDIS Secor	Mechanical	6 X 1.4	45	Bolus (1 or 3 ml)	12	No	No	No

EW = Empty wt.
RV = Rerservoir Vol.
A = Alarm
P = Prgramable
S = Sideport

c.   The electro-mechanical pulsatile solenoid pumps, manufactured by
PACESETTER[+++] (e), uses a chamber which is activated by an alternate coming and going movement produced by the solenoid. Two feed-check valves
move the drug out toward the catheter. Energy is provided by a lithium
battery. The pump measures 2 cm high and has a diameter of 8.1 cm. The
empty weight is 170 grams, and it has a reservoir capacity of 7.2 ml. The
system is controlled by a microprocessor-based circuitry which permits
programation and interrogation by telemetry. This systems has only been
used as a prototype.
    d.   The totally mechanical pumps. The "SECOR" pump designed by
CORDIS represents the first implantable pump activated by a simple manual
gesture (22). It is entirely mechanical, including no electronic features
nor battery; thus, it is not a programable system. The working mechanism
consists of three one-way valves which control and deliver doses of a constant volume. The disk-shaped pump has a diameter of 6 cm and a height of
1.4 cm. Its empty weight is 45 grams. On the top of the pump you can see
2 push-buttons which are activated transcutaneously. They must be pressed
sequentially and in the correct order before a dose is delivered. A center self-sealing refill dome made of silicone elastomer permits percutaneous emptying and refilling. It includes a safety valve and a needle stop
which prevents the needle from completely passing through the dome and entering the reservoir. The bottom of the pump includes a supple reservoir
composed of teflonreinforced silicone with a working capacity of 12-15 ml.
    2)   If we consider the various pumps with respect to security and
prescriptions, we can distinguish between the following:
    a.   Constant-flow pumps INFUSAID. Considering the pump is activated

by a gaseous pressure, fixed according to a given temperature, the flow is relatively stable but precalibrated during manufacturing. Having been set between 2 and 6 mg/24 hours, it is impossible to change the flow rate after implantation. In order to modify the prescription, you need to change the drug concentration. One other inconvenience with this system is that the flow increases with changes in body temperature and diminishes with the atmospheric pressure. Moreover, it is impossible to immediately stop perfusion other than by emptying the drug reservoir percutaneously which entails a risk in the event of serious side effects. The 400 model includes a side outlet which can be used to administer another drug and to check the catheters permeability.

b. The "multidose" pumps (CORDIS "SECOR" model). The external manipulation of the 2 push-buttons releases a 0.1 ml (+ or - 10%) bolus. These buttons must be pressed sequentially and in a correct order before a dose is delivered so that they cannot be activated accidentally. To modify the flow, you simply increase or diminish the number of boluses. A new SECOR generation will have pop-up push-buttons and make a clicking sound to assure the manipulator that the bolus has been released.

c. The multiprogramable pump (MEDTRONIC'S DAD model). This pump has three programable infusion parameters that can be set or changed by telemetry: 1) a choice of measurements (microgram, milligram, milliliters, micromoles, etc.), 2) a variety of infusion modes (continuous hourly infusion, infusion with a specified delay, multi-step dose over programed interval, or bolus infusion) and 3) a range of infusion rates (approx. 0.09 ml/hour to 0.9 ml/hr).

Telemetry permits the clinician to non-invasively program the pump to a specific prescription, to control the DAD's operation and to interrogate the different alarm systems. In case of emergency, the programer can be used to stop the pump. In order to do so, the patient must be transported to the hospital where the implanation took place. There exists portable programers similar to those used for diabetics, however they are expensive and not everyone can afford them. To overcome this handicap, we hope that a simplified version with only an on-off control will be developed soon. There are also auditory alarms that indicate the reservoir capacity, the lifespan of the battery, and an eventual electronic breakdown.

The priniciple characteristics of these different implantable systems are summerized in Table 1 (above).

2. IMPLANTATION TECHNIQUE

The implantation is normally done percutaneously under local anesthetics or neuroleptanalgesia (19,20,21,22).

2.1 Catheter placement

Catheter placement depends on the drug administration action site: spinal, intraventricular or intra-arterial. The catheter must be passed under radioscopic-control to determine its exact location.

*CORDIS EUROPA, PO Box 38, AA 9300 RODEN, The Netherlands.
**PHARMACIA FRANCE SA, 8 square Newton, 78391 BOIS D'ARCY.
(+) MEDTRONIC INC., 3055 Old Hwy., PO Box 53, MINNEAPOLIS MN 55450 USA.
(++) SIEMENS CORP., 5310 North Siemens Court, Rosemont, IL 60018.
(+++) PACESETTER SYST., 12884 Bradley Av., SYLMAR CA 91342 USA.
(***) INFUSAID CORP., 1400 Providence Hwy., Norwood, MA 02620, USA.

We use a radio-opaque silicone catheter with an outer diameter of 1.6 mm and an inner diameter of 0.75 mm (CORDIS) for intraspinal and intraventricular placement.

A 14 G Touhy needle permitted us to place the intra-spinal catheter into the subarachnoid or epidural space. We used a percutaneous lumbar latero-median approach so that the puncture pathway was as oblique as possible in order to avoid catheter kinkage during interlaminar penetration of the vertebral canal. The pump connection can either be made at the site of the paravertebral incision or close to the subcutaneous pocket which will house the reservoir. It is extremely important that the connection be leak-free to prevent CSF fistulas and subcutaneous drug leakage.

In only 3 cases was the subarachnoid catheter inserted under visual control during a laminectomy and securely sutured to the dura mater.

The intraventricular method was done via a classical ventricular puncture. The distal tip of the catheter is either placed in the frontal horn of the right lateral ventricle opposite the foreman of Monro or in the third ventricle.

When using an implantable system for intra-arterial chemotheraphy treatment, we prefer a radio-opaque silicone catheter whose outer diameter is 2.29 mm and whose inner diameter is 0.72 mm. The distal end is equipped with a suture ring which permits catheter fixation (PHARMACIA). This extremity is placed in the external carotid artery and catheterized going backwards to the carotid bifurcation.

2.2. Implantation of a drug administration system

Regardless of whether you are using a reservoir or a micropump you must make a subcutaneous pocket to house the system. Make sure that the pocket is situated 2-3 cm beyond the incision not directly on top of it but yet close enough to facilitate fixation and to control the catheter connection. The subcutaneous surface must be thick enough to prevent skin necrosis especially with large-size pumps; but on the other hand, the system must not be implanted too deeply in order to facilitate transcutaneous palpation. Each system has its own particularities.

a. The reservoir-injector "UNIDOSE" by CORDIS for intraspinal and intraventricular drug administration. To simplify injection procedures, we normally place the unidose on a hard surface: either the external iliac fossa or on the cranial cavity nearest the action site. The entire system (catheter-connector reservoir) should be as straight as possible in order to avoid kinks and assure optimal permeability. Before fixing the reservoir in the subcutaneous pocket, pump it up to test the permeability. The reservoir puncture technique is identical to the lumbar puncture; a 25 G or smaller tuohy needle will preserve the self-sealing properties of the silicone dome. During drug administration, we can test the permeability of the system by observing a CSF reflex and take CSF samples for bacteriological analysis. Drug injection must be done slowly; once the needle is removed, the dome is pushed down so that the bolus is progressively ejected into the subarachnoid space. You can rinse the reservoir with an additional 1-2 ml bolus of CSF which has been drawn prior to injection of the drug.

b. The "PORT-A-CATH" intra-arterial systems is placed in a subcutaneous subclavicular pocket. The chamber must be flushed with a heparin solution of 500 µ/ml. After cutting the catheter at the desired length you connect it to the drug chamber. This chamber is then attached to the fascia with 4 nonabsorbable suture ligatures. It is important to test the permeability of the system by injecting a heparin solution using a 22 G needle. Perfusion can be done either with a syringe or with a portable pump (minimum flow rate of 5 cc/mn). To withdraw the needle, you must at the same time hold the chamber down between 2 fingers to avoid pulling out the suture stitches and continue injecting to avoid blood reflux at the catheter tip. An anti-coagulant treatment is continued with daily injections of 3-5 ml of heparin at 500 µ/ml for the first three days. The eighth day, we make another injection then once every week until treatment is completely discontinued.

    c. The "SECOR" (CORDIS) multidose reservoir. It's fairly large size requires implantation on the lower latero-thoracic level for intra-spinal administration, while the subclavicular level is more suitable for intraventricular administration. Before connecting the reservoir, you must purge it of all air bubbles by filling it with a sterile saline solu-tion. The pump must be pre-operatively calibrated to check the bolus volume and filled with the drug solution. With a bolus volume of 0.1 ml (+ or - 10%) and a morphine concentration of 5 mg/ml, the bolus will correspond to 0.5 mg (+ or - 0.05) of morphine.

    d. The "Drug Administration Device" (DAD MEDTRONIC). Prior to imp-lantation, remove all water in the reservoir and fill it up with 20 cc of drug solution in a sterile manner. Using the programer under sterile conditions, you can then proceed with the examination and programation. You must feed in data concerning the patient, the metrology and the nature of the drug to be administered (morphine, antimitotics, saline solution, etc.). The limits of the "empty reservoir" alarm must then be set. In practice, according to the pumps specific flow rate, you must program the quantity of drug that can be consumed before the audible alarm rings. At this point, the pump is submerged in 37°C water to check if all the bubbles have been completely evacuated. Considering the pumps large size, it is preferable to make the subcutaneous pocket in the flank or in the para-umbilical abdominal area. The DAD is now ready to be programed. The programer includes a computer-type console television screen, keyboard and transmission head. Programation is simplified by the fact that the software guides the manipulator, eliminating any chance of error.

    Since 1978 we have implanted 62 "Unidose" reservoirs of which 46 were connected to intra-spinal catheters and 16 were connected to ventricular catheter. During the same period we implanted 5 multiprogrammable DAD pumps and 6 multidose SECOR systems for clinical investigation purposes in conjection with the French authorization committee.

    2.3 <u>Incidents and complications due to implantation</u>

Catheter disconnection occurred in 3 cases. The diagnosis was made after observing the subsequent inefficiency of the injections and after-wards visualizing the leak through opacification. In each of the 3 cases, surgery repaired the connection and therapy continued normally. To pre-vent incidents of this sort, we now overlap the silicone catheter ends and make a ligature before suturing the metal connector to the fascia.

    Two patients had local infections and the systems had to be removed. One case involved a cachectic patient (with multiple urinary tract and respiratory infections) who developed sceptic skin necrosis with the unidose system. Another case developed a late (3rd month) post-operative hematoma infection with a SECOR pump. This risk of infection imposes certain preventive measures and eliminates patients with underlying infec-tion. One must insure a thorough subcutaneous hemostasis and select an implantation site where cutaneous and subcutaneous layers are adequate. Finally, strict aseptic precautions must be observed while puncturing, emptying and refilling the reservoir. Hence the value of pumps with a sufficient storage capacity, reducing manoeuvres of this type to a minimum.

Only one case of purulent meningitis was seen, this being the most serious complication. In this case where it was not possible to isolate the germ, recovery occurred spontaneously by injecting antibiotics intrathecally via the reservoir. The reservoir remained in place and continued functioning normally for another 8 months.

With regard to implantable pumps we did not observe any specific complication. In the first SECOR multidose generation, it was difficult to transcutaneously palpate the push-buttons. This inconvenience was rectified with the second generation which includes a pop-up action. None of the 5 Medtronic (DAD) programmable systems had any electronic failures and the flow-rate checks were always accurate.

3.   PRESENT DAY APPLICATIONS.   PRELIMINARY RESULTS

  3.1 <u>Chronic pain and intrathecal opioids</u>

This method is based on neurobiological, experimental and clinical data:

  a.   Opiate receptor sites have been discovered in the central nervous system and in particular in the most superficial layers of the dorsal horns of the spinal cord (34).

  b.   In vertebrates, we have observed a direct spinal action mechanism after morphine had been injected intravenously (5) and after micro-iontophoretic injections of morphine in the gelatinous substance (10).

  c.   Morphine administered directly into the lumbar CSF in the rat produces a powerful prolonged analgesia which is limited to the caudal extremity (45). These effects suggest that specific opiate receptors are involved since they are dose-dependent, stereospecific and naloxone-reversible.

  d.   An intensive, selective and prolonged (average of 24 hrs.) analgesic effect was observed in patients suffering from chronic pain who received small doses of morphine (0.5-3 mg) injected both intrathecally (46) and epidurally (3). The works of Yaksh emphasize the considerable importance of this type of drug delivery both from a fundamental standpoint and its clinical applications.

This technique essentially applies to chronic pain secondary to inoperative cancer. The incapacitating pain which is not relieved by conservative medical techniques, in particular by administering oral opiates, generally has a midline bilateral or diffuse topography. Consequently, both open and percutaneous surgical procedures designed to interrupt the nociceptive pathways are ineffective.

If we compare the indications, we can distinguish 2 complementary drug administration sites:

  a.   Intrathecal lumbar administration of morphine is essentially recommended for pain with a sub-diaphragmatic topography. This well known technique has become a routine treatment in analgesic therapy for cancer patients. The terminal cancer patient who has a life expectancy of only a few weeks can be effectively relieved with epidural morphine injections. The epidural catheter is tunnelized and connected to either a millipore filter or a portable external pump. The inconveniences of an external catheter for chronic pain relief are: the risks of catheter migration; a great risk of infection in an immuno-depressive population; and the numerous restraints that a strict supervision implies, above all on an out patient basis. For these reasons, when the patients life expectancy is sufficient, the use of a totally implantable system is more suitable.

Since 1978, we have implanted the following systems: 44 Unidose reservoirs, 6 Multidose "SECOR" pumps and 3 DAD micropumps (1980, 1982, 1983).

TABLE 2. SPINAL MORPHINE FOR CANCER PAIN

| | Ref. | Devices | | Site | | Dose | Follow-up |
		R	P	EPI	I-TH	(Mg/24 h)	(Months)
Wang JK	(47)	–	4	–	4	2	–
Poletti CH	(37)	2	–	2	–	2	6 - 7
Onofrio B	(30,31)	–	8	–	8	1 - 4.8	3 - 34
Leavens M	(23)	2	–	–	2	1 - 4	4 - 7
Saunders R	(40)	–	12	8	4	0.5 - 50	2 - 8
Penn R	(33)	–	14	2	12	1.5 - 8	1 - 9
Lazorthes Y		43	9	4	48	1 - 10	1 - 14
& Verdie JC						Mean = 2.5	Mean = 4

Table II is a summary of our experience, as well as that of other authors in this particular field of drug administration. We prefer using hyperosmotic preservative-free morphine. The daily dose is minimal (between 1 and 5 mg with an average of 2.3 mg per day). We had a patient follow-up of 1 to 14 months with an average of 4 months. Clinical evaluation was based on three criteria: the degree of analgesia obtained using a subjective pain-rating scale; consequences concerning the patients functional activities; and analgesic consumption. All totaled, we had 75% positive results. Repeated bolus injections on demand seems to be a better choice than continuous intrathecal perfusion due to the variable evolving nature of pain. The most frequent side effect is transient nausea. We had two cases of respiratory depression accompanied by drowniness and myosis; these were among our first patients and the complications occurred during the percutaneous pre-testing period after normo-osmotic morphine administration. For this reason, we now prefer using a hyperosomtic morphine solution and require the patient to remain in a half seated position 2 to 4 hours after the injection. Moderate tolerance developed in 6 of our patients but we did not need to interrupt treatment.

    b.   Intraventricular administration of morphine. More recently, different authors (23,39) showed that intraventricular morphine injections in the lateral ventricle produced 12 to 52 hours of pain relief with only 0.1 to 2 mg/hrs of morphine in patients with pain of cephalic or diffuse topography due to ear-nose-throat cancer. Pain relief was not associated with neurological changes or central depression. In fact, very few cases of respiratory depression have been reported with intraventricular injections. Euphoria and transient confusional hallucintation syndromes are two side effects specific to this particular injection site. The activating mechanism is probably directly at the supraspinal level, but there is controversial discussion that it might complement action at the spinal level. The problem of tolerance did not interrupt treatment. Major publications are summarized on Table 3. Our present-day experience with 14 patients corresponds with the other authors' observations.

TABLE 3.   INTRAVENTRICULAR MORPHINE FOR CANCER PAIN

	Ref.	Systems		Dosis (Mg/24 h)	Follow-up (Days)
		R	P		
Roquefeuil B	(39)	8	-	0.2 - 7	8 - 120
Leavens ME	(23)	4	-	0.5 - 7	2 - 90
Lobato R	(24)	17	-	0.25 - 16	15 - 120
Nurchi G	(29)	6	-	0.33 - 4	-
Thiebaud JB	(44)	32	-	0.12 - 5	4 - 230
Lazorthes Y & Verdie JC		16	-	0.12 - 1.5 Mean = 0.66	12 - 140 Mean = 68

In practice, these two injection sites appear complementary in that lumbar administration is indicated for pain of a subdiaphragmatic topography, whereas intra-ventricular administration is effective and justified when pain is diffuse or located above the diaphragm. Other than being extremely effective, other advantages of this method are it's conservative, scarcely invasive nature and the fact that when undesirable side effects do occur they are immediately totaly naloxone-reversible. Morphine which is a mu receptor agonist, remains the opiate of choice, but several studies are underway concerning the use of other opiates such as pentazocine, dynorphine or the enkephalines which are also receptor agonists. The future prospects of this approach are numerous and, for the most part, related to the development of the drug-release systems and their capability to adapt to the needs of the cancer patient. One of the limitations we are facing is the high cost of such implantable systems. Repeated bolus injections on demand appear to be more effective and easier to control than continuous perfusion.

3.2 Spasticity Control through intrathecal drug administration
The applications in this field are more recent and the neurobiological, experimental and clinical basis are still somewhat limited:

a.   J.C. Willer demonstrated that intravenous morphine injections (0.2 to 0.3 mg/kg) in volunteer paraplegic patients produced a significant, prolonged depression of nociceptive reflexes without modifying monosynaptic reflexes. Moreover, this was verified clinically with a significant reduction in spasticity (48).

b.   Rabbit studies with intrathecal lumbar administration of baclofen induced hind-foot flaccidity with small doses of 5 micrograms, whereas from 20 μg onwards, the front feet were also affected even though the animal remained alert (18). This dose/effect relationship coincides with T.Yaksh studies.

c.   H. Muller, through a lumbar injection, successfully treated a spastic strychnine induced cat with benzodiazepine, midazolan (0.15 mg/kg) together with intrathecal morphine administration.

A 2 mg dose of intrathecal morphine (11) and a 10-30 mg dose of epidural morphine (43) significantly improved both the pain and the spasticity of patients stricken with post-traumatic paraplegia and multiple sclerosis.

Currently clinical experience is limited to intrathecal administration of endogenous and exogenous ligands involved in the spinal motor reflex arc. These include morphine which is a mu-receptor agonist: Baclofen which is a GABA B receptor agonist; and the benzodiazepines which are essentially GABA A agonists. Preliminary trials are summarized on Table 4.

TABLE 4. INTRATHECAL SPINAL DRUG DELIVERY FOR CONTROL OF SPASTICITY

Authors	Ref.	Etiology	N Tested	Implanted	Drug	Systems R	P
Erickson D	(11)	Post Trauma	15	8	Morphine	-	8
		Demyelinating D	1	-			
Muller H	(26)	Demyelinating D	3	-	Midazolan	-	-
Penn R	(32)	Post Trauma	2	-	Baclofen	-	-
Lazorthes Y	(21)	Post Trauma	6	2		1	1
& Verdie JC		Demyelinating D	5	2	Morphine	2	-
		Cerebral Palsy	2	2	Baclofen	1	1

D. Erickson's experience is the most important, especially in the use of implantable pumps functioning at a continuous flow rate. This same author tested 16 patients, implanting 8 continuous-flow pumps (INFUSAID) in a 6 post-traumatic quadriplegic patients. A daily average dose of 2 mg controlled spasticity. There was a 1 to 17 month follow-up with no tolerance in those patients having isolated spasticity (11).

In 1984, R. Penn (26) reported his clinical experiences on two paraplegic patients after injecting 25-50 micrograms of baclofen. They suggest using implantable pumps for chronic intrathecal drug administration in these cases.

We have had experience with different spasticities of medullar and central origin (21). Post-traumatic spasticities and spasticities secondary to demyelination and cerebral motor disability were tested. Six patients received implants; 4 with reservoirs and 2 with programmable DAD pumps. Baclofen proved to be the most efficient drug for small dosage, however, the lack of a specific antagonist limited its applications. In fact, one of our patients received two serious baclofen overdoses causing loss of consciousness and hypoventilation which led us to discontinue its prescription. Small doses of morphine administered for chronic pain relief has proven extremely effective and much easier to control due to the fact that its effects are completely naloxone-reversible. Nevertheless, there are always the long-term risks with chronic opiate administration for patients having a long life expectancy.

Our interest in this method is based on its remarkable efficiency and its non-invasive, conservative, selective nature since it reduces spasticity without causing residual deficiencies in motor function. The future prospects for this method are undoubtedly very promising but we need further proof provided by rigorous, quantitative studies on spasticity, in particular double-blind and objective evaluations. Continuous drug administration require extremely precise dosages that can be perfectly programed; this is the advantage of programable micropumps such as DAD. The inconvenience of this system however is that it is impossible to immediately stop perfusion in case of undesirable side effects. Nevertheless, the need for an implantable system permitting repeated bolus injections on demand is obvious, providing you can use weakly diluted solutions particularly with drugs as active as Baclofen.

3.3 Intracarotid chemotherapy for malignant glioma

The cytotoxicity of antimitotics depends upon the duration of drug administration beyond a critical threshold. The brain and the cerebrospinal fluid are limited access sites and drugs delivered systemically do not reach the central nervous system in high concentrations. The carotid artery is the principle afferent for the majority of the subtentorial gliomas. It seems logical to use loco-regional antimitotic perfusion such as those done in monkeys by injecting equal amounts of BCNU marked with 14 carbon both intravenously and in the carotid artery (7, 12). Results showed that with the intra-carotid approach the concentration was three times greater in the homolateral brain than with the intravenous approach. In addition, the cerebral hemisphere that was perfused received 4 to 5 times the dosage that the controlateral hemisphere received.

The advantage of local chemotherapy treatment is that it not only avoids dispersing cytotoxic chemotherapy agents, but also avoids increasing their local plasmatic peak concentration. The indications are essentially cerebral malignant glioma (III and IV grade astrocytoma) with a unilateral hemispheric topography and secondary diffuse metastasis. Prior to chemotherapy surgical exeresis and conventional radiotherapy are performed. Chemotherapy is either given systemically, following radiotherapy, or only when there is a recurrence. Taking this concept and these indications as a basis initial results of intra-arterial chemotherapy using various chemical agents were reported (14,15,35). Some of these preliminary experiences are on Table 5.

TABLE 5. REGIONAL CHEMOTHERAPY FOR MAGLIGNANT BRAIN TUMORS

Authors	Ref.	Patients GL	M	Technic Cath	P	Site	Drug
Greenberg H.S.	(14,15)	30	–	30	–	I-A.	BCNU
Dakhil S.	(8)	7	–	–	7	I-V.	Methotrexate
Philips T. W.	(35)	6	–	–	6	I-A.	BCNU, FUDR, Cisplatin
Feun L.G.	(13)	20	10	30	–	I-A.	Cisplatin
Stewart D.J.	(42)	16	16	32		I-A.	BCNU, Cisplatin
Beck D.O.	(2)	–	3	–	3	I-Th.	Methotrexate
Morantz R.A.	(25)	11	–	–	11	I-T.	Bleomycin

(GL = Gliomas grades III and IV; M = Metastasis; CATH = Femoral Catheterism; P = Pump; I-A = Intraarterial; I-V = Intraeventricular; I-T = Intratumoral; I-Th = Intrathecal).

Most of the authors used the femoral approach with intra-arterial catheterisms during each chemotherapy session (normally every 2 to 3 months). The advantage of the percutaneous catheterism is to be as selective as possible (supra-ophtalmic), thus limiting the risks of neurotoxic retinal effects. Prior to chemotherapy, you may breakdown the blood-brain barrier by intravenous or even intra-arterial hypertonic mannitol perfusion followed by a rapid BCNU or cisplatinum perfusion (28).

Few authors have used implantable pumps for this indication. In 1982, Philips proposed a protocol which included a slow, continuous FUDR perfusion (4.8 - 6.5 mg/day) using an Infusaid 400 model pump for a 14-70 day period. A sideport permitted repeated bolus injections of either BCNU or of cisplatinum. There were no iatrogenic complications such as internal carotid thrombosis or transient ischemia encountered during continuous external carotid perfusion. The risk of ocular toxicity is the major complication with this method (15). It seems to be related to the alcoholic concentration of the BCNU solution; thus the importance of supra -ophtalmic catheterisms which reduce the risks of retinal toxicity. The second toxic risk is of a neurological sort, the risk being identical whether perfusion is done via the intra or the supra-carotid approach and regardless of which perfusion system is used. Nevertheless implantable, continuous-flow perfusion pumps permit silmultaneous perfusion of such "cell-cycle-specific" chemical agents as FUDR or even radio-sensitizers (BudR). Another advantage of these slow continous-flow pumps is to be able to maintain a high tissue concentration of a drug as necessary. Perhaps in the future we will be able to connect a slow-flow perfusion pump to an intra-arterial, supra-ophtalamic catheter without encounter-ing any iatrogenic complications.

Intraventricular chemotherapy has also been considered (8). Last of all, there is the direct intratumoral approach to chemotherapy whereby the catheter is implanted at the tumor site. There have been studies with rate as reported by Kroin (17) administering cisplatin locally; however, it seems that tissue diffusion (maximum of 2 cm) limits such applications. the concept of local chemotherapy is tempting because it reduces the neurotoxic, neurological, ocular and more general risks to a minimum. Local micro-infusion may be the technique of the future. Clinical tests with man have already been performed using bleomycine in glioma cases (25).

3.4 Additional applications

Progress made in our knowledge of neurochemical mechanisms concerning degenerative central nervous system diseases in the presence of a neurome-diator deficit has led to the development of new applications.

1) Alzheimer's disease (16). Recent data suggests there is a re-duction in cholinergic cerebral activity in patients stricken with Alzheimer's disease (A.D.).

Concurrently, cerebral biopsies of A.D. patients showed a decrease in choline acetyl transpherase (ChAT) the specific cellular tracer of the cholinergic neurones, as well as a decrease in the acetylcholine synthesis (6,9).

Based on this cholinergic hypothesis of a decrease in muscarinic re-ceptor activity in A.D. patients, Harbaugh and coll. (16) suggested a new therapy which consists of perfusing small doses of the muscarin agonist directly into the ventricular cerebrospinal fluid.

After analyzing toxic studies on dogs, we subjected four A.D. patients to a preliminary feasibility test followed by a cerebral biopsy. A constant-flow pump (INFUSAID) was connected to a catheter placed three times in the lateral ventricle and once in the great cistern. Bethanecolchloride was gradually perfused until the optimal therapeutic dose for each patient was obtained (between 0.05 and 0.7 mg/day). After an eight-month follow-up, we observed some spontaneous, reversible complications: initial nausea, and in one case, transient parkinsonian syndrome which retroceded after reducing the dose (0.6 to 0.4 mg/day). The therapeutic effects are encouraging, but we are still insufficiently documented. Subjective family reports noted improvement in the cogni-tive functions as well as in the patients functional activity. Patients returned to their initial state after placebo perfusion. The efficiency of this treatment has yet to be confirmed by a longer follow-up, a quantitative evaluation of mental functions using standarized scales and a placebo controlled double-blind study. The prospects of this new thera-

peutic approach are essentially neuropharmacological; for example, in the
case of Alzheimer's disease, our goal is to find a product capable of
reestablishing the cholinergic activity there where only one correction is
needed (49).

2)   The intrathecal administration of thyrotropine releasing hormone
(TRH) in degenerative neurological diseases such as amyotrophic lateral
sclerosis was proposed by T.L. Munsat (27). It appears to be less toxic
with a longer lasting effect than intravenous administration.

3)   According to P. Balentine (1) the intraventricular administration of lithium has potential psychiatric applications. Kinetic animal
studies showed that intraventricular drug delivery can be used to reduce
extra-cerebral toxicity and the caudal neurotoxicity of lithium.

4)   The intrathecal perfusion of glial GABA uptake inhibitors such
as THPO was suggested in the treatment of obstinate epilepsy (4).

5)   Lastly, D. W. Roberts (38) proposed using intracerebral drug
administration at a precise action site through stereotaxy, not only for
local chemotherapy as R. Penn did with cisplatinum, but also for the
treatment of motor disorders affecting the nuclei of the base.

4.   DISCUSSION
We will limit this discussion to implantable drug delivery systems
and the standards of choice with respect to their applications for
neurosurgery. As a general rule, regardless of the intended application,
it is preferable to use implantable systems rather than portable external
systems. No matter how small they may be external pumps are poorly
adapted to neurological indications due to their inherent restrictions on
patients who are often disabled and highly susceptible to injection. The
implantable system to be utilized must be:
1)   Easy to implant and manipulate
2)   Composed of biocompatible material which does not modify the
chemical stability of the drug being administered (22).

Drugs contained in the pump reservoirs will remain there for various
lengths of time, eventually beyond several months if necessary. During
this period, the drug solution will be in contact with the different
materials that constitute the pump. The materials mentioned on Table VI
have been selected for their biocompatibility qualities.

TABLE 6.   BIOCOMPATIBLES MATERIALS FOR IMPLANTABLE DRUG DELIVERY SYSTEMS

1.	Metal =	Titanium, Stainless steel
2.	Plastic =	Polysulfone, Teflon
3.	Filters =	Porus Titanium
4.	Wrapping =	Silicon elastomer

Titanium is a noble metal widely used for cardiac and neurological stimulator cases. It has been the material of choice for most of the
implantable pump cases because it not only prevents corrosion, but also
polymerization. Polysulfon resin is a plastic widely used for medical
instruments because its specifications meet their stringent requirements.
In fact, it has replaced all other plastics, in particular in the construction of implantable pumps due to its exceptional physical properties.
Polysulfon resin is extremely inert and durable, notably resistant to
autoclave (121°C) and ethylene oxide sterilization. It can be molded in
complex shapes without additional assembly work which cuts costs
considerably compared to the manufacture of metal products. Finally,

most chemical agents have no effect on polysulfon. Medical-grade silicone elastomer is also highly appreciated for its biocompatibility and easy handling.

All these materials may cause the degradation of the drug solution being administered regardless of what their physiochemical qualities might be. For this reason drug stability tests must be performed on each implantable system. For our part, we have tested for morphine stability in solutions destined for intratecal administration using high-pressure liquid chromatography analysis (22).

3) The system must be reliable not only from a programation stand-point, but also from a security standpoint.

4) The pump should have a reservoir capacity sufficiently large to permit the patient significant autonomy.

5) An integral anti-bacterial filter must be included.

6) Its life expectancy must be sufficient, in partuciluar if the energy source is also implanted.

7) The working mechanisms should avoid all risks of involuntary administration.

8) Finally, the price should be acceptable, that is adapted to the patients life expectancy.

Other standards of choice are specific with respect to the particular indication, the administration site, and the drug to be delivered. Thus, concerning chemotherapy, the continuous flow pumps are perfectly suitable because they include a sideport which permits polychemotherapy in conjunc-tion with continuous infusion of sequential bolus, in spite of their relatively imprecise flow rate. This type of pump is much less suitable in cases requiring a precise delivery rate variable in time, because the flow rate cannot be modified. To compensate, you must change the concentration of the drug to be delivered.

For antalgic purposes implantable mechanical pumps permitting the delivery of opiates "on demand' by repeated bolus injections are all the more appropriate given their low cost. The SECOR (Cordis) multidose res-ervoir which permits sequential bolus injections is an interesting solu-tion. It would be the best solution if the reservoir was larger and if a sideport was incorporated, providing the cost remains low.

Implantable multiprogrammable electronic pumps provide the greatest precision and are perfectly suitable every time an active neuromediator drug is used entailing risks of side effects. Programable pumps are appropriate for chronotherapy but, for the most part, their present-day use is limited due to their high cost; especially if we want to give the patient himself the means to stop perfusion in the event of undesirable side effects.

Be that as it may, the future prospects of local pharmacological neu-rosurgery appear very promising. They will develop parallel with progress concerning the methods of action of endogenous and exogenous ligands in the neurophysiological mechanisms and their implications with degernera-tive cerebral disease. In our speciality, the progress of the future will be in the field of neurochemistry. From the biotechnological standpoint the development of implantable drug delivery systems must be adapted to the patients needs, striving to improve their reliability and security while reducing their costs.

REFERENCES

1. Ballantine P: Intraventricular lithium infusion and potential applications in psychiatry. In: A Professional Briefing on "Totally Implantable Pumps", Isle of Palms, South Carolina, Sept. 19-22, 1984.
2. Beck, DO: Continuous infusion of methotrexate therapy of meningeal carcinomatosis. In: A Professional Briefing on "Totally Implantable Pumps", Isle of Palms, South Carolina, Sept. 19-22, 1984.
3. Behar M, Olshwang D, Magora F, Davidson JT: Epidural morphine in treatment of pain. The Lancet, 1: 527-528, 1979.
4. Blackshear P: Implantable drug delivery systems. Scientific American, 241: 66-73, 1979.
5. Conseiller C, Menetrey D, Le Bars D, Besson JM: Effet de la morphine sur les activites des interneurones de la couche V de Rexed de la corne dorsale chez le chat spinal. J Physiol (Paris) 65:220, 1972.
6. Coyle JT, Price DL, Delong MR: Alzeihmer's disease: a disorder of cortical cholinergic innervation. Science 219:1184-1190, 1983.
7. Crafts DC, Levin VA, Nielsen SA: Intracarotid BCNU (NSC-409962): a toxicyti study in six rhesus monkeys. Cancer Treat Rep 60:541-545, 1976.
8. Dakhil S, Ensminger W, Kindt G, Niedorhuber J, Chandler W, Greenberg H, Wheeler R: Implanted system for intraventricular drug infusion in central nervous system tumors. Cancer Treat Rep 65:401-411, 1981.
9. Davies P: Neurotransmitter-related enzymes in senile dementia of the Alzherimer type. Brain Res 171:319-327, 1979.
10. Duggan AW, Hall JG, Headley PM: Suppression of transmission of nociceptive impulses by morphine: selective effects of morphine administered in the region of the substantia gelatinosa. Brit J Pharmacol 61: 65-76, 1979.
11. Erickson DL, Blacklock JB, Michaelson M, Sperling KB, Lo JN: Control of spasticity by implantable continuous flow morphine pump. Neurosurgery 16:216-217, 1985.
12. Fenstermacher JD, Cowles AL: Theoretic limitation of intracarotid infusions in brain tumor chemotherapy. Cancer Treat Rep 61:519-526, 1977.
13. Feun LG, Wallace S, Stewart DJ, Chuang WP, Yung WKA, Leavens ME, Burgess MA, Savaraj N, Benjamin RS, Young SE, Tang RA, Handel S, Mavligit G, Fields WS: Intracarotid infusion of cis-diamminedichloroplastinum in the treatment of recurrent malignant brain tumors. Cancer 54:794-799, 1984.
14. Greenberg HS, Ensminger WD, Seeger JF, Kindt GW, Chandler F, Doan K, Dakhil SR: Intra-arterial BCNU chemotherapy for the treatment of malignant gliomas of the central nervous system: a preliminary report. Cancer Treat Rep 65: 803-810, 1984.
15. Greenberg HS: Intra-arterial chemotherapy for malignant tumors of the central nervous system. In: A Professional Briefing on "Totally Implantable Pumps", Isle of Palms, South Carolina, Sept, 19-22, (1984).
16. Harbaugh RD, Roberts DW, Coombs DW, Saunders RL, Reeder TM: Preliminary report: Intracranial cholinergic drug infusion in patients with Alzheimer's disease. Neurosurgery 15:514-518, (1984).
17. Kroin JS, Penn RD: Intracerebral chemotherapy: chronic microinfusion of cisplatin. Neurosurgery 10: 349-354, (1982).

18. Kroin JS, Penn RD, Beissinger RL, Arzbaecher RC: Reduced spinal reflexes following intrathecal baclofen in the rabbit. Exp Brain Res 54: 191-194, (1984).
19. Lazorthes Y, Gouarderes Ch, Verdie JC, Montsarrat B, Bastide R, Campan L, Cros J: Analgesie par injection intrathecale de morphine. Etude pharmacocinetique et application aux douleurs irreductibles. Neurochirurgie 26A:159-164, (1980).

POTENTIAL USEFULNESS OF INTELLIGENT DRUG ADMINISTRATION SYSTEMS IN IMPROV-
ING ANTIARRHYTHMIC THERAPY

Ph. SCHOENFELD

1. INTRODUCTION
    Progress in experimental and clinical cardiac electrophysiology has
greatly improved the understanding of the mechanisms of normal and abnormal cardiac impulse formation and propagation, as well as the modes of
action of antiarhythmic drugs. However, common clinical experience has
shown that insufficient attention has been paid to the interactions
between spontaneous and drug-induced variations of the electrical activity
of the heart on one hand, and the timing of administration of antiarhythmic drugs on the other hand. Routine drug administration schedules that
do not take into account the aforementioned interactions often result in
inefficacy or even unwanted effects of otherwise potentially useful antiarrhythmic agents.
    From these preliminary considerations, we will discuss how arrhyth-
mia pharmacologic management could be optimized by intelligent drug-delivery systems capable of integrating significant dynamic and morphologic ECG
parameters. "Dynamic" parameters essentially are the variations of sinus
rate on one hand, and the degree of arrhythmia suppression on the other
hand. "Morphologic" parameters refer to beat-to-beat variations in ECG
morphology, reflecting useful or potentially toxic effects of the drug on
electrogenesis.

2. DRUG ADMINISTRATION IN FUNCTION OF DYNAMIC ECG PARAMETERS
    a. Basic sinus rate
    It is well known that the basic sinus rate undergoes circadian varia-
tion which are mainly related to autonomic influences (1-4). Several antiarrhythmic compounds more or less profoundly depress sinus nodal activity,
with considerable patient to patient variability. So, dosage schedules
which ignore the underlying variations of heart rate are a major cause of
unwanted effects, often leading to drug withdrawal. Initial assessment of
the patient response using a temporary rate-response delivery system,
could be of help in delineating optimal administration schedules for
chronic treatment.
    Careful monitoring of sinus rate is not only useful in avoiding bra-
dycardia per se. Several authors have studied the relationship between
the incidence and severity of supraventricular and ventricular arrhythmias, and the underlying variability of sinus rate is mainly related to
autonomic influences. This holds true, for instance, in cases of paroxys-
mal artrial fibrillation, "torsades de pointe", ventricular tachycardia
and fibrillation, atrial vagal arrhythmia (5-8). Conceivably, antiarrhythmic compounds of various types may exert deleterious rather than beneficial effects when administered at arbitrarily predetermined intervals
which do not take into account the underlying heart rate at the time of
administration. As a first approach, we believe that in intensive care

patients prone to developing dangerous arrhythmias, temporary closed-loop drug delivery devices integrating the variations of heart rate during antiarrhythmic drug infusion should be evaluated as a possibility of optimizing the pharmacologic management of these patients.

    b. Assessment of the therapeutic response

    Computerized analysis of atrial and ventricular activity, atrioventricular conduction ratio and degree of ventricular ectopy is already available in Holter monitoring systems providing arrhythmia reports on an automated basis. The administration of antiarrhythmic drugs on the basis of feedback systems integrating the degree of reduction of ventricular ectopies, the slowing of ventricular response in case of atrial fibrillation should be evaluated in order to avoid excessive, as well as insufficient drug delivery, in the initial, or even perhaps in the chronic stage of pharmacologic antiarrhythmic therapy.

3.   DRUG ADMINISTRATION IN FUNCTION OF MORPHOLOGIC ECG PARAMETERS

    As already mentioned, "morphologic" ECG parameters refer to beat to beat variations of electrocardiographic parameters that essentially reflect how electrical depolarization followed by repolarization progresses in the normal or diseased myocardium. Of special interest is the fact that specific drug actions at specific cardiac sites are reflected by variations of these parameters, much more significantly than variations in plasma levels of the drug, which however are currently used as indicators of so-called "therapeutic" or "toxic" levels of drug treatment. In our view, good clinical practice in monitoring the effects of a given antiarrhythmic compound basically relies upon closely monitoring the changes in morphologic parameters induced by the drug, rather than simply adapting daily dosages to variations of plasma levels; plasma levels simply do not reflect tissue impregnation. This is well illustrated by the frequent occurrence of digitalis intoxication in the presence of so-called "therapeutic" plasma levels of the drug. the ECG parameters that have to be monitored in order to optimize antiarrhythmic drug administration mainly consist of three "intervals" that can be readily identified on the standard ECG: PR, QRS and QT intervals. PR interval is a measurement of the time of transmission of the electrical influx from the atria to the ventricles; QRS interval reflects the total time of ventricular depolarization (and, in fact, corresponds to phase zero of the ventricular monophasic action potential); QT interval corresponds to total electrical systole and provides a good evaluation of the duration of ventricular refractoriness, and important determinant of ventricular arrhythmogenicity. Several of presently available "classifications" of antiarrhythmic drugs are at least partially based upon drug effect on morphologic ECG parameters (9,10). Unfortunately, considerable overlap exists between the subclasses of these classifications. Several compounds in fact belong to more than one class, the clinical effects may be contradictory to the theoretical classes developed from animal studies based on healthy atrial tissue, whereas clinical applications often refer to diseased ventricular myocardium. Considerable patient to patient classifications are encountered. Rather than blindly refering to the existing classifications in order to predict the effect of a given drug on a given patient presenting with a given electrical status at the time of drug administration, we find great potential improvement in the use of antiarrhythmic compounds. However, care must be taken to modulate their dosage schedules by way of feedback systems integrating the alterations of ECG parameters induced during drug administration.

As an example, the degree of prolongation of PR interval during pharmacologic impregnation by digitalis, verapamil and amiodarone is an useful marker of drug efficacy, as well as an indicator of potential overdosage. Important patient to patient variability exists regarding the degree of PR prolongation for similar dosage schedules. So, modulating drug administration in order to maintain PR prolongation at a desired level could prove of value in improving toxic to therapeutic ratio of these compounds.

Interval monitoring of QT could be especially useful in preventing the incidence of one of the most severe unwanted arrhythmogenic effects of antiarrhythmic drugs: "torsades de point". This iatrogenic arrhythmia results from prolongation of ventricular repolarization, inducible by several antiarrhythmic compounds; this is reflected on the surface ECG by QT lengthening (11,12). Important patient to patient variability exists in the magnitude of QT lengthening induced by a given dosage, which explains the impossibility of predicting the risk of developing "torsades de pointe" in a given patient when therapy is started. On the other hand, lengthening of ventricular refractoriness to a certain degree probably represents a major determinant of antiarrhythmic drug action in ventricular arrhythmias. So, progressive achievement of a limited degree of QT lengthening during loading dose schedules could be utilized as an useful criterion of sufficient or excessive myocardial drug impregnation.

Ideally, several ECG parameters should be simultaneously monitored and integrated in order to optimize the initial (and possibly chronic) dosage schedules of antiarrhythmic compounds. It is well known that many antiarrhythmic drugs exert more than one electrophysiologic action, some or even all of them being reflected by ECG morphologic criteria. The different electrophysiologic effects may not develop at the same pace, in other words, they manifest different apparent pharmacokinetics, manifested by the fact that a given effect may be absent or barely detectable while, at the same moment, another one may be present in a sufficient or even toxic level. This holds true, for instance, when amiodarone therapy is initiated. During initial rapid intravenous infusion, some acceleration of sinus rate may be induced; thereafter, PR interval will lengthen, and sinus rate will slow down. At more pronounced impregnation, the drug alters repolarization in a typical fashion. Finally, after important, prolonged impregnation, QRS widening may be observed (13). Flecainide also induces several electrophysiologic changes (14-15) the appearance of which can be usefully monitored by observing dynamic and morphologic ECG changes.

Table 1 gives an example of the various sequential electrophysiologic effects induced by intravenous flecainide loading doses.

TABLE 1.

Rate (mg/m)	Time	Dose	A cycle	V cycle	QRS
			320	640	0.10
6.70	0.5	200	390	780	0.10
0.54	4	130	430	610	0.12
0.18	24	260	400	800	0.11
0.83	4	200	475	475!	0.16
0.14	24	200	440	880	0.14
			420	700	0.13
4.30	0.5	130	540	540!	0.18 STOP

(See text for legend and discussion).

Each dosage regimen is characterized by the rate of administration (in mg/minute), the duration of administration (in hours) and the total amount delivered. The effect of such dosage regimen is shown in terms of atrial cycle and ventricular cycle (in msec) and width of the QRS complex. As can be seen, the initial arrhythmia consists of an atrial tachycardia with a cycle length of 320 msec, followed by 2/1 atrioventricular transmission resulting in a ventricular cycle length of 640 msec. The QRS complex was basically moderately prolonged (0.10 sec). The initial bolus of 200 mg. induced definite slowing of the atrial rate, without change in the atrioventricular transmission, and no effect on QRS. Further administration of the drug at slow rate (130 mg in 4 hours) induced further lengthening of the atrial cycle, but this in turn allowed episodes of 1/1 a-v conduction alternating with 2/1 ratio, which resulted in mean ventricular cycle of 610 msec. QRs widening appeared at that stage. Further attempts of different modes of administration resulted in different degrees of slowing of the atrial arrhythmia, which eventually reached a cycle length of 540 msec but at that stage, 1/1 permanent a-v conduction ratio remained present, resulting in a ventricular response that was faster than the basic one. Simultaneously, QRS widening alarmingly increased, and drug administration was stopped. Thus, in this peculiar case, several electrophysiologic properties of the antiarrhythmic compound, with different chronological dose-action relationships, were evidenced by means of careful ECG monitoring during various rates of infusion. Progressive beneficial effect during various rates of infusion. Progressive beneficial effect on the atrial arrthythmia itself was demonstratable, but at the final stage of impregnation, the magnitude of intraventricular conduction disturbance (manifested by QRS widening) prompted us to stop the therpeutic trial.

In conclusion, we believe the the pharmacologic management of arrhythmias could be optimized, at least during the initiation of therapy using complex drugs, by intelligent drug-delivery systems which are capable of integrating dynamic and morphologic ECG parameters. Some of the technology already in use (in sophisticated pace-makers including telemetry, computerized ECG analysis, arrhythmia reports in Holter systems) can be utilized in research and development of this potential new area of biotechnology. Theoretically, the application of closed-loop delivery systems in the field of antiarrhythmic therapy should be extremely helpful in improving the toxic to therapeutic ratio of several efficaceous but potentially dangerous antiarrhythmic compounds. One must be aware, however, that much remains to be done in order to evaluate the technical feasibility and the clinical applicability of such antiarrhythmic drug administration devices.

4. SUMMARY

The variability of sinus nodal activity under autonomic and other influences plays an important role in the incidence and severity of supraventricular and ventricular dysrhythmias. Hence, monitoring of spontaneous and drug-induced variations of sinus rate could usefully be integrated into the evaluation of apparent drug efficacy (arrhythmia suppression, slowing of ventricular response). Feedback loops influencing the delivery of antiarrhythmic drugs should also take into account other electrocardiographic parameters. The PR, QRS and QT intervals all reflect some aspects of tissue impregnation by antiarrhythmic drugs. As an example, some degree of QT lengthening can be desirably achieved (reflecting potential antiarrhythmic efficacy by prolonging ventricular refractoriness); however, excessive lengthening should be avoided (potential arrhythmogenic effect). Similarly, the degree of PR and QRS lengthening can indicate useful impregnation or potential toxicity, and could thus be integrated into the feedback loop of a drug delivery system in order to adequately increase or decrease the rate of administration.

We believe that arrhythmia management can be optimized by sophisticated drug-delivery systems that are capable of integrating dynamic and morphologic ECG parameters - reflecting the degree of arrhythmia suppression, the variations of basal sinus rate and progressive tissue impregnation as well as potential toxicity. Technology is already in use in other fields (high performance Holter analysis, computerized ECG protocols, sophisticated implantable pace-makers including telemetry) and could be 'useful in orienting future developments in this new area of research.

REFERENCES

1. Dighton D H: Sinus bradycardia: Autonomic influences and clinical assessment Br Heart J 36:791, 1974.
2. Agruss N S, Rosin E Y, Adolph R J, et al: Significance of chronic sinus bradycardia in elderly people. Circulation 46:924, 1972.
3. Bjerregaard P: Premature beats in healthy subjects 40-79 years of age. Eur Heart J 3:493, 1982.
4. Brodsky M, Wu D, Denes P, et al: Arrhythmias documented by 24 hour continuous electrocardiographic monitoring in 50 male medical students without apparent heart disease. Am J Cardiol 39:390, 1977.
5. Verrier R L: Neural factors in ventricular electrical instability, in Kulbertus H E, Wellens H J J (eds): Sudden Death. Boston/London, Martinus Nijhoff, 1980. pp. 137-155.
6. Coumel Ph, Attuel P, Leclercq, J F, et al: Arythmies auriculaires d' origine vagale ou catecholergique. Effet compare du traitement beta-bloquant et phenomene d'echappement. Arch Mal Coeur 75:373, 1982.
7. Coumel Ph, Fidelle J, Lucet et al: Catecholamine-induced severe ventricular arrhythmias with Adams-Stokes syndrome in children. Br Heart J 40:28, 1978 (supplement).
8. Coumel Ph: Heart rate trend analysis: Patterns and clnical significance, in Roelandt J, Hugenholtz PG (eds): Long-term Ambulatory Electrocardiography. The Hague, Martinus Nijhoff, 1982, p. 51.
9. Vaughan Williams, E M: Classification of antiarrhythmic drugs. In Sandoe, et al. (eds): Symposium on Cardiac Arrhythmias. Sodertalji, Sweden, A. B. Astra, 1970.
10. Keefe, D L, Kates, R E and Harrison, D C: New antiarrhythmic drugs: Their place in therapy. Drugs, 22:363-400, 1970.
11. Motte G. Coumel Ph. Abitbol G. Dessertenne F. Slama R: Le syndrome QT long et syncopes par "torsade de pointes". Arch Mal Coeur 63:831-853. 1970.
12. Krikler D M, Curry PVL: Torsade de pointes, an atypical ventricular tachcardia. Br Heart J 38: 117-120, 1976.
13. Heger J.J., Prystowsky E.N., Miles W. N. and Zipes D. P.: Clinical use and pharmacology of amiodarone - Med. Clins. North Amer. 68: 1339, 1984.
14. Mark Estes N A, Garan H, Ruskin J N. The electrophysiologic properties of flecainide acetate in man. Am J Cardiol 1984; 53: 26B-9B.
15. Hellestrand, K J, Bexton, R S, Nathan, A W, et al.: Acute electrophysiological effects of flecainide acetate on cardiac conduction and refractoriness in man. Br. Heart J., 48:140-148, 1982.

Endocrine disorders: need for new instrumentation

Mortimer B. Lipsett* and Franz Halberg**
*National Institute for Arthritis, Diabetes, Digestive and Kidney Diseases, NIH, Bethesda, MD, USA
**Chronobiology Laboratories, University of Minnesota, Minneapolis, MN, USA

Two textbooks describe the loss of bioperiodicity in serum cortisol in association with Cushing's disease (1,2). This finding continues to be reported in research papers as well (3), apart from an increase in serum cortisol concentration in this disease. There are, however, reported cases of the persistence of circadian changes in this condition (see 4 for review) and also in hypercortisolemia without any stigmata of Cushing's syndrome (5).

2 subjects, a father and his son, described as having primary cortisol resistance, provided blood samples over 24 hours at 30-min intervals for cortisol determination. A circadian rhythm with a similar timing of high values (acrophase) is present in both cases ($P \leq .05$), although around a much lower mean in the son as compared to his father, Figure 1. The circadian amplitudes of 5.5 and 4.6 µg/dl do not differ with statistical significance between the 2 subjects. In keeping with the higher MESOR (rhythm-adjusted mean) observed for the father, a statistically significant difference in the amplitude/MESOR ratio (relative amplitude) is found between the 2 patients ($P < .05$), Figure 1.

The data provided by the two subjects were compared to reference standards, Figure 2, computed as time-specified tolerance limits (including at least 90% of the reference distribution with 90% confidence; top) and as prediction limits (including, on the average, 90% of the reference distribution; bottom). The reference population consists of 10 clinically healthy men 16-28 years of age, providing a total of 25 data series at 4-h intervals for 24 hours. Against these reference limits, it can be seen that the data from the father are elevated (Figure 2, right), while only few

Figure 1.

Comparison of Circadian Rhythm in Serum Cortisol in a Father and Son with long-term "Hypercortisolism"
(samples every 30 minutes for 24 hours)

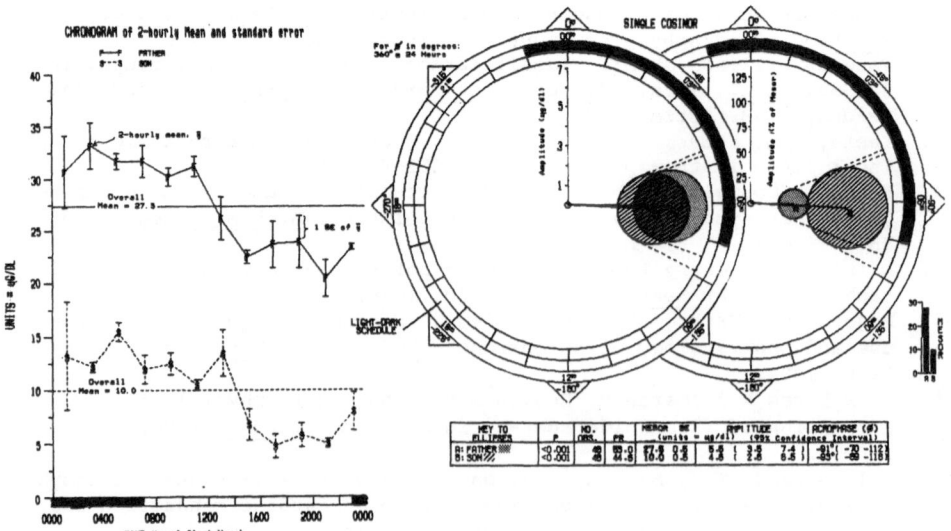

Figure 2.

SERUM CORTISOL IN A FATHER AND SON WITH LONG-TERM "HYPERCORTISOLISM"
Compared with Chronodesm (time-qualified reference limits*) Calculated from 25 Series of Cortisol
obtained from 10 Clinically-Healthy men, 16-28 years of age

data fall outside the reference standard for the son (Figure 2, middle). These 2 patients' circadian parameters were compared against a reference region for the (amplitude, acrophase) pair, constructed as a 90% prediction region from the reference population. The circadian characteristics of the father and son are found to lie outside the reference region, as a result primarily of an earlier acrophase, but also because of a reduced relative amplitude in the case of the father.

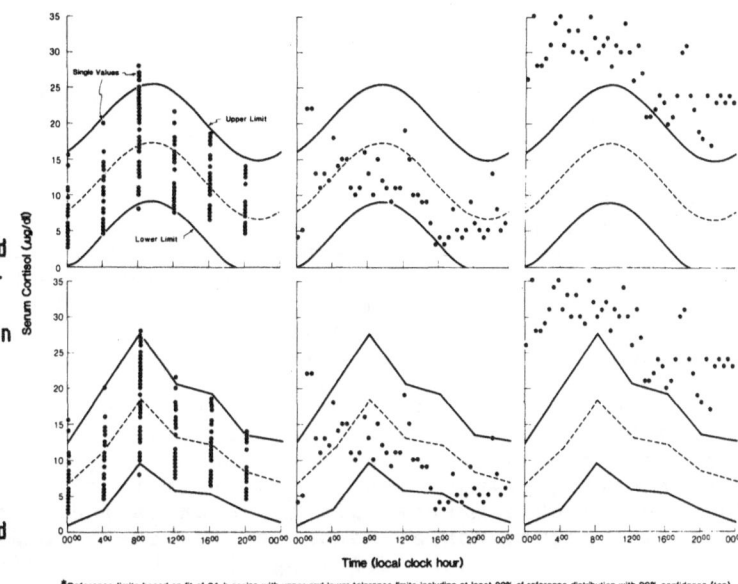

*Reference limits based on fit of 24-h cosine with upper and lower tolerance limits including at least 90% of reference distribution with 90% confidence (top), or consisting of time-specified prediction limits including 90% of reference distribution (bottom)

Admittedly, the reference standards used herein have grave shortcomings, resulting primarily from the lack of proper data bases. Nonetheless, the results presented above, placed in the broader context of a statistically significant cortisol rhythm alteration found in a population of 28 patients with adenoma, carcinoma, diffuse or macronodular hyperplasia of the adrenal cortex, providing a total of 47 data series (6), indicate the need for a more systematic assessment of the rhythmic structure of cortisol. Modern technology has a crucial role to play to achieve such a goal, by rendering more practical the serial drawing of blood for hormonal determination followed by chronobiologic data analysis. Such an instrumentation would help investigate problems such as receptor defects in the absence of Cushing's syndrome.

References

1. Krieger D.T.: Rhythms in CRF, ACTH and corticosteroids. In: Krieger D.T. (ed.): Endocrine Rhythms, Raven Press, New York, 1979, p. 123.
2. Liddle G.W.: The adrenals. In: Williams R.H. (ed.): Textbook of Endocrinology, Saunders, Philadelphia, 1981 (6th ed)., p. 269.
3. Kreze A., Spirova E., Putz Z.: Cirkadiánny rytmus plasmatického kortizolu v diagnostike Cushingovho syndrómu. Lek. Obzor. 32: 11-16, 1983.
4. Lipsett M., Halberg F.: Circadian serum cortisol rhythm characteristics in a father and son, reportedly with long-term hypercortisolism. Proc. 2nd Int. Conf. Medico-Social Aspects of Chronobiology, Florence, Oct. 2, 1984, in press.
5. Chrousos G.P., Vingerhoeds A., Brandon D., de Regt J., Pugeat M., Eil C., Loriaux D.L., Lipsett M.B.: Primary cortisol resistance: a glucocorticoid receptor-mediated disease. 63rd Ann. Mtg. Endocrine Society, Cincinnati, OH, 1981, abstract 773.
6. Kreze A., Spirová E., Sánchez de la Peña S., Halberg F.: Circadian pattern of circulating human cortisol in health and Cushing's syndrome. Chronobiologia 12: 255, 1985.

CHRONOBIOLOGIC DATA ANALYSIS SYSTEMS WITH EMPHASIS IN CHRONO-THERAPEUTIC MARKER RHYTHMOMETRY AND CHRONOEPIDEMIOLOGIC RISK ASSESSMENT

Ramón C. Hermida

Chronobiology Labs., Univ. of Minnesota, Minneapolis, MN 55455

1. RHYTHMOMETRY.

1.1. Introduction.

Certain phenomena can be readily recognized by the naked eye as involving changes repeating themselves in a regular predictable fashion. A macroscopic approach is based on the inspection of original data or of averages and of dispersion indices, tabulated or plotted as a function of time. Statistical tests such as a t- and F-tests, complementing tables or plots of data as a function of time (Halberg & Visscher, 1950; Halberg et al., 1953), do not provide, in themselves, information concerning the characteristics of a bioperiodicity--a term that we use for recurring changes not tested statistically for periodicity. Although such a macroscopic approach is indispensable to visualize the phenomenon at hand, it is best complemented by a microscopic approach allowing for the provision of point and interval estimates of rhythm characteristics, thereby also allowing for further statistical testing.

A rhythm is a component of a biologic time series, formulated algoritmically as a recurrent phenomenon and demonstrated as being periodic by inferential statistical means. This demonstration may be achieved by testing the null-hypothesis of zero-amplitude of a cosine function fitted to the data by least squares. By rejecting this assumption, a rhythm is described and concomitantly certain parameters are determined.

When the rhythm departs from sinusoidality, a plexogram gives valuable information concerning its waveform, which also can be described statistically by adding harmonic components in the model. Plexograms display, along an abscissa of a single period, original data covering spans longer than the period of a rhythm investigated, with these data stacked into the single idealized period. The plexogram, in itself, constitutes a macroscopic way of looking at the waveform of a phenomenon. It is best combined with computer programs for an analysis of variance, as has also been done with desk calculators (Halberg et al., 1953).

Objective methods available to obtain estimates of timing of high values on non-sinusoidal rhythms include: 1) Harmonic interpolation, a method applicable to equidistant data covering an integral number of cycles with the period assumed to be known. This method provides the detailed shape of the waveform (by the fit of harmonics) and permits an estimation of the rhythm's high values, called the paraphase (De Prins et al., 1981). 2) The computation of orthophase, based on the fitting of multiple components that are statistically and biologically significant (Tong et al., 1977).

These methods account for non-sinusoidal waveforms and provide parameters characterizing them. When the data are non-
sinusoidal, the least-squares fit of a cosine curve to the data
may be used for rhythm detection, although this approach may
not be as powerful as the simultaneous fit of all statistically
significant components. The P-value obtained in testing the
zero-amplitude assumption should thus be regarded as reflecting
whether the data are better approximated by a cosine curve than
by a horizontal line.

To summarize, 1) for a phenomenon to qualify as a rhythm,
the hypothesis of "no rhythm" (zero-amplitude) must be objectively rejected. Moreover, whenever possible, 2) the phenomenon
should be objectively quantified in terms of point-and-interval
estimates of all pertinent components. In this discussion, the
period has been assumed to be known. This is often justified
under synchronized conditions. When the period is unknown,
linear least squares have to be replaced by nonlinear least
squares, allowing for the estimation of the period as well as
the amplitude and acrophase of each component. In short and
sparse series, the estimate of the period may, however, be
questioned and tested (Bingham et al., 1984).

1.2. Early background of biological time series analysis.

Figure 1 shows a flowchart with particular reference to some
of the procedures developed for the analysis of unequidistant
data. A plot of the raw data (chronogram) and a histogram of
the raw data are invariably useful but not sufficient. The histogram is best prepared with an estimation of parameters such
as the mean and the variance. In the case of a normal distribution, one can also derive, for a given parameter (such as the
mean), a confidence interval at a desired probability level.

To gain a better impression of the shape of the rhythm from
time series with a length covering several cycles, one can fold
the data within one idealized cycle to obtain a plexogram. For
each interval along the time scale covering a single period of
the rhythm investigated, a mean and standard deviation or standard error are displayed to show the likely individual or group
variabilities.

For period estimations, Schuster's periodogram (1898) was
extensively used in the early 1950's (Halberg, 1954; Halberg &
Visscher, 1954); its computation was illustrated in detail with
the analysis of body temperature series (Koehler et al., 1956).
This method served originally to quantify a consistent circadian desynchronization of the rectal temperature rhythm in blinded mice (Halberg, 1953, 1960; Halberg & Visscher, 1954). The
autocorrelogram (Halberg, 1960) and power spectra consisting of
a first autocorrelation followed by generalized harmonic
analysis (Halberg & Panofsky, 1961; Panofsky & Halberg, 1961)
were used for noisy data.

From variance spectral analysis, a circadian quotient (CQ)
can be derived. The CQ can be the sum of the smooth spectral
estimate of the period equal to 24 hours plus the two adjacent
such estimates, divided by the total variance. The latter is
obtained by adding all the spectral estimates. All of these
procedures required equidistant data. Frequently, however,
biologic data are available only at unequidistant intervals.

90

This limitation was particularly vexing in the study of time
series characterized by circadian rhythms from subjects kept in
isolation. It became clear that new procedures were needed for
work on unequispaced data.

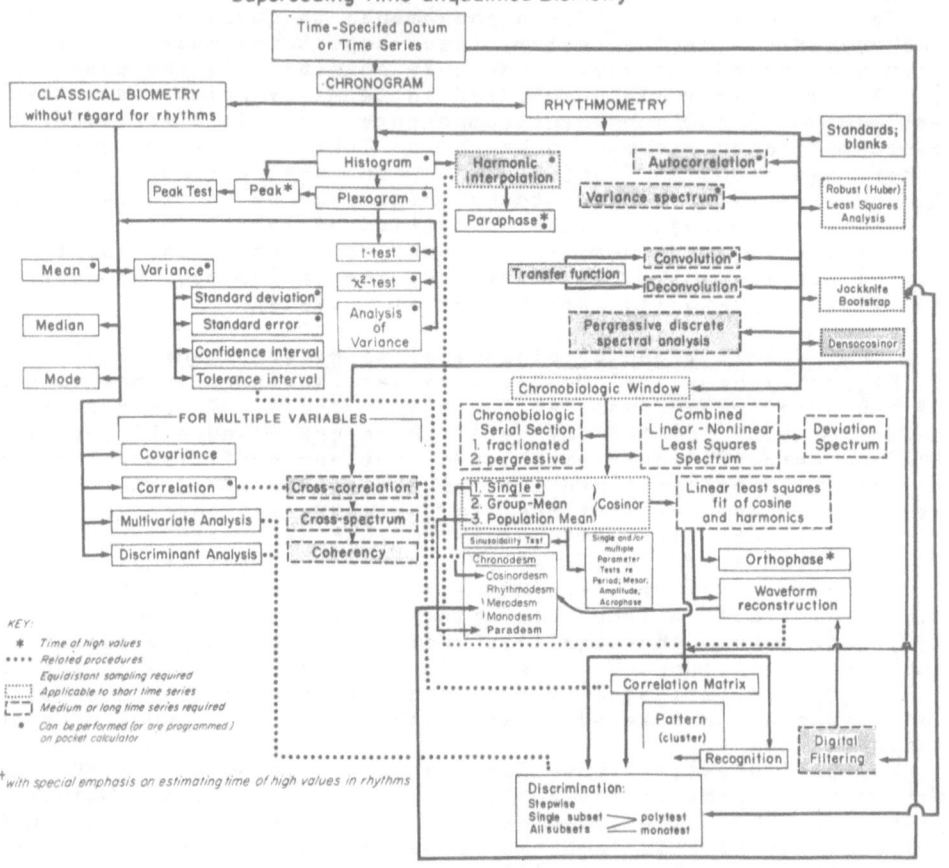

FIGURE 1

1.3. Least-squares rhythmometry

This approach is based on regression techniques. As such, it
is applicable (at least operationally) to the analysis of unequidistant data. The procedure consists of fitting, one at a
time, a set of cosine curves to the data--with the analyst
choosing the domain of trial periods to be analyzed and the
distance between consecutive trial periods. Thus, one obtains
an estimate of the MESOR (midline estimating statistic of
rhythm, M), a rhythm-adjusted mean, and also, at each period

considered, estimates of the amplitude (A=half the extent of rhythmic change in a cycle approximated by the fitted cosine curve) and the acrophase (Ø=lag from a defined reference timepoint of the crest time in the cosine curve fitted to the data). This approach is generally used to determine periodic components characterized by a large A and, correspondingly, by a (local) minimal residual sum of squares. Physiologically pertinent and statistically significant components in the time series are thus detected and their A and Ø objectively quantified. A prominent peak in the least-squares spectrum (plot of As as a function of frequency) is indicative of a rhythmic component at that frequency.

Depending on whether the periods are assumed to be known or unknown, linear (LLS, Halberg et al., 1965) or nonlinear least squares (NLLS; Marquardt, 1963) rhythmometry can be applied.

When multiple components that are distant from each other in their spectral location characterize a time series, the LLS is often satisfactory, notably if provisions are made to account for multiple testing and for any correlations in the data (Halberg and Panofsky, 1961; Cornelissen et al., 1982). When a time series of appropriate length is available, we can estimate parameters by repeatedly fitting the cosinor model to the data, incrementing and/or decrementing the period of the cosine function over an appropriate range, and performing tests for statistical significance at each period. The choice of trial periods usually involves first the scanning of a broad spectral region. Whenever the length and density of the series permits it, the scanning of several domains--ultradian to infradian--is recommended. Quite often in the case of prominent components, the LLS method yields satisfactory results. Sometimes, however, the LLS method may detect pseudoperiods or fail to detect true periods close to each other (say periods of 24 and 24.8 hours).

These problems are partly resolved by combining the LLS method with the NLLS procedure (Halberg et al., 1977a). Apart from the resolving power of NLLS, this approach also presents the advantage of being able to estimate all parameters concomitantly, allowing the parameters to vary in the parameter space in order to minimize the residual sum of squares (Rummel et al., 1974). The NLLS method performs as follows: Initial values for all the parameters in the model are first estimated by LLS. These are usually the overall M and the period, and the A and Ø of each component with a period found to be statistically significant by LLS. The NLLS method then converges to the parameters resulting in the minimal residual sum of squares and provides confidence limits for the M and for each period, as well as for the corresponding As and Øs.

The nonlinear approach, as a complement to the LLS approach, combined with biologic considerations, represents an important step forward: it renders an analysis more reliable. This approach may eliminate undue focus on spurious peaks in the spectrum (so-called side lobes) and directly estimates the period along with its confidence interval. As an added check, in long time series, the analyses can be repeated for different parts of the same total observation span.

1.4. Chronobiologic serial section.

This method is also applicable to time series covering several cycles of the component of interest. For this kind of analysis, we first define a data section of fixed length, called an interval. Thereafter, we displace that interval throughout the time series, in increments, also chosen a priori by the analyst. At the outset, the interval may be equal to the period fitted and the increment to the longest time interval between consecutive observations. The interval may have to be manipulated--shortened to reveal a pattern, e.g., of Øs, and lengthened, e.g., until statistical significance (P<.05 in zero-A test) is reached in a majority (>50%) of the intervals, so as to ascertain stability in the parameter estimates. A single cosine with a constant period is fitted to the data in each interval, providing rhythm parameter estimates which can be displayed in parallel with the original data, along an appropriate time scale. If the intervals chosen overlap, the resulting analyses are not statistically independent but useful for a macroscopic check of the microscopic results. Overlapping analyses of this kind have been called "pergressive" (Halberg et al., 1965) and non-overlapping ones "fractionated" (Halberg et al., 1965, 1977a).

This method is in keeping with an approach introduced as a "moving" A and phase by Stumpf (1937) and comparable, in results, to complex demodulation (Bingham et al., 1967). The display of moving rhythm parameters as a function of time, primarily in a pergressive approach, reminds one of the smoothness resulting from a moving average. This procedure provides valuable information, e.g., when rhythm parameters are slowly varying with time or when, at a given instant, the synchronizer schedule and/or the organism's time structure are altered. Additional information concerning the best fitting period in each interval should complement the chronobiologic serial section. This information could then be used to perform a second "frequency-locked" serial section to obtain a better estimate of the A sequence (De Prins & Cornelissen, 1979). In any event, one can perform a second serial section on the results of a first serial section (the so-called serial section on the serial section), to quantify the time course of the characteristics of the rhythms with several periods that are likely to characterize most biologic data series, if they are of sufficient length and density (Arbogast et al., 1983).

1.5. Plexo-serial-linear-nonlinear rhythmometry.
This approach involves a combination of the foregoing procedures (E. Halberg et al., 1981). It is applicable when dense and long time series are available. The procedure starts with the computation of a least-squares spectrum to obtain candidate periods and corresponding rhythm characteristics. These are used as initial values in the NLLS program for the concomitant assessment of all statistically significant components in the selected model. Each component is then examined by chronobiologic serial sections to check on the stability of its (rhythm) characteristics. Depending on the results, data from different subspans are reanalyzed separately. Once a component rhythm has been isolated as being statistically significant and satisfying all assumptions underlying the applicability of the model,

point and confidence interval estimates of characteristics are
provided and waveforms visualized by plexogram.

This approach combines the merits of microscopic analyses
with the macroscopic viewing of a plexogram and of classical
analyses of variance (Halberg et al., 1953). It can be perfected further by the calculation of deviation spectra (Halberg et
al., 1977a). This procedure involves, after the removal of components that have been found to be statistically significant, a
further spectral analysis of the residuals (Halberg & Panofsky,
1961; Panofsky & Halberg, 1961). This step augments resolving
power and permits the detection of signals with a small A. It
can be repeated as often as needed. Once all components have
been detected, the complete model should be applied to the original data for concomitant fitting of all pertinent parameters.
The examination of residuals by spectral analysis and digital
filtering (Laraña et al., 1984, in press) allows for the study
of the different kinds of noise characterizing the time series.

1.6. Cosinor methods.

The cosinor procedures involve both an analytical method and
a graphic presentation of results. The graphical part is a convenient and useful way of presenting the results of statistical
analyses. A polar plot serves to illustrate two of the rhythm
parameters of the cosine fitted to the data. In this presentation, the A and Ø are represented as a directed line (vector).
The length of that line indicates the A of the rhythm. The
orientation of the line, i.e., its direction with respect to
the circular scale, indicates the Ø of the rhythm. The circular
scale covers one period or 360 angular degrees. A 95% confidence region for (A,Ø) is shown by an error ellipse around the
tip of the vector. An ellipse not overlapping the center of the
circle indicates that the A differs from zero; hence, the
rhythm is statistically significant (Halberg et al., 1967,
1972, 1977a). Three kinds of cosinor procedures have been
designed in an integrated routine, each appropriate to a different task:

1a) Single cosinor as a definitive statistic: a cosinor procedure applicable to single biologic time series anticipated to
be rhythmic with a given period (Halberg et al., 1972). This
procedure amounts to fit a cosine function of fixed period to
the data by least squares. This method can now be implemented
on pocket calculators (Cornelissen et al., 1980; Monk & Fort,
1983; Vokac, 1984). Series amenable to cosinor analysis may be
sampled with serial dependence from an individual or with serial independence from a group (Halberg et al., 1981). Sometimes, a single cosinor can be computed on data derived from
different individuals, each sampled at a different time.
Methods for comparing individual rhythm parameters, jointly or
separately, have also been developed (Bingham et al., 1982).

1b) Single cosinor for imputation purposes (a particular
single cosinor procedure, used a priori as an intermediate
statistic for the sole purpose of using results as a basis for
definitive statistics): a tentative estimation from limited or
insufficient evidence, such as a procedure for deriving from a
short and sparse time series endpoints for use in further analyses. Even when a cosinor curve describes the data well, the

brevity of a series constitutes a real shortcoming. Thus, when no prior information is available on a certain bioperiodicity in a given species, and curve fitting is done on short series, the rhythm parameters thus obtained are regarded as imputations. Methods such as the population-mean cosinor can then be applied on the basis of rhythm characteristics imputed from single cosinor analyses to test for a rhythm characterizing a given population.

2) Population-mean cosinor: the original cosinor procedure applicable to parameter estimates from 3 or more series for assessing the rhythm characteristics of a population. The parameter estimates are based on the means of estimates obtained from individuals in the sample, and their confidence intervals depend on the variability among individual parameter estimates.

3) Group-mean cosinor: a cosinor procedure applicable to data series from 2 or more individuals for characterizing a rhythm in that particular group only. The group parameter estimates are based on averages of estimates obtained from individual series, weighted either equally or by the number of observations in each series. Confidence regions or intervals for the group-mean cosinor are derived by pooling the error term from all individual fittings.

2. STUDY OF MARKER RHYTHMS.
2.1. Introduction.

Chronopharmacology and chronotherapy (Halberg, 1969, 1982; Halberg & Halberg, 1984; Reinberg & Halberg, 1971, 1979; Takahashi et al., 1982; Walker et al., 1981) have demonstrated value in experimental cancer treatment, experimental chemotherapy in particular. Furthermore, in a double-blind test of clinical chronoradiotherapy, carried out with marker rhythmometry, a gain of 2 from the timing of treatment at the circadian peak of tumor temperature was recorded (Deka et al., 1976; Halberg et al., 1977b). Nonetheless for practical reasons and for both diagnostic and therapeutic aims, most chemotherapists, radiotherapists and those in nuclear medicine continue to regard the body as a constant; thereby, often unwittingly, they swell the ranks of those who draw a curtain of ignorance over the physiologic range of variability by subscribing to a temporally unqualified concept of homeostasis. This clinical status quo prevails while, from the viewpoint of basic science, chronobiologic teamwork has already lifted this curtain of ignorance. The next task on hand is to render the basic information useful. This task, in health science, revolves, first, around prevention and, only in the face of disease, around screening, diagnosis, prognosis and therapy. In all chronobiologic tasks of these areas, monitoring by measurement and proper data analyses are desirable or indispensable.

A marker rhythm (MR) is defined as a rhythm in a readily-measured variable, used to monitor a corresponding rhythm in a related but less accessible variable for purposes of prophylaxis, diagnosis and therapy (Halberg et al., 1977a). MRs in basic or applied physiologic and pharmacologic work have been defined and discussed (Halberg et al., 1977c). They have many potential applications in preventive health maintenance (prophylactic MRs), risk monitoring (risk MRs), for diagnostic purposes (diagnostic or screening MRs), and for timing therapy (chronotherapeutic MRs yielding treatment time markers), for assessing therapeutic response (response MRs) or for both of the latter purposes (double chronotherapeutic MRs). Such rhythms may be used without any implication of causal relations between the process being monitored for its rhythmic marker, and a given treatment. When such relations exist, however, they certainly constitute an advantage and should lead to the preference of a specific MR over an unspecific one. Apart from any specificity, a multiple chronotherapeutic marker should possess several characteristics, documented by inferential statistical means: 1) the property of being a reference for the timing of treatment leading to an appreciable benefit and/or 2) the property of being an index of critical toxicity to one or several targets, e.g., to the bone marrow, kidney or heart, and/or 3) the property of being an index of the desired effect(s). To document such possibilities on the proper scale, it is extremely important that the index be applicable on a large scale or be rendered applicable with currently available technology.

Moreover, information on MRs, that indicate the best time for treatment, can also serve to establish reference standards that are time-specified, so-called chronodesms, for the interpretation of time-specified single samples, e.g., to gauge toxicity. The circadian $\emptyset$s of white blood cell counts (WBC) and of potassium excretion are both treatment-time markers; the $\emptyset$ of the WBC serves in addition to evaluate an undesired response such as bone marrow toxicity.

Once one examines a potential marker variable, one must try to answer several methodologic questions at the outset: What are the distributions of a global index of the timing of the marker variable, such as the $\emptyset$ of a time series, as compared to those of a local index, such as a peak in the series, the macrophase, Ψ? It can be anticipated that the $\emptyset$ is more stable than the Ψ, since the latter is more sensitive than the former to random fluctuations in the data series. Moreover, a global rather than a local index may be less flexible in reflecting a change in best timing. Thus, stability throughout a treatment course may be a disadvantage as well as an advantage. When stability is a lasting advantage, i.e., when it reflects a basic periodic (marker) process, rather than an artefact, the $\emptyset$ may be determined only once for a given patient, before the first treatment. When the best timing is variable, the $\emptyset$ should be determined accordingly with some optimal frequency preferably, yet perhaps not necessarily, before each treatment.

Other questions to be raised concern the sampling span required to determine a trustworthy $\emptyset$ and the matter of modulation of a $\emptyset$ with a given frequency by rhythms with a lower frequency, such as circannual, circaseptan or other infradian modulations of a circadian $\emptyset$. Since very many potential MRs indeed exhibit about-yearly changes (Halberg et al., 1983), still another question to be examined is the possibility of circannual changes in circadian characteristics which has been explored for the WBC by Halberg et al. (1977c).

2.2. White blood cell counts and chronochemotherapy.

The WBC is an admittedly indirect and unrefined, yet often practical, marker of drug effects (Halberg, 1953). It serves to gauge the dramatic circadian changes that characterize the bone marrow's response to toxic agents, including carcinostatic drugs (Halberg et al., 1973; Haus et al., 1972; Scheving et al., 1976, 1983). The use of the WBC as an index of bone marrow toxicity has to be qualified by the fact that the WBC undergoes circadian and other changes of large extent. These changes are a vexing source of variability when ignored but may be valuable new endpoints when exploited by time-specification based preferably on around-the-clock measurements.

Against the background of around-the-clock masurements, Hrushesky et al. (1981) have documented circadian-circannual aspects of WBC depression and recovery in patients given dox-orubicin (and cisplatin). These patients with advanced-stage ovarian and bladder cancer were treated about monthly with 60 mg/m^2 of each doxorubicin and cisplatin, the latter 12 hrs after the former. In a first stage, patients were randomized to receive their chemotherapy beginning either 1 hour before their habitual awakening (at 06:00; schedule A) or 13 hrs after habi-tual awakening (at 18:00; schedule B), and then crossed over to the other schedule at the following treatment, with a continu-ing alternation of schedules A and B throughout the treatment span, usually consisting of 9 about-monthly courses. In a second study stage, patients were randomly assigned to either schedule A or B consistently throughout the treatment span, so that the alternation of treatment no longer confounded the time course of cumulative myelotoxicity associated with a given schedule. When results on schedule A obtained during the first stage of the study were compared with those on schedule B, about one month after each treatment, recovery of the WBC was greater with schedule A in spring, summer and fall, but worse in winter. A 3-way analysis of variance on weekly total WBC as a gauge of myelosuppression reveals as main effects the (cir-cadian) difference between schedules A and B and the effect of the day after treatment; both are statistically significant below the 1 per mil level. While this same analysis does not detect any added effect of circannual rhythm stage (DF=3; F=0.559; P=0.642), there is indeed a statistically highly significant interaction between circannual rhythm stage and schedule A vs. B (DF=3; F=4.773; P=0.003).

The circadian $\emptyset$ and Ψ of the WBC are both candidate treatment-time markers. Ψ may not serve as well as $\emptyset$ for treatment-time optimization, even if the computation of $\emptyset$ is more costly, in that it requires an added, though simple, cosi-nor computation. A lesser pertinence of Ψ may possibly result in part from its greater variability. The Ψ and $\emptyset$ were calcu-lated from data covering a 24-hr span at 4-hr intervals (by six WBCs). These counts were made on each of 59 patients with ad-vanced ovarian or bladder cancer, before each combination treatment (Rx), with up to 60 mg/m^2 of doxorubicin followed after 12 hrs by up to 60 mg/m^2 of cisplatin in a sequence of up to 11 about-monthly courses. The six values were fitted with a 24-hr cosine curve to obtain the single-cosinor $\emptyset$. A computer program for the so-called macro-micro comparison by serial section (Hermida et al., in press a, b), was then used to compute the mean Ψ, found at 17:30, and the mean Ø, found at 18:30, and to compare them in a first step, for a total of 29 patients who had received 8 or more Rxs. For these patients, paired t-tests show no difference between the mean Ψ and Ø of the profiles before each Rx course in a given patient, whether one considers all Rxs (P=.83) or only schedule A (doxorubicin Rx at 06:00, 1 hr before awakening or 12 hrs after the WBC Ø; P=.43), or only B (doxorubicin Rx at 18:00, near the WBC Ø; P=.31 for the null hypothesis of no difference between mean Ψ and Ø) (Hermida et al., in press a). The largest differences between the mean Ψ and mean Ø are found for Rx B. A high (angular-angular) correlation (r=.52) is found between the mean Ψ and Ø when all 29 subjets are considered, irrespective of Rx timing. The correlation is higher (r=.65) for Rx A than for Rx B (r=.39).

By comparing Ψ and Ø variances in all profiles for these 29 patients with 8 or more courses, paired t-tests show a large reduction in variance by the use of Ø rather than Ψ. The smallest, but still significant (P=.02) differences between Ψ and Ø variances are found for Rx A. Even in this case, 85% of the cases had a higher Ψ variance as compared to the Ø variance. No statistically significant correlation is found between the Ψ and Ø variances whether one considers all Rxs (r=.02) or only schedule A (r=.01) or only B (r=.08) (Hermida et al., in press a).

The equality of variance in Ψ and Ø was also tested for the set and 2 subsets (Rx A or B separately) of 386 series from 59 patients and for the set and 2 subsets of the 55 means of these series for those 55 patients with at least two series (Table 1). In all cases (except for the means from 28 patients under Rx A) the test of equal variances for Ψ and Ø allows the rejection of the null hypothesis at the 1% level.

TABLE 1: Test of equal variances for Ψ and Ø of white blood cell count (WBC) profiles of patients receiving timed therapy (Rx)*

Kinds of series (Rx)	# of cases	Standard Deviation of Ψ	Ø	For Ψ versus Ø F	P
		(hours)			
Indiv. -(All)	386	81.64	68.51	1.42	<<.001
" -(A)	188	83.98	70.54	1.42	.009
" -(B)	198	79.46	66.40	1.43	.006
Mean -(All)	55	74.54	54.95	1.84	.013
" -(A)	28	50.25	48.59	1.07	.430
" -(B)	27	99.67	60.47	2.72	.006

*A=doxorubicin Rx at 06:00, 1 hr before awakening or about 12 hrs after the population WBC Ø, followed by cisplatin 12 hrs later; B=doxorubicin Rx at 18:00, near the population WBC Ø, followed by cisplatin 12 hrs later.

2.3. Urinary potassium in health.

MRs may be needed during spans of 5 weeks, as for radiotherapy (Deka et al., 1976; Halberg et al., 1977b; Halberg,

1983), or for many months, in chemotherapy. In either case, information on any infradian, e.g., circaseptan or circannual, changes in a variable considered for marker rhythmometry is highly desirable if not indispensable. A problem arises, however, when such marker rhythmometry is to be carried out on patients whose treatment is to be urgently initiated. Cancer patients in advanced stages of the disease are cases in point. In such patients, the effects of treatment timed along the circadian scale can exhibit changes with a lower-than-circadian frequency. Thus, the effect ot treatment with doxorubicin at 06:00 is advantageous in some, but not in all seasons. Moreover, treatment effects may also differ with the stage of about 7-day (circaseptan) rhythms. Since the best treatment time exhibits changes that are predictable with an infradian frequency, it follows that candidate MRs for use in chronotherapy must be sought that also undergo an infradian modulation of their circadian characteristics, such as the $\emptyset$. In the patient with cancer, treatment can not be postponed until infradian, notably about-yearly, changes are evaluated; in other words, treatment must not be withheld for a year in order to assess with serial dependence any circannual change in the circadian urinary potassium (K) rhythm of patients scheduled to receive potentially nephrotoxic therapy.

Instead of studying cancer patients, data gathered in health may be explored. In so doing, one realizes very well that any results are at best approximations, since a disease may accentuate an existing rhythm or may induce a rhythm that is not otherwise observed, or it may alter rhythm characteristics or obscure an otherwise prominent rhythm.

We analyzed K in 2860 samples of an apparently healthy man, 21 years of age when he started collecting 5-7 urine samples on most days for 18 months (Hermida et al., in press b). Samples at 3-5 hrs are more readily collected for long series covering years than are collections at shorter intervals. The latter are preferred, however, when a Ψ or a $\emptyset$ is to be reliably estimated. In any event, a 24-hr cosine curve was fitted by the single-cosinor method to consecutive non-overlapping data sections of 1-14 days in length using the macro-micro-comparison by serial section (Hermida et al., in press b). This was done in order to seek the minimal length of a time series (with the given sampling rate) that would allow the rejection of the zero-A assumption. Accordingly, a more reliable estimation of timing of high values in most, though not all, time series available with a given length can be obtained. The total number of series varied from 513 (for 1-day-long series) to 39 (for 14-day-long series). It can be seen from Table 2 that, as a rule, series of 1-day length do not allow the inferential statistical documentation of a rhythm: of 513 consecutive series on the same subject, only 15% are significant below the 5% level by cosinor. The resolution of the rhythm, i.e., the % of series that allow rejection of the A=O assumption, increases as the duration of the data section analyzed lengthens. Up to a length of 6 days, the gain from each added day is large. With series covering 6 days, 80% allow rejection of the zero-A assumption. Only relatively small further gains in rhythm description are associated with spans of 7-10 days. There seems

to be a further gain, however, with spans longer than 10 days,
Table 2. A lack of gain from the increment in the length of the
urinary K record may be attributted to the obscuring effect of
an infradian modulation of the waveform, which cancels, in
records of a length between 6 and 10 days, gains from the increment in record length.

TABLE 2: Relation of series length to demonstrability and quan-
tifiability of circadian rhythm in human urinary potassium
excretion in health*

Series length (days)	1	2	3	4	5	6	7	8	9	10	11	12	13	14
% series with P<.05	15	37	45	63	66	80	81	85	87	82	94	96	98	97
N " " "	76	97	81	85	71	72	62	57	52	45	47	43	41	38

*By rejection of zero-amplitude assumption in single-cosinor
procedure.

As noted above, for practicability, the sampling in this
study (actually covering 15 years) was sparse, with individual
samples (5-7/day) covering, on the average, about 4 hrs. For
future work it will be more efficient to increase sampling
rate, e.g., from 4 to 2 hrs during waking, e.g., for 2 days,
rather than to sample longer spans at a lower rate, unless
there is a suggestion of desynchronization. Series based on
about 2-hourly samples, at least during wakefulness, covering a
few days are recommended to render the description of a 24-hr
synchronized rhythm more efficient. Longer series are needed
for an estimation of the period in its own right by NLLS.

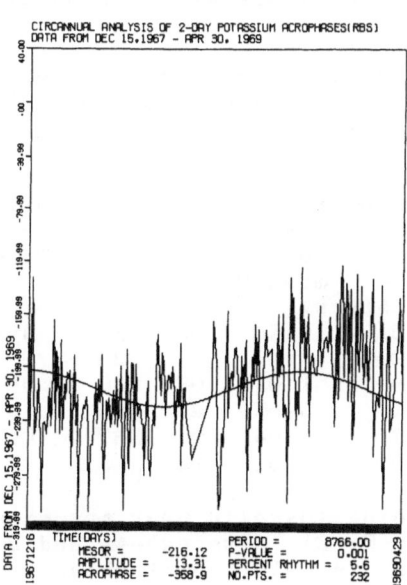

FIGURE 2

The cosinor analysis of
original K values (mEq/hr)
shows not only a circadian
but also a circannual rhythm
(P<.001, M=3.15±0.03;
A=0.19±0.04 and Ø at -27±14°
from December 22 with
360°=365.25 days). The variability of the circadian K Ø
along the scale of a year is
particularly pertinent to
treatment-timing, as shown
in Figure 2. This figure
shows time on the abscissa
(from Dec. 16, 1967, to
April 29, 1969). On the
ordinate, the circadian Ø is
shown with earlier values on
top and later ones at the
bottom. These Øs can be seen
to extend from nearly 300°
from local midnight to 130°
from midnight, a considerable variability which (only
to a very small extent) is
accounted for by a circannual rhythm.

In view of the density of the series consisting of circadian characteristics, the zero circannual A assumption can be tested. A 365.25-day cosine curve was fitted to the 240 circadian K Øs computed separately for consecutive 2-day spans (by reference to 00:00 and with a 1-hr correction for daylight saving time); Øs obtained within consecutive 4-day spans were considered as replicates for the sinusoidality test. By excluding 8 outliers, a circannual Ø rhythm is found (P=.001; Fig. 2) without any violation of the assumptions underlying the use of the single-cosinor model (normality of the residuals, sinusoidality and variance homogeneity). For at least one serially-dependent (longitudinal) series in health, a circannual modulation of the circadian K Ø is thus documented on the basis of dense sampling. Any (possibly larger than 2-hr) circannual change in circadian K Ø of cancer patients, as a potential marker for chronotherapy, can be studied only with serial independence.

2.4. Urinary potassium excretion in cancer patients.

Since unquestionably a circannual rhythm characterizes the circadian Ø and other characteristics of urinary K excretion in a clinically healthy subject, it is conceivable that such a rhythm persists and even that it may perhaps be amplified and/or changed in frequency in patients of different kinds, including those with cancer here under discussion. For 53 patients with advanced ovarian or bladder cancer, the circadian Ø of urinary K before a first 60 mg/m^2 cisplatin treatment (Rx) was compared with the mean Ø of all profiles in a sequence of up to 10 about-montly courses (of a combination treatment with 60 mg/m^2 doxorubicin, the latter given 12 hrs before cisplatin, Table 3).

TABLE 3: Similarity between the circadian acrophase (Ø) of urinary potassium excretion before a first treatment and mean Ø of all profiles of patients receiving timed therapy (Rx)1

Kinds of Rx (# of cases)	D= (1st Ø−Mean Ø) % with neg. D (delay)	Paired t-test mean D (hours)	SD of mean D	P	Correlation r	P<.05
All (53)	62	-0.33	0.48	.50	.39	yes
"* (50)	60	-0.02	0.48	.96	.38	"
Alternate (15)	40	1.94	1.07	.09	.08	no
A (18)	61	-0.81	0.67	.24	.43	"
B (20)	80	-1.60	0.64	.02	.69	yes
"* (17)	76	-0.92	0.61	.15	.70	"

1 A=Rx with cisplatin in the evening (usually near pre-Rx Ø); B=Rx in the morning (~180 from pre-Rx Ø); Alternate=A and B in alternation, in consecutive courses. * Deletion of three cases with mean calculated by averaging over only two Rxs.

No difference is seen by paired t-test between the Ø before the first Rx and the average Ø of all profiles before each Rx

course in a given patient (including profile before first Rx).
A high (angular-angular) correlation is found between the first
and average Øs when all subjects are considered, irrespective
of Rx timing. The correlation is maintained for Rx B but not
for Rx A (Hermida et al., in press b, c).

Figure 3 (lower right) compares the Ø before the first Rx
and the average Ø of all profiles (before each of the subsequent Rx courses) in 50 cancer patients. In comparing the
dispersions for all patients, one can conclude that the mean Ø
is more stable than the Ø before the first Rx. Indeed, the distribution for the mean Ø of the 50 patients has a high peak
with 42% of the total values around 13:00-15:00.

The top rows and the 4th row left indicate the differences
between the two Øs for each patient, classified as a function
of Rx mode. A comparison of the two lines connecting the
corresponding Øs for the 18 patients on schedule A (top left)
and the 17 patients on schedule B (top left of bottom half)
shows no large differences between the Ø before the first Rx
and the mean Ø. The remainder of the figure consists of frequency histograms for the Ø before the first Rx and the mean Ø,
respectively, in each of these groups.

The top right of Figure 3 shows a similar comparison for 15
cancer patients receiving Rx alternating between schedules A
and B. The differences in timing, shown in the top row, are big
but not systematic; the mean Ø randomly appears before or after
the Ø found in the profile before the first treatment. A paired
t-test shows no significant differences (P=.09). The peak in
the distribution of the mean Ø of each patient is around
14:00-16:00 (lower third of the upper half in the left part of
the graph).

Smaller differences can be observed for the 18 cancer patients consistently receiving Rx A (upper third of Figure 3,
left). In fact, the hypothesis of no difference is supported by
a paired t-test (P=.24, Table 3). In this case, a greater variability can be observed for the mean Ø, with a peak in its distribution of only 27.7% of the total situated around
15:00-17:00.

For 17 cancer patients receiving Rx B, Figure 3, there is
again only a small difference between the Ø before the first Rx
and the mean Ø of urinary K. A shift in Ø after Rx B is suggested by a high (80) percentage of unidirectional differences
in Ø (delays), corresponding perhaps to the organism's endeavor
to adjust its Ø after an inappropriately timed Rx (Rx at the
"right" time may not displace the Ø, whereas Rx at the "wrong"
time does so).

2.5. Discussion.

On the basis of the prospective use of a Ψ, a clear advantage from timing radiotherapy has already been reported (Deka
et al., 1976). Tumor temperature was the MR used in that case,
prospectively for timing treatment. In the study with WBC here
discussed, however, prospective timing was by clock-hour rather
than MR. Marker rhythmometry was done prospectively, but its
effects were evaluated retrospectively; hence, the merit of Ψ
over Ø cannot be assessed on the basis of outcomes and thus of
direct pertinence. The first conclusion drawn, however, is

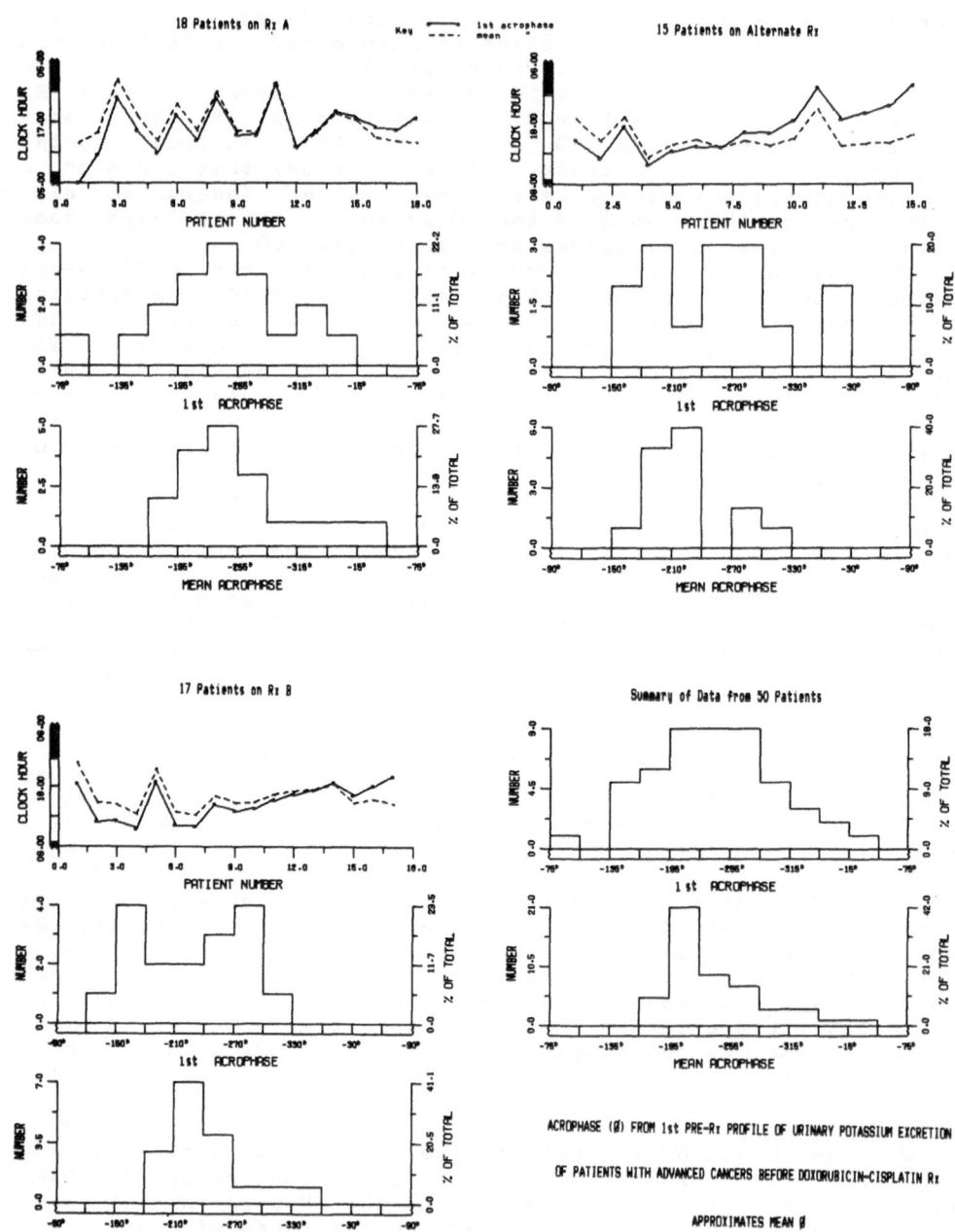

FIGURE 3

based on evidence in Table 1, showing that the Ø is the more stable endpoint. Greater stability, of course, does not necessarily imply greater pertinence. The problem of pertinence has been examined separately. More specifically, the WBC M before treatment was equated to 100%, and weekly WBCs during the month following treatment were expressed as percentages of this M. The area between the horizontal line corresponding to 100% and any depressed weekly WBC was then computed. These areas were assigned on the one hand to the time of WBC Ø (tØ) and on the other hand to the time of Ψ (tΨ). With Ø, but not Ψ, the zero-A assumption of no circadian rhythm in toxic response was rejected. Moreover, when the areas with treatment within 2 hrs of tØ were compared with those obtained with treatment within 2 hrs of a timepoint at 12 hrs from tØ the difference was statistically significant. This was not the case for the areas in the case of treatment at tΨ and 12 hrs from the tΨ. Pertinence can be established on such a basis. Hereafter, primary focus is to be placed upon the behavior of the Ø. Further work should focus upon the sampling requirements for the determination of the Ø rather than the Ψ. Sampling for a reliable circadian Ψ must be denser than that for a circadian Ø. Moreover, an answer to the question whether the determination of a circadian Ø before each treatment course is indispensable, must await the results of pertinent prospective studies on cost-effectiveness. Moreover, urinary K excretion exhibits also a more stable circadian Ø as compared to a Ψ (Hermida et al., in press b).

In view of the fact that the results of the two schedules tested, A and B, differ with the seasons, the added condition to be met by a MR is that it exhibits a circannual change in Ø. Since the data at hand did not suffice to demonstrate such a change, with serial independence in cancer patients for K, the availability of a longitudinal series on human K was exploited and a circannual rhythm in circadian Ø, albeit of small A, was demonstrated. For the case of K, the initial Ø was compared with the mean Ø, to explore the possibility that the former could be substituted for the latter. While a statistically significant difference for K between the first and the mean Ø could not be established in the data available, a larger sample may be needed to ascertain the lack of a difference. If such a lack should be established, this could indicate that a single K Ø taken before the first treatment may be satisfactory for a contribution by this MR. The use of this MR under such circumstances, however, for gauging kinds of toxicity that change in a circannual rhythmic fashion, may not be satisfactory. Clearly, this chapter on MRs in cancer patients can only introduce methodologic considerations. Figure 4 provides a scheme for programming further research along this line on larger sets of samples on these and other MR variables. The scheme corresponds to the macro-micro comparison by serial section program, allowing analyses on an unlimited number of data and the graphic representation of results (see Figure 3) comparing two of the parameters computed from the data. At this point, a question can be raised whether or not the circadian Ø suffices as a proper MR, specially in dealing with non-sinusoidal rhythms. Objective methods available to obtain estimates of timing of high values on non-sinusoidal rhythms have already

been discussed previously; they include the determination of
the paraphase by harmonic interpolation (De Prins et al., 1981)
and the computation of the orthophase (Tong et al., 1977).

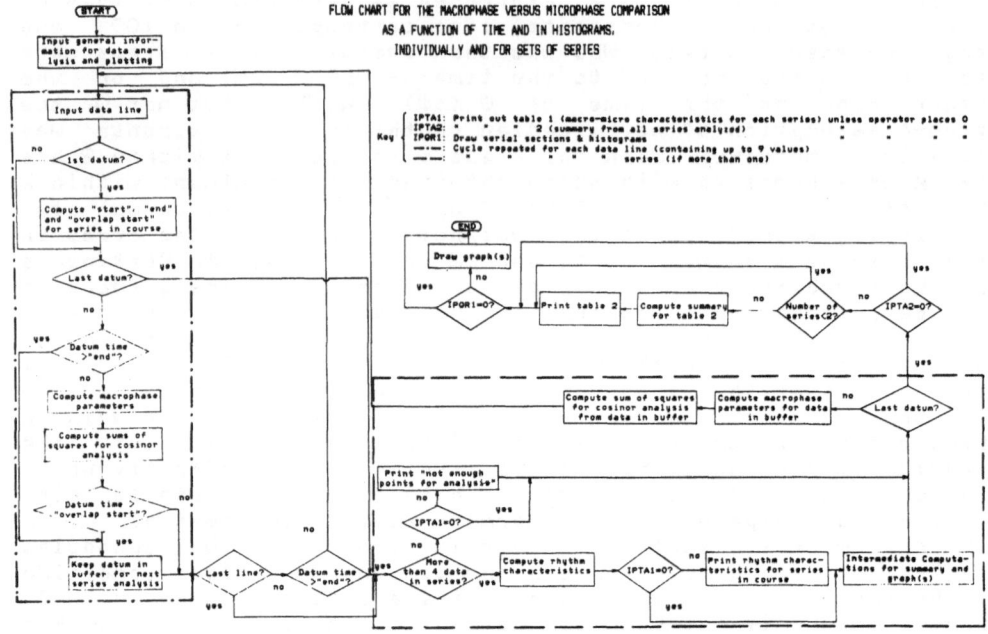

FIGURE 4

An adaptive filtering method also was proposed (Laraña et
al., 1984, in press) to cope with some features that are often
present in biologic time series, namely: scarce a priori
knowledge of the signals; a low signal to noise ratio; the
presence of multiple related harmonic components and above all,
the expected occurrence of oscillations with varying frequency
that introduces nonstationarities that cannot be treated with
classic methods of spectral estimation. Results described elsewhere have shown the ability of adaptive filtering to detect
and reconstruct periodic components in noise and to track their
changes in frequency. Since this method requires less information about the signal than other methods of spectral analysis,
it seems specially suited for chronobiologic applications.

3. CHRONOEPIDEMIOLOGIC RISK ASSESSMENT.
3.1. Introduction.

Once predictable rhythms and trends have been shown to contribute a large proportion of the variability seen in laboratory and clinical data, judgment will be refined when data are
time-coded and interpreted in the light of time-specified
reference intervals or "chronodesms" (from chronos=time and
desmos=bound) (Halberg et al., 1977a, 1982). This time-

specification may be implemented along a wide range of scales corresponding to pertinent rhythms and trends; e.g., a circadian chronodesm specifies the "normal range" or, rather, the range of usual values along the scale of a day. It should be noted that reference values (collected under standardized conditions) or "normal ranges" (based on "usual conditions") may also be specified in terms of parameters describing various rhythms and trends. Thus one may obtain "second-order" chronodesms. For example, given estimates of circadian Ms for n individuals, one may construct reference intervals for this particular parameter. In the case of parameters which vary jointly, as do the A and Ø of a cosine model, one may construct multivariate reference intervals along analogous lines (Halberg, 1983; Nelson et al., 1983).

A chronopsy has been defined as the collection of a time-specified datum or data series for comparison with an appropriate chronodesm for an individual or for a group. The term has been coined by analogy to biopsy, from chronos (time) and opsis (appearance); the term is preferred to "chronobiopsy" since it is shorter and because "biopsy" implies removal of tissue, hence a compound new word should restrict it to this particular use. A chronopsy can be carried out on different materials: blood = hemopsy; urine = uropsy; saliva = sialopsy; temperature = thermopsy; blood pressure = tensopsy; tissue = chronobiopsy.

Chronobiologic methods define health by accounting for the dynamics of values remaining within time-specified physiologic ranges and standards of variation, with each time-specified test value interpreted singly or as part of a computer-analyzed series, characterized by novel dynamic objective and quantitative endpoints. This approach is positive (as compared to a negative ruling out of disease for the assessment of health). The chronobiologic approach is personalized, instead of relying on the % morbidity or % mortality of a population. The alteration of one or several chronobiologic (rhythm) characteristics in one or several variables quantifies vulnerability or risk, prior to the occurrence of overt disease. Once such alterations are charted, one seeks to gauge cost-effectively rhythm alterations on just this one or a few variables determined on but one or a few time-specified samples, interpreted in the light of time-specified reference standards.

With these aims, a small number of selected (rather than randomly picked) women of three age groups was extensively sampled in two geographic locations (Halberg et al., 1981). Blood was drawn for hormone determinations and several other physiologic systems were monitored around the clock, several times a year on subjects with different ethnic backgrounds and with different known risks of developing certain diseases. More specifically, the variation of 12 circulating hormones and systolic (S) and diastolic (D) blood pressure (BP) was assessed--along the 24-hour, menstrual cycle (when pertinent), and 1-year scales--for clinically healthy women on a standardized routine. Methods used to separate groups of subjects at different risk included linear regression and correlation analysis (Halberg et al., 1981), cluster analysis and pattern discrimination (Hermida et al., 1983, 1984b). Results demonstrate that the circannual A of prolactin is negatively correlated with the risk of

developing breast cancer (RDBC) (Halberg et al., 1981). By contrast, the circannual A of plasma TSH was positively correlated
with the RDBC. Moreover, relations were sought with focus upon
the risk of developing diseases associated with a high circadian M of BP, i.e., with the risk of M-hypertension (RMH). RMH
correlated with 1) the circannual A and M of plasma aldosterone, and with 2) the circadian as well as circannual M of S
and D BP (Halberg et al., 1981; Hermida et al., 1983). The
time-specified circadian BP profile awaited scrutiny, however,
as predictor of RMH in conjunction with a cost-effective endocrine spotcheck on one or two plasma samples of aldosterone and
a few co-classifiers that differ in kind and circadian timing
from season to season.

3.2. Subjects investigated.
     Adolescent (15-21 years; I); young adult (29-36 years; II);
and post-menopausal (44-59 years; III) women in Japan and in
the United States at initial (physical and psychologic) and
subsequent examinations were found to be in good health; no
oral contraceptives had been taken for at least 6 months
preceding and during study. Subjects were admitted to a clinical research center for 24-hour profiles once in each season
(Halberg et al., 1981). Throughout each profile, one ml blood
was withdrawn once every 20 min for radioimmunoassay of prolactin and cortisol and an additional 12.5 ml every 100 min for
analysis of other hormones. BP was automatically monitored
about every 10 minutes in the same profiles (Halberg et al.,
1981). Some subjects had to be replaced partway through the
study. Different seasons are documented in part by different
subjects. Age effects upon rhythm parameters were found (Nelson et al., 1980). Accordingly, earlier work with methods for
pattern discrimination revealed bias from age effects (Hermida
et al., 1982a, 1984c). The data on the 12 most extensively
documented hormones in plasma (out of a larger total of hormones sampled) here summarized stem mainly from the young adult
subjects. Data from the two other age groups were analyzed for
those variables that did not exhibit an age effect. Data on
certain additional hormones in blood or urine not here considered were sparse and/or described only few subjects.

3.3. Pattern discrimination method: the monotest.
     Two steps were carried out for pattern discrimination: 1)
dimension reduction, to identify the minimal number of variables needed for classification; and 2) classification, i.e.,
assignment of each individual to one of two classes being considered.
     Original data from each of four seasons were handled
separately for dimension reduction by a so-called "monotest"
(Hermida, 1984; Hermida et al., 1982b; 1983; 1984b; 1984d), an
all-subsets variable selection technique for allocation (MaKay
& Campbell, 1982). The test sought classifiers from among an
initial set of 24 variables which consists of original values
on 12 hormones at 08:00 and the absolute difference between the
values at 08:00 and at 00:00 for these same 12 hormones. A
second comparative study was also carried out; in it, the
paired item (an original or transformed variable or set of

variables picked for classification) used for all subjects and variables consists of the 08:00 and 00:00 values as such. Preference for the difference between the 08:00 and midnight values stems from the circumstance that for some hormones this difference approximates the circadian A while the 08:00 value approximates the circadian M for that hormone. The value at 08:00 is invariably included in a first test since it corresponds to the current sampling routine of many hospitals.

For a particular combination of variables (hormones & times), the monotest performed as many steps of separate analyses as the total number of subjects, each subject's data being compared as a set with those of all others (leave-one-out approach; Hermida, 1984; McKay & Campbell, 1982), taking into account all criteria chosen for classification. Two classes, both of healthy subjects, yet one regarded epidemiologically as being at a relatively low RMH, the other as being at a high RMH, are available a priori for classification (Halberg et al., 1981). In each analysis, a single subject is considered as the "test" subject and the remainder as "reference" subjects.

The test subject is classified by comparison with the reference subjects, according to three different classification rules: a) the shortest average Euclidean distance to each class in the reference set, the low or high risk classes, respectively; b) the shortest single Euclidean distance to the nearest neighbor in the reference set (Cover & Hart, 1967); c) The 2 or 3 shortest (single) Euclidean distances to the nearest neighbors in the reference set. Thus, one obtains for each determination three different results, one corresponding to each classification criterion. These results are summarized as the extent of agreement for the given test subject of the a posteriori obtained and the a priori assigned classifications. The final result is expressed as the percentage of equivalent a priori and a posteriori classifications (PEC), the total number of subjects in each of 3 comparisons being 100%. This PEC indicates whether a better discrimination is obtained with a given "constellation" of hormones and times, as compared to all other possible combinations. The procedure aims at the best possible classification (maximal PEC value) with the smallest number of items, which we describe as a pertinent constellation of items (hormones & times) or as an "equivalent classifier".

The equivalent classifiers selected in the dimension reduction step from original values at 08:00 and 00:00 can now be studied for their classifying ability around the clock. A discriminant timing (DT) is sought for each constellation and season as a suitable time for a subsequent classification of new subjects. The DT must represent a peak of equivalent classification and must separate populations of low and high RMH in terms of the mean and standard error of hormone concentration at the corresponding sampling time.

3.4. Pattern discrimination results.

For diurnally active, nocturnally (~22:30 to ~7:30) resting young adult women, certain selected endocrine tests for detecting and assessing RMH in four seasons can be tentatively specified in Table 4. The clock-hours and seasons here picked as a first approximation, are valid only for young adult women with an indication of the rest-activity schedule and geographic location. Eventually, reference to the complete spectrum of pertinent (ultradian, circadian and infradian) marker rhythms should be considered for the timing of tests for risk assessment.

TABLE 4: Kinds and times of endocrine sampling recommended for further tests of diseases associated with high blood pressure*

	SEASON							
	SUMMER		FALL		WINTER		SPRING	
TEST TIMES	00:00	08:00	00:00	08:00	00:00	08:00	00:00	08:00
HORMONES								
1=Prolactin					$\overline{\$}$(3,7)			
2=Cortisol		{$}(3,4)						
3=Aldosterone	{$}(2,4)		{$}↔{$}		{$}(1,7)			
4=TSH		{$}(2,3)					$(6)	{$}(5)
5=Estrone							$ ↔ $(4)	
6=LH								$(4)
7=DHEA-S					$\underline{\$}$(1,3)			

*Overlined symbol indicates direct relation, underlined symbol inverse relation, between risk and hormone concentration at certain clock hours examined. Symbol in {} when a Student t-test (done solely for ordering) yields a P<.05 for the inter-risk-group difference. Double-headed arrow connecting symbols at 2 clock hours indicates sampling at both time points listed; numbers in parentheses after symbol refer to hormone(s) to be considered concomitantly for classification.

The best classifiers differ among seasons. Moreover, even when the classifying hormone is the same in several seasons, the recommended sampling time can differ considerably, as is the case for aldosterone. Table 4 reveals that in summer as in spring TSH is a classifier. In the fall, the best classifier is the difference in original values (irrespective of sign) between the aldosterone concentrations at 08:00 and 00:00. In the winter the appropiate classifier includes prolactin and dehydro-epi-androsterone sulfate (DHEA-S) concomitantly with the 00:00 sample of aldosterone. The relation between plasma aldosterone and RMH is an indirect one in the three seasons, namely the low RMH subjects have the higher aldosterone M in winter, summer and fall. This relationship is not found, however, in the spring (Figure 5; Hermida et al., 1984c).

3.5. Inferential considerations: bootstrapping.
The method of pattern discrimination described above is deterministic assuming that 1) we know the a priori classification for each subject and 2) the classification is "correct". For a given combination of variables concerning a given subject, an a posteriori classification can be obtained with uncertainty relating only to the "correctness" of the a priori classification. Inferential statistics must now check the results obtained with the monotest. Bootstrapping (Efron, 1981)

introduces inferential considerations in the monotest and validates results obtained with a limited sample size, as is the
case herein with respect to the number of subjects. Further
study is even more warranted since the large number of determinations on any one variable per subject, the number of variables so documented, and the systematic placement of test times
along the scales of the year and the day render the data set
unique.

Common and fundamental to biology and statistics is variability. Biologic data usually are generated by a process with
both stochastic and deterministic features. Let V be a quantity
computed from the data, an estimator or statistic. Because of
stochastic components and as a first approximation V can be
regarded as a random variable; one may think of an observed
value of V as being randomly selected from a population of possible values. The distribution of values of V in the population is known as the sampling distribution of V. The sampling
distribution is determined by the distributions $F(x)$ of the
random quantities contributing to the data. When the distributions of these quantities are known, in principle, mathematical
analysis can determine the sampling distribution of V. This
procedure may be intractable, however, especially if V is a
complicated function of the data and/or if errors are not normally distributed. Again, in principle, if it were possible to
generate an arbitrarily large number N of data sets, all by the
same random mechanism, one could then compute V for each set,
and the values obtained would be a random sample from the sampling distribution of V. Its sample statistics would then
estimate the corresponding population quantities. The larger
the value of N, limited only by considerations of cost or time
required, the more accurate these estimates would be. This process of repeated empirical sampling is feasible only when one
completely specifies the distributions $F(x)$ generating the
data, in which case the entire process may be simulated on a
computer. This computer-use to generate artificial data sets
with a specified random structure is a particular form of the
Monte Carlo method, fundamental to the usual bootstrap application.

Bootstrapping (Efron, 1981) is a fairly general, usually
computer-intensive technique for estimating the sampling distribution of V--for gaining information about its bias and
standard error--without assuming a particular form for the distributions $F(x)$ of the data. It can use certain assumptions (as
to symmetry, independence, normality, etc.) when appropriate,
but ordinarily does not do so. The fundamental bootstrapping
paradigm consists of two steps: 1) Use the data (and any assumptions in which one has confidence) to estimate the
distribution(s) in the data-generating model; designate the
estimated distributions by $\hat{F}$. 2) Based on $\hat{F}$ determined in 1),
compute the sampling distribution of V. By this we mean the
sampling distribution of V when data are sampled from $\hat{F}$. This
distribution is called the bootstrap distribution of V. For
bootstrapping one here assumes: 1) A subject has a given probability to remain in the study from one season to the next; we
also assume that this probability remains the same during the
year for all subjects and estimate it by the ratio between the

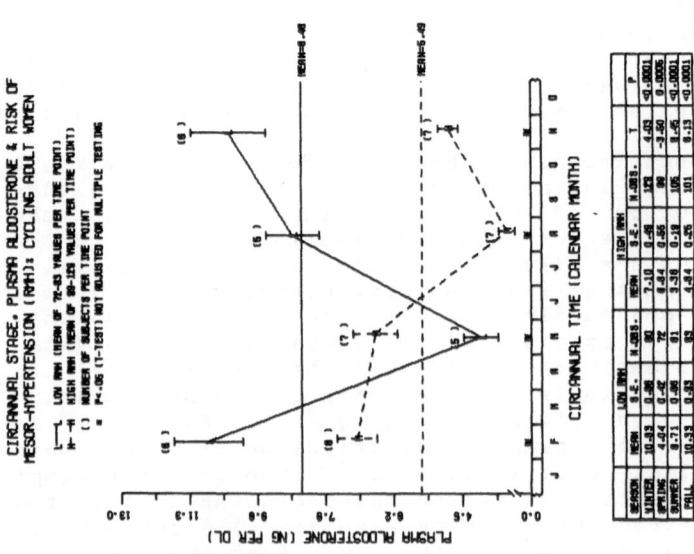

FIGURE 6

FIGURE 5

number of subjects in the study and the possible total sample
size when nobody withdraws. 2) Circadian Ms are correlated for
a subject from season to season. And 3) deviations of each
circadian M from the average are random. Monte Carlo simulation
then estimates the bootstrap distribution of the difference in
circannual characteristics betwen the low and high RMH groups
for the hormonal classifier considered (Hermida et al., 1984a,
in press d, e, f).

3.6. Bootstrapping results.
    The findings of neuroendocrine chronobiologic markers in
data from adult menstrually cycling women, providing the Figure
5 data, were re-analyzed by bootstrapping. The results thus
obtained are summarized in Table 5.   A percentile confidence
interval (CI; Efron, 1981) can be computed for the inter-risk-
group difference in circannual M, given that this difference is
median unbiased and symmetrically distributed, using the
bootstrap distribution of the difference, computed in all cases
with 2000 bootstrap replications. The 90% CI differs from zero
for aldosterone (Fig. 7) and TSH (Table 5). Moreover, by a
two-way analysis of variance, a RMH effect is seen for aldosterone and TSH, and a time effect and interaction also are seen
for aldosterone (P<.01).   These results are also validated by
bootstrapping in that a difference is seen in circannual A
(1.81 ng/dl) and Ø (98°; 360°=1 year) between the low and high
RMH groups.   For DHEA-S a difference is reproduced by
bootstrapping (Table 5) but its CI overlaps zero and hence the
role of DHEA-S remains uncertain, although an analysis of variance reveals a risk effect of borderline statistical significance.

TABLE 5: Bootstrapping of endocrine data from women--young
adults (set I) and all ages (set II; 1)--at low (L) and high
(H) risk of MESOR-hypertension (RMH).

Variable Units	Set #	RMH Group	MESOR 2	Inter- groupΔ	P from 3 RMH effect	90% CI 4
Aldosterone ng/dl	I	L	8.65	3.64	<.001	(1.96, 5.55)
	"	H	5.01			
	II	L	7.80	3.04	<.001	(1.96, 4.15)
	"	H	4.76			
TSH μIU/ml	I	L	8.58	5.02	<.001	(1.72, 8.40)
	"	H	3.56			
	II	L	6.90	2.78	<.001	(0.79, 4.74)
	"	H	4.12			
Cortisol μg/dl	I	L	8.94	0.06	.902	(-0.81, 1.02)
	"	H	8.88			
	II	L	8.83	0.22	.569	(-0.67, 1.07)
	"	H	9.05			
DHEA-S μg/cl	I	L	18.17	4.50	.056	(-1.80,10.69)
	"	H	13.67			

    1. Including adolescent and post-menopausal women for a total
of 21 H and 9 L subjects (set I including 7 H and 6 L subjects).   Except for 2 cases, each subject provided 4 circadian

MESORs. Moreover, MESORs were each based upon usually 15
values, except for cortisol MESORs based in most cases upon 72
values each. Thus the number of actual determinations underlying this analysis is about 35000.
  2. Midline estimating statistic of rhythm, M. This circannual
M is the result of fitting by least squares a 1-year cosine
curve to the circadian Ms obtained in each season, assigned to
February 15, May 15, August 15 & November 15, respectively.
  3. Obtained by 2-way analysis of variance.
  4. Percentile confidence interval (Efron, 1981) computed from
the .05 and .95 centiles of bootstrap distribution of difference in circannual M between groups at L & H RMH. In all cases
this distribution was computed using 2000 bootstrap replicates.

     Herein, we also extended the approach by the bootstrap to
a further analysis of a larger pool including endocrine data
from clinically healthy adolescent and post-menopausal women--
for those variables that do not undergo statistically significant changes within the age-span examined (Nelson et al.,
1980), namely aldosterone, TSH and cortisol. Earlier findings
on a single age-group of women for aldosterone (Hermida et al.,
1984b) are complemented by Figure 6, extending the difference
in circannual rhythm characteristics of this hormone between
women at high and low RMH to a pool of subjects from several
age-groups. The difference in circulating aldosterone again
stands out clearly in several seasons but not in spring (Hermida et al., in press e). The question as to whether aldosterone
classifies in spring deserves further scrutiny. Until proof is
offered to the contrary, it is assumed that it is not a classifier in this particular season. Apart from aldosterone, it
will be desirable to check whether women at a high RMH, as compared to women at low RMH exhibit a higher plasma cortisol M in
spring, a lower M in summer, while there is no M difference in
other seasons. Overall, however, there is no difference in cortisol M and none emerges from bootstrapping (Table 5). The
main results (Table 5) consist of support for an inverse relation between RMH and the hormone concentration of aldosterone
(Fig. 8) and TSH. In the case of aldosterone this indirect
relation is circannual stage-dependent, being apparent only in
three seasons.

3.7. Discussion.
     The role of aldosterone in clinically healthy and presum-
ably MESOR-hypertensive subjects is extensively discussed in
the literature (Cugini et al., 1981; Gordon et al., 1967;
Laragh et al., 1966). It is hardly surprising, thus, that
aldosterone, with other hormones, is one of the primary classifiers for RMH. Figure 5 shows, for the composite of the four
seasons, the circannual change in the relation between aldosterone concentration and RMH. This inverse relation in summer,
fall and winter is validated by different approaches to the
same data. A validated inverse relation to RMH of 1) the circannual aldosterone A, and of 2) the circannual aldosterone M
and possibly added differences in $\emptyset$ and waveform of aldosterone, all contribute to the seasonal change in the sign of an
endocrine relation to RMH. This change renders mandatory the

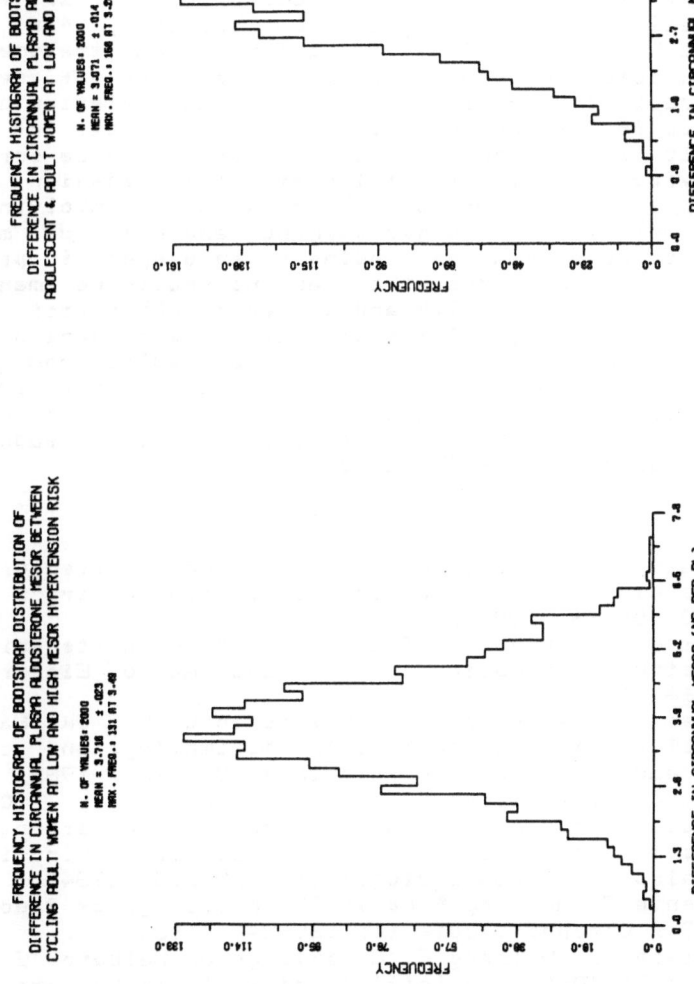

FIGURE 7

FIGURE 8

specification as to clock-hour and season of any spotcheck for risk assessment, whether it is based upon a single sample or several of them. The raison d'être of this study is a facilitation of meaningful sampling by time-specification for assessment of RMH and of underlying mechanisms.

The findings on circulating hormones, now based on the consideration of more extensive data, corroborate inferences drawn originally from the more restricted sample. Moreover, the results of the added bootstrapping of the greater data pool render a heretofore confusing physiologic variability, notably around the scale of a year, into a potentially useful risk assessment modality and a tool for the study of mechanisms underlying risk. As soon as RMH is recognized, combined chronobiologic BP and neuroendocrine approaches may help to arrive at early decisions concerning the need for preventive intervention and the kind of measure(s) required, quite apart from novel chronobiologic dimensions to the screening for high BP (Carandente & Halberg, 1984), its diagnosis and treatment.

In the specific case of an elevated risk of developing diseases related to a high BP, hygienic manipulation has documented value for prevention. Moreover, any effects of manipulating salt intake and/or dietary calories can be scrutinized in an individualized inferential statistical fashion (Lee et al., 1982). In some cases, such as a chronopsy involving aldosterone (as well as a few other hormones and BP), we might be dealing with more than the finding of an unspecific predictor. We may identify a mechanism that can and should be manipulated in order to optimize health and to reduce chronorisk (Tarquini et al., 1979). The major limitation of the work herein is that it has to relate hormone patterns to results from questionnaires. The former will have to be evaluated in due time in the light of morbidity and mortality statistics of each individual in larger cohorts, if we are to deal in a rational fashion with major diseases of our civilization.

REFERENCES

1. Arbogast B, Lubanovic W, Halberg F, Cornelissen G, Bingham C: "Chronobiologic serial sections of several orders". Chronobiologia 10: 59-68, 1983.
2. Bingham C, Godfrey MD, Tukey JW: "Modern techniques of power spectrum estimation". IEEE Trans. Audio. Electroacoust. AU-15: 56-66, 1967.
3. Bingham C, Arbogast B, Cornelissen G, Lee JK, Halberg F: "Inferential statistical methods for estimating and comparing cosinor parameters". Chronobiologia 9: 397-439, 1982.
4. Bingham C, Cornelissen G, Halberg E, Halberg F: "Circadian cardiovascular rhythmicity on ordinary routine: extent of 24-h synchronization revealed by testing an assumed period in single cosinor analysis". Chronobiologia 11: 263-274, 1984.
5. Carandente F, Halberg F(eds): Chronobiology of Blood Pressure in 1985, Chronobiologia 11: 189-341, 1984.
6. Cornelissen G, Halberg F, Stebblings J, Halberg E, Carandente F, Hsi B: "Data acquisition and analysis by computers and pocket calculators". La Ricerca Clin. Lab. 10: 333-385, 1980.
7. Cornelissen G, Halberg F, Fanning R, Kanabrocki EL,

Scheving LE, Pauly JE, Redmond DP, Carandente F: "Analysis of circadian rhythms in human rectal temperature and motor activity in dense and short series with correlated residuals". Biomedical Thermology. New York: Alan R. Liss, Inc., pp. 167-184, 1982.

8. Cover TM, Hart PE: "Nearest neighbor pattern classification". IEEE Trans. Inf. Theory IT-13: 21-27, 1967.

9. Cugini P, Scavo D, Cornelissen G, Lee JY, Meucci T, Halberg F: "Circadian rhythms of plasma renin, aldosterone and cortisol on habitual and low dietary sodium intake". Hormone Res. 15: 7-27, 1981.

10. Deka AC, Chatterjee B, Gupta BD, Balakrishnan C, Dutta TK: "Temperature rhythm--an index of tumour regression and mucositis during the radiation treatment of oral cancers". Ind. J. Cancer 13: 44-50, 1976.

11. De Prins J, Cornelissen G: "Complex demodulation and double demodulation". Bull. de l'Acad. des Sc. de Belgique, 5 serie, LXV: 445-455, 1979.

12. De Prins J, Cornelissen G, Hillman D, Halberg F, Van Dyck C: "Harmonic interpolation yields paraphases and orthophases for biologic rhythms". In: Chronobiology, Proc. XIII Int. Soc. Chronobiol., Pavia, Italy, Sept. 4-7, 1977. F. Halberg, L.E. Scheving, E.W. Powell, D.K. Hayes (eds.). Milan: Il Ponte, pp. 333-344, 1981.

13. Efron B: "Nonparametric estimates of standard error: The jackknife, the bootstrap and other methods". Biometrika 68: 589-599, 1981.

14. Gordon RD, Kuchel O, Liddle GW, Island DP: "Role of the sympathetic nervous system in regulating renin and aldosterone production in man". J. Clin. Invest. 46: 599-605, 1967.

15. Halberg E, Halberg F, Shankaraiah K: "Plexo-serial linear-nonlinear rhythmometry of blood pressure, pulse and motor activity by a couple in their sixties". Chronobiologia 8: 351-366, 1981.

16. Halberg F: "Some physiological and clinical aspects of 24-hour periodicity". J. Lancet 73: 20-32, 1953.

17. Halberg F: "Beobachtungen uber 24 Stunden-Periodik in standard-isierter Versuchsanordnung vor und nach Epinephrektomic und bilateraler optischer Enukleation". 20th meeting of the German Physiologic Society, Homburg/Saar, Sep., 1953. In: Berichte uber die gesamte Physiologie 162: 354-355, 1954.

18. Halberg F: "Temporal coordination of physiologic function". Cold Spr. Harb. Symp. Quant. Biol. 25: 289-310, 1960.

19. Halberg F: "Chronobiology". Ann. Rev. Physiol. 31: 675-725, 1969.

20. Halberg F: "Chronopharmacology and chronotherapy". In: Cellular Pacemakers. D.O. Carpenter (ed). New York: John Wiley & Sons, pp. 261-297, 1982.

21. Halberg F: "Quo vadis basic and clinical chronobiology: promise for health maintenance". Am. J. Anat. 168: 543-594, 1983.

22. Halberg F, Visscher MB: "Regular diurnal physiological variation in eosinophil levels in five stocks of mice". Proc. Soc. Exp. Biol. and Med. 75: 846-847, 1950.

23. Halberg F, Engel R, Treloar AE, Gully RJ: "Endogenous eosinopenia in institutionalized patients with mental

deficiency". AMA Arch. Neurol. Psychiat. 69: 462-469, 1953.

24. Halberg F, Visscher MB: "Some physiologic effects of lighting". Proc. 1st Int. Photobiological Congress, Amsterdam, pp. 396-398, 1954.

25. Halberg F, Panofsky H: "I. Thermo-variance spectra; method and clinical illustrations". Exp. Med. Surg. 19: 284-309, 1961.

26. Halberg F, Engeli M, Hamburger C, Hillman D: "Spectral resolution of low frequency, small-amplitude rhythms in excreted 17-ketosteroid; probable androgen-induced circaseptan desynchronization". Acta Endocrinol. 50 (Suppl. 103): 5-54, 1965.

27. Halberg F, Tong YL, Johnson EA: "Circadian system phase-- an aspect of temporal morphology; procedures and illustrative examples". Proc. International Congress of Anatomists. In: The Cellular Aspects of Biorhythms. Symposium on Biorhythms, Springer-Verlag, pp. 20-48, 1967.

28. Halberg F, Johnson EA, Nelson W, Runge W, Sothern R: "Autorhythmometry--procedures for physiologic self-measurements and their analysis". Physiology Teacher 1: 1-11, 1972.

29. Halberg F, Haus E, Cardoso SS, Scheving LE, Kuhl JFW, Shiotsuka R, Rosene G, Pauly JE, Runge W, Spalding JF, Lee JK, Good RA: "Toward a chronotherapy of neoplasia: Tolerance of treatment depends upon host rhythms". Experientia (Basel) 29: 909-934, 1973.

30. Halberg F, Carandente F, Cornelissen G, Katinas GS: "Glossary of chronobiology". Chronobiologia 4, Suppl. 1, 1977a.

31. Halberg F, Gupta BD, Haus E, Halberg E, Deka AC, Nelson W, Sothern RB, Cornelissen G, Lee JK, Lakatua DJ, Scheving LE, Burns ER: "Steps toward a cancer chronopolytherapy". Proc. XIVth International Congress of Therapeutics, Montpellier, France; L'Expansion Scientifique Francaise, pp. 151-196, 1977b.

32. Halberg F, Sothern RB, Roitman B, Halberg E, Halberg Fr, Mayersbach Hv, Haus E, Scheving LE, Kanabrocki EL, Bartter FC, Delea C, Simpson HW, Tavadia HB, Fleming KA, Hume P, Wilson C: "Agreement of circadian characteristics for total leucocyte counts in different geographic locations". Proc. XII Int. Conf. Int. Soc. Chronobiol., Washington, August 10-13, 1975. Milan: Il Ponte, pp. 3-17, 1977c.

33. Halberg F, Cornelissen G, Sothern RB, Wallach LA, Halberg E, Ahlgren A, Kuzel M, Radke A, Barbosa J, Goetz F, Buckley J, Mandel J, Schuman L, Haus E, Lakatua D, Sackett L, Berg H, Kawasaki T, Ueno M, Uezono K, Matsuoka M, Omae T, Tarquini B, Cagnoni M, Garcia Sainz M, Griffiths K, Wilson D, Wetterberg L, Donatti L, Tatti P, Vasta M, Locatelli I, Camagna A, Lauro R, Tritsch G, Wendt H: "International geographic studies of oncological interest on chronobiological variables". In: Neoplasm--Comparative Pathology of Growth in Animals, Plants and Man. H. Kaiser (ed). Baltimore: Williams and Wilkins, pp. 553-596, 1981.

34. Halberg F, Halberg E, Nelson W, Teslow T, Montalbetti N: "Chronobiology and laboratory medicine in developing areas". In: Proc. 1st African and Mediterranean Congress for Clinical Chemistry. N. Montalbetti (ed). Milan, Nov. 11-15, 1980, pp. 113-156, 1982.

35. Halberg F, Lagoguey JM, Reinberg A: "Human circannual rhythms in a broad spectral structure". Int. J. Chronobiol. 8: 225-268, 1983.

225–268, 1983.
36. Halberg F, Halberg E: "Chronopharmacology and further steps toward chronotherapy". In: Pharmacokinetic Basis for Drug Treatment. L. Z. Benet, N. Massoud, J. G. Gambertoglio (eds). New York: Raven Press, pp. 221–248, 1984.
37. Haus E, Halberg F, Scheving L, Cardoso S, Kühl JFW, Sothern RB, Shiotsuka RN, Hwang DS, Pauly JE: "Increased tolerance of leukemic mice to arabinosyl cytosine given on schedule adjusted to circadian system". Science 177: 80–82, 1972.
38. Hermida RC: Variable Selection Approach to the Chronoendocrine Epidemiologic Assessment of an Expansive Personality. Master Thesis. School of Statistics, Univ. Minn., Minneapolis, MN, 225 pp., 1984.
39. Hermida RC, Del Pozo F, Halberg F: "Endocrine chronorisk of developing breast cancer assessed individually by pattern recognition". Chronobiologia 9: 341–342, 1982a.
40. Hermida RC, Halberg F, Halberg E, Del Pozo F: "Toward a psychoneuroendocrine hemopsy". Clin. Chem. Newsletter 2: 191–198, 1982b.
41. Hermida RC, Halberg F, Halberg E, Del Pozo F: "Cost-effective potential classifiers of the risk of developing high-blood-pressure-associated disease". IEEE Frontiers of Engineering and Computing in Health Care—1983. Proc. 5th An. Conf. IEEE/EMBS; Columbus, Ohio, Sep. 10–12, 1983, pp. 296–301.
42. Hermida RC, Bingham C, Halberg F: "Software system for chronoepidemiologic risk assessment". Proc. 37th IEEE/ACEMB An. Conf.; Los Angeles, Cal., Sep. 17–19, 1984a, pag. 223.
43. Hermida RC, Halberg F: "Assessment of the risk of mesor-hypertension". In: Chronobiology of Blood Pressure in 1985. F. Carandente, F. Halberg (eds). Chronobiologia 11: 249–262, 1984b.
44. Hermida RC, Halberg F, Del Pozo F, Chavarria F: "Pattern discrimination and the risk of developing breast cancer". In: Chronobiology 1982–1983. Proc. XV Int. Conf. Int. Soc. Chronobiol., Minneapolis, MN, Sep. 14–17, 1981. E. Haus, H. Kabat (eds). New York: S. Karger Publishers, Inc., pp. 399–412, 1984c.
45. Hermida RC, Halberg F, Halberg E, Haus E, Lakatua D, Uezono K, Kawasaki T, Mandel J, Del Pozo F: "Endocrine chronorisk of mesor-hypertension in clinically healthy women sought by circadian and circannual pattern discrimination". SIRMCE Congress 1982: Influence of Environment on Man. Vienna, Nov. 17–20, 1982, pp. 74–163, 1984d.
46. Hermida RC, Halberg F, Langevin TR: "Serial white blood cell counts and chronochemotherapy according to highest values (macrophases) or by model characteristics (acrophases)". Proc. 2nd Int. Conf. Medico-Social Aspects of Chronobiol., Florence, October 2, 1984, in press a.
47. Hermida RC, Sothern RB, Halberg F, Langevin TR: "Variability of circadian acrophase of urinary potassium excretion as a potential marker for cancer chronotherapy". Proc. 2nd Int. Conf. Medico-Social Aspects of Chronobiol., Florence, October 2, 1984, in press b.
48. Hermida RC, Halberg F, Langevin TR, Hrushesky W: "Circadian stage-dependent response to cisplatin of urinary potassium

acrophase--A cost-effective chronotherapeutic marker". Chronobiologia, 1985, in press c.

49. Hermida RC, Halberg F: "Bootstrapped circannual endocrine
and blood pressure markers of vascular disease risk". IEEE
Frontiers of Engineering and Computing in Health Care--1985.
Proc. 7th An. Conf. IEEE/EMBS. Chicago, Illinois, Sep. 28-30,
1985, in press d.

50. Hermida RC, Halberg F: "Bootstrapping and added data
discriminate, at low blood pressures, neuroendocrine risk of
developing mesor-hypertension". Chronobiologia, 1985, in press
e.

51. Hermida RC, Halberg F, Bingham C, Del Pozo F: "Bootstrapping validates recommended cost-effective use of endocrine data
bases for cardiovascular risk assessment". Proc. 9th Annual
Symposium on Computer Applications in Medical Care (SCAMC);
Baltimore, Maryland, Nov. 10-13, 1985, in press f.

52. Hrushesky W, Halberg F, Levi F, Langevin T, Kennedy BJ,
Gergen J, Goetz F, Theologides A: "Optimal circadian treatment
time reduces cis-diamminedichloro-platinum-induced vomiting".
Int. J. Chronobiol. 7: 257, 1981.

53. Koehler F, Okano FK, Elveback LR, Halberg F, Bittner JJ:
"Periodograms for the study of physiologic daily periodicity in
mice and in man". Exp. Med. Surg. 14: 5-30, 1956.

54. Laragh JH, Sealey JE, Sommers SC: "Patterns of adrenal
secretion and urinary excretion of aldosterone and plasma renin
activity in normal and hypertensive subjects". Circ. Res. 18/19
(Suppl. 1): 158-174, 1966.

55. Laraña M, Del Pozo F, Sanchez C, Halberg F: "Adaptive
filtering to detect oscillations in biomedical signals". Proc.
37th ACEMB An. Conf., Los Angeles, Cal., Sep. 17-19, 1984; pag.
232.

56. Laraña M, Del Pozo F, Cornelissen G, Halberg E, Hermida
RC, Halberg F: "Ultradian rhythmometry by adaptive line enhanc-
er (ALE)". Proc. XVII Int. Conf. Int. Soc. Chronobiol., Little
Rock, AK, Nov. 3-6, 1985, in press.

57. Lee JY, Gillum RF, Cornelissen G, Koga Y, Halberg F:
"Individualized assessment of circadian rhythm characteristics
of human blood pressure and pulse after moderate salt and
weight restriction". In: Toward Chrono-Pharmacology. R.
Takahashi, F. Halberg, C.A. Walker (eds). Oxford: Pergamon
Press, pp. 375-390, 1982.

58. Marquardt DW: "An algorithm for least squares estimation
of nonlinear parameters". J. Soc. Indust. Appl. Math. 11:
431-441, 1963.

59. McKay RJ, Campbell NA: "Variable selection techniques in
discriminant analysis. II. Allocation". British J. Math. Stat.
Phychol. 35: 30-41, 1982.

60. Monk TH, Fort A: "'Cosina': A cosine curve fitting program
suitable for small computers". International Journal of Chronobiology 8: 193-224, 1983.

61. Nelson W, Bingham C, Haus E, Lakatua DJ, Kawasaki T, Halberg F: "Rhythm-adjusted age effects in a concomitant study of
twelve hormones in blood plasma of women". J. Gerontol. 35:
512-519, 1980.

62. Nelson W, Cornelissen G, Hinkley D, Bingham C, Halberg F:
"Construction of rhythm-specified reference intervals and

regions, with emphasis on 'hybrid' data, illustrated for plasma cortisol". Chronobiologia 10: 179-193, 1983.

63. Panofsky H, Halberg F: "II. Thermo-variance spectra; simplified computational example and other methodology". Exp. Med. Surg. 19: 323-338, 1961.

64. Reinberg A, Halberg F: "Circadian chronopharmacology". Ann. Rev. Pharmacol. 2: 455-492, 1971.

65. Reinberg A, Halberg F(eds): Chronopharmacology. Proc. Satellite Symp. 7th Int. Cong. Pharmacol. New York: Pergamon Press, 1979.

66. Rummel JA, Lee JK, Halberg F: "Combined linear-nonlinear chronobiologic windows by least squares resolve neighboring components in a physiologic rhythm spectrum". In: Biorhythms and Human Reproduction. M. Ferin, F. Halberg, R.M. Richart, R. Vande Wiele (eds.). New York: John Wiley & Sons, pp. 53-82, 1974.

67. Scheving LE, Haus E, Kühl JFW, Pauly JE, Halberg F, Cardoso S: "Close reproduction by different laboratories of characteristics of circadian rhythm in 1-β-D-arabinofuranosyl cytosine tolerance by mice". Cancer Res. 36: 1133-1137, 1976.

68. Scheving LE, Tsai TS, Pauly JE, Halberg F: "Circadian effect of ACTH 1-17 on mitotic index of the corneal epithelium of BALB/c mice". Peptides 4: 183-190, 1983.

69. Schuster A: "On the investigation of hidden periodicities with application to a supposed 26-day period of meteorological phenomena". Terrestrial Magnetism 3: 13-41, 1898.

70. Stumpf K: Grundlagen und Methoden der Periodenforschung. Berlin: Springer-Verlag, 332 pp., 1937.

71. Takahashi R, Halberg F, Walker E(eds): Toward Chrono-Pharmacology. Oxford: Pergamon Press, 1982.

72. Tarquini B, Benvenuti B, Moretti R, Neri B, Cagnoni M, Halberg F: "Atherosclerotic chronorisk--recognized by autorhythmometry combined with hemopsies as a step toward chronophylaxis". Chronobiologia 6: 162-163, 1979.

73. Tong YL, Nelson WL, Sothern RB, Halberg F: "Estimation of the orthophase--timing of the high values on a non-sinusoidal rhythm--illustrated by the best timing for experimental cancer chronotherapy". In: Proc. XII Int. Conf. Int. Soc. Chronobiol., Wash., D.C. Milan: Il Ponte, pp. 765-769, 1977.

74. Vokac M: "A comprehensive system of cosinor treatment programs written for the Apple II microcomputer". Chronobiology International 1: 87-92, 1984.

75. Walker CA, Winget CM, Soliman KFA(eds): Chronopharmacology and Chronotherapeutics. Tallahassee: Florida A & M University Foundation, 1981.

SELECTION OF DATA ANALYSIS METHODS IN CHRONOBIOLOGY

Jean DE PRINS, University of Brussels, Belgium.
Germaine CORNELISSEN, University of Minnesota, USA.

Introduction

The purpose of this manuscript is to consider data acquired by automatic monitoring devices, i.e., to consider the
case of dense and (mostly) equidistant measurements. It is
easy to state that in order to obtain good results and a valid
interpretation of the data, both adequate instrumentation and
appropriate data analysis methods are needed. But it is more
difficult to actually implement these two requirements. This
paper attempts to examine the complexities of the problem and
to give some recommendations on how to avoid pitfalls in data
analysis.

Experimental conditions

In order to understand the diversity of methods of
analysis, it is important to first review some concepts associated with the acquisition of data:

1) The biological system under study is usually represented
by one or several variables. These variables are essentially
conceptual, in the sense that they are gauged through a justi-
fying theory allowing their quantification (or measurement).
2) Transducers assign to these conceptual variables a
scalar function that varies with time and that is easily
"readable". For instance, the concept of temperature is based
on the theory of thermodynamics. An adequate electronic circuit delivers an electric current proportional to the temperature of a site adjacent to the probe. The resulting function
Y(t) constitutes the only accessible "reality".
3) A sampler controlled by a clock provides at regular time
intervals (θ) numerical values (Ym) of the function Y(t). A
finite number (N) of such measurements can be obtained,
corresponding to a total observation span $T=N\theta$. The set of
values Y_0, Y_1, ..., Y_{N-1} constitutes the sequence Y[N].

In order to be able to reconstruct the variation of the
biological variable as a function of time on the basis of the
sequence Y[N], the instrumentation used to measure Y(t) has to
follow certain criteria, reviewed below.
No biological system responds "instantaneously". Any
variation requires a certain amount of time. As a result, the
spectral density of measurable variations is limited to an

upper frequency f_B. When a reasonably regular biological rhythm is studied over several cycles, the spectrum is approximated by a series of equidistant spectral lines. The lowest frequency representing a significant line generally corresponds to the inverse of the period of the rhythm.

The transducer is also characterized by a response time, associated with a cut-off frequency f_A, and acts as a low-pass filter. In order to correctly represent the biological phenomenon by the function Y(t), the transducer has to be as neutral as possible with respect to the biological phenomenon and have a cut-off frequency f_A much higher than f_B. A major difficulty is that only Y(t) is accessible so that f_B cannot be measured directly.

As for the sampler, according to the theory, a necessary condition for reconstructing all the information of Y(t) on the basis of the sequence Y[N] is given by:

$$\theta \leqslant \frac{1}{n f_A}$$

where n lies between 2 and 4 (De Prins and Lechien, 1977).

The different noises affecting the biological signal also have to be defined:
- Type I noises are fluctuations of the biological system, considered not to be part of the deterministic portion of the signal. The corresponding noise spectrum is also characterized by the cut-off frequency f_B.
- Type II noises are fluctuations, external to the system, measured by the transducer. They are filtered by the transducer and are limited in frequency by f_A.
- Type III noises originate from the transducer and the sampler. These noises are not filtered but eventually are redistributed over the whole frequency range (folding effect) because of the sampling procedure and its interpretation.

In principle, in the absence of the biological system, it is possible to evaluate the characteristics of type II and III noises. The following table summarizes some of the effects likely to affect the biological signal and the different noises.

	"Conceptual" freq. limit	Filtering through a "good" transducer	Folding effect – "good" sampling	Possibility of "leakage"
BS	yes	no	no	yes
NT I	yes	no	no	yes
NT II	---	yes	no	yes
NT III	---	---	yes	yes

BS=Biological Signal; NT=Noise Type.

Let P_I, P_{II}, and P_{III} be the power of type I, II, and III noises, respectively, and let P_S be the power of the biological signal. Ideal measurement conditions are of course present when

$$P_S > P_I \geqslant P_{II} > P_{III} \ .$$

It is obvious that in most cases, such ideal conditions are not met. Well adapted data analysis methods have then to be used.

Justification of the plurality of methods

Mathematical theories, on which data analysis is based, rely on simplifying hypotheses. It is important to examine to what extent such hypotheses are likely to be verified in the most favorable case, as described above:

- "Normally" distributed noise: This hypothesis is rarely verified and constitutes in our opinion an "educative myth" (see Preface of Tables of Lindley and Scott, 1984). Usually, the distribution of errors is not known a priori and is diffi-cult to estimate. For these reasons, the use of nonparametric tests and of resampling methods is recommended.

- Independence of errors: An adequate sampling rate neces-sarily implies important correlations ($\cong 0.7!$) between consecu-tive errors in the case of type I and II noises. Any computa-tion of confidence limits not accounting for this aspect may be grossly erroneous. These limits can be corrected by es-timating correlations (Malbecq and De Prins, 1981; Cornelissen et al., 1982), or by decimation ("desperate" solution!).

- Stationarity (or actually ergodicity): This condition has to be seriously tested, since most instruments and biological systems are characterized by "drifts" of the zero point, and by variations in the power of the noise as a function of time. Let us also note that biological systems are often less stable than measuring instruments, and present important fluctuations of their global characteristics (e.g., fever effects). When-ever possible, non-stationary effects have to be "corrected" prior to data analysis itself.

Since computation methods have to be adapted to the vari-ous experimental conditions, there will be numerous methods as well. Let us briefly review some of them.

When a functional model exists, the biologist is able to predict some of the characteristics of the biological signal. The values of the parameters remain to be estimated. In this case, one can proceed with tests and statistical fits concomi-tantly with an analysis of residuals allowing to check the validity of the model. Often, prior knowledge of the model is not available in chronobiology, and rhythms have to be empiri-cally sought.

If the sampling rate is adequate, and noises have a low power, the biological signal can be reconstructed and analyzed by relying on all resources of signal analysis and spectral methods. By contrast, if the above-mentioned conditions are not met, data have to be considered as a statistical sample and analyzed by means of statistical procedures, with a cau-tious use of spectral analysis techniques.

The rhythm investigated can be very stable, in which case the use of Fourier analysis (Discrete Fourier Transform, DFT) and certain kinds of filtering procedures (averaging, complex demodulation, etc.) are recommended. When the rhythm is ir-regular, linear or nonlinear methods can be used, such as ARMA processes (so-called "modern" spectral methods; Haykin, 1983).

The characteristics of the noises also influence the selection of the analysis methods. For instance, if the bio-logical signal has a power comparable to or smaller than that of the noises, but the biological signal predominates in a given frequency band, the different filtering procedures may be successfully applied (optimal or non optimal filters; Boz-ic, 1979; Szentirmai, 1973). If fortunately the noises are normally distributed and errors are independent, (linear or nonlinear) least squares methods can be used efficiently. If the distribution is not normal, robust methods can be applied.

These few examples illustrate that in view of the dif-ferent experimental conditions, an array of methods, each with its own domain of applicability, have to be considered. It is illusory to search for "the best" universal method, each ex-periment being unique. But it is always advisable to use several acceptable procedures concomitantly, and to compare with "common sense" the results obtained by each of them. Let us also note that methods having different domains of applica-bility should not necessarily be compared.
Finally, it is important, particularly with respect to empirical research, to ask the right questions and to select methods likely to provide a good answer. Let us consider the case of the determination of the maximum of a rhythm. So stated, the question is not valid. What do we really want to know: During which time interval (how long) does the signal assume a significantly higher value? What is its most likely time of occurrence? What is the prediction for the future (e.g., following days)? What is the highest predictable value taken by the variable? Once the problem is correctly stated, the methods best adapted to the experimental conditions and to the question being asked have to be selected. For instance, adequate methods for fitting data correctly do not necessarily provide a valid answer to the above questions.

Conclusions

According to Altman (1980) in his excellent article on pitfalls of data analysis, some of the well known principal sources of error are:
1) incomplete choice of variables;
2) inadequate measurement of variables: poor modelling of the measurement technique;
3) presence of systematic errors;
4) incorrect treatment of outliers: too small or too large weights assigned to these values;
5) unnecessary complexity of the model, rendering the in-terpretation of results needlessly arduous.

Other difficulties are not so apparent and are usually not discussed in great enough detail:

1) Premature stop in the analysis: for instance, neglect of analyzing the residuals.

2) Erroneous causality attribution amounting to consider as a direct causal relation either a fortuitous correlation, or a relation due to an external cause. Causality and its rules have been studied for centuries by both philosophers and scientists (for instance, see Bynum et al., 1981). Difficulties related to the attribution of causality are well covered in most textbooks and courses. Nevertheless, examples of this kind of error are unfortunately numerous.

3) Operational insignificance: This is a very delicate topic! It is related to the concept of usefulness for the biologist. Often in numerical analyses, there is a tendency to believe that any statistically significant difference is of operational value. But in some instances such a difference does not provide any useful information to the biologist. It is then said to be operationally insignificant. Only the biologist can decide what is operationally significant or not. For instance, if the mathematician assures, by statistical means, the validity of a 7-day rhythm in temperature with an amplitude of $0.01°C$, it is to the biologist to decide whether this rhythm is operationally significant or not. Obviously, its importance may lie in terms of the understanding of underlying biological mechanisms.

When examining mistakes and errors related to data analysis, it is rare that they result from a lack of rigor of the mathematical methods used. They are generally due to the inadequacy between the underlying assumptions and the "real" conditions of the experiment. There is then a lack of "rigor of correspondance". This drawback often results from the desire to safeguard a certain mathematical "easiness of use". This is the case for instance when postulating a normal distribution of errors. Unfortunately, it is not easy by means of test procedures to correctly reject this hypothesis (risk of type II error). For instance, it is known that correlated errors lead to important errors in deriving confidence limits and in hypothesis testing well before such correlations can be actually detected. Against this background, common sense dictates to give preference to nonparametric methods (Conover, 1980) or to resampling methods (Efron, 1982), even at the cost of a more complex procedure of analysis.

Numerous criteria exist to determine the rigor inside the mathematical model. It is much more difficult to check the rigor of correspondance. Like many other authors, we are tempted to refer to relatively vague concepts such as "common sense, judgment, invention, imagination, critical mind, ingenuity". But, as noted by Archibald (1980), when and where are these concepts taught? Are we even in agreement with what these concepts cover? In our opinion, this rigor of correspondance relates to a real need, and the efforts of data analysis should also tend to clarify this concept and its needs.

These considerations lead to a fundamental question: what is the usefulness of data analysis methods for the biologist. We would like to provide two answers.

If a model exists, previously set by the biologist, and which is functional, explicative and quantitative, methods of data analysis are extremely valuable to specify the model and eventually to invalidate it if need be.

By contrast, in the case of empirical research, methods of data analysis (including statistical methods) should be used with great caution. For instance, 95% or 99% confidence levels do not correspond to certainties and remain conjectures. Moreover, when these conjectures are obtained on the basis of a single data set, it is mandatory to proceed with new experiments to test them, and eventually to invalidate them if need be. In any event, from an epistemological point of view (Bynum et al., 1981), it seems "presumptuous" to present these results as being "demonstrated" by the experiment.

Once these limitations are well understood, data analysis methods constitute extremely valuable tools for chronobiologic research.

References

1. Altman SA: Pitfalls of data analysis. In: Pitfalls of analysis. G. Majone, ES Quade, eds., Wiley & Sons, 1980.
2. Archibald KA: The pitfalls of language, or analysis through the looking-glass. In: Pitfalls of analysis. G. Majone, ES Quade, eds., Wiley & Sons, 1980.
3. Bozic SM: Digital and Kalman filtering. Arnold, 1979.
4. Bynum WF, EJ Browe, R Porter (eds): Dictionary of the history of science. Mac Millan Press Ltd., 1981.
5. Conover WJ: Practical nonparametric statistics. Wiley & Sons, 2nd ed., 1980.
6. Cornelissen G, F Halberg, R Fanning et al.: Differences in internal and external timing of circadian rhythms in human rectal temperature and motor activity. Biomedical Thermology, M Gautherie, E Albert, eds., Alan R Liss Inc., 1982: 167-184.
7. De Prins J, JP Lechien: Echantillonnage et analyse spectrale. Cahiers du Centre d'Etudes de Recherches Opérationnelle 19: 357-364, 1977.
8. Efron B: The jackknife, the bootstrap and other resampling plans. CBMS-NSF Regional Conference series in applied mathematics. SIAM, 1982.
9. Haykin S (ed.): Nonlinear methods of spectral analysis. Springer-Verlag, 2nd ed., 1983.
10. Lindley DV, WF Scott: New Cambridge Elementary Statistical Tables. Cambridge University Press, 1984.
11. Malbecq W, J De Prins: Applications of maximum entropy methods to cosinor analysis. Journal of Interdisc. Cycle Res. 12: 97-107, 1981.
12. Szentirmai (ed.): Computer-aided filter design. IEEE Press, 1973.

A BIODATA ACQUISITION RECORDING SYSTEM (BIDARS)

R. M. GOODMAN, Department of Physiology and Biophysics, Hahnemann
University, Broad and Vine Streets, Philadelphia, PA

1. INTRODUCTION

Workers in the fields of chronobiology, the clinical sciences, biological and biomedial research all have needed the means to observe preselected parameters in their subjects for extended periods of time (chronic
studies). To date, instrumentation which will acquire such data for weeks
or months (or longer) and which is appropriate for use with free-roaming
subjects, particularly humans, has not been available. BIDARS addresses
this problem area.

2. DISCUSSION

Instrumentation for subject surveillance which uses telemetric
approaches is simply inappropriate for free-roaming subjects. Such systems
are primarily effective when operating within a controlled environment such
as one floor of a hospital etc. Problems involving signal loss, transmitter power, etc. preclude telemetry for the applications discussed herein.

Chronic applications usually have several characteristics in common:
one wishes to acquire parametric data (one or more parameters) in digital
form for long periods of time: weeks to months. One wishes the subjects
to be free to go about their daily life without the interference which
might be introduced by massive or awkard instrument packets, and/or
devices obvious to a third party.

One finds it desireable for acquired data to be held in non-volatile
form - a form in which the original repository may be filed itself, or
have its contents transferred to a large permanent file (very large magnetic tape storage, or very large hard-disk storage) and in a form which
can be fed to a computer system in an uncomplicated way. In view of the
present state-of-the-art for non-volatile, solid-state memory systems, we
have selected the microcassette as the memory medium of choice. In passing
one must note that the BIDARS techniques are equally appropriate to
minicassettes, standard cassettes, large 0.25 inch tape cassettes and very
large reel-to-reel systems.

Since we can store on the order of 5000 bpi per track, the capacity
of these larger tape systems is extremely large. Since we are dealing
with devices for application to human subjects, the microcassette was
selected so that criteria for size and weight could be met.

Obvious applications for such a data acquisition systems include:
single or multiple localized temperature data, cardiac arrhythmia data,
occurrence of petit-mal seizures, heart rate and temperature data,
occurrence of episodic panic (or severe anxiety), accumulation of cause
of death data from ambulatory cardiac patients, pre-stress/stress/post-
stress data, etc. The parameters to be recorded must be digitizible and
of course, sensors must exist or be possible to fabricate. We note here
that the BIDARS system is based on incremental recording. It is not

designed to record continuously - a capability often not needed when dealing with biologic parameters. The system (refer to Figure 1) can be
described as follows: A parameter(s) is sensed; the system is not limited
to the recording of a single parameter. In any case, when a datum is
sensed it is then conditioned and standardized for conversion to digital
form. The analog-to-digital converter makes the conversion and the datum,
via the microprocessor is held in the microprocessor memory, or in a buffer
R/W memory. At an appropriate time the processor sends the datum to the
magnetic tape head and a record is made on the tape.

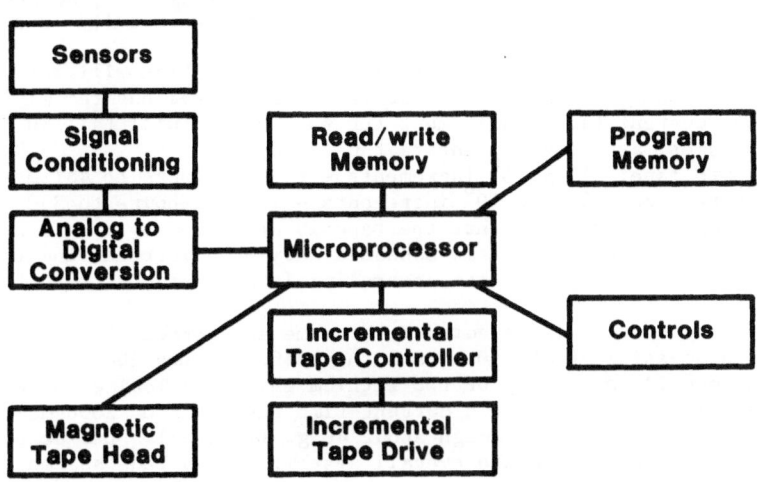

Figure 1. FUNCTIONAL DIAGRAM, BIODATA ACQUISITION RECORDING SYSTEM

Since we expect to use a 4-track head, it is apparent that for a byte
to be recorded, the tape must be incremented between nibbles.
This is accomplished by initiation, from the processor, of the incremental tape controller and the incremental tape drive. Input control
information may be built into the program memory of the microprocessor
(ROM) and/or be entered via external controls. For example, one may be
interested in recording several seconds of ECG should the heart rate fall
below a preset value, or exceed a preset value.
Such settings may be adjustable via subminiature switches available
to the user. Or in addition to recording the ECG when limits are
exceeded, the subject may initiate a record by pressing a control switch.
Another simple example would be the periodic recording of say, heart rate
and temperature.
The non-volatile memory medium is the microcassette magnetic tape.
Standard microcassettes capable of 90 minute or 60 minute record
time at 1.2 cm/s have the following characteristics with our system:

Microcassettes	Tape Length (cm)	Tape Capacity (bits, 4 track)	Tape Capacity Theoretical Bytes
90 min.	6480	52×10^6	6.5×10^6
60 min.	4320	34.7×10^6	4.34×10^6

It is interesting to observe that the pulse-packing factor indicated above was obtained with a 4-track audio read/write head. We believe that special read/write heads with gaps smaller than 65 uinches could further increase the tape storage capacity - however, the cost of such a head is substantially greater than desirable for our system. If one assumed that every bit position on the tape were written, the following represents the write current-time required in milliampere-hours:

90 minute tape: 52×10^6 bits - 7.65 ma-hrs (max.)
60 minute tape: 34.7×10^6 bits - 5.1 ma-hrs (max.)

The indicated current-time requirement for writing in every possible position on a given tape represents a fraction of the capacity of a very small hearing aid battery.

The tape is incremented by a special mechanism which will introduce an accurately controlled motion on the order of several hundred microinches. inches. The current-time requirement for this action will fall in the following ranges, assuming the entire tape is used:

90 minute tape: 13×10^6 increments - 1950 ma-hours to 487 ma-hrs
60 minute tape: 8.68×10^6 increments - 1320 ma-hours to 330 ma-hrs

It is important to note that the tape is not moved by a rotating motor; power for tape movement is consumed only when incrementing occurs and not between increments. Also, recording is accomplished with the tape at rest.

The microprocessor is expected to consume an average of less than 100 uA; signal processing about 150 uA and the buffer memory about 5uA.

If one considers the use of two lithium thionyl chloride AA cells in series, we will have available a current-time reservoir of 2000 ma-hours, (Tadrian) and the cells will weigh about 40 g. ($\approx$1.4 oz). Let us assume an 80% efficiency factor in the overall system; we may thus assume that 1600 ma-hours are available, in this example, for BIDARS operation.

For the purposes of this example, let us suppose that one wishes to record body temperature each 10 minutes, 24 hours a day for an extended time (using only the two original lithium cells). Since one can assume that the microprocessor will power-down circuits not in use and power-up circuits as necessary and that the buffer memory will not be needed, one may approximate the use of available battery energy for a study duration of 3 years as follows:

-157,680 data will be recorded.
-a total of 473,040 tape increments will be stepped this will require 73.6 ma-hrs.
-the microprocessor will require 1314. ma-hrs.
-the ADC will require 1.1 ma-hrs.
-the signal processor will require 6.6 ma-hrs.

Thus, if data are taken each 10 minutes, the system will accumulate information over a period of 26,280 hrs. (3 years). A total of 1395 ma-hours will be used from an available 1600 ma-hrs. - a 13% safety factor.

The foregoing are essentially the simplest and worst-case analysis. With control by the BIDARS microprocessor, the ADC will be powered down a substantial fraction of the time as will the signal processor. By such a design, the system will easily operate for 3 years and will use only about 6% of the available tape in the microcassette. If one assumes a more complex assignment as, say, recording groups of 200 bytes at a periodicity of 10 min., one will collect 10,000 such groups over a period of 1667 hrs. which is about 10 weeks. During that time we will have recorded 24×10^6 bits (2×10^6 bytes) and the device will have incremented 6×10^6 times.

It is estimated that a total of 1268 ma-hrs. will be required to accomplish the foregoing with a 21% safety factor.

I note that this particular example could easily represent the recording of the occurrence of a number of ECG waveforms recorded when heart rate exceeds or falls below given limits, also recorded would be average heart rate per hour and of course, date and time of day when ECG's are recorded.

It is part of the beauty of the BIDAR design that as a function of the problem (specific sort of data acquisition) assigned, the system can be programmed to optimize the energy use-factor of each functional component of the system. Now with specific examples of data acquisition behind us, let us look at Figure 2 which will give one an idea of the capacity of a 90-minute microcassette tape.

Datum (bit words)	Sample Freq. (min)	Total No. of Data Groups	Duration to Full Tape
1-8	5	3.99×10^6	38.0 yrs
10-8	1	3.99×10^5	9.1 mos
"	5	"	3.8 yrs
"	10	"	7.6 yrs
30-8	5	1.33×10^5	1.26 yrs
"	10	"	2.52 yrs
"	30	"	7.56 yrs
200-8	10 (est.)	1.99×10^4	4.56 mos

Figure 2. ESTIMATED CAPACITY FOR STANDARD 90-MINUTE CASSETTE

One must remember that in certain cases the two AA - lithium cells we plan to use in our standard unit may not suffice. Certainly, we do not have batteries with 38-year lifetimes.

Figure 3 shows a tracing of a raw playback from a microcassette tape where the data were recorded at 4700 bpi. Signal level and S/N ratio is extremely good. Figure 4 illustrates seven nibbles after amplification and squaring. Figure 5 represents our estimates of the shape and size of the developed BIDARS package. As one can see it is about 160 cc and is expected to weigh about 150 g. (5.4 oz)

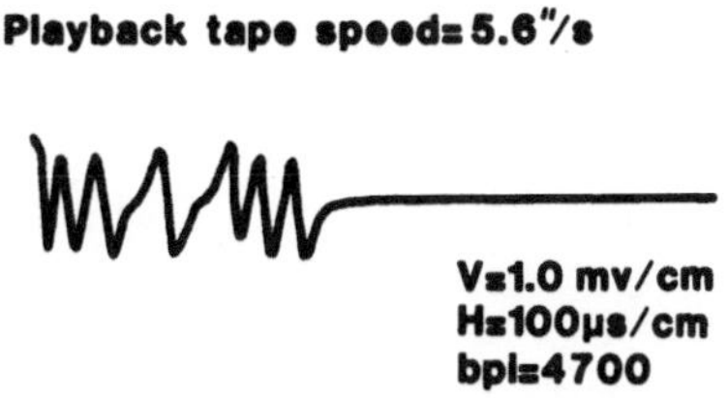

Playback tape speed= 5.6"/s

V=1.0 mv/cm
H=100µs/cm
bpi=4700

Figure 3. RAW PLAYBACK SIGNAL
1 Mv, pk-pk (1-track shown)

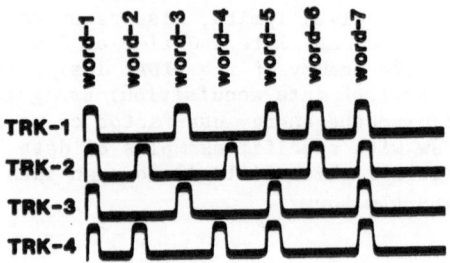

Figure 4.   7-NIBBLE PLAYBACK AFTER GAIN AND SQUARING

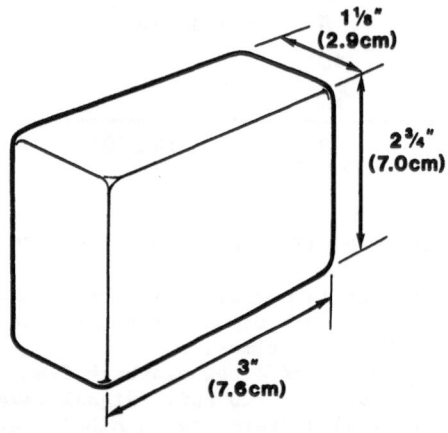

Figure 5.   PROJECTED FORM-FACTOR FOR BIDARS

Computing in Medical Chronobiology; practical aspects of data collection, analysis and instrumentation.

Knapp, Martin S./Gordon, K.
Unit of Medical Information Technology
Department of Obstetrics and Gynaecology and
Department of Mathematics
University Hospital, Nottingham, U.K.

Introduction

Investigations of rhythmic events in biology and medicine involve the study of individuals. Adequate account of this fact must be taken when planning studies to consider the importance of rhythms, espcially in pharmacology and in therapeutics, so that the rhythmic information can be used to improve the treatment of individuals (Knapp, 1984).

Consideration of data from groups of subjects studied to consider whether rhythms are present, or to establish whether rhythms are an influence on drug absorption, activity, excretion, toxicity or on the effectiveness of treatment involve, as a first step, the study of individuals. In such studies there is usually more data collected than can easily be considered using manual methods of data collection, presentation and analysis. In medical care the emphasis has always been on the individual about whom decisions must be made. Group information, collected earlier, is used to help make these decisions, but it is the set of data from one individual that is of most relevance to patient care.

A feature of monitoring, that is becoming increasingly common, is that more facts are collected than can be presented or analysed using current methods. Neither people or equipment using biological signals in control mechanisms take little account of rhythmicity, partly because they are already swamped by an excess of unanalysed or inadequately analysed data. Consideration of rhythmicity can be of great importance when information is to be used to influence, or even control, treatment. Computers should now be used to store information, collected "on line" whenever possible, and to analyse, present it and use it. A search for rhythms graphically coupled with the appropriate analysis is now feasible "on-line", making applied chronobiology a more practical possibility, and the use of equipment on a closed 'feed back' loop is a feasibility.

132

Certain aspects of how best to use computers to assist in chronobiology have taken much of our attention, and form the material for this paper. The difficulty of resolving certain problems, that arose in the analysis of time series with the use of statistical methods currently used by chronobiologists, led us to develop new methods for analysis and for presentation. These are now available for use, "on-line" in certain situations. An outline of some of these new methods are included in this summary of techniques, both old and new, that we feel are useful in the consideration of time series, whether for rhythms or for event detection or both.

Fig. 1. Plasma Creatinine (P.Cr) improves after kidney transplantation. Results are best considered as the reciprocal (1/P.Cr), as P.Cr is inversely related to renal function. Weight changes, due to changes of body fluid (dehydration and rehydration), cause dilution and concentration of plasma creatinine: these can be "corrected" for by calculations when P.Cr is used to indicate renal function (as on right), allowing timing of the event. Kidney graft rejection is detected on day 23. If an event can be timed correctly, by graphical presentation or by stistical analysis as a time series it can be considered chronobiologically.

Fig. 1

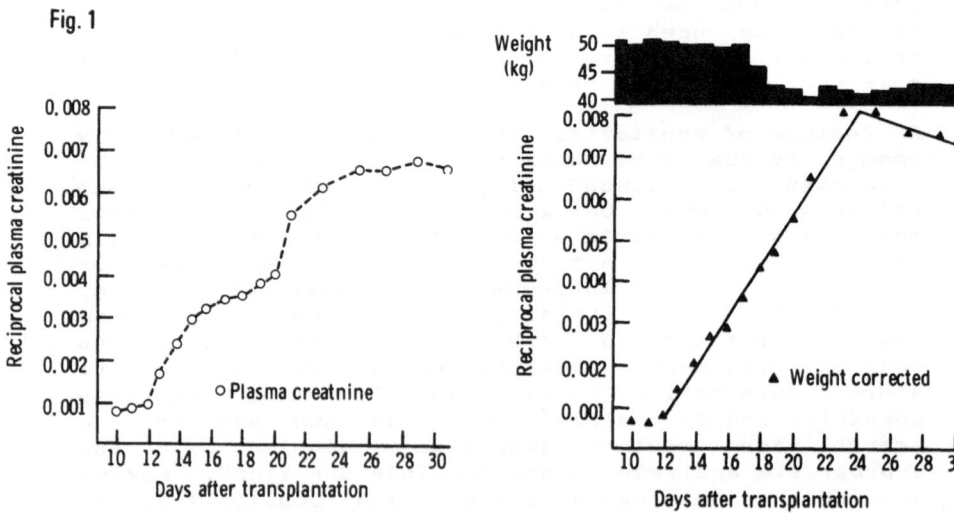

Relationships between time and the displayed data may
be seen, and these may then call for statistical
validation. The patterns observed may bring rhythmic
or episodic events to the attention of the observer.
The potential to consider presentations of data after
different transformations, or modifications, is
sometimes essential, e.g. to the logarithm or to the
reciprocal as in fig 1(Gore, 1982), by factoring (e.g.
by dividing plasma urea by plasma creatinine to
identify catabolic events) or by some adjustment to
reduce the influence of another variable as (e.g.
weight adjustments to allow for changing body fluid
content as in fig 1 (Knapp et al, 1979 and 1983)).
Data interpretation becomes a great deal easier when
the use of such an adjustment reduces "noise", and so
the true patterns in the data become more plainly
visible (fig 1).

Fig. 2

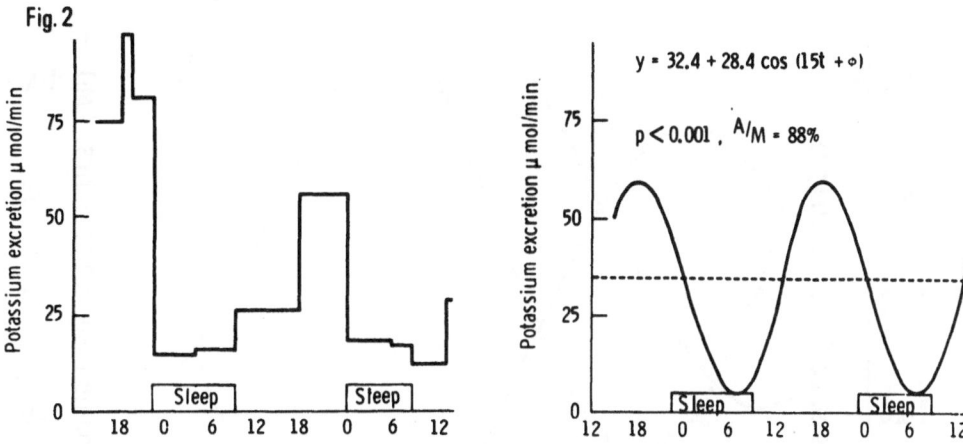

Fig. 2. Potassium excretion data, from urine collected
every four hours, is shown as a histogram display.
This shows excretion as the average flow over each 4
hour period. Cosinor analysis provides high
probability (p< 0.001) of the data fitting a fitted
sine wave, and the fitted curve appears to imply a
smooth rhythmic output with a rhythm of equal amplitude
each day (A/M is the value for the mesor (M), dotted
line, as a percentage of the amplitude (A) of the best
fitting sine wave with a period of 24 hours. Displays
of the actual data demonstrate visually day to day
variations in pattern. Neither presentation reflects
the true pattern which would require continuous
recording of both urine excretion and of potassium.

The ability to create a model of a rhythm, statistically validated as a fit to the data, allows interrelationships to be considered.

Fig 3. Data of Pownall, Knapp and others presenting three calculated "best-fit" sine waves, to demonstrate three variables collected as time-series and studied for rhythms and their interrelationships.

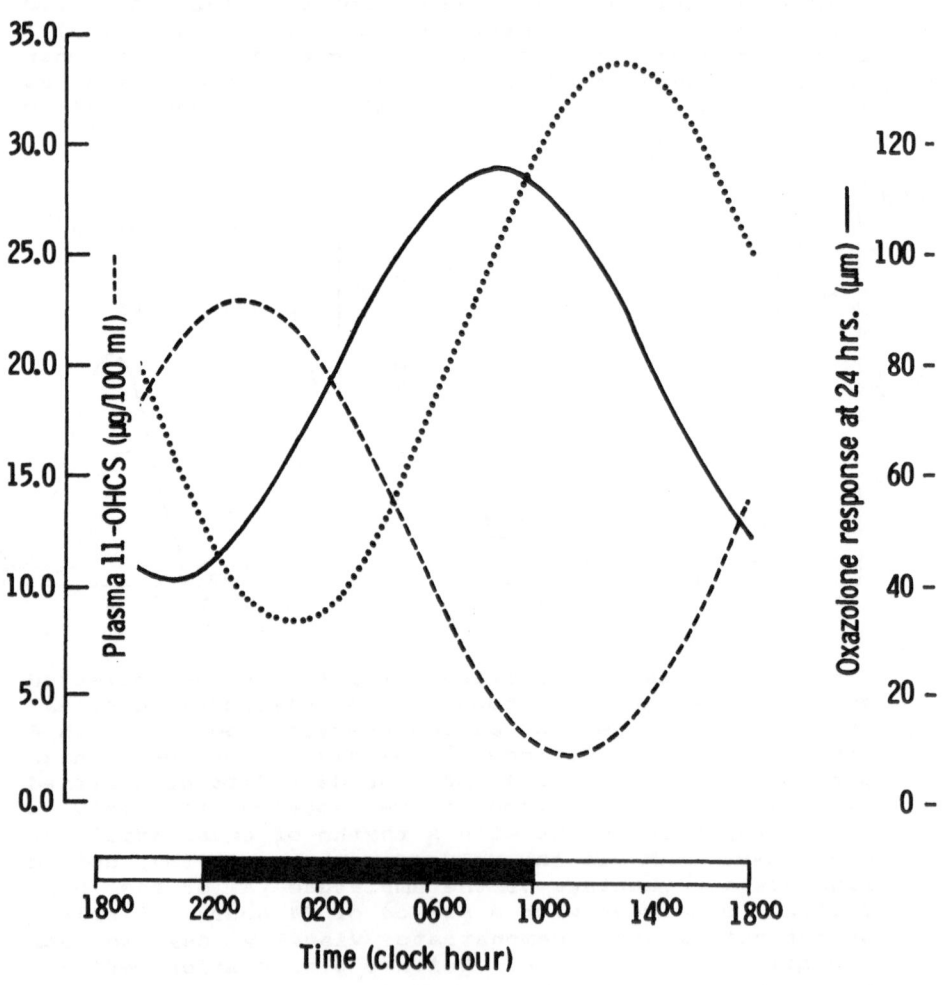

Microcomputer Systems

Programmes are now available that allow physicians to use chronobiological methods, but usually only in units where an interest in medical chronobiology has developed alongside an interest in computing methods. It is when systems incoporate graphical & statistical methods that practical systems for clinicians result. Such systems have been developed by our team by an experienced clinician and chronobiologist (MSK), a statistician (KG) and a systems analyst/computer programmer (G. Dowling), all with an interest in rhythm analysis and clinical care. The system design is for the BBC microcomputer, but can be transferred, & is based on experiences gained by two decades of using main frame computing facilities to analyse clinical data, and 5 years of using a mini-computer for data handling in renal units, with subsequent experience in other specialised units, wards and clinics; incorporating, when appropriate, chronobiological methods. These points are made to emphasise that providing computer software that is functional and useful takes a great deal of time. Clinical users, research workers and systems analysts need familiarity with the problems of computing in a clinical setting.

Statistical Modelling and Event Detection incorporating Chronobiology

There are still rather few examples of modelling and statistical filtering techniques in practical use in medicine. An experienced team is again needed to make techniques effective in clinical situations

Our experience has been in collaboration with Prof. A. F. M. Smith, and has now involved over ten years of mathematical research, and further time in programme writing and testing. This is only one of many experiences that illustrate the importance of starting new programming projects on the basis of existing knowledge and not with a "blank" sheet of paper or "blank" computer disc. From this base we anticipate that problems in many specialties can be tackled using a similar approach, but with a careful initial analysis for similarities and differences. The next phase of development could be the transferrable "package". As with the Cosinor, which is an early example of a retrospective method based on modelling, there will be problems if new methods are used without some understanding of the objectives and limitations.

Fig 4. On-line event detection should consider each new incoming item of information, and consider statistically if it could reasonably be expected from previous information on the patterns of information; taking into account the variability ('noise') in previous data. Change points with rhythm change, if instantaneous, may be indicated by as few as two points in a sequence of incoming information if in an unexpected, but anticipated, relationship to the previous pattern. Statistical methods that when first developed took no account of rhythmicity have now been modified to incorporate the reality that clinically important sequences of data are rhythmic(Knapp, Smith,Trimble,Pownall,Gordon, 1983).

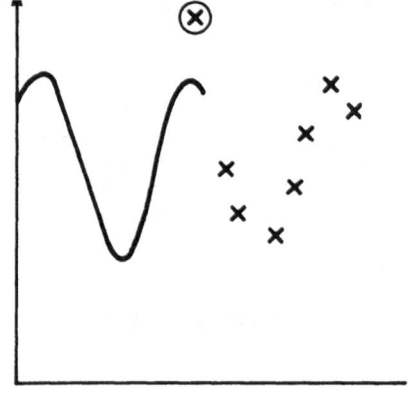

Simulated data illustrating change points when a rhythm changes, detectable with a calculated probability value using recent modifications of the Kalman Filter technique.

Transient

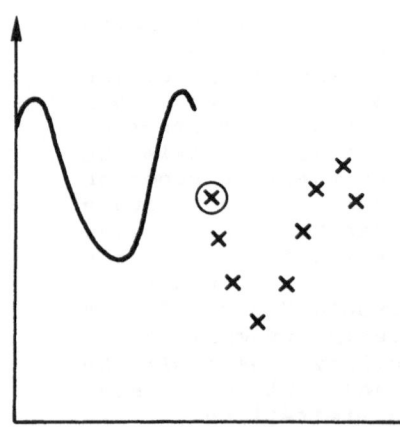

Level change

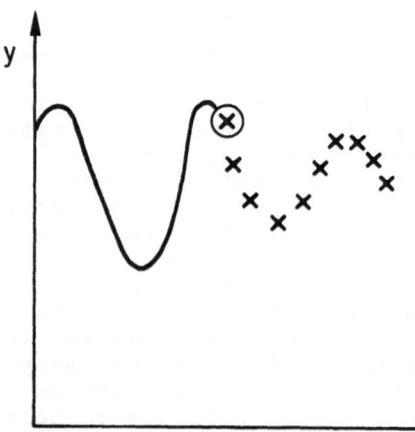

Amplitude change

Practical aspects of Chronobiological Computing

Those who embark on creating their own system need to
be aware of the problems, and the use of programmes
already created by others is almost always the most
cost effective route to take. In this case, the
programmes can be available on desk top microcomputers
in the range of £1,000 to £5,000, for less than 10% of
the cost of the equipment, but the cost of creating a
functional system using a local programming team can
easily extend to the £10-100,000 price bracket if time
is costed.

Some groups, including our own, have a long experience
of using more expensive mini-computers for analysis,
and one of the most suitable comprehensive systems for
this purpose that we recommend continues to improve
beyond that which has already been well documented
(Gordon et al 1982), and needs funds of over £25,000 to
implement. There will, it can be anticipated, be an
increasing number of easily portable and transferrable
chronobiological computer "packages" available, but
other than those with which we are associated, only
that of Viteck is known to us at the present time. Our
own programmes are to be expanded and made available
for a range of computers and for boards to incorporate
as part of instrumentation.

Those micro systems described are among rather few
available incorporating rhythm analysis for those who
cannot afford larger comprehensive systems. The mini
systems described by Gordon et al has, in the opinion
of the author, the most potential of the systems in the
intermediate price-ranges i.e. in the mini-computer
range. The sophistication of the data organisation and
graphical programmes used by Gordon and his colleagues,
now further developed by his group and ours, provides a
system to store a large proportion of all the data
about patients and can now incorporate chronobiological
presentations. This makes that system one that can be
considered to have a very wide potential, after linkage
to appropriate statistical programmes to supply the
needs of chronobiologists. This computer system is now
installed in the majority of U.K. Dialysis and
Transplant Units and in many specialty units ranging
from cardiothoracic units to oncology and bone marrow
transplantation units. In intensive care units and in
obstetrics clinics there are obvious advantages in
having such systems, and they have now been adapted for
these situations. Now that there is extensive clinical
experience of computer use for non-chronobiological
functions there is an obvious need to use methods that
analyse, chronobiologically.

Progress in monitoring function in most clinical situations allows analyses for rhythms of those variables that are important in the disorder or condition being monitored. The data exists in clinical databases, and the techniques are now available to analyse it. It is time and motivation that is lacking - so few doctors have an interest or an expertise in chronobiology, and those that do often work without relevant on-site computing.

Statistics and computer graphics, both chronobiological and non-chronobiological, have usually only been available by arrangement with Research units or University Departments. This has restricted their use mainly to research, when the real contribution could be in the day to day care of patients. Technical developments make this next phase both practical and, with good decisions, inexpensive. A major contribution of chronobiologists to clinical care could be to encourage and help clinical teams to acquire appropriate computer based information systems, and so help to bring more awareness of the relevance of clinical chronobiology; and also to incorporate a chronobiological awareness into devices used for therapy especially "closed loop" feedbacks from physiological signals.

Small effective computer systems, located in the laboratory or the office, can perform many other functions besides generating graphs and computing retrospective statistics of group data. They make available considerable computational power, and a substantial amount of computer 'memory' for storing both programmes and data. Improvements in technology now make it feasible to provide on-line statistical monitoring of individuals. These facilities seem to be the minimum needed if clinical teams are to incorporate the more graphically and mathematically based approaches to considering data into the daily care of their patients. These approaches are now being described as useful by chronobiologists and have been accepted, by some as being of value in the care of certain groups of patients; the most convincing examples, perhaps, being in rheumatology, oncology, respiratory medicine and in the consideration of data on psychological testing & in organ and tissue transplantation monitoring. The administration of treatment after transplantation, has been one of our main interests, and monitoring of the fetal allograft (i.e. a pregnancy) is now also a major area of potential exploration.

Fig 5. A three dimensional presentation that displays
the result of statistical chronobiological analysis of
sequential sets of data. The picture can be sen at a
glance to be "jagged", or multimodal. This indicates an
uncertainty as to the 'true' whereabouts of the phase
(on the 24 hour clock). The uncertainty persists even
after 100 sets of data points had been considered,
suggesting that a sinusoidal model was a poor fit to
the data; display created by KG, using University of
Nottingham computer (Pownall, Gordon, Smith & Knapp,
1984). An example of how a picture can give information
at a glance, as with the Cosinor plots of Halberg.

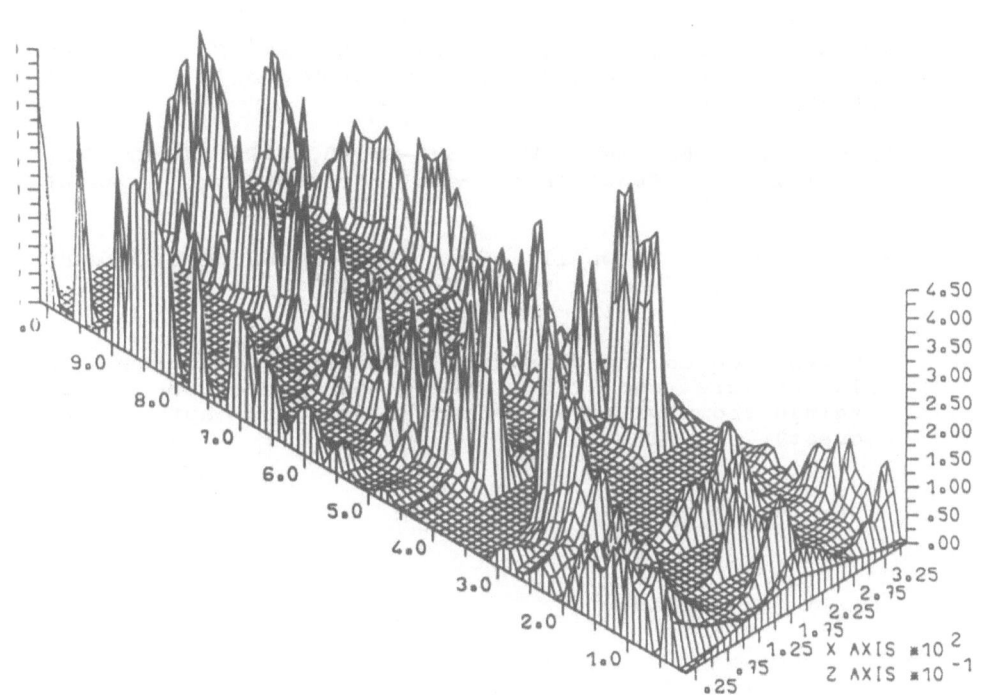

References:

Knapp, M.S., Chronotherepeutics - the importance of the individual and the need for an individual approach in therapeutic trials and in therapy, in Annual Review of Chronopharmacology, Biological Rhythms and Medications (Editors: Reinberg, A., Smolensky, M., Labrecque, G.,) Pergamon, Osford: Vol 1: 365-368 1984.

Knapp, M.S., Chronobiology: a subject of importance to the rheumatologist? Br. J. Clin Pract. Symp. Suppl. 33, (Chronobiology and Chronotherapeutics): 1-7 1984.

Gordon, J.M., Venn, C., Gower, P.E., de Wardener H.E., Experience in the computer handling of clinical data for dialysis and transplantation units: Kidney Int. Vol. 24: 455-463 1983.

Perkins, W.J., Green, R.J., Three-dimensional reconstruction of Biological Sections. J. Biomed. Eng. 4, 37-43. 1982.

Nelson, W., Tong, Y.L., Lee J.K., Halberg, F. Methods for cosinor-rhythmometry. Chronobiologia 6 (4): 305-323 1979.

Knapp, M.S., Blamey, R.W., Cove-Smith, J.R., Heath, M., Monitoring the function of renal transplants: Lancet 2: 1183, 1977.

Knapp, M.S., Pownall, R., Time of day of allograft rejection: Br. Med J. 1 : 749-753 1979.

(Information on the Computer Programmes described in this article and fact sheets on where they can be obtained from will be provided by the authors on request).

HUMAN THERMOMETRY IN HEALTH AND DISEASE

THE CHRONOBIOLOGIST'S PERSPECTIVE

(A) SELECTED EVENTS IN THE CHRONOLOGY OF INSTRUMENTATION AND OBSERVATION.

(B) AMBULATORY INSTRUMENTS

    (I) Introduction

    (II) A tabulation of characteristics

(C) APPENDIX

    (I) Subcutaneous temperature measurement by microwave thermography (by Dr. D.V. Land).

    (II) Factors in the interpretation of human circadian temperature data.

        (i) Physiological
        (ii) Pathological

        Compiled by H.W. Simpson (Glasgow)
           in collaboration with:

W. Gruen	(New York)
E. Halberg	(Minneapolis)
F. Halberg	(Minneapolis)
P. Knauth	(Dortmund)*
D.V. Land	(Glasgow)
R. Moog	(Marburg)**
J. + J. Nougier	(Paris)
A. Reinberg	(Paris)
M. Smolensky	(Houston)
D. Wilson	(Cardiff)

* Representing Laboratory of Professor Rutenfranz

** Representing Laboratory of Professor Hildebrandt

(A)   SELECTED EVENTS IN THE CHRONOLOGY OF
      INSTRUMENTATION AND OBSERVATION
      (Observations in **BOLD** type)

1592-97
      The invention of a graduated air expansion thermometer
by Galilei of Padua University. This consisted of a glass
bulb to which was attached a graduated glass tube. The end
of this tube was inserted into a container of coloured
liquid. The liquid rose up the tube (presumably a partial
vacuum had been created in the bulb by heat beforehand).
On exposure to a higher temperature, the air in the bulb
expanded and the fluid was driven back downwards into the
reservoir. This instrument, which was the forerunner of
the modern liquid in glass clinical thermometer was,
however, not entirely satisfactory because variations in
atmospheric pressure from day to day altered the "zero"
setting.

1611
      **Sauctorius Justipolatauus used the Galilei thermometer
to observe temperature changes in fever patients at Padua
University.**

1632-1641
      From Galilei's invention it was a comparatively small
step to contain the liquid in a hermetically sealed glass
bulb with a fine tube attached. This thermometer was first
brought into general use by the Grand Duke Ferdinand II of
Tuscany. Alcohol was the liquid first employed and
"degrees" were marked as small beads of enamel fused on the
stem. The problem was that if somebody elsewhere made a
thermometer it could not be comparable.

1694
      Renaldini proposed the temperature of freezing and
boiling of water as the fixed points on the scale.

1709-1714
      Fahrenheit built alcohol and mercury (in glass)
thermometers. Following Renaldini's proposal these were
scaled 32° and 212° for freezing and boiling water. (His
idea was that body temperature at 100° should be a key
value. Perhaps his subjects were slightly fevered or his
thermometers inaccurate because normal body temperature on
the Fahrenheit scale is about 98°F).

1736   **de Gorter made what are probably the first
descriptions of the variation in human body temperature
throughout the day.**

1743

The centigrade scale was established where 0° was the freezing and 100° the boiling point of water respectively.

1799

Herschell detects radiation (now known as infra-red) beyond the red end of the sun's visible spectrum.

1821

Seebeck discovers that junctions at different temperatures in an electric circuit generate an E.M.F. - the so-called thermoelectric effect.

1836

Pouillet exploits the thermoelectric effect to measure temperature. He used an iron platinum thermocouple and tangent galvanometer to measure temperature.

1839 Hunter; 1842 Gierse; 1844 Halman and 1845 Davie

All these scientists made physiological measurements of body core temperature and its variation. Davie made particularly detailed studies under relatively controlled conditions. He measured his body temperature every 3 hours throughout the day and stayed indoors and kept his physical activity fairly constant. Under these conditions he found that his temperature varied from 97.6°F at 0.7^{00} to 98.9°F at 16^{00}. Particularly, he noticed that the body temperature when he went to bed was often colder than that recorded during the day in spite of the fact that the room was often warmer.

1852

Baerensprung measured body temperature in man and concluded that the lowest body temperature was at 04^{00} and a maximum at about 18^{00}. (If a contemporary chronobiologist was asked to give the expected maximum and minimum of temperature for man on diurnal activity these would probably be the figures he would give today).

1853

Damrosch observed that body temperature rose from 07^{00} until 10^{00} fell until 13^{00} to reach a maximum at 17^{00}.

1866 Ogle undertook detailed observations of the daily body temperature rhythm in man. He noted that the morning rise of body temperature occurred when the subject was still asleep and that the fall in the evening occurred when he was still awake. He deduced that the changes in the resting individual were not immediately driven by the environment but were probably induced by periodic variations in the activity of organic function. Ogle also discovered that the rhythm persisted during bed rest throughout the day and that the morning rise still occurred when light was excluded.

<u>1871</u> - Seimens used resistance thermometers for temperature measurement. These dependend on a new principle namely that electrical resistance (of a pure metal) increases as the temperature is raised.

<u>1887</u>
Mosso made temperature observations before and for a few days after changing from day to night work. His data suggested there was only a gradual "adaptation" to the new schedule.

<u>1888</u> - Chappuis uses a hydrogen gas thermometer for precision calibration of mercury in glass thermometers.

<u>1893</u> - Wein formulated the displacement law for thermal radiation.

<u>1901</u> - Planck described the radiation formula for black body radiation.

<u>1906</u> - Northrock used electrical resistance thermometry to make continuous recordings of body temperature.

<u>1913</u> - Lindhard studying explorers in Greenland found (sometimes) a rise in rectal temperature during the night in the Arctic winter.

<u>1915</u>   Du Bois first determined total body heat production by indirect calorimetry. The respiration calorimeter sited at the Russell Sage Institute of Pathology, also measured heat loss by the direct method. Vapourisation was measured by absorbing the water vapour in bottles of sulphuric acid which were weighed. Heat loss by radiation and convection were measured by the temperature changes in the measured stream of cold water flowing in the pipes near the top of the calorimeter. The method, however, did not distinguish between convection and radiation.

<u>1920</u> - Recording thermometers for clinical work became available. These were a resistance thermometer of the usual pattern, namely platinum wire wound on a microcross and enclosed in a silver sheath.

1920 cont'd.

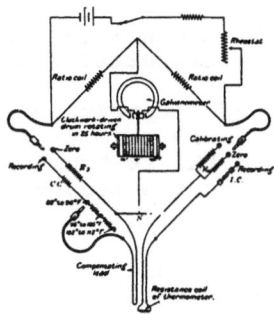

Recording thermometer for clinical work described by Mr.
R.S. Whipple in a paper to the Journal of the Institution
of Electrical Engineers.

1922 - Description of temperature changes in women during
the menstrual cycle (Cullis, Oppenheimer and
Ross-Johnson).

1924   Moll observed that the surface temperature of the
lactating breast was higher than the axillary temperature.
If the milk secretion stops, the breast temperature falls.
When one beast secretes milk and the other does not, the
temperature of the secreting breast is higher than the
non-lactating breast.

1925   Heusler discovered that the temperature of the breast
in normal non-pregnant women was lower than axillary
temperature. In pregnant women the temperature was either
the same or higher than the axillary temperature.

1934. Hardie devised a radiometer. It consisted of 8 black
and tinfoil receiving elements made up of 8 bismuth alloy
thermocouples and 8 compensating thermocouples. Radiation
heat was focussed by means of a silver cone so that all
radiation heat fell on a blackened disc. Hardie's data
indicated that in the resting human subject, 58% of heat
was lost by radiation, 15% by convection and 27% by
vapourisation.

1939. Kleitman published "Sleep and Wakefulness". He made
important observations on what was then called the "diurnal
variation" of body temperature. The word diurnal is, of
course confusing because it can mean a 24 hour cycle.
Alternatively, it can be the antithesis of nocturnal. In
much physiological writing, the word diurnal is ambiguous,
the writer leaving it an open question as to whether the
observed cyclical changes are due to the diurnal activities

of the subject e.g. muscular activity, diet and posture, or that the observed 24 hour cycle is to some extent endogenous. Kleitman's observations included the following.

1. Posture effect. If a man lies down after standing for 1 hour his body temperature may drop by 0.2°C.

2. The 24 hour rhythm of temperature appears in the second year of life. In view of the posture effects, Kleitman interpreted the 24 hour rhythm of temperature as being mainly due to the assumption of the upright posture and walking.

3. He studied body temperature in human subjects subjected to day/night cycle lengths totalling 12, 21, 28 and 48 hours. He found that the usual 24 hour cycle of temperature was modified in some but in others it was not changed at all.

4. He lived in the Mammoth cave, Kentucky, with an associate for one month. This was an important experimental breakthrough because it meant that certain diurnal factors such as temperature and light could be controlled. Obviously such methodological points were important if one was to understand the factors in the 24 hour temperature rhythm (of course in the 17th century, cellars had been used to provide steady environmental conditions for the study of the 24 hour leaf movements in plants, and in them this is how endogeneity was proved). Kleitman and his colleague adopted a 28 hour day (19 awake hours; 9 hours in bed). In one subject the observed temperature cycle corresponded to 28 hours but in the other subject, a 24 hour cycle persisted.

5. His Scandinavian travels prompted him to suggest that the Arctic might be a natural laboratory for those wishing to study non-24 hour environments.

1954 Halberg described the effect of optic enucleation on the daily temperature rhythm of mice. Rectal temperatures were measured every 4 hours using mercury and glass thermometers for 48 days in sham-operated controls and test animals deprived of light perception. Whereas the controls had an invariable group mean temperature peak at 20.30 in the 12:12 lighting conditions, the test animal group mean peak occurred systematically earlier each day. In other words the periodicity of their temperature rhythm had become shorter than 24 hours. By day 22/23 after operation, it had accumulated a 12 hour lead so that the animals deprived of light perception were in temperature antiphase with their litter mates. (See following figure).

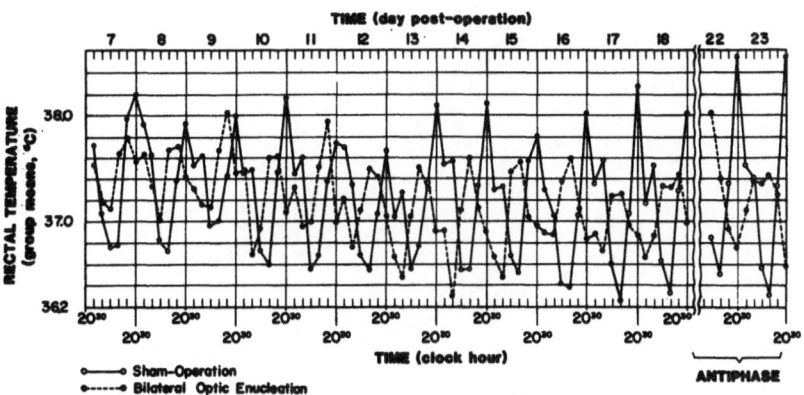

CIRCADIAN DESYNCHRONIZATION AFTER BILATERAL OPTIC ENUCLEATION

This study, more than any other, led the way to our contemporary understanding of the control of the 24 hour rhythm in mammals. Earlier observations had provided hints about the endogeneity of temperature rhythms (e.g. the 1840 observation by Davie that body temperature was cooler on retiring to bed in the evening than during the day, even though the room temperature was generally warmer). Classical physiology had a reactionary effect on the acceptance of an endogenous temperature rhythm; observed changes were dismissed and interpreted as reactions to the diurnal environment such as the effects of food, sleep, posture (see discussion by du Bois 1940). When one reads the establishment literature on body temperature, there is always a tendency to adhere to the homeostatic concept i.e. of an average temperature with deviations from that average for reasons of environmental effect e.g. meals, posture, exercise or, of course, fever.

1956. Lawson establishes a link between breast cancer and heat emission. This led to widespread interest in a cheap thermographic screening process especially since the infra red technology was common to the missile detectors being produced in the arms race.

1959. Halberg introduces the word "circadian".

1970. The Zenith of clinical thermography using instruments such as the AGA thermovision camera scan below.

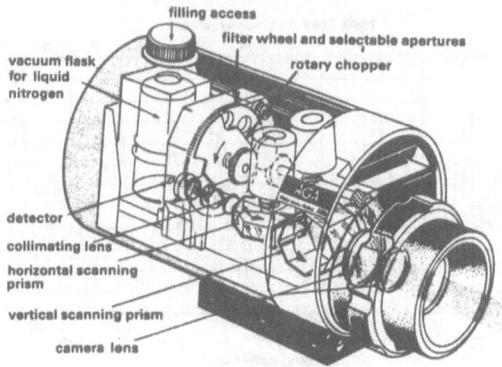

1971. Fox and Solman described the transcutaneous measurement of deep body temperature. The methodology is illustrated in the following diagram.

Cross section of the sensing probe

1. Electrically heated layer.
2. Thermistors.
3. Insulating layer.

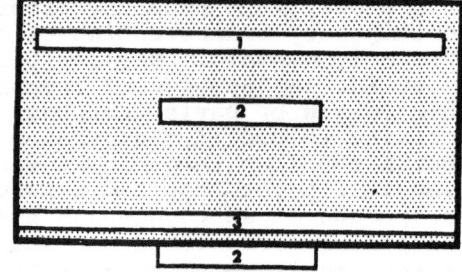

The two thermistors in the probe are connected to a comparator. If the outer sensor records a lower temperature than the inner skin sensor, the comparator switches on the heating circuit until the two signals become identical. This on and off cycling of the heater unit results in the net flow of heat across the probe approximating to zero. The inner skin thermostat is also wired via an amplifier to a recording meter which has a range from 29 to 42°C. The equilibration time is reduced by allowing the heating element to be switched on continuously until 37°C is achieved, thereafter the on and off cycling is continued until equilibrium takes place.

1972. First reports of the effects of suprachiasmatic nucleus ablation on circadian rhythms (Moore and Eichler, 1972; Stephen and Zucker, 1972). These and other studies which followed from them prompted discussion by some that the suprachiasmatic nucleus might be the circadian pacemaker. (These suggestions led to many more investigations which refuted the pacemaking role of the suprachiasmatic nucleus - see entry under Halberg 1977 and Fuller et al 1981).

1973. Mansfield, Carabasi, Wells and Borman make the first descriptions of the circadian rhythm of breast surface temperature overlying breast cancer. They concluded: (1) the non-cancerous breast (the control side) exhibits a phase and frequency synchronised rhythm with a period at or close to 24 hours and an acrophase in the late evening or early morning hours; and (2) the cancerous breast also exhibits a phase and frequency synchronised rhythm (at or close to 24 hours), but the acrophase is earlier and the amplitude is less. These observations were confirmed in 1975 by Gautherie and Gross.

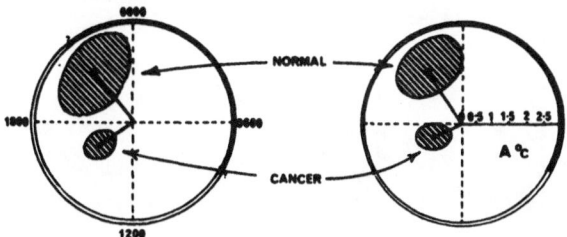

TRANSVERSE COSINOR CHRONOTHERMOGRAPHY OF HUMAN BREAST CANCER: circadian acrophase differences between surface temperatures over the tumour and from a matched contralateral site.

AUTHORS:	Mansfield, Carabasi, Wells & Borman (1973)	Gautherie & Gross (1975)
PATIENTS:	N = 14♀ (△ advanced or recurrent ca.)	N = 11♀ (37–63y) Selected by criteria for slow growth

Cosine vector diagrams summarizing published temperature acrophase differences between the circadian temperature changes over the cancerous breast versus that obtained from the contralateral breast over a matched anatomical site. The normal acrophases agree with that found in normal subjects. The sensor over the cancer detects a phase lead in the circadian rhythm and also a diminished amplitude.

1976. The Solicorder, the first commercial ambulatory solid state temperature recorder became available. This was marketed by W. Gruen of Ambulatory Monitoring Incorporated, New York.

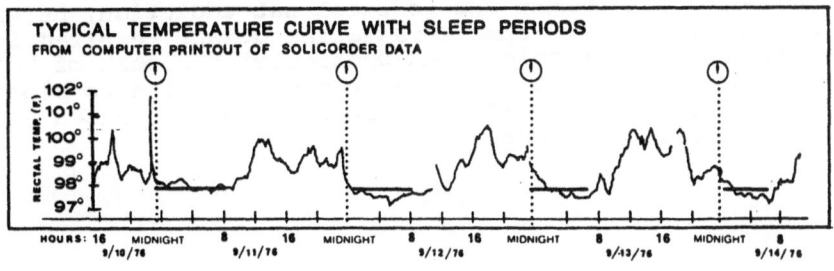

TYPICAL TEMPERATURE CURVE WITH SLEEP PERIODS
FROM COMPUTER PRINTOUT OF SOLICORDER DATA

150

1977. Halberg published data on the intercession of the
suprachiasmatic nucleus on the circadian rhythm of
temperature. His studies indicated that there were changes
in amplitude and acrophase of the temperature rhythm after
ablation of the suprachiasmatic nuclei but not cessation of
the rhythm. Halberg's data cast serious doubt on the
supposition that the circadian rhythm of temperature in
mammals (and also presumably man) was initiated from a
pacemaker in the nuclei.

TELEMETERED CORE TEMPERATURE OF SHAM-OPERATED RAT (C)
AND RAT WITH VALIDATED BILATERAL SUPRACHIASMATIC LESION (L)·

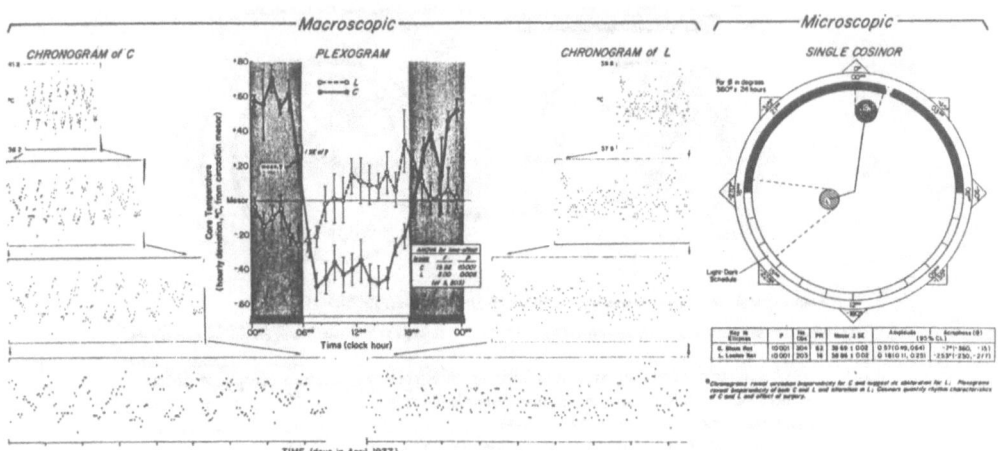

Halberg optimises radiotherapy by exploiting the
circadian rhythm of body temperature to achieve maximum
therapeutic effect. Taking advantage of the special
conditions in India where superficial squamous carcinomas
of the mouth are common due to betel nut addiction, he was
able to show that the same X-radiation dosage resulted in a
greater tumour regression when applied at the peak of body
temperature. Presumably this effect was related to blood
supply and the availability of oxygen which are known to
enhance radiation effect.

1977 cont'd.

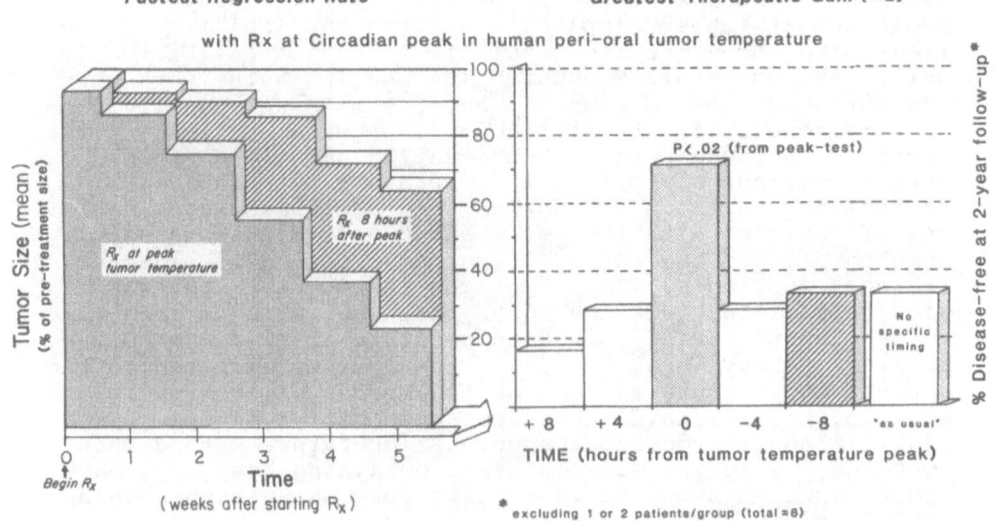

CHRONORADIOTHERAPY (Rx)

Fastest Regression Rate   *Greatest Therapeutic Gain (=2)*

with Rx at Circadian peak in human peri-oral tumor temperature

Chronoradiotherapy.   See script above.   (Data of Halberg, Gupta, Haus and many others 1977).

1981.   Fuller, Sulzman and Moore-Ede report persistence of the circadian rhythm of core temperature in primates with suprachiasmatic lesions.

(B) AMBULATORY INSTRUMENTS

I. Introduction

      The traditional clinical mercury-in-glass thermometer
is eminently portable and of high utility in fever
medicine. Its sheer simplicity and the availability in the
1960s of a more accurate "ovulation" version calibrated in
0.1°F instead of 0.2°F ensured its use in rhythm work then
and for some time to come.   The oral site was usually used
in time zone shift studies though many were critical of the
accuracy because personal observation sometimes showed
them a continuously climbing temperature with the
thermometer in the mouth for as long as 10 minutes !   This
was at variance with the recommended half minute in-situ.
Some complained the thermometer took too long to register.
In these instances, it was not the thermometer that was
slow to register, but the mouth that was taking a long time
to warm up to carotid blood temperature after a bout of
talking or heavy breathing. The thermometer will record the
correct temperature as soon as the mercury is thermally
equilibrated and this takes less than half a minute.   In
1969 Simpson introduced the urine temperature method when
confronted with the difficulty of obtaining body
temperature rhythm data in a North Pole Expedition.   This
method produced good data in explorers on the North Polar
pack in an ambient temperature of -50°C.

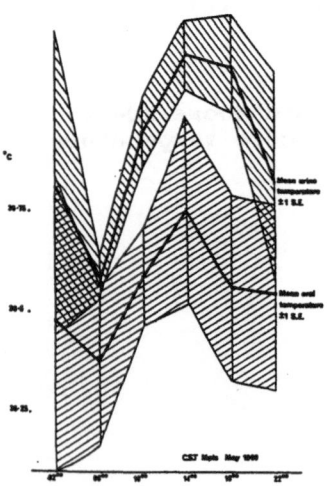

The figure illustrates 73 synoptic measurements of urine
and oral temperature in one adult male over 13 days.

Laboratory type instruments were also used at this time.

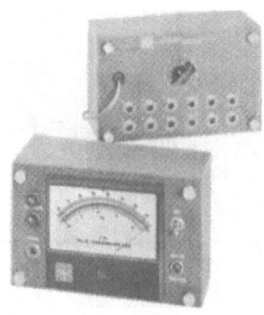

YSI Model 4002
YSI Model 43

These Yellow Springs thermometers were reliable and could
be linked to multiple thermistors (see top part of
Figure).

The model 43 illustrated had a temperature range from 30 -
41°C an accuracy of 0.1°C and a readability of 0.05°C. The
instrument was large, 19 x 9 x 12cm and weighed 1kg. Never
theless, it had its usefulness. The reason was that the
thermistors could be taped in position on the surface of
the body, and the wires led down the subject's sleeve. The
instrument was then carried round by the subject e.g. in a
handbag, and to obtain readings the subject had merely to
plug in the jack-plugs emerging from the sleeve into the
instrument and record the reading.
        Interest in circadian rhythms in the 1960s and early
1970s led to many different types of study. Bunker
isolation studies of Aschoff, Cave studies of Siffre,
Arctic studies of Lobban, and many trans-meridian flight
studies. All of these had in common a large number of
data.
        The real inadequacy of the traditional methods lay in
the labour involved in obtaining one datum and the fact
that all figures had then to be entered into the computer
by hand for time series analysis. This situation is
exemplified by the following figure:-

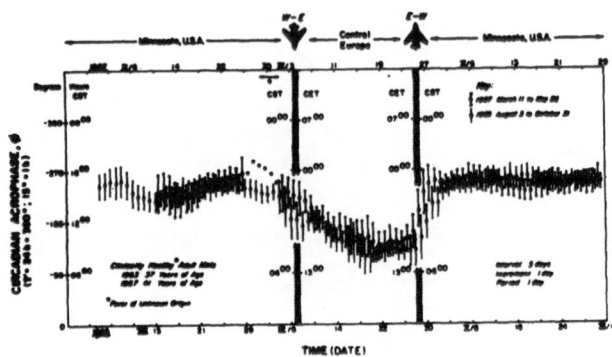

The figure illustrates phase-shifts of the circadian rhythm
in oral temperature as a result of 2 inter-continental
flights by the same subject in 1963 and 1967. Notice that
the subject adapts slowly after the east bound flight to
Europe, whereas on the return flight westward to the United
States there is a relatively rapid phase adjustment (data
of Haus and Halberg).

From such data the science could be seen to have important
practical applications to, e.g. the training of rapid
deployment forces, athletic practice, international
businessmen and airline pilot schedules. More in the
future Halberg foresaw that chronothermometry would be the
phase reference for the new chronotherapeutics especially
the drug and radiation treatment of neoplasia. Others such
as Miles and Weitzman saw that ambulatory instrumentation
was an important adjunct to the study of sleep disorders
whereas Simpson saw chronothermometry of the breast -
especially its menstrual and circadian heat rhythm - as a
means of quantifying the phenotypic abnormality in the high
risk gland that heralds neoplasia i.e. pre-emptive breast
screening. In addition, Reinberg in Paris and the Dortmund
School of Rutenfranz and Knauth had a particular interest
in optimising shift work. They all found that they needed
an ambulatory instrument which was not then available.

This pressure and the availability of solid state
technology in the late 1970s led to the host of ambulatory
devices available today.

All this sounds straightforward. Those who were
involved in the actual electronic development of the
instruments and those who bought commercial instruments
and then tried them, were beset with problems. They were
always driven forward by the lure of high data density and
the minimum handling necessary before the data were in the
computer. Time and time again after expensive trans-
atlantic flight studies there were no data on board when

the instrument reached the lab. These difficulties not only occurred with the solid state instruments, but also with the Medilog - a mini taperecording instrument which became available slightly before the solid state versions (1972).

The Medilog was evaluated in detail by Marks and Smolensky in 1976. During their ambulatory study, numerous deficiencies and difficulties were encountered. The most serious ones were:

1. Drift in calibration.
2. Variability in capstan drive speed due to battery drain, resulting in incorrect recording of events in time.
3. Data loss, especially when batteries were weak.
4. Fragility and frequent servicing required due to continual malfunction.
5. Special equipment requirement for data analysis.

These authors concluded that ambulatory recorders should have the following features:

(1) Clock for time-coding data.

(2) Inclusion of an alarm system for failing batteries or malfunction.

(3) Better calibration retention to prevent or minimise drift.

(4) Stronger construction to resist the rigor of field use.

(5) Strong lightweight materials and small size.

Halberg, too, also had many comments about the Medilog. He noted in the late 70s that the checking of tapes and the entire system of operation required some specialised engineering support. Moreover, he found that 24 hours of operation cost $10 in batteries and the audible noise of the Medilog was a drawback. In the early recorders Halberg had trouble from environmental electrical noise. This appeared to arise from such sources as hospital paging systems and static electricity.

This was also the problem with another system that was used at this time, namely FM telemetry. Mansfield at the Jefferson and Gautherie in Strasbourg both used frequency modulated telemetry to monitor human breast temperatures. Unfortunately, the hospital environment is an extremely noisy one electrically, and though the system had advantages, it is not now the general practice to use this system for human studies; but for animal studies (e.g. with intraperitoneal thermistors) it has continued to be useful in view of better environmental control.

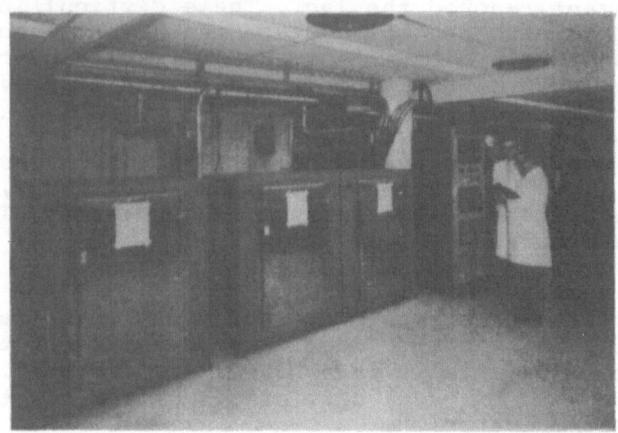

The figure shows Halbergs F.M. thermo-telemetry units for
rodents in the late 1960s. Dr. Nelson and Dr. Runge
checking the units. Data acquisition computer to right
funded by NASA for biosatellite work.

In general, designers knew that electrical noise can be
minimised by having the analogue to digital conversion
close to the point of acquisition of the temperature.

     A perennial problem with "body temperature" is to
define the variable and to identify a representative site
for its measurement. Oral temperature is about 0.6°C lower
than rectal temperature. Intra-arterial catheters have
obtained a temperature of 36°C in the brachial artery.When
the arm was exposed to cold conditions it fell to 31°C.
This means that arterial blood can cool several °C in its
rapid progress towards the periphery. With a view to
ambulatory monitoring, many sites have been assessed for
satisfactoryness in the field situation. Probably, rectal
temperature is the one that has been most commonly employed
and indeed is still employed. For some reason, subjects
are becoming increasingly intolerant of sensors in this
site, and indeed it has been difficult to obtain one which
remained in-situ and did not cause local irritation. These
problems have not been solved and hence the search for
at other possibilities e.g.,the aural cavity. Methods have
been developed to measure the colour temperature of the
eardrum, also an aural thermometer has been used to measure
deep body temperature by monitoring the actual temperature
of the cavity itself. In the latter method, a probe is
inserted into the canal and it is then plugged with cotton
wool. Since the cavity temperature then approximates to
that of the carotid blood, the method has a distinct
attraction. However it does involve wires attached to the
head and many subjects find instrumentation in the ear
uncomfortable. Reinberg has tried to overcome the problem
by monitoring body temperature with an insulated sensor on
the medial axillary wall. This has the advantage of

simplicity and that the wiring is on the trunk where it is relatively well tolerated.

What would, however, seem to be the best technology has not yet been incorporated into an ambulatory instrument. This would involve the integration of the so-called "deep body thermometer" with one of the solid state ambulatory instruments already described. The deep body thermometer works on the principle of a heated element over the sensor measuring the skin temperature. This provides just sufficient heat to zero heat flow (across the skin surface of the body) just under the sensor. This means that the surface temperature obtained is in fact a deep temperature. The latest development of this instrument is sold by Deep Body Thermometers Limited, Little Everston, Cambridge, CB3 7HE, England. The instrument is illustrated below. In terms of magnitude it gives values very close to those obtained from the ear cavity or from the rectum.

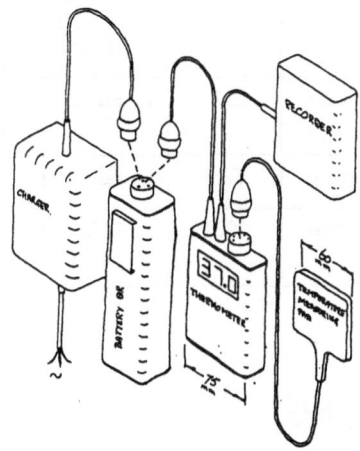

The 1985 'deep body thermometer'. An accurate reading takes about 20 mins.

(B) AMBULATORY INSTRUMENTS

(II) A tabulation of characteristics.

| NAME OF DEVICE | GENERAL DESIGN | LAUNCH DATE | ORIGINATORS | | PLACE OF ORIGIN |
			(Chrono) Biologist	Detailed design etc.	
Chronothermograph	Clockwork/ mechanical	1968	F. Halberg	K. Large	Minneapolis
Medilog	C-120 mini tape recorder	1972	F. Stott	Oxford Insts (U.K.)	Abingdon
Solicorder	Solid state	1976	E.D. Weitzman	Ambulatory Monitoring	New York
Thermolog TML 2	Solid state	1978	L. Miles	Vitalog	Palo Alto
Chronobra	Solid state	1979*	H.W. Simpson (D.W. Wilson)	D. Green	Glasgow
Dortmund Recorder	Solid state	1979	P. Knauth	H. Otto P. Dillman	Dortmund
The Collectron	Solid state	1979	(F. Halberg)	K. Veil	Zurich
Chronotherm	Solid state	1984	A. Reinberg	J. and J. Nougier	Paris

* Patented 1973

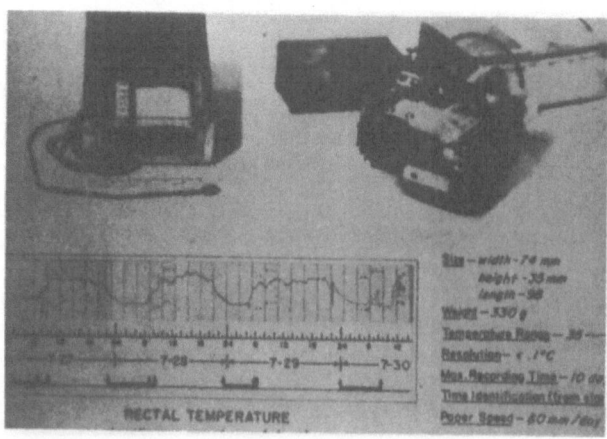

The 1968 Chronothermograph, the original ambulatory device of Halberg and Large

(II) A tabulation of characteristics cont'd.

NAME OF DEVICE	SIZE (mm)	VOLUME CM^3	WEIGHT (g)	MEMORY	ACCURACY °C
Chronothermograph	98 x 74 x 75	254	330	Direct print-out	0.10°
Medilog	121 x 90 x 39	425	ca.400	Very large indeed	0.02°
Solicorder	140 x 76 x 38	404	400	4K-16K	0.025°
Thermolog TML2	152 x 97 x 36	531	402	2K	0.20°
Chrondbra	140 x 65 x 20	182	176	4K	0.05°
Dortmund Recorder	140 x 70 x 20	196	274	2K	0.01°
The Collectron	Relatively small	INFORMATION NOT AVAILABLE			
Chronotherm	155 x 88 x 45	614	Not avail	4K	0.04°
Polychronor	Information not available at time of going to press				

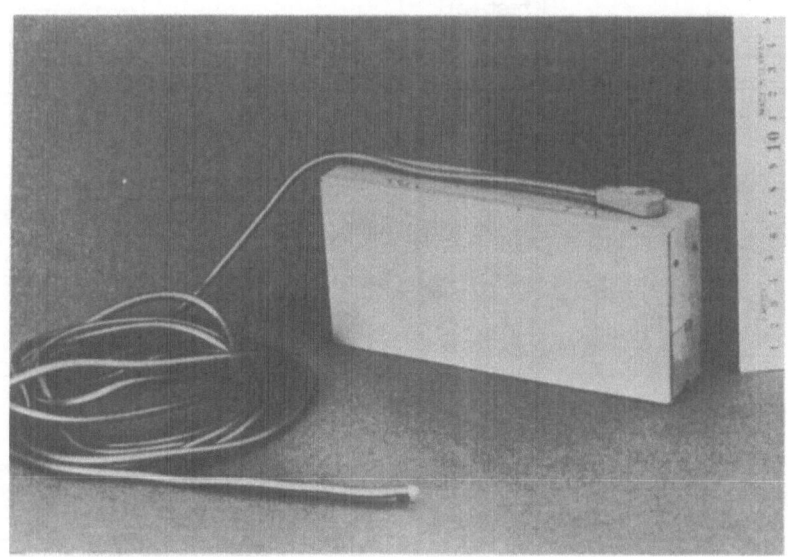

the 1979 Dortmund recorder designed by Otto and Dillman
and used in shift work studies by Knauth and Rutenfranz.

(II) A tabulation of characteristics cont'd.

NAME OF DEVICE	RECOMMENDED PROBE	USUAL SITE OF MEASUREMENTS	RANGE OF Δt OF DATA	POWER ON / STAND BY
Chronothermograph	YSI Thermistor	Rectal	Continuous data	Clockwork
Medilog	YSI 400 series	Surface or rectal	6/7 or slower	78 m w
Solicorder	YSI 400 Thermistor 44032	Usually rectal	15 sec to 12 min	Not known.3.6v lamp/hour battery.
Thermolog	YSI 702	Rectal	0.93 sec to 2 min	5 m w / 3 m w
Chronobra	Customised semi conductor junction	Breast surface	64 secs to 1.13 hours	20 m w / 1.5 m w
Dortmund Recorder	YSI Thermistor	Rectum	1 sec to 90 min	1.2 m w / 0.12 m w
The Collectron	Not available	Rectum	NO INFORMATION	
Chronotherm	YSI 409	Skin surface Chest wall	1 min – 15 min	3 m w at 180 records/hour
Polychronor	Custom	Rectum	10 mins	9v UCAR battery

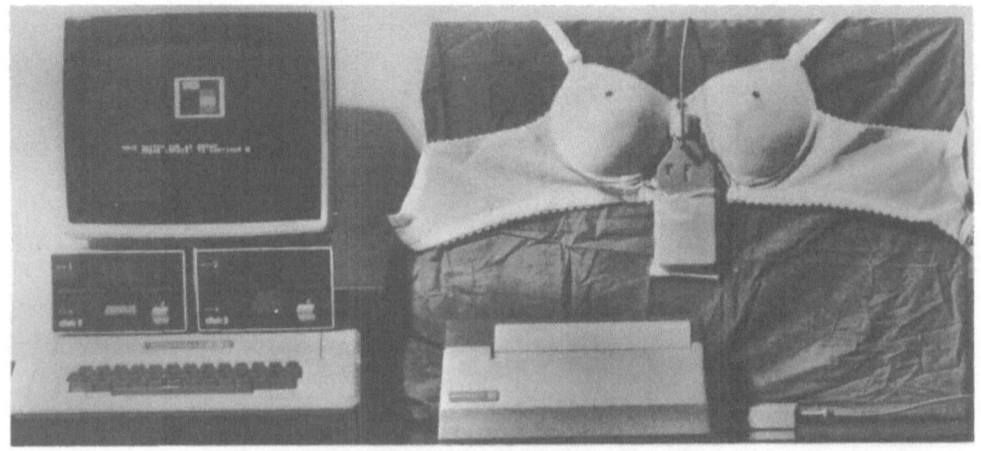

the 16 Channel Chronobra seen in the replay mode

(II) A tabulation of characteristics cont'd and finished.

NAME OF DEVICE	REPLAY	OTHER CHANNELS	SPECIAL FEATURES	RANGE ° C
Chronothermograph	Not necessary	None	Mech. Chart recorder	35-40
Medilog	Bench cassette	ECG;EEG.	Large data storage	36-38
Solicorder	Field read out device + computer interface	Actograph pulse respiration rate etc.	Commercially available 10 y.	34-40
Thermolog	Special micro replay system or PDP-11	Actograph	Carrying belt	35.5 - 42.9
Chronobra	Interface to apple computer	None	15 channels located in custom bra	c.28-37
Dortumund Recorder	Commodore SX64 infield. Also computer interface.	No	Accuracy	30-40
The Collectron	NO INFORMATION AVAILABLE			
The Chronotherm	On board or M. frame	Wrist actograph	MC 146805 low power CPU. 4K byte CMOS static RAM.	34-41
The Polychronor	Personal or mainframe	No	NOT KNOWN	

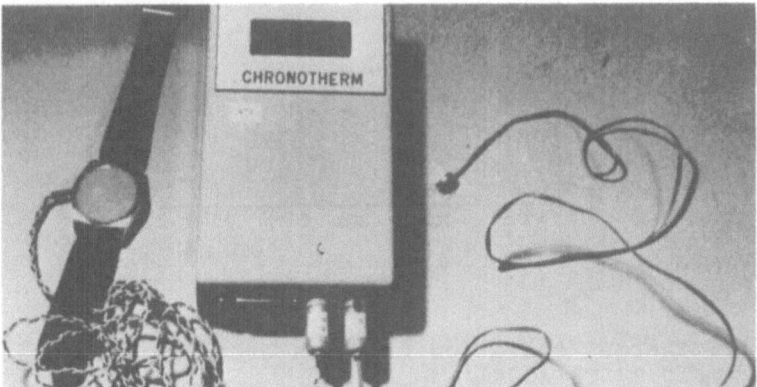

the 1985 Reinberg and Nougier's Chronotherm.
The black window on the front of the recorder displays successively a set of particulars allowing the subject to know the last figures recorded, the time, etc. On the left, the actometer in form of a wrist watch. On the right the thermal probe.

HUMAN THERMOMETRY IN HEALTH AND DISEASE   CONT'd.

(c)   Appendix

    (1)   Subcutaneous temperature measurement by
        microwave thermography by D. V. Land.

1. Introduction

    Microwave thermography is the technique of measuring
the natural thermal radiation of the tissues of the body in
the microwave or centimetric wavelength region of the
electromagnetic spectrum (Fig. 1).

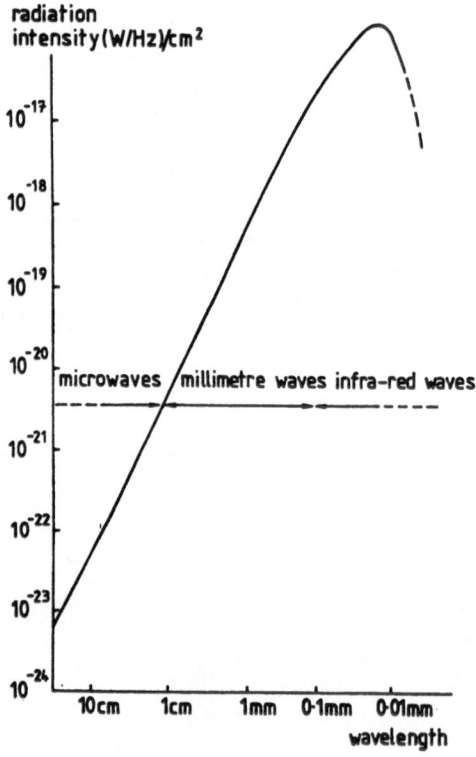

Fig. 1.   Thermal radiation from a source at a temperature
        of 37°C (310K).

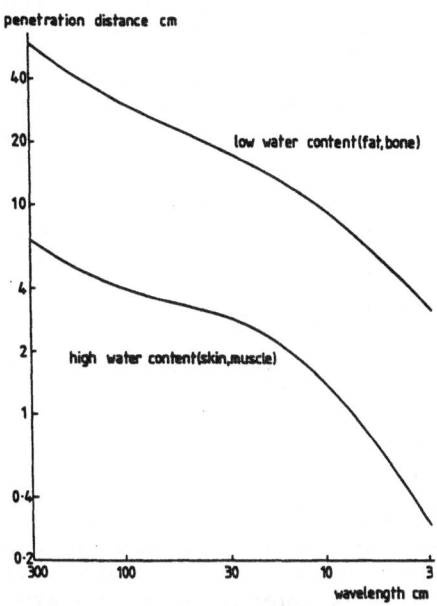

Fig. 2.   Transmission of microwave radiation through body
          tissues.

At the centimetric wavelengths electromagnetic
radiation can penetrate medically useful distances of the
order of several centi-metres through body tissues (1)
Fig. 2). The intensity of the microwave thermal radiation
is proportional to the absolute temperature of the source
tissue and this, combined with the microwave transmission
through tissue, makes possible the observation of the
subcutaneous temperature patterns of the body by radiation
measurements made at the skin surface. Since measurement
is made of entirely natural radiation at the body surface,
microwave thermography is a passive, non-invasive technique
which is inherently completely safe.

The penetration of tissue by the measured radiation
makes the technique of microwave thermography fundamentally
different from that of infra-red thermography. At infra-red
wavelengths tissue penetration distances are extremely
small and observable radiations can come essentially from
only the surface of the skin. The infra-red skin
temperature pattern which is observed is the result of
thermal conduction from internal sources through the
subcutaneous tissues, the state of perfusion of the
cutaneous tissue, and a delicate thermal balance at the
skin surface. Microwave thermography attempts to observe
directly the thermal radiation from internal body sources.

Microwave thermography equipment using the concepts
described in this paper has been used in major Glasgow
Hospitals for clinical assessments of the technique since
1983. The performance of the equipment and some of the
potential applications of the technique will be illustrated
by results from these assessment programmes.

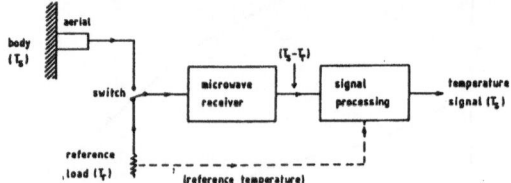

Fig. 3. Arrangement of Dicke radiometer type microwave
thermography equipment.

2. Equipment Design

The essential elements of a microwave thermography system
are a microwave antenna, of special design for operation in
contact with the body, and a radiometer type of microwave
radio receiver for thermal signal intensity measurement
(2,3) (Fig.3). The frequency of microwave radiation chosen
for measurement by the system has to be a compromise
between the requirement for adequate tissue penetration
distances to obtain temperature information from useful
depths within the body, and the requirement to achieve
adequate spatial resolution to observe temperature
patterns. Penetration distances, the distances over which
the radiation intensity is reduced by the factor $e^{-1}(0.37)$,
useful for many clinical applications can be obtained at
frequencies up to about 6GHz, corresponding to a radiation
wavelength in air of 5cm. At frequencies higher than this
the tissues of the skin become the most important source of
the thermal radiation and the information obtained will be
very similar to that given by infra-red thermography
(Fig.4).

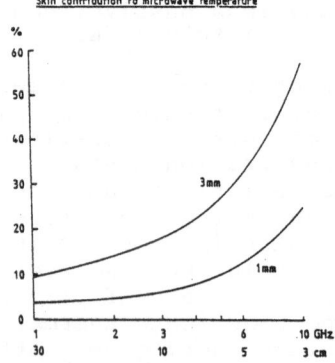

Fig. 4. Contribution of skin tissues to total microwave
thermal signal.

At all frequencies in the microwave range the attenuation
of the radiation is, however, such that the major part of
the signal observed comes from tissue within a distance of
only a few wavelengths from the antenna. In this situation
the spatial resolution which can be achieved is of the
order of one half of a radiation wavelength in the tissue
viewed by the antenna. At microwave frequencies tissue
dielectric constants are relatively high, between approximately 6 and 45 (Table 1). The radiation wavelength in
the tissue, varying as the inverse of the square-root of
the dielectric constant, is considerably reduced from the
in-air value which enables good spatial resolution to be
achieved when using suitable body contact antennas
operating at frequencies which give good tissue
penetration. The Glasgow microwave thermography systems
have been designed to measure the intensity of thermal
radiation at frequencies from 3.0 to 3.5 GHz, corresponding
to wavelengths in air from 10 to 8.6 cm. At these
frequencies penetration distances are about 1.6cm and 10cm
in high and low water content tissues respectively, and
spatial resolution is between 0.7 and 2.0cm near the
antenna.

Table 1.

Tissue properties at 3Ghz, 10cm wavelength in air

	High water content (skin, muscle)	Low water content (fat, bone)
Dielectric constant	43 - 48	5.5 - 7
Wavelength in tissue	1.5cm	4cm
Penetration distance (power attenuation length)	1.6cm	10cm
Tissue wave impedance	55 ohms	150 ohms
Reflection coefficient at air boundary		

In the microwave region the high tissue dielectric
constants reduce the tissue electromagnetic wave impedance
significantly from the air value of 377 ohms to values
between approximately 55 ohms and 150 ohms. The large
discontinuity in impedance at the tissue to air boundary
then causes a large fraction of the emerging microwave
radiation to be reflected back into the body (Table 1)
(Section 3 below). The microwave antenna is designed to
simulate the mean body tissue wave impedance to reduce this
reflection to a level which will permit accurate measurement
of the radiation intensity where the antenna is in contact
with the body.

To provide medically useful information the microwave thermography equipment must have a temperature resolution of about 0.1°C and have a measurement stability of the order of a few tenths of a degree Celsius. Since the tissues of the body at temperatures close to 37°C are seen radiometrically as sources at absolute temperatures close to 310K measurement resolution of about 0.03% and stability of better than 0.1% are normally required. To meet these requirements a Dicke comparison type of radiometer microwave receiver is used (3) in which the radiation signal being measured is compared with the similar thermally generated signal from a source of known temperature (Fig.3). The optimum temperature resolution achievable with a radiometer receiver is given by the Gabor relationship which can be written in the form:

$$\Delta T = Q(T_r + T_s)/\sqrt{Bt}$$

(1)

where Q is the radiometer receiver constant in the range 4.6 to 6.6 (2), T_r is the effective noise temperature of the measuring system at the antenna input, T_s is the source temperature, here close to 310K, B is the receiver pre-detection noise signal bandwidth, and it is the receiver post-detection signal filter response time. Practical microwave receivers for this application can have input noise temperatures in the region of 300K and pre-detection bandwidths of 500 MHz. A temperature resolution of 0.1K can then be achieved for a measurement response time of about 2 seconds (Fig. 5).

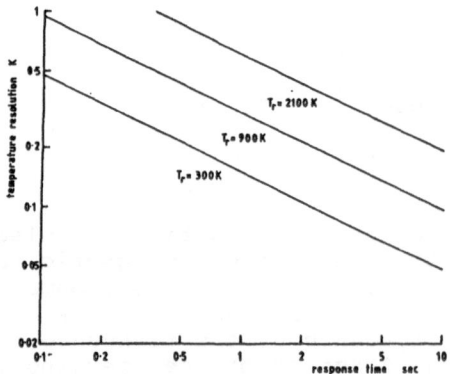

Fig. 5.   Temperature resolution and response time performance of radiometer receivers for microwave thermography.

Accurate measurement of the radiometric temperature is dependent also on the proper designs of the microwave receiver input circuits (4). The residual antenna to body reflection coefficient and the signal losses in the antenna receiver input circuits are the factors of importance. The Dicke radiometer input circuit of Fig. 3 when analysed in terms of these factors is found to give an error in the measurement of the radiometric source temperature given by:

$$S - T_s = -\rho T_s + \rho \dot{A}_1 T_i + (G-1)(1+\rho A_1) T_i$$
$$- G(1 - A_2) T_2 + (1 - G A_2) T_R \qquad (2)$$

$$\text{with } G A_1 = 1$$

Here S is the temperature equivalent receiver output, T_s is the true source temperature, P is the antenna to body reflection coefficient, G is the receiver gain, A_1 and A_2 are respectively the antenna to comparator switch and reference source to switch circuit power transmission, T_1 and T_2 are the temperatures of these signal paths, T_1 is the receiver input noise temperature, and TR is the reference source temperature.

With the input circuits maintained at the same temperature, $T_1 = T_2 = T_0$, and circuit losses equalised to give $A_1 = A_2 = A$, the measurement error is:

$$s - T_s = \rho(- T_{os} + A T_{oi}) \qquad (3)$$

with $T_s = T_0 + T_{os}$ and $T_i = T_0 + T_{oi}$

With the proper choice of T_{oi} for a given input circuit loss the measurement error can be minimised for a given range of source temperatures. Fig. 6 illustrates this relationship and shows the importance of minimising both antenna to body impedance mismatch and circuit losses. If the receiver gain condition GA = 1 is not met then if GA = 1+g the measurement error is:

$$s - T_s = \rho(1+g)(- T_{os} + A T_{oi}) + g(T_{os} - T_{oR}) \qquad (4)$$

168

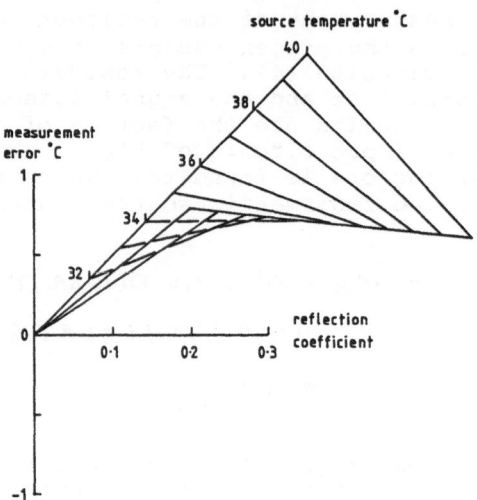

Fig. 6. Microwave temperature measurement error due to
        antenna-body reflection for a circuit loss of 1.5
        dB (circuit signal transmission A = 0.7).

with reference temperature $T_R = T_O + T_{OR}$
This source of error is minimised by setting the reference
temperature close to the source temperature.

     The Glasgow microwave thermography equipment has been
designed in accordance with these requirements to permit
body radiometric temperatures to be measured substantially
independently of the type of tissue viewed by the antenna
and without disturbance from ambient temperature changes.

(3) <u>Microwave radiation from body tissues</u>

     The contribution to the radiometric temperature signal
from a thin element of material is proportional to the
temperature of the material and the radiation loss or
attenuation in passing through the element.

If the element is 'dz' thick and has a temperature T(z) and
the material has an attenuation constant 'd' nepers per
unit length the signal contribution at z is:

$$dS = T(z) \alpha\, dz \qquad\qquad (5)$$

If this signal is observed some distance away such that the transmission from the element is 't' the contribution will be:

$$t \, dS = t \, T(z) \alpha \, dz \tag{6}$$

In a uniform material the transmission factor will be $t = e^{-\alpha z}$ over a distance z. The contribution to the radiation signal from a uniform material region from z = 0 to z = d, observed at z = 0, is then:

$$S = \alpha \int_{0}^{d} T(z) e^{-\alpha z} dz \tag{7}$$

For modelling purposes some simple variations of temperatures (Tz) are normally assured.

(i) Region of uniform temperature, $T(z) = T_1$

$$S = T_1 \left(1 - e^{-\alpha d} \right). \tag{8}$$

(ii) Linear variation of temperature with depth

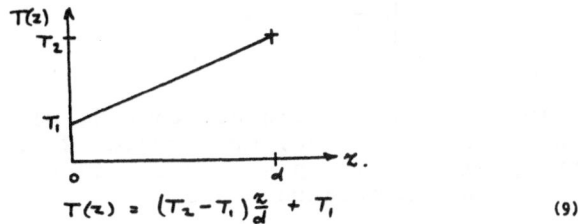

$$T(z) = (T_2 - T_1) \frac{z}{d} + T_1 \tag{9}$$

$$S = \left(\frac{T_2 - T_1}{\alpha d} \right) \left[1 - (\alpha d + 1) e^{-\alpha d} \right] + T_1 \left(1 - e^{-\alpha d} \right) \tag{10}$$

(iii) Exponential variation of temperature with depth.

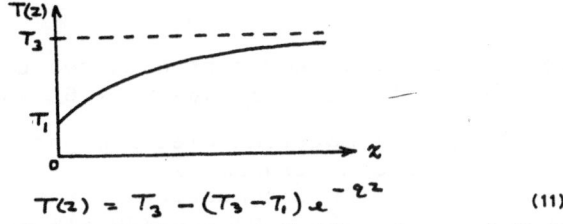

$$T(z) = T_3 - (T_3 - T_1) e^{-qz} \tag{11}$$

This form of temperature variation is useful for representing the final region when modelling inwards from the body surface, when T3 is taken as the body core temperature. The factor 'q' is given by the rate with which the temperature rises with increasing depth.

$$S = T_3 (1 - e^{-\alpha z}) - \left(\frac{\alpha}{q + \alpha} \right) (T_3 - T_1) \left[1 - e^{-(q + \alpha) z} \right] \tag{12}$$

For thick region of material we take $z \rightarrow \infty$ giving

$$S = \frac{\frac{q}{\alpha} T_2 + T_1}{\left(\frac{q}{\alpha} + 1\right)} \qquad (13)$$

If $q = \alpha$, often a reasonable approximation, then

$$S = \frac{T_1 + T_3}{2}$$ (14), the average of core and surface temperatures.

     The effective radiation temperature signal seen by the aerial viewing the source will be the sum of the signals at the aerial due to all the elements of the source:

From region 1 have temperature signal $T_{ei} = S_1$ with S_1 appropriately evaluated as above. From region 2 we have signal $T_{e2} = t_1 S_2$ with again S_2 appropriately evaluated. The overall effective temperature signal is then:

$$T_e = T_{e1} + T_{e2}$$
$$= S_1 + t_1 S_2 \qquad (15)$$

For a three region model this would be extended to give $T_e = T_{e1} + T_{e2} + T_{e3}$ with $T_{ei} = S_1$, $T_{e2} = t_1 S_2$ and $T_{e3} = t_1 t_2 S_3$
Where there are changes of material electromagnetic properties between the signal transmission factors, t_1, t_2 etc., will depend on both the attenuation of the radiation across the width of each uniform region and also on the reflection of radiation at the boundaries of the region. The magnitude of the reflection depends on the degree of change of properties of the materials across a boundary, the change in wave impedance seen by the radiation, and also the importance of multiple reflections of the radiation between the discontinuities of the boundaries of the region.

The reflection coefficient at the junction of the two
materials with wave impedance Z1 and Z2 is

$$\rho_{12} = \left(\frac{Z_1 - Z_2}{Z_1 + Z_2} \right)^2 \qquad (16)$$

The wave impedance is in general complex and dependent on
the real and imaginary parts of the dielectric constant and
the conductivity of the material. For biological materials
at microwave frequencies, however, the wave impedance can
be given with more than adequate accuracy for these
calculations simply by

$$Z = \frac{Z_0}{\sqrt{K}} \qquad (17)$$

where Z_0 is the vacuum wave impedance, 377ohms, and K is
the real part of the dielectric constant of the material.

    The importance of multiple reflections between the
boundaries of a region, which will set up a standing-wave
or interference pattern across the region, will depend on
the reflection coefficients at the boundaries and the
wavelength and wave attenuation across the region. If the
region is relatively thin, reflections from the two
surfaces of a region may tend to cancel. If the region is
relatively thick, attenuation will absorb reflected
radiation. In practice multiple reflections producing
standing-waves are only likely to be significant in
intermediate thicknesses of subcutaneous fat layers and
here can be reduced by proper choice of measuring aerial
impedance and the use of reflection compensating techniques
in the receiver.

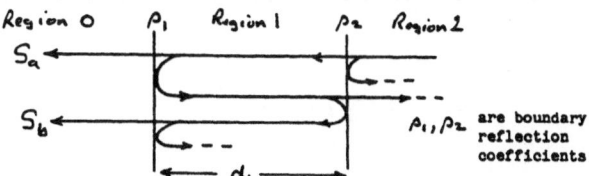

ρ_1, ρ_2 are boundary reflection coefficients

The relative values of the components of the signal emitted from the surface of region 1 are:

$$S_a = t_1' (1-\rho_1)(1-\rho_2) \quad \text{where } t_1' = e^{-\alpha_1 d_1}$$

and

$$S_b = t_1'^3 \rho_1 \rho_2 (1-\rho_1)(1-\rho_2) \quad \text{, neglecting interference of the waves,}$$

giving

$$\frac{S_b}{S_a} = t_1'^2 \rho_1 \rho_2 \tag{18}$$

If wave impedances of the regions are 150 ohms, typical of fat, and 55 ohms, typical of skin and muscle, then reflection coefficients $\rho 1$ and $\rho 2$ would be typically 0.21. For a standing-wave pattern in a fat layer the maximum multiply reflected signal will occur with t'_1 at about 0.8 giving a maximum value of S_b/S_a of about 2.8%.
The transmission factors across different tissue regions within the body can thus usually be calculated with sufficient accuracy from the attenuation across each region and the reflection coefficient of the appropriate boundary between regions giving, for example,

$$t_1 = (1-\rho_1) e^{-\alpha_1 d_1} \tag{19}$$

The effect of reflection at an inner boundary between regions may not, however, be negligible when considering what happens to radiation coming from the measuring system.

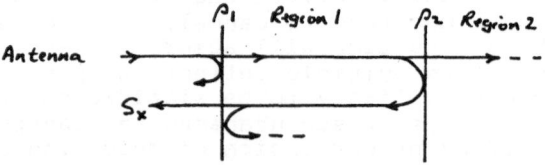

The relative value of reflected signal from the inner boundary is

$$S_x = t_1'^2 (1-\rho_1)^2 \rho_2 \tag{20}$$

If $\rho_1 \sim \rho_2$ compared to the first boundary reflection this is $t_1'^2 (1-\rho_1)^2$ and compared to the signal coming from the inner region this is $t_1^1 \rho_1$.

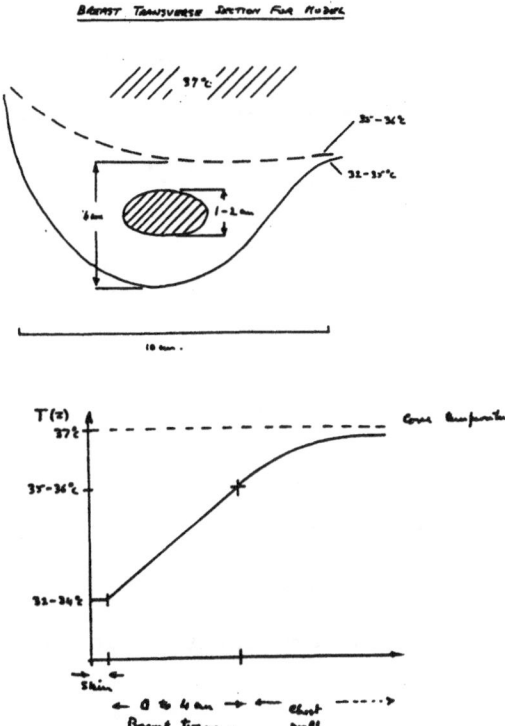

Fig. 7. Thermal model transverse section of female breast
for microwave temperature calculations.

These modelling techniques are illustrated for the
simple model of the female breast shown in Fig. 7. The
form of the temperature variation with depth within the
breast has been confirmed by direct temperature
measurements with thermocouple probes. Fig. 8 shows the
microwave temperature profiles expected from this modelling
for two different values of breast tissue radiation
attenuation constants considered to be representative of
the young and post menopausal breast with different sizes
and temperatures of tumour embedded within the breast. The
tumour size and temperatures used for the modelling are
again typical of measured values. The calculated profiles
of Fig. 8 for the higher attenuation tissue can be seen to
be in good agreement with the profiles of Fig. 9 measured
across the breasts of a 34 year old woman with a 1.5cm
diameter carcinoma situated approximately centrally within
the left breast.

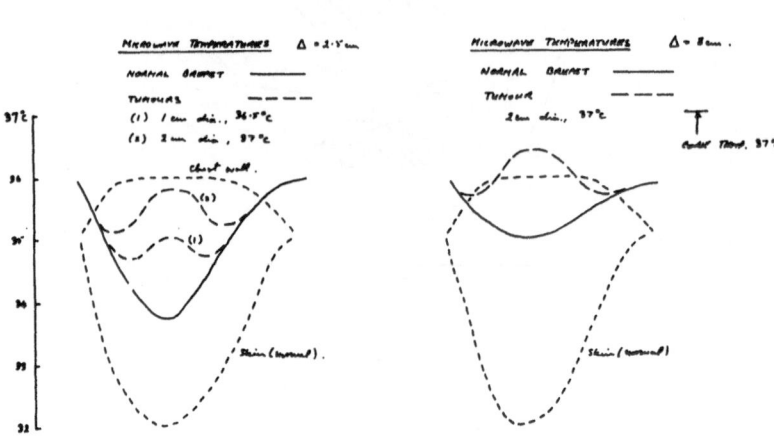

Fig. 8. Calculated temperature profiles for breast models.

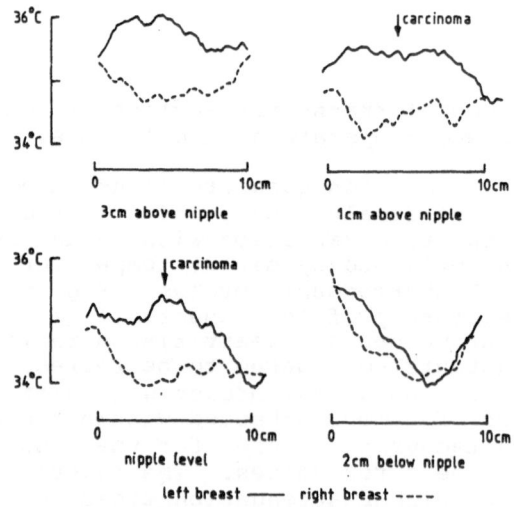

Fig. 9. Microwave temperature profiles taken transversely across left and right breasts of a patient with a carcinoma in the left breast.

4. Clinical Performance

The performance of the equipment in clinical use is illustrated briefly with measurements taken during the clinical assessment programmes in progress in Glasgow Hospitals. The equipment is shown in Fig. 10. It is compact, simple to use, and does not require the provision of any special facilities.

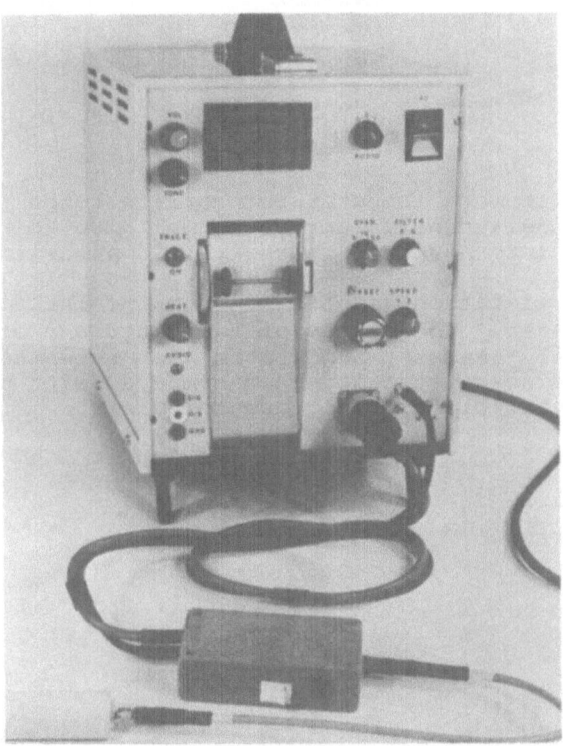

Fig. 10.   Microwave thermography equipment for clinical use.

Fig. 9, which has already been referred to above, shows four of a set of microwave temperature profiles taken across the left and right breasts of a woman with 1.5cm diameter carcinoma in the left breast slightly above the nipple level. Below the nipple level there is seen to be good profile symmetry. The temperature elevation associated with the tumour is clearly seen. The left breast temperature elevation is also seen to extend into the upper inner quadrant, this most probably showing a region of markedly increased blood supply.

Fig.11 shows microwave temperature profiles taken longitudinally across normal knee joints and across knee joints suffering from rheumatoid arthritis. The

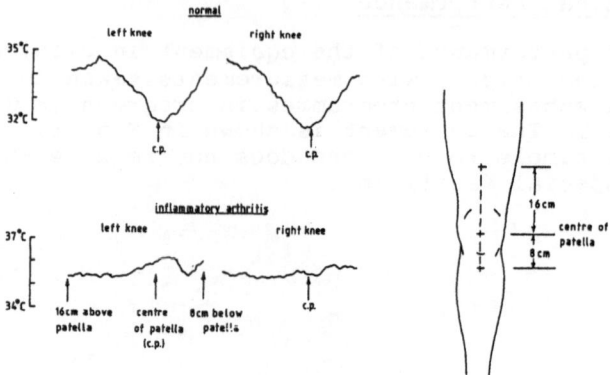

Fig. 11.   Microwave temperature profiles taken
            longitudinally across normal knee joints and knee
            joints affected by rheumatoid arthritis.

temperature elevation associated with the inflammed joints
is clearly seen.   The change of temperature profile can be
quantitatively assessed and it has been shown to be a good
measure of disease activity when compared with measures
currently available to the rheumatologist.

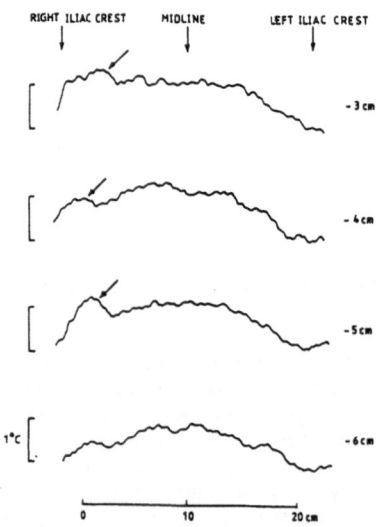

Fig. 12. Microwave temperature profiles taken trans-
          versely across the lower anterior abdominal wall
          of a patient with appendicitis.

Fig. 12 shows a series of scans taken transversely across the lower anterior abdominal wall of a patient with appendicitis. The temperature elevated region marked overlies the inflammed appendix exactly and indicates a temperature rise of 1.5°C to 2°C within the appendix relative to the surrounding tissues.

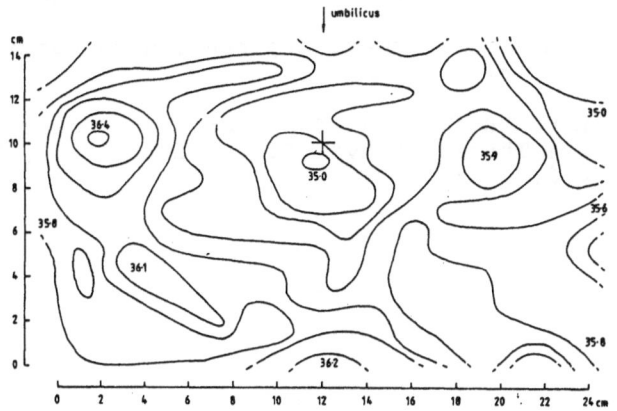

Fig. 13. Microwave isothermal plot constructed from temperature profiles taken across the anterior abdominal wall of a healthy 27 year old woman.

Fig. 13 is chosen to illustrate the temperature and spatial resolution being achieved with the Glasgow equipment. This isothermal plot has been constructed from a series of profiles taken transversely across the central region of the anterior abdominal wall of a healthy 27 year old female. Thermal features approximately 1 to 2cm in extent are being detected.

5. Conclusions

Microwave thermography equipment has been developed which is suitable for routine clinical use. The temperature resolution, spatial resolution and speed of response of the equipment permit the recording of continuous temperature profiles over body regions of interest. It has been demonstrated that the technique of microwave thermography, when using appropriately designed equipment, can provide clinically valuable information about body internal temperature variations. The technique is passive, non-invasive and inherently completely safe.

178

References

1. SCHWAN, H.P., FOSTER, K.R. "Microwave Dialectric Properties of Tissue" Biophys J. 1977, 17, 193-197.

2. LAND, D.V. "Radiometer Receivers for Microwave Thermography" Microwave J. 1983, 26, 196-201.

3. HARVEY, A.F. "Microwave Engineering" Academic Press, 1963, ch. 16.

4. LAND, D.V. "Radiometer Input Circuit Requirements for Microwave Thermography" Elect. Lett. 1983, 19, 1040-1042.

HUMAN THERMOMETRY IN HEALTH AND DISEASE (Continued)

(C) APPENDIX

II. Factors in the interpretation of human circadian
    temperature data.

(i) Physiological factors.

There has been a traditional tendency by some to
intepret human circadian temperature data exclusively in
terms of environmental effects (diurnal variations in
posture, exercise, diet and ambient temperature); in
contrast, others have exaggerated the endogenous element
and have applied cosine-wave fits to environmentally noisy
circadian data with little regard to the fact that the
rhythm parameters may be severely distorted.

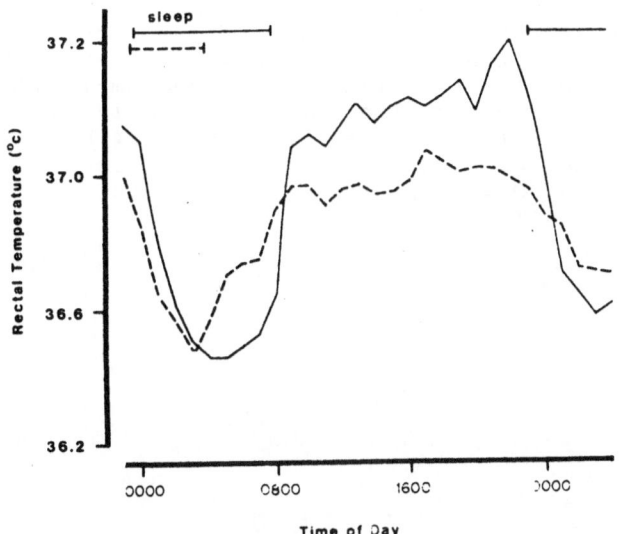

The above data of Minors and Waterhouse (1985)
illustrate the point. The solid line indicates the mean
temperature in 8 subjects living their normal sleep-
wakefulness routine. The interrupted line represents the
average temperature in the same subjects awoken at 04^{00}.
Thereafter, for the subsequent 24 hours, they were awake,
in constant light and the diet consisted of hourly
identical snacks. Examination of the differences between
these 2 avergaged sets of temperature data, reveals the
effect of this environment. It increases the amplitude and
delays the phase of the circadian rhythm.

180

The relative importance of environmental versus intrinsic effects may be quantified by studying human subjects on a 21 hour day system. The data below are illustrative of this technique. Five adult subjects participated in the study. Their data, the temperature of voided urine, is seen in the top rectangle of the figure. The subjects were living in an isolated locale in the high arctic around mid-summer. There was a regular schedule in the camp e.g. reveille 0730, breakfast at 0800, lunch 1300 etc. The experimental protocol dictated that subjects should take short walks around the camp studying the arctic birds and the flowers between observations and meals i.e. light exercise. Clocks in the camp had had the hairspring shortened so that when 24 hours had appeared to elapse, only 21 hours of time had really passed. Temperature data were collected 2 hourly on the clocks, that is every 1.75 hours of elapsed time. The pooled data (1.5 weeks) have been subjected to the least square spectral analysis with trial periods extending from 18 hours to 26 hours.(Courtesy of Professor Franz Halberg). The bottom rectangle of the figure illustrates the amplitudes of the fits of the trial periods and also the residual errors after the fit has been applied. Using the criterion of maximum amplitude and minimum residual error, the analysis reveals two real periodicities in the data, one at around 24 hours and the other at around 21 hours. The former represents the endogenous rhythmic component and the latter the environmental component.

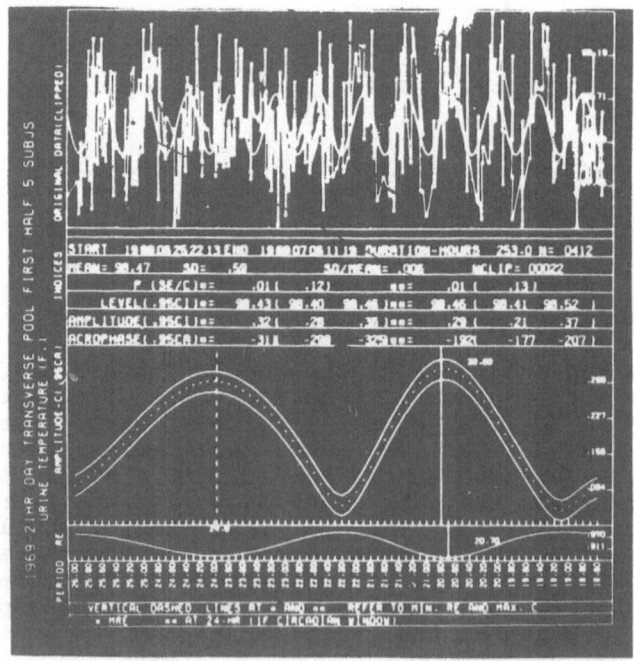

It is seen that the strength of the environmental component

is very similar to the endogenous component i.e. the
amplitude ratio is close to one. This method was introduced
to quantify the relative importance of rhythmic components
(see Simpson Halberg & Lobban 1970). Another of the
subjects in this study, a child aged 8, who was inclined to
take a minimum interpretation of the exercise prescribed,
showed an about 24 hour component but no 21 hour
component. The data illustrated are from the first 1½ weeks
of exposure to a 21 hour day. Subsequent data over the
second 1½ weeks of 21 hour exposure indicated that the 24
and 21 hour amplitude ratio did not change materially. In
other words, there was no apparent learning effect.

Moog and Hildebrandt have made a particular study of
these "masking" effects. For example, it has been
suggested that (1) a deep body temperature fall is
triggered by sleep onset, and (2) that the phenomenon of
awakening is associated with a rise of temperature. On
their so-called "control" days, the subjects remained
recumbent over 24 hours in a sound-proof climatic chamber
and received an equidistant 3 hour low protein diet. After
over 500 control day studies they failed to find a
consistent decrease in rectal temperature triggered by
sleep onset. Equally, there was no triggered increase of
temperature at awakening.

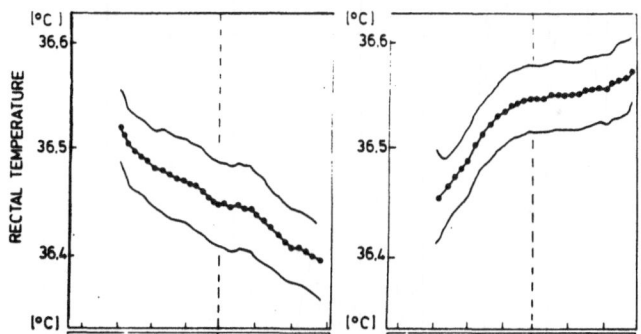

On the left sleep onset indicated by interrupted vertical
line; on the right time of awakening. Both EEG
controlled. Mean temperature based on 500 studies. Neither
the event of falling asleep nor awakening triggered a
change in rectal temperature.
(Data of Moog and Hildebrandt).

It has also been suggested that the temperature microclimate on the surface of the body is a factor in the
setting of deep body temperature. For example, in the warm
climate between bedclothes (34 - 35°C) an increase of
peripheral temperature has been reported leading to a
decrease of deep body temperature (Vokac and Jeltnes 1981).
To investigate this effect, Moog had his subjects dressed
in night attire, exposed to alternations of bedclothes for

45 minutes, removal for 30 minutes, and so on. He found no
significant change of body temperature (maximum deviation
from the baseline; 0.15°C). He concluded that masking
effects due to this microclimate are minor if, indeed,
there are any.

The third type of masking effect studied by Moog was
that due to physical exercise. He first observed rectal
temperature of 12 subjects during control days (see
description above) in order to obtain a circadian rhythm
reference day. Then the control routine was broken by
bursts of physical activitiy made up of 5 minutes each of
25 watts, 50 watts and 75 watts and then 15 minutes
workload at 100 pedal revolutions per minute. Rectal
temperature was increased for 70 minutes after the end of
the exercise. The average increase in temperature relative
to the control days was 0.56°C. This indicates that even
moderate physical work is able to obscure the circadian
temperature rhythm.

Another physiological factor that can affect the
interpretation of circadian temperature data is the
menstrual cycle.

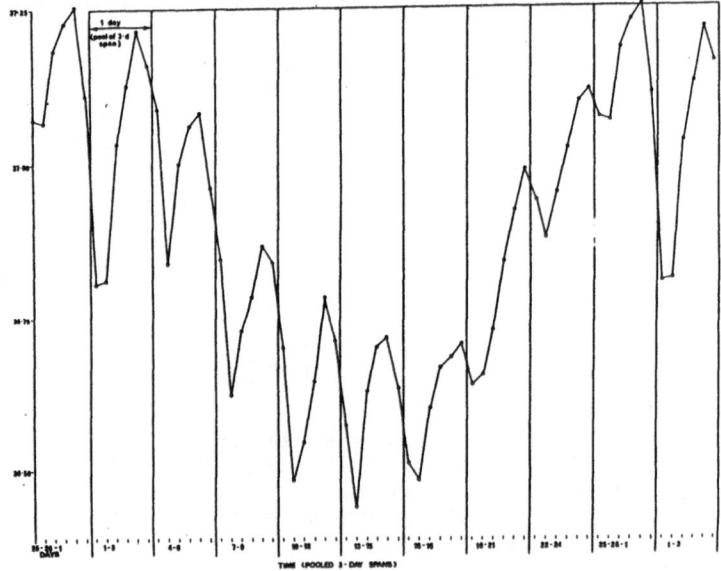

The above data are based on urine temperature measurements
collected over 8 concurrent menstrual cycles in one woman
and then plexogrammed to give the one idealised cycle shown
in the graph. Note that the cycle results in a
lopsidedness of the circadian rhythm and an interesting
point is that in the first 15 days of the cycle the highest
temperatures are recorded some 4 hours before

local midnight whereas on the second part of the cycle, when the temperatures are rising, the peak temperatures are very close to midnight. Our interpreptation of these data is that there is a super position of menstrual and circadian rhythms (Simpson & Halberg 1972).

(ii) Pathological factors.

Halberg has made some interesting findings on the effect of a pyrexial illness on the circadian rhythm of rectal temperature. The data are summarised in the amplitude and phase diagram given below.

CIRCADIAN CHARACTERISTICS – HARBINGERS OF NOSOCOMIAL INFECTION

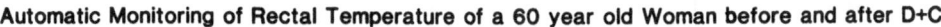

Automatic Monitoring of Rectal Temperature of a 60 year old Woman before and after D+C

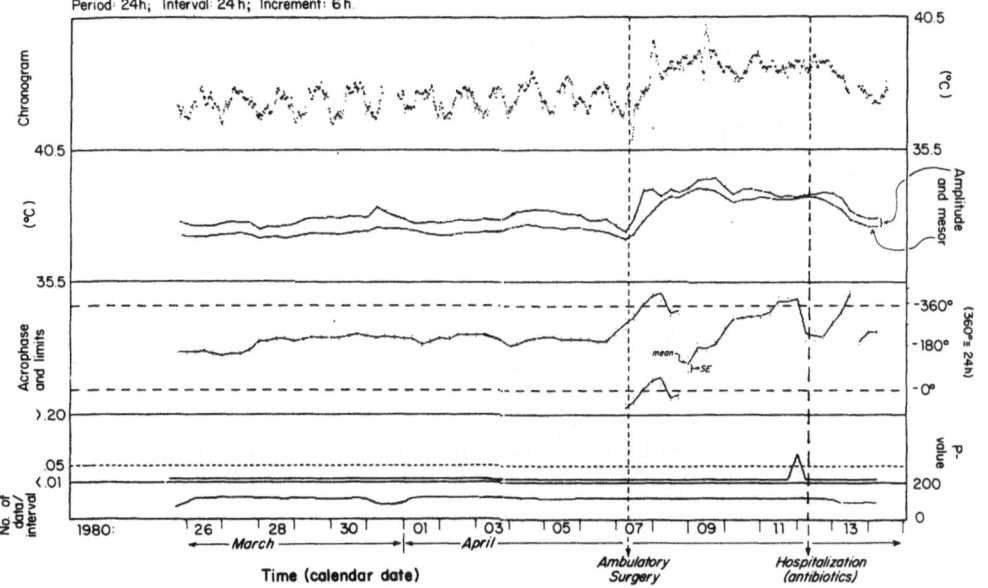

Note the clear circadian cycles in the chronogram in the top rectangle of the figure. Note also that when a pyrexial illness supervened the rhythm is much less apparent in the gross data though it remains significant in terms of the statistical analysis.   There is a drift of acrophase.

An interesting phenomenon in breast cancer was

originally described by Mansfield and now is being further investigated by ourselves. Below is a representative set of data from a cancerous breast and a matched site on the contralateral breast. Four days of data are shown with readings every 15 minutes. Note that over the cancerous breast there is a higher mesor, smaller amplitude and earlier circadian phase than over the contralateral breast.

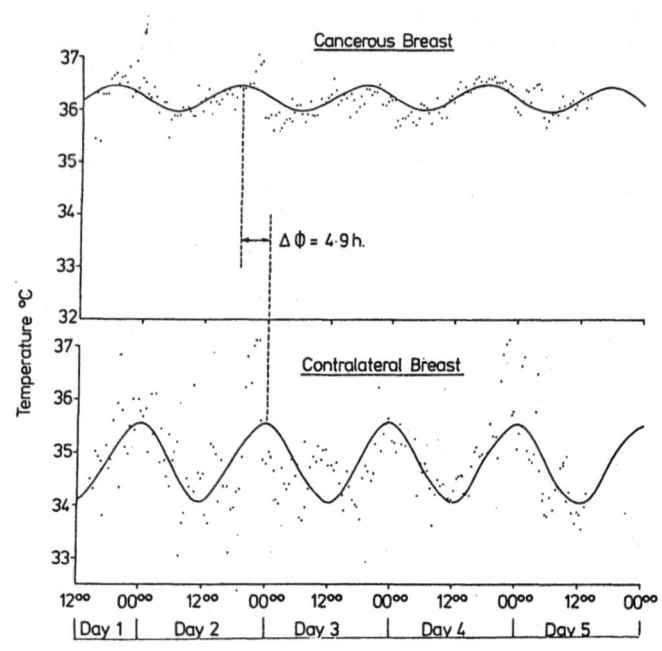

1978 Data of Wilson, Simpson, Blamey and Griffiths. See text.

How can this phase shift be explained ? Below, in a further figure, the surface temperature of the cancerous breast and the normal breast are compared along with the oral temperature. It can be seen that the surface temperature over the cancer approximates to that of the oral temperature (i.e. the deep temperature of the body) whereas the normal breast has a later phase. These data suggest that the reason that the surface temperature of the cancerous breast leads in phase that of a matched site on the other side is that the hypervascularity in the cancer allows the deep body temperature to come to the surface so quickly that the cancer temperature approximates that of

that of the deep body. It is well established that under
normal conditions, the surface of the body has a later
temperature circadian phase than that of the deep body.

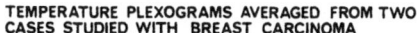

TEMPERATURE PLEXOGRAMS AVERAGED FROM TWO
CASES STUDIED WITH BREAST CARCINOMA

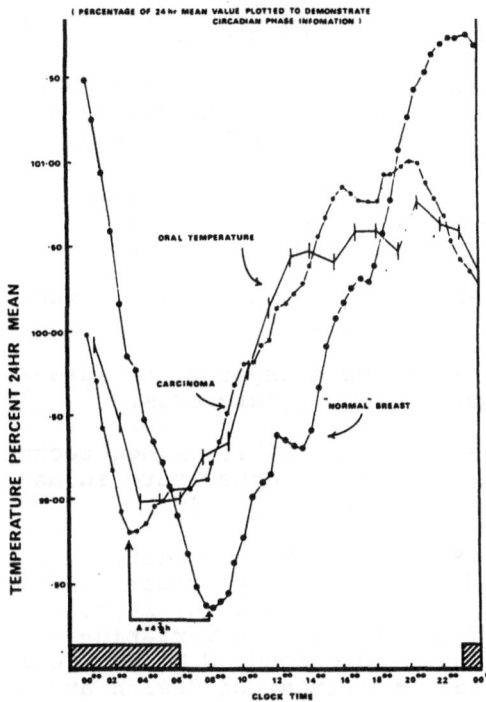

1978 Data of Simpson, Wilson, Blamey and Griffiths. See
text.

REFERENCES (except those in the article by D. V. Land)

Baerensprung, F. 1852. Untersuchungen uber die temperatur verhaltnisse des menschen im gesunden und kranken zustande. Archives of Anatomy and Physiology. U Wissensch. Med. 3: 217-286.

Ball, S.G., Chalmers, D.Mc.M., Morgan A.G., Solman A.J. and Losowsky, M.S. 1973. A clinical appraisal of transcutaneous deep body temperature. Biomedicine, 18, 290-294.

Cullis, W.C., Oppenheimer, E.M., Ross-Johnston, M. 1922. Temperature and other changes in woman during the menstrual cycle. Lancet 2: 954-956.

Damrosch, L. 1853. Uber die taglichen schwankungen der menschlichen eignwarme in normalen zustande. Journal of D.T. Sch. Klin. 5: 317-319.

Davie, J. 1845. On the temperature of man. Philosophical transactions 319-333.

De Gorter, J. 1736. De perspiratione insensibili - (2nd edition) Vander ed lugd., Batavorum.

Fox R.H. and Solman A.J. 1971. A new technique for monitoring the deep body temperature in man from the intact skin surface. J. Physiol. 212, 8p.

Fuller, C.A., Sulzman, F.M. and Moore-Ede, M.C. 1981. Shift-work and the jet-lag syndrome: conflicts between environmental and body time. In: 24 hour workday: Proceedings of a Symposium on Variation in Street (Johnson, L.C., Tepas, D.I., Colquhoun, W.P. and Colligan, M.J. Eds) Cincinnati: U.S. Department of Health and Human Services (National Institute for Occupational Safety and Health) Publication No. 81-127. 305-320.

Gautherie, M., Gros, C. Anarchic ultradian rhythms of skin temperature in breast cancers. Presentation at the Annual Congress in Biological Systems. Vienna, Austria, September 11th 1975.

Gierse. 1842. Cited by Marotte, H., Doctor of Science thesis. Lyons University 1979.

Halberg, F., Visscher, M.B., Bittner, J.J. 1954. Am J Physiol 179: 229-235.

Halberg, F. 1959. Z. Vitamin-, Hormon-u. Fermentforsch 10, 225-296.

Halberg, F., Gupta, B.D., Haus, E., Halberg, E., Deka, A,C., Nelson, W., Sothern, R.B., Cornelissen, G., Lee, J.J., Lakatua, D.J., Scheving, L.E., Burns E.R. 1977. Steps towards a cancer polychronopolytherapy. In: XIV Int. Cong. Therapeutics, Montpellier, France. L'Expansion Scientifique Francaise, 151-196.

Halman. 1844. Ueber eine zweckmassige behaudlung des typhus. Berlin.

Hardy, J.D. 1934. The radiation of heat from the human body. J Clin Invest 15 593.

Heusler, K. 1925. Temperaturehohungen der laktierenden Mamma. Zentralbl. f. Gynak 49: 204.

Hunter, J. Chapter VIII. 1839. de la chaleur des animaux. Oeuvres completes (traduction de l'edition du Dr. J.F. Palmer). Firmin Didot, Paris 8: 330.

Kleitman, N. 1939. Sleep and Wakefulness. Univ. of Chicago press.

Lawson, R. 1956. Implications of surface temperatures in the diagnosis of breast cancer. Cand M.A.J. 75 309-310.

Lindhard, J. 1913. Contribution to the physiology of respiration under the Arctic climate. Meddelesler om Gronland, 41: 78-81.

Marotte, H. 1979. Doctor of Science Thesis entitled "Etudes des rythmes biologiques par analyse de varience". Lyon University.

Mansfield, C.M., Wallace, J.D., Curley, R., Kramer, S., Southard, M., Driscoll, D. 1970. A comparison of the temperature curves recorded over normal and abnormal breasts. Radiology, 94; 697.

Mansfield, C.M., Carabasi, A., Wells, W., Borman, K. 1973. Circadian rhythm in skin temperature of normal and cancerous breasts. International Journal of Chronobiology, 1; 235.

Moll, L. 1924. Die erhohte temperatur der laktierenden Mamma als gradmesser ihre funktions. Wien. Med. Wchnschr., 74: 1059.

Moore, R.Y. and Eichler, V.B. 1972. Loss of circadian adrenal corticosterone rhythm following suprachiasmatic lesions in the rat. Brain Research, 42: 201-206.

Mosso, U. 1887. Recherches sur l'inversion des oscillations diurnes de la temperature chez l'homme normal. Archives Britallion Biology 8: 177-185.

Ogle, J.W. 1866. On the diurnal variations in the temperature of the human body in health. St. George's Hospital 1: 220-245.

Simpson, H.W. 1970. The urine temperature measurements in human circadian rhythm studies. J Physiol Proc. 25p-27p.

Simpson, H.W., Halberg, F., Lobban, M. 1970. Near 24-hour rhythms in subjects living on a 21-hour routine in the Arctic summer at 78°N revealed by circadian amplitude ratios. Arctic Anthropology VII, 144-164.

Simpson, H.W., Halberg, E. 1972. Investigation of possible amplitude or phase modulation of the circadian and menstrual temperature rhythms in a woman. Chapt. 36 in Biorhythms and human reproduction. Ed. M. Ferin, F. Halberg, R.M. Richart, R. Vande Wiele. J. Wiley, New York.

Stephan, F.K. and Zucker, I. 1972. Circadian rhythms in drinking behaviour and locomotor activity in rats are eliminated by hypothalamic lesions. Proceedings : The National Academy of Sciences U.S.A. 69: 1583-1586.

Vokac, Z., Jeltnes, H. Core-peripheral heat redistribution during sleep and its effect on rectal temperature. In: Night and Shift Work: Biological and Social Aspects. Ed. Reinberg, A., Vieux, N and Andlauer. Pergamon Press. 1982.

THE MEASUREMENT OF CIRCADIAN RHYTHMS IN PSYCHOLOGICAL FUNCTIONS

S. FOLKARD AND T. H. MONK   MRC Perceptual and Cognitive Experimental
Psychology, The University of Sussex, Falmer, Brighton and Department
of Chronobiology, Cornell Medical Center, White Plains, N.Y.

1. INTRODUCTION

There is now a wealth of physiological evidence that man's internal body chemistry changes predictably as a function of time of day.   It is thus hardly surprising that there are equivalent predictable changes in his mood and performance efficiency, and it is to these psychological circadian rhythms that the present chapter is primarily addressed. In particular, it will be concerned with circadian performance rhythms, the history of their study, the methodological problems connected with measuring them, the forms of rhythms usually found, and the arousal model conventionally used to explain them.   A final section is then concerned with some of the practicalities of measuring psychological rhythms, and the direction in which future developments might be expected to lead.

At an intuitive level, there are two reasons why psychological processes should vary over the day, and indeed these have long been recognised.   First, as Michelson (1897) realised, there are variations in people's level of sleepiness over the day.   On awakening in the morning we typically feel fairly drowsy, and only wake up properly as the day progresses;   then at some point later during the day, we stop becoming more wakeful and start to feel more drowsy again.   The time at which this peak occurs varies from day to day, depending on our activities, and also from one individual to the next.   Nevertheless, Michelson (1897) proposed an average hypothetical function relating the level of sleepiness to time of day.   According to this, people's level of sleepiness is highest at about midnight, decreases rapidly until about 07.00, and then more gradually to reach a minimum level of sleepiness (or maximum level of wakefulness), in the evening at about 17.00.

Michelson thus viewed the level of sleepiness as varying fairly smoothly throughout the 24 hour period, rather than simply reflecting a dual state of being asleep or awake. Indeed, it would appear from more recent studies (e.g.Froberg, 1977) that this variation may be partially independent of whether or not people actually sleep during the night hours. In contrast, the second 'obvious' reason why psychological processes should vary over the day is linked rather more closely to the occurrence of sleep.   It can again be traced back to the turn of the century when a number of researchers were concerned with the problem of 'mental fatigue'.

Fatigue was assumed to be at a minimum on awakening in the morning, to accumulate over the day, and to result more or less directly in the onset of sleep. Sleep was thus viewed as having a recuperative or refreshing function. While there was some debate as to whether or not this build up of mental fatigue over the day was independent of the amount of work done (e.g. Thorndike, 1900), it seems to have been generally accepted that such fatigue was dissipated by sleep.

The early workers in this area thus viewed time of day effects in psychological functions as due to either a cycle of 'sleepiness', or a build up of mental fatigue. While both these ideas seem intuitively reasonable, more recent theorists have tended to ignore the influence of mental fatigue, and have concentrated on the idea of a sleepiness cycle, or, more usually, its inverse, referred to as 'the arousal rhythm' which is held to parallel the circadian rhythm in body temperature. The reason for this concentration should become clear to the reader later on in this chapter. Nevertheless, it is worth noting that some recent evidence suggests that there may be more than one factor responsible for time of day effects in performance, and it seems possible that one of these factors may correspond to the early notion of mental fatigue (cf. Borbely, 1982).

2. TIME OF DAY EFFECTS IN PERFORMANCE
2.1. Historical origins
Research on the effects of time of day on performance efficiency has two early roots. One of these stems from the work of Lombard at Clark University in the USA. Lombard was interested in the time of day effect in the magnitude of the 'knee jerk' and published the results of his pioneering investigations in 1887. This led two students of his, Dressler and Bergstrum, to look for time of day effects in performance efficiency per se. Like many early psychologists, Dressler (1892) used the speed with which he could tap a morse-key as his measure of performance and found it to steadily improve with practice over the first four weeks. However, in the last two weeks of his six-week study, his tapping got faster from 08.00 to 12.00, was rather slower again after lunch at 14.00, but then improved again up to 18.00. This trend over the day is fairly typical for studies using this type of task.

Lombard's other student, Bergstrum (1894), was more concerned with 'mental activity' and examined performance on tasks such as memory, mental arithmetic and reading, as well as simpler tasks similar to that used by Dressler. Bergstrum found time of day effects in the performance scores, but these were "....not of a single type such as would be required if a natural inherited rhythm of activity exists". In other words, Bergstrum found that the trend in performance over the day differed from one person to another, and from one type of task to another. Subsequently, this lack of consistency in Bergstrum's results has sometimes been attributed to his failure to practise his subjects adequately, although there is now ample evidence that the trend in per-

formance over the day is affected by both the type of individual and the type of task. Rather surprisingly, Bergstrum's most important finding has been almost totally ignored
by subsequent researchers in this area: namely that performance on more complex mental tasks shows a bigger variation
over the day than that on simple tasks.

This early research by Lombard and his students appears
to have been motivated primarily by theoretical interest
rather than by any specific practical problems. In contrast,
the other main root of research in this area developed from
consideration of the best way to organise or schedule school
timetables. This problem was being discussed in Prague
as early as 1889 (see Halberg, 1973) although it was some
years later that the first experimental studies in this
area were published. Among the earlier of these pedagogical
studies was that of a German called Baade (1907) who examined
children's speed at solving arithmetical problems at different
times of day. Similar studies were also conducted in Britain
(e.g. Winch, 1912a, b) and the United States (e.g. Gates,
1916a, b; Laird, 1925).

This early research on the effects of time of day on performance was reviewed by Freeman and Hovland (1934) who concluded that "the balance of evidence apparently favours an
afternoon superiority for sensory and motor performance,
but there is little agreement as to the time when complicated
mental work can be done most efficiently" (p.786). Subsequently, and perhaps consequently, research in this area
has, until very recently, tended to concentrate on the fairly
simple performance measures for which Freeman and Hovland
claimed some consistency.

2.2. Methodological problems

Before considering more recent studies of the effects
of time of day on performance it is worth considering the
methodological and statistical techniques that have been
used to study circadian performance rhythms since they are
often very different from those conventionally used by the
physiologist. The main difference is due to a number of
problems encountered in obtaining the long sequences of frequent observations which are so often used by the physiologist
to produce either a power spectrum or a cosinor plot for
a particular measure.

First, performance differs from most physiological measures
in that there is nearly always a marked practice effect.
This means that subjects will (almost invariably) tend to
perform better on a given trial than they did on the trials
preceding it. Unfortunately, such practice effects are
extremely hard to eradicate, even when dozens (or hundreds)
or trials are given and discarded prior to the actual experiment. Failure to realise this can result in totally spurious
conclusions about the timing of peak performance. Thus,
in his pioneering study, Dressler (1892) had to discard the
data from the first four weeks of his six-week study in order
to obtain a time of day function that was relatively uncontaminated by practice effects. More recently, the usual

192

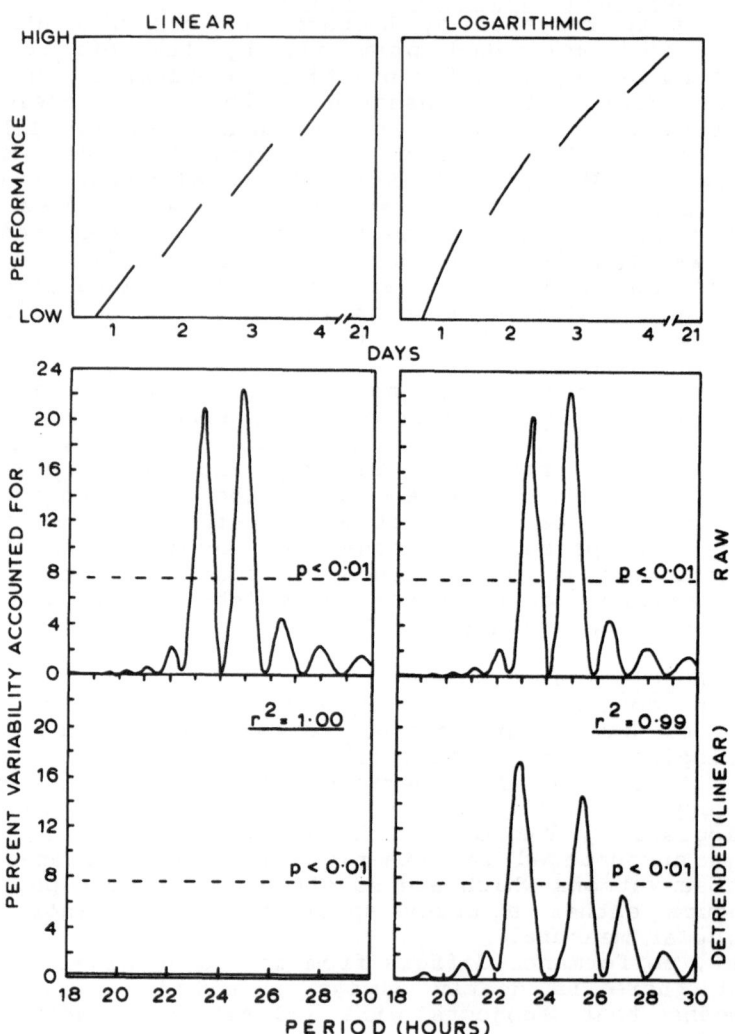

FIGURE 1. Examples of "Simon's artefact". The top panels show artificial linear and logarithmic 'practice' effects, the middle panels the results of period analyses based on these raw scores, and the bottom panels the results of parallel analyses after a linear trend had been removed.

technique used to circumvent this problem has been to either
have a separate group of unpractised subjects at each time
of day (e.g. Folkard & Monk, 1979), or to have different
groups of subjects experiencing the time of day conditions
in different orders (thus for one group, for example, the
11.00 session may be their first, whilst for another it is
their fifth, etc.) (e.g. Folkard, 1975). By combining groups
one can then 'balance out' any practice effects and obtain
an accurate circadian performance rhythm for the sample as
a whole (although no subject in the sample will actually
have shown such a rhythm).

Secondly, performance measurement is almost always intru-
sive, in that subjects are required to interrupt their ongoing activity for performance to be measured. This means
(a) that sampling can seldom be more frequent than once every
two or three hours at best, and (b) that sampling has to
be either reduced or suspended during sleep hours since otherwise either sleep deprivation effects or 'sudden waking'
effects might outweigh any truly circadian ones. In practice
this means that performance measurement is very often restricted to comparatively few (e.g. 6 or less) times during the
'normal waking' day.

One of us has recently discovered that the combination
of a long-term trend in a time series (e.g. due to 'practice',
'motivational', or even menstrual effects) and relatively
regularly occurring 'gaps' in the data (e.g. due to sleep)
can result in totally spurious 'peaks' in the power spectrum
when a period analysis is performed. "Simon's artefact"
is illustrated in Figure 1 for two artificial, 3-week, time
series of 6 readings per day. The top panels show the first
few 'days' of data assuming either a linear (left-hand panel)
or logarithmic (right-hand panel) increasing trend over
successive trials. The middle panel shows the percent of
variability accounted for by cosine curves of different
periods, while the bottom panel shows the results following
a linear de-trending of the data. Note that despite the
fact that a linear trend accounted for 99% of the variability
in the logarithmic time series, it did not remove the arte-
factual peaks in the 'power spectrum'.

The inadequacy of a linear de-trending process is further
illustrated in Figure 2. This shows the power spectra derived from the performance data of two subjects living on
a constant 24-hour day for three weeks. The top panel shows
the 'power spectra' derived from the raw data, the middle
panel shows the results following linear de-trending, and
the bottom panel the results following de-trending by means
of multiple regression analysis that extracted all trends
up to X^7. Clearly totally spurious conclusions would be
drawn from this data if only the raw, or linearly de-trended,
time series had been analysed. Finally, it is important
to note (a) that "Simon's artefact" occurs when non-cosinor
forms of period analysis are used, and (b) that the nature
and magnitude of the artefact varies according to the length
of the time series, the duration of the gaps in the data,
and the precise nature of the long-term trend. Monotonic

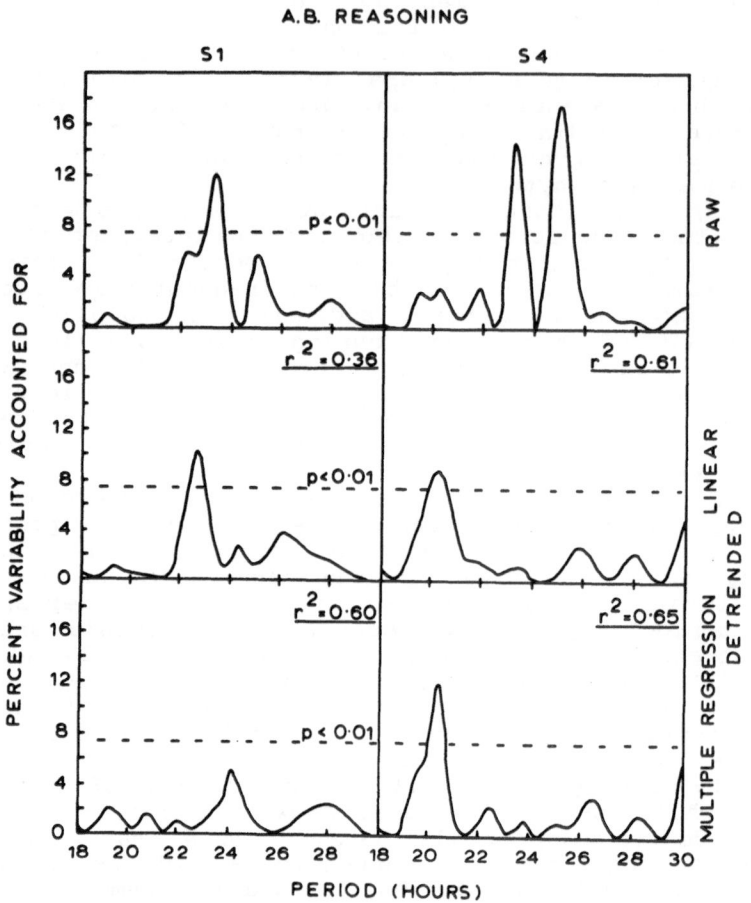

A.B. REASONING

FIGURE 2. The occurrence of "Simon's artefact" in the AB reasoning performance data of two subjects living on a constant 24h routine for three weeks (data collected in collaboration with Drs D. S. Minors & J. M. Waterhouse).

trends usually produce two 'peaks', but non-monotonic trends can produce a single peak that may be indistinguishable from a 'real' rhythm unless a sophisticated de-trending of the data is performed. Another problem with psychological measurement is that it can be notoriously inaccurate in comparison with physiological measures. Psychological measures reflect a number of chance factors such as differences in the motivation of the subject, his perception of the task, and whether or not he is distracted by some non-task event.

This means that one can't, for example, take a single performance reading and feel that one has meaningfully 'measured
performance'. The only way that circadian performance rhythms
can be accurately measured is by using designs which employ
sufficient replications for such inaccuracies to be evened
out. Thus each trial should contain a large number of measured events (e.g. reactions) and each time of day should
be associated with a large number of trials, coming either
from different subjects, or from different days, or, preferably, from both.

An example of the care needed to circumvent all these
problems (and several more) is provided by an early study
of scholastic performance carried out by Laird (1925).
Laird used 112 subjects divided into 7 squads, matched for
intelligence. Six weeks of experimentation were necessary,
with each squad attending at six times of day, in a design
which enabled both time of day and day of week to be studied
independently of each other and uncontaminated by either
practice effects or the actual material given. At each
session a battery of nine different tasks was given, with
tasks often being represented by several different instances
(e.g. about 50 computations for the 'simple additions' task).
To avoid contamination due to personal prejudices, the subjects were misled into believing that the experiment was
a study of temperature changes.

It is, perhaps, rather chastening to realise that even
in this present age of electronic data analysis and on-line
experiment control, the care and elegance of Laird's study
has seldom been approached, let alone surpassed. All too
often performance measures (sometimes of the most trivial
sort) have simply been "lumped in" as part of a battery of
otherwise physiological tests, without their special needs
and controls being taken into account.

2.3. Trends over the day

Despite the problems discussed above, considerable progress
has been made in describing and accounting for the pattern
of some psychological functions over the normal waking day.
The trends for some of the more consistent of these are shown
in Figure 3. It should be noted that these "time of day"
patterns reflect the effects of 'masking' factors, such as
fatigue and time since getting up, as well as any endogenous
circadian rhythm in the parameter being observed. In summary,
it appears that for performance the shape of the curve, and
the timing of peaks and troughs, depends on the particular
mix of cognitive functions which are required to perform
the task under consideration. This is assumed to reflect
differences in the trend over the day for different components
of the human cognitive system (Marks & Folkard, 1984).

On a comparatively simple cognitive task such as serial
search, performance gets progressively faster over the day
to peak at around 20.00 (e.g. Blake, 1967). This pattern
parallels that of the temperature rhythm and led to the notion
of a causal link between the temperature and performance
rhythms. However, there is some indication that the trend

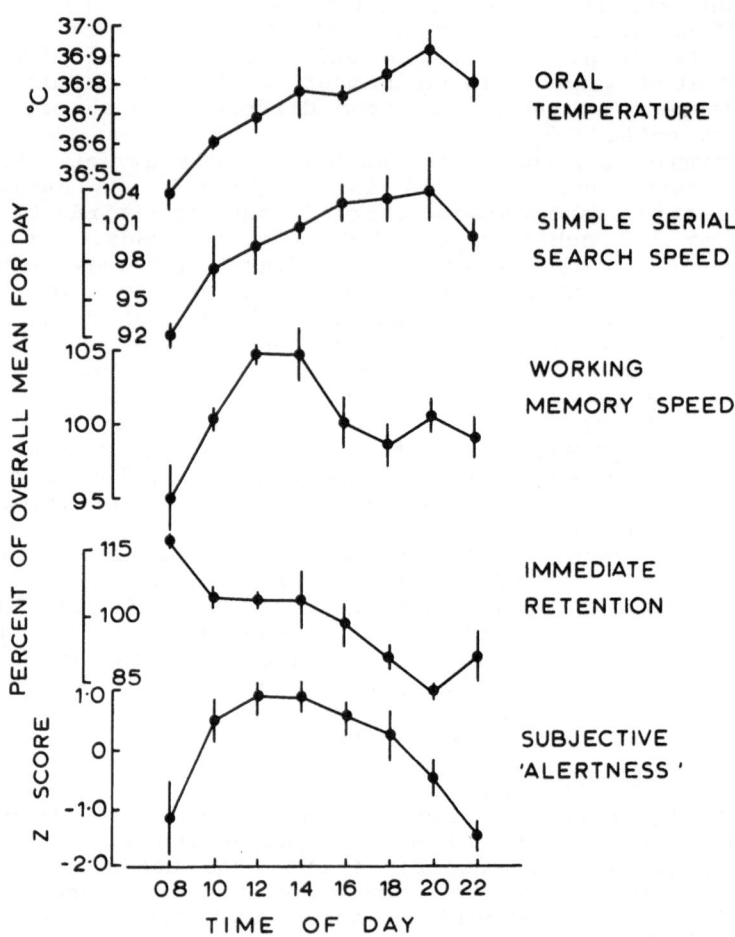

FIGURE 3.   The normal trend over the day in oral temperature, three different performance measures, and subjective ratings of alertness.   Each plot represents the mean and standard deviation of 3 - 5 average trends from independent studies. See Folkard (1983) for details of the individual studies.

over the day for a given task may depend on the short-term memory load involved in carrying out that task.   Simple serial search involves little, if any, memory component.

When we add a memory load to this task we find that as memory
load is increased peak performance moves to an earlier time
in the day (Folkard et al., 1976). On more complex (working
memory) tasks, such as logical reasoning, performance tends
to improve to about mid-day and then declines. The logical
reasoning task is said to require the use of a working memory
system which involves a number of different cognitive sub-
systems (e.g. short term storage, processing throughput,
etc.). It is likely that the rhythm observed for this task,
and others involving working memory, is the outcome of a
combination of different trends associated with the different
cognitive mechanisms involved. When the task is one of
'immediate retention' which emphasises memory mechanisms,
such as that required to memorise digit strings or even pass-
ages of text, then immediate recall of this material tends
to be best early in the day and then steadily declines (Folkard & Monk, 1980).

The link between performance on simple tasks and the temperature rhythm led to the view that either the circadian
variation in temperature was responsible for circadian variations in performance (Kleitman, 1939), or that there was
some other mechanism which controlled both temperature and
performance rhythms, for example, an underlying rhythm in
base level arousal or sleepiness (Colquhoun, 1971). The
direct performance temperature link was discounted on the
basis that when time of day is controlled for, correlations
between temperature and performance disappear (Rutenfranz,
Aschoff & Mann, 1972). It was then thought that the results
could be explained in terms of increasing arousal over the
day, and that increasing temperature was merely an indicator
of diurnal variations in arousal.

One reason that the arousal explanation was so enthusias-
tically adopted was that it could account for the many different trends observed. This model invokes the Yerkes-
Dodson inverted U-function relating performance to arousal
which states that as arousal increases, performance on a
given task improves until some optimal level of arousal is
reached when performance then starts to decline. In addition
there are different functions for different levels of task
difficulty, namely as task difficulty increases, the optimal
arousal level for that task declines. Thus the arousal
model can account for the three performance trends shown
in Figure 3 if it is assumed that task complexity increases
from 'serial search' through 'working memory' to 'immediate
retention'. Unfortunately, this explanatory power of the
arousal model was also its downfall: any set of data could
be explained away by invoking a particular point on the inverted U.

Furthermore, when we consider findings from studies involving a phase shift relative to the external zeitgebers, as
a result of time-zone transitions or working at night, a
unidimensional model proves inadequate. When the zeitgebers
are shifted it usually takes some time for the circadian
system to become synchronised to the new 24-hour routine,
and the rhythms in various psychological functions adjust

to this new routine at different rates (see review by Monk
& Folkard, 1985).   This finding emphasises the importance
of measuring as wide a range of different psychological functions as possible.   There is not a single 'psychological
rhythm', just as there is not a single 'physiological rhythm'.
As is the case for physiological processes, different psychological processes appear to be controlled by different underlying circadian control processes (Monk et al, 1983; Folkard
et al., 1983, 1985).

3. THE MEASUREMENT OF PSYCHOLOGICAL VARIABLES

The problems discussed above associated with the inaccuracy
of psychological measures are unfortunately often compounded
by the use of badly designed measures.   There are a number
of criteria which a psychological measure, and, in particular,
one of performance, should meet.   First, the measure should
be as pure a measure of the particular function under consideration as possible.   Thus, for example, in the case
of serial search measures we favour requiring subjects to
search through random letters, line by line, searching for
the occurrence of a particular letter.   However, in the
literature one can find examples of serial search tasks based
on text, where the serial search component is confounded
with a reading component, or on abstract symbols, where the
unfamiliarity of the material will increase the magnitude
and duration of the 'learning' or 'practice' effect.

Secondly, a large number of equivalent versions of each
measure are needed for the monitoring of circadian rhythms.
If a particular version is repeated too soon after its original presentation, then the responses obtained may reflect
the subjects' memory for their previous responses rather
than their ability on the task per se.   This problem is
particularly serious in the case of more cognitive measures
of performance, and indeed, to date, has effectively ruled
out the long-term monitoring of some types of performance.
For example, the immediate retention curve shown in Figure
3 is based on studies in which subjects were presented with
information in text or short films and then required to recall
it at the end of the presentation.   Clearly, a different
text/film had to be used for each presentation in order to
avoid confounding by memory for an earlier presentation of
the same material.   In addition, potential differences between the texts/films had to be counterbalanced over the
different times of day.   In order to monitor this type of
performance function over a prolonged period, a very large
number of identically difficult texts or films would have
to be produced.   In view of the fact that different subjects
will inevitably find different texts or films more or less
difficult, this requirement seems unattainable. Consequently,
the measurement   of immediate retention   has normally been
limited to that for random lists of digits or words which
shows a rather different trend over the day (see Folkard
& Monk, 1980).   While lacking realism, this procedure does
allow a large number of equivalent tests to be produced.

Thirdly, the response required of the subject should be

as simple as possible, compatible with the stimulus material, and highly practised. If this is not achieved, then response times may be a better reflection of motor speed and response uncertainty than they are of the task under consideration. Thus, for example, it would be fairly pointless trying to test a subject's memory for a list of words by requiring them to type the words on a computer keyboard unless the subject happened to be an extremely competent typist. Most subjects would spend so long searching for and depressing each key that they may well have forgotten the rest of the list of words by the time they had typed in the first one! A tape recording of a spoken recall, or even a written recall, would reveal a rather higher memory score. This is, of course, an extreme example, but the basic principle of using simple, compatible, highly practised responses holds for most performance tests. In general, we try to limit responses to a simple left- or right-hand key press, or a tick or cross in an appropriate position, although some tasks, such as mental arithmetic, usually require slightly more complex responses.

Most of the criteria described above can be met using minimal equipment, and, indeed, in many cases, require only paper, pencil, and a stopwatch. It is difficult to imagine how such 'paper and pencil' tests can be improved upon in terms of their portability. However, they do suffer from the disadvantage that the results have to be scored by hand, and this can prove extremely time-consuming. In addition, some types of performance function, such as vigilance performance, choice reaction time, or manual dexterity, are not amenable to this type of approach. To overcome this problem, portable equipment based on cassette recorders has been developed (e.g. Wilkinson & Houghton, 1982), but such equipment is usually restricted to the testing of a single psychological function.

Microprocessor-based 'test batteries' are potentially capable of overcoming all these restrictions, and, indeed, some progress has already been made in this direction. We are currently using such computer-based 'test batteries' in laboratory 'temporal isolation' studies (Monk et al., 1983; Folkard et al., 1985). With the rapidly decreasing size (and increasing power) of microprocessors, data storage facilities, and monitors, there is no reason why such test batteries should not become truly portable in the near future.

REFERENCES

1. Bergstrum FG: An experimental study of some of the conditions of mental activity. American Journal of Psychology, 6, 1894.
2. Blake MJF: Time of day effects on performance in a range of tasks. Psychonomic Science, 9, 1967.
3. Borbely AA: A two process model of sleep regulation. Human Neurobiology, 1, 1982.

4. Colquhoun WP: Circadian variations in mental efficiency. Biological Rhythms and Human Performance. London: Academic Press, 1971.
5. Dressler FB: Some influences which affect the rapidity of voluntary mnovements. American Journal of Psychology, 4, 1892.
6. Folkard S: Diurnal variation in logical reasoning. British Journal of Psychology, 66, 1975.
7. Folkard S: Diurnal variation. Stress and Fatigue in Human Performance. Chichester: Wiley, 1983.
8. Folkard S, Hume KI, Minors DS, Waterhouse JM & Watson FL: Independence of the circadian rhythm in alertness from the sleep/wake cycle. Nature, 313, 1985.
9. Folkard S, Knauth P, Monk TH & Rutenfranz J: The effect of memory load on the circadian variation in performance efficiency under a rapidly rotating shift system. Ergonomics, 19, 1976.
10. Folkard S & Monk TH: Time of day and processing strategy in free recall. Quarterly Journal of Experimental Psychology, 31, 1979.
11. Folkard S & Monk TH: Circadian rhythms in human memory. British Journal of Psychology, 71, 1980.
12. Folkard S, Wever RA & Wildgruber CM: Multioscillatory control of circadian rhythms in human performance. Nature, 305, 1983.
13. Freeman GL & Hovland CI: Diurnal variations in performance and related physiological processes. Psychological Bulletin, 31, 1934.
14. Froberg, JE: Twenty-four-hour patterns in human performance, subjective and physiological variables and differences between morning and evening active subjects. Biological Psychology, 5, 1977.
15. Gates, AI: Diurnal variations in memory and association. University of California Publications in Psychology, 1, 1916a.
16. Gates AI: Variations in efficiency during the day, together with practice effects,sex differences, and correlations. University of California Publications in Psychology,d 2, 1916b.
17. Halberg F: More on educative chronobiology, health and the computer. International Journal of Chronobiology, 2, 1973.
18. Kleitman N: (Revised and enlarged 1963) Sleep and Wakefulness. Chicago: University of Chicago Press, 1939.
19. Laird DA: Relative performance of college students as conditioned by time of day and day of week. Journal of Experimental Psychology, 8, 1925.
20. Lombard WP: The variations of the normal knee jerk, and their relation to the activity of the central nervous system. American Journal of Psychology, 1, 1887.
21. Marks M & Folkard S: Diurnal rhythms in cognitive performance. Psychology Survey 5. Leicester: British Psychological Society, 1984.
22. Michelson M: Ueuber die Tiefe des Schlafes. Psychol. Arbeiten, 2, 1897.

23. Monk H & Folkard S: Shiftwork and Performance. Hours of Work: Temporal Factors in Work Scheduling. Chichester: Wiley & Sons Ltd, 1985.
24. Monk TH, Weitzman ED, Fookson JE, Moline ML, Kronauer RE & Gander PH: Task variables determine which biological clock controls circadian rhythms in human performance. Nature, 304, 1983.
25. Rutenfranz J, Aschoff J & Mann H: The effects of a cumulative sleep deficit, duration of preceding sleep period and body temperature on multiple choice reaction time. Aspects of Human Efficiency: Diurnal Rhythm and Loss of Sleep. London: English Universities Press, 1972.
26. Thorndike E: Mental fatigue. Psychological Review, 7, 1900.
27. Winch WH: Mental fatigue in day school children as measured by immediate memory, Part I. Journal of Educational Psychology, 3, 1912a.
28. Winch WH: Mental fatigue in day school children as measured by immediate memory, Part II. Journal of Educational Psychology, 3, 1912b.
29. Wilkinson RT & Houghton D: Field test of arousal: a portable reaction timer with data storage. Human Factors, 24, 1982.

THE DESIGN OF HUMAN ACTIVITY MONITORS

D. P. REDMOND AND F. W. HEGGE, Biomedical Measurement and Instrumentation Research, Walter Reed Army Institute of Research, Washington, DC

1.INTRODUCTION

Devices which record human motility are used to produce data indexing the daily cycle of rest and activity, variations in that circadian rhythm, relative activity within days (ultradian effects) and across days (infradian effects), and the timing, duration, and disruption of sleep. Such data have proved important to assessment of shift-work schedules, continuous operations scenarios, time-zone changes, hyperactivity and motor disorders in children, unipolar, bipolar, and seasonal affective disorders, and hypnotic, anxiolytic, and anti-depressive drug effects.

Over the last 20 years, the design technology of self-contained, non-restrictive activity monitors has improved considerably. Initial designs were simply modified wrist watches which reported an accumulated count of movements (Bell, 1968). In 1972, an electronic telemetric device which permitted continuous recording was introduced, albeit restricted by the location of the receiver/recording apparatus (Foster et al., 1972). By the mid-seventies, these monitors had been refined into truly self-contained activity counters, with integrated circuitry and memory to provide both internal control and timing, and off-line data retrieval (McPartland et al., 1976). Concurrently, Colburn and others (1976) produced a similar system with different transducer and timing characteristics, and 256 bytes of memory. Other activity monitors have also been in common use, consisting of transducers (wrist-worn or otherwise) connected by cable to light-weight tape recorders (Kripke et al., 1978) or solid-state memory packages (Taylor et al., 1982). A careful engineering analysis by Wong, Webster, Montoye and Washburn (1981) clarified the design issues surrounding accelerometric transducers used in this application. And most recently, Gueuning and Eugene (1985) described a design which uses microprocessor, read-only memory (ROM), and random-access memory (RAM) chips for programmable timing and storage functions, along with a novel transducer design.

It is a main goal of this laboratory to study the rest/activity cycles of soldiers in sustained operations and other conditions which adversely affect sleep and performance. Large numbers of individuals are involved simultaneously, and operations occur in rugged field environments. For several years we have used activity monitors of various designs, both home-made and commercially available. Success was sharply limited by inconsistency and narrow dynamic range of the data, by artifact sensitivity, and by maintenance problems with the devices. About three years ago, we undertook a program to optimize the design and to assure the utility of our activity monitoring system. First, a review of existing devices led to the conclusion that there were serious flaws in design concept, as well as technological limitations. We then studied the fundamental characteristics of the wrist movement signal from which a motor activity index is derived. Next, we examined transducers, their response to movements, methods of analog signal processing, and signal-to-count transforms -- an extension of work previously done by Kripke and his colleagues (Webster, Messin, Mullaney, & Kripke, 1982). Finally, we outlined and specified a design which satisfied our purposes at the same time that it exploited current electrical engineering technology.

This paper summarizes that program, and describes the new Walter Reed Activity Monitoring System. Using descriptive data exemplifying the several issues, our observations and the resulting design specifications are presented. Key issues center on the transduction of motion and management of the signal leading to digitization. Analog recordings of human activity were obtained and studied, leading to a discussion of these issues as follows:

a. Fundamental Nature and Source of the Signal
b. Frequency Characteristics of the Signal
c. Vibration Artifact
d. Sensitivity and Dynamic Range
e. Directionality of Movements
f. Non-Linear Motion Sensors
g. Analog-to-Digital Transformation
h. Calibration
i. Memory Capacity

2.ANALOG RECORDINGS OF WRIST ACTIVITY

2.1.Method

To acquire raw, undigitized movement signals for examination of signal properties, commercially acquired miniature accelerometers were mounted within wrist-watch cases, worn on the subjects' wrist, with the leads threaded down to a belt-worn miniature tape recorder (Oxford Medilog Model 4-24). Time base was provided by a 60 Hz signal recorded on one channel.

Preliminary studies indicated that greater than 99% of signal power was produced in the frequency band below 5 Hz with the majority of signal power in the sub-Hertz frequencies. Wrist activity was thereafter sensed using transducers and recording amplifiers with an overall frequency response of DC to 8.3 Hz on playback. Calibration was achieved simply by rotating the transducer 90 degrees, from horizontal to vertical, for a 1 g output change. Triple axis recordings utilized three identical recording channels. Orthogonal x,y, and z axes of the transducer were aligned such that the x-axis was transverse (or medial-lateral), the y-axis transecting (or anterior-posterior), and the z-axis longitudinal with respect to the wrist.

2.2.Data Acquisition and Computations

The activity signals retrieved on playback were filtered and coupled to the inputs of a 4-channel, programmable digital oscilloscope, with 128K-word buffer memory for each channel (Norland Model 3001A). Programmability of the oscilloscope includes a variety of mathematical and statistical functions such as root-mean-square (RMS), power spectral density (PSD) functions, mean, standard deviation, and linear correlations. In a typical usage, a 15 Hz sampling rate produced 128K samples (or 145.64 minutes of activity recording). In blocks of 1024 (or 1K) samples, RMS was computed for each 68.3 seconds of data. As an estimate of total power in the voltage waveform, these RMS values were used as activity scores for each block or epoch, and served as a standard against which other activity indices were compared. PSD functions were likewise computed from 1K-sized blocks of data, and averaged by summing for successive blocks.

2.3.Studies of Wrist Activity

The recording system described has been used in a variety of studies, including those of soldiers in training exercises, temporal isolation ("free running") experiments, and work-motion studies. Over two hundred of these tapes have been examined for signal characteristics, but to summarize the variety of surveys performed on these data over the last three years, a special 2-hour study was performed, using one subject engaged in a set schedule of activities, ranging from bed rest to reading, typing, walking, jogging, and vigorous calisthenics. The purpose was to encompass a range of activity observed typically within a period convenient to the analytical and graphic methods applied in this report. Figure 1 depicts that 2-hour session and the activities involved.

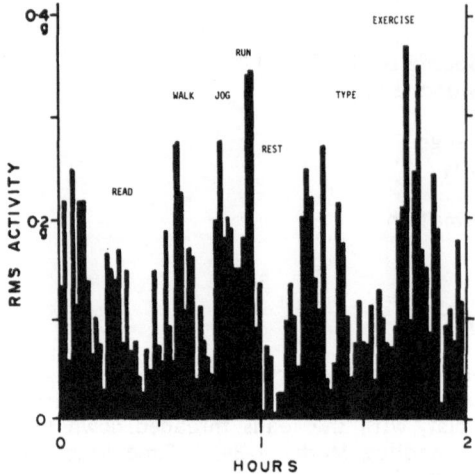

FIGURE 1. Two-hour Session of Activity. Levels represent the Root-Mean-Square (RMS) value for each 68-sec. epoch.

3.DESIGN ISSUES AND RESULTS
3.1.Sources of the Wrist Activity Signal

An accelerometric signal derived from the wrist emanates from several sources: 1) rotation of the transducer in relation to the vertical gravitational force; 2) changing velocity of the transducer in space due to displacement of the arm; 3) abrupt accelerations due to bouncing or bumping of the transducer against other objects; 4) excitation of an undamped transducer at its frequency of mechanical resonance, also associated with bumping or jolting; 5) external vibrations and sounds coupled to the transducer; 6) electromagnetic noise interference; and 7) non-linearities introduced by a viscous or freely moving objects within the transducer (e.g., balls of mercury or steel). Of these, only the first two seem directly related to movement of the wrist (except insofar as proximity to or generation of noise might be considered an index of normal human activity). In bench-testing of several candidate transducers, sources 3-7 were commonly observed to dominate their response, even among devices in standard usage. The analog recording system used here rejected or attenuated such sources, and thus was useful for examining characteristics of the signal associated with movement per se.

Figure 2 illustrates the complexity of the activity signal taken from the wrist. This 68-second block of data was recorded in three axes while the subject was walking at 2 paces per second; as well as his arms swinging with his gait, he was observed to move his arm about, checking his wrist-watch, and wiping his brow. In the last half of the tracing, the walking cadence is most discernible (component A) in the Y-axis, fluctuating about a baseline of about -1 g, with an amplitude of one half to one g. This component reflects a combination of both displacement and rotation. Shifts in baseline, both abrupt and gradual, are discernible as changes in the order of 2 g (component B), lasting several seconds. This component, often of very low frequency, most probably represents 90-180 degree rotations in the position of the transducer with respect to the vertical. A third component (C) consists of transient deflections, occasionally greater than 2 g, which probably represent bumping of the transducer against the body; these deflections, in this damped system, contribute little to the over-all power of the sampled signal.

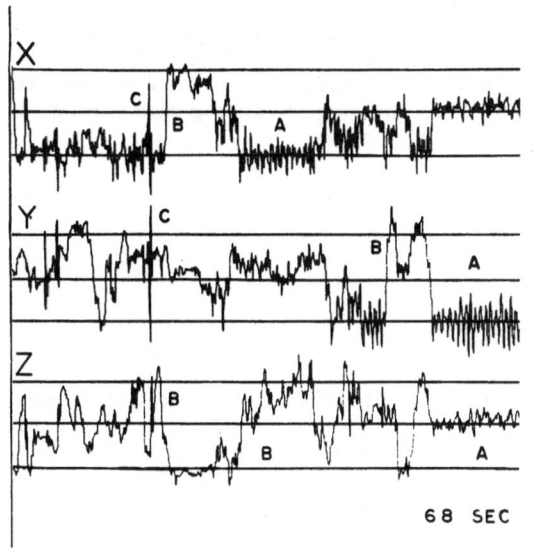

FIGURE 2. Wrist activity signal in three axes. Horizontal lines represent +/- 1 g accelerations (see text).

68 SEC

3.2. Frequency Characteristics of the Activity Signal

The first design problem is to assure that the transduction system is appropriately responsive to the frequency characteristics of the naturally occurring wrist activity signal. Figure 3 depicts the averaged PSD functions from 105 sixty-eight second data blocks. First, it is clear that very low frequency components dominate the spectrum. Second, the contributions to power at frequencies above 1 Hz appear to be quite small. Virtually all devices in the literature are unresponsive to low frequency, and generally, the passband is not specified or even described.

3.2.1. Desirable high pass characteristics are not easily resolved by inspection of the Spectral Density curve. Since the wrist is limited in the distance it can travel, displacement accelerations which are very slow (low frequency) must also be very low in amplitude; conversely, large accelerations must be of high frequency. In contrast, rotational changes may be quite high (up to 2 g), irrespective of their rapidity. If one assumes that displacement measures have more to do with the "energetics" of motility than mere rotation in gravity, then it would seem desirable to separate displacement and rotational components. Although it is possible to do so, using point-by-point analysis of triaxial data, such analyses seem impractical for inexpensive portable devices, especially in the absence of evidence that it would be fruitful to do so. (Such evidence might be obtainable in a weightless state). Nevertheless, it is desirable to reject the DC and very low frequencies, if only to prevent baseline shifts from "swamping" the detection of higher frequency movements. Wong et al. (1981), for instance, chose 0.125 Hz as a high-pass corner frequency with that rationale. For some designs, (e.g. Colburn et al. (1976)), the passband is well above the area of interest - above 10 Hz or so.

A pertinent basis for this choice resides in practical engineering concerns. DC-responsive accelerometric strain gages, of the type used in our studies, are extremely expensive and difficult to fabricate in laboratory shops. An economical approach has been to construct transducers from cantilevered piezoelectric ceramic plates, or bender elements (Gulton, Inc). (Alternatives such as mercury switches are discussed further below). As analyzed by Wong et al. (1981), such transducers are electrically capacitive; as such, their low frequency response is restricted by tradeoffs between physical size of circuit components, pre-amplifier input impedance and offset, and over-all sensitivity. Thus, these practical considerations limit low frequency response to around 0.1 Hz.

Given the discussion above, and observing that the spectrum in Figure 3 appears to have a "shoulder" in the region of 0.25 Hz, we have chosen to specify a range between 0.1 to 0.5 Hz (to give an octave leeway about 0.25 Hz). Figure 4 represents the same 105-spectra average as Figure 3, after filtering the analog data through a high pass filter set at 0.25 Hz, with rolloff of 48 dB/octave.

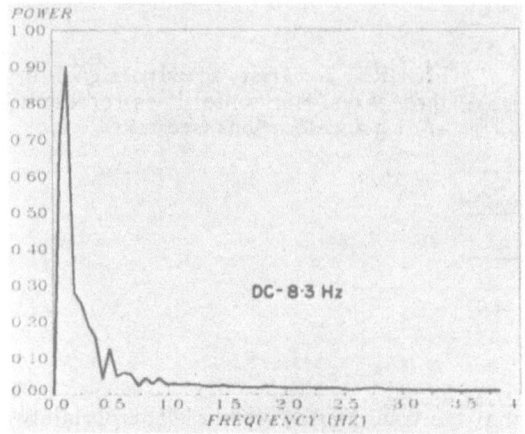

FIGURE 3. Averaged Power Spectrum from 105 blocks of 68-second signal data. Passband is D.C. to 8.3 Hz.

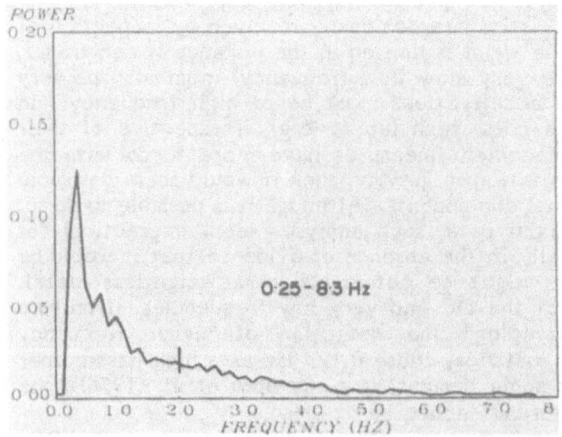

FIGURE 4. Same as Fig. 3, with passband of .25 - 8.3 Hz.

3.2.2. Desirable low pass characteristics are selected to admit the majority of residual power (after high pass filtration) of the activity signal for downline processing or counting. According to Foster, McPartland, and Kupfer (1978), intentional human movements do not occur at a rate greater than about 200 per minute (3.3 Hz), which might serve as a useful cutoff point. It is assumed here that it is desirable to reject higher frequency movements, such as fine tremor and shivering, which occur in a range greater than 5 movements/second.

Low pass filtering provides rejection of high frequency components of the signal other than movement, which are important potential sources of noise. Sensitivity to audio-frequency (50 Hz or higher) and electromagnetic noise (usually 50 or 60 Hz) should be eliminated, along with transients associated with large amplitude rotations and impacts (B and C in Figure 2, respectively).

3.2.3.Vibration artifact may be both internal and external. Transducers built from cantilevered piezoelectric plates or phonograph pick-ups pose a special problem. These devices are not fluid damped, and possess a mechanical resonance of less than a few hundred Hertz (Wong et al, 1981). On excitation by movement or impact, a significant part of the signal will consist of this resonant component, potentially swamping any downline counting process. Thus it is necessary to attenuate such internal transducer vibration signals by analog filtering well below the resonant frequency of the transducer. Such filtering is absent from several designs.

External vibration artifacts result from contact of the transducer or the subject with vibrating objects. In our own applications, involving subjects riding in vehicles or operating machinery, such artifact is a major problem. In former designs, this artifact was due to the absence of low pass filtering, since the vibrations involved were well above 10 Hertz. However, when the frequency of vibration is near the frequency of human movements, the problem persists, as Figure 5 exemplifies. In Fig. 5a, the subject was first shaking his wrist as fast as he could (about 4 Hz), and then grasped the handle of a power lawn mower (about 5.5 Hz). Although the PSD curve (Fig. 5c) clearly discriminates between the two signal sources, low pass filtering set to admit the movement component did not entirely eliminate the vibration artifact (Fig. 5b).

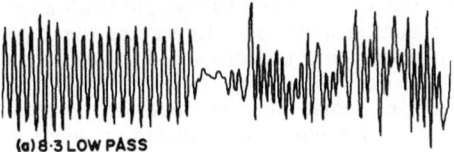
(a) 8·3 LOW PASS

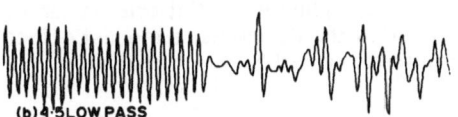
(b) 4·5 LOW PASS

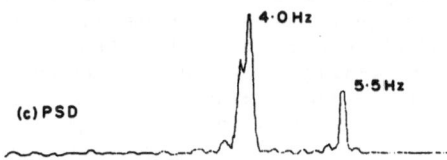
(c) PSD

FIGURE 5. Low pass filtering of vibration artifact. a) Signal in the left half is from intentional shaking of the wrist, followed by grasping a power lawn mower. b) The same signal, filtered below 4.5 Hz. c) PSD function of original signal.

3.2.4.Selection of low pass cut-off frequency is made on empirical grounds. Since the 4 Hertz movements shown in Figure 5 represent a rare extreme, and since vibrational artifacts appear potentially more harmful than the loss of high frequency data, a cutoff of 2 Hertz was chosen for our specification, yielding a final passband of 0.25 to 2 Hz, and accounting for more than 80% of the power displayed in Figure 4. Figure 6 displays a segment of the signal similar to that in Figure 2, but subjected to analog bandpass filtering in the specified range.

208

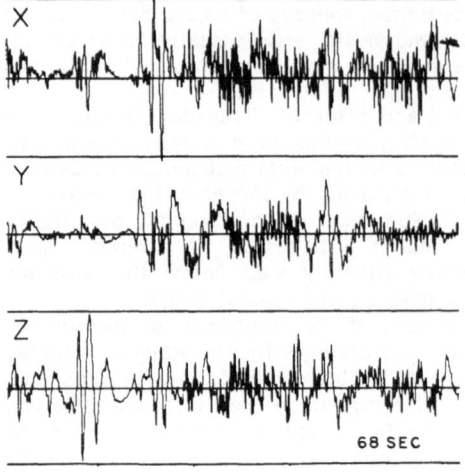

X

Y

FIGURE 6. Band-passed activity signal
similar to Fig. 1. Passband = 0.25 -
2.0 Hz.

Z

68 SEC

3.3. Sensitivity and Dynamic Range

In the two hour recording of Figure 1, the maximum deflection observed was the equivalent of 1.2 g acceleration, and maximum RMS acceleration for any 68-second interval in the recording was about 0.4 g. In other observations, deflections above 1.5 g are exceedingly rare and transient. With the transducer at rest, the RMS level for this system is about 0.01 g, representing a background noise figure for the tape recorder. A minimum sensitivity specification, indicating the threshold above which a deflection should be counted as movement and not noise, was chosen to be in the range of 0.05 - 0.10 g, to provide rejection of noise in the face of possible temperature drift. Accelerations between 0.05 - 1.5 g indicates a dynamic range in the order of 15 dB. In terms of displacement acceleration, 0.05 g represents (roughly) a rather low value of 50 cm/sec/sec. In terms of rotation, 0.05 g change would occur from a change of 20 degrees or less, depending on initial orientation of the transducer. The actual threshold level realized in the design has a modest effect on the fidelity of the analog to digital transform used, as will be described below.

3.4. Directionality of Motion Transduction

On its face, it would seem advantageous to use transducers sensitive in three axes. Figures 1 and 6 indicate that the _instantaneous_ accelerations in axes x, y, and z are quite different from one another. For the single piezoelectric bender element, the use of an mass weight offset from the central axis, as described by Wong et al (1981), provides some sensitivity outside the bending axis, due to tortional movements of the plate. However, using a multi-axis sensing scheme, Webster et al. (1982) showed, at least grossly, that the signal from one axis was about as good as another. Our data confirm this. Movement detection occurs not instantaneously, but is counted over a period of time; thus data from each axis are summated over each epoch, reducing the difference between axes. Figure 7 indicates that this reduction is a function of epoch length, so that by 1 second or so, each axis provides a fair index of the signal in the others. This conforms to a notion that any given movement will only rarely be monoaxial, and that within seconds there will occur a counter-movement involving other axes. Only sustained, repetitious movements in a single axis might escape detection in a monoaxial system. With that warning, the ability to use one axis of motion sensing considerably reduces the expense, space, and complexity of electronic design of the specified system.

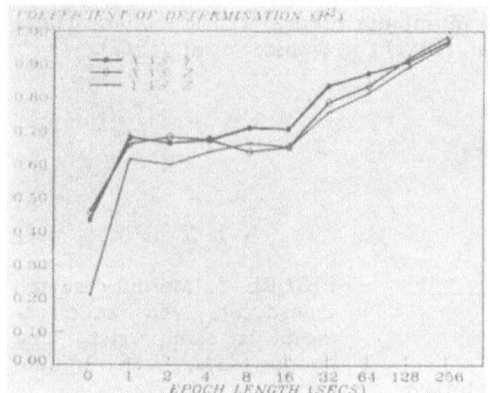

FIGURE 7. Interaction of triaxial signals as a function of epoch length. RMS values/epoch for one axis are correlated with those of other axes at and above Epoch = 1 sec.

3.5.Non-Linear Motion Sensors

The present discussion has emphasized the use of an accelerometer largely because such a transducer provides a linear transformation of physical movement into an electronic signal, and thus lends itself to analog processing, filtration, calibration and adjustment using standard linear circuitry. It should be understood that the overall system relating movement to signal is very complex, involving the nervous system, the tissue beneath the wrist-worn monitor, the rigidity and mass of the case strapped to the wrist, and of course the mechanical and electrical characteristics of the transducer. Such a system is probably replete with sources of distortion and non-linearity. Relationships between the raw signal and higher order measures of physiology and behavior, such as psychomotor activation or energy consumption depend on empirical information, which is very meager at present.

Nevertheless, it seems parsimonious to maintain simplicity of the movement/signal transform to any extent that this is possible. Other transducer systems have been implemented which do not do so, but instead introduce an additional response sub-system to an already complex system, a subsystem which is non-linear in concept. These transducers have in common a mass which moves within a confined space or chamber: either a self-winding watch movement (Bell, 1968), a metal ball (Foster et al., 1972; Gueuning & Eugene, 1985), or a globule of mercury (McPartland et al., 1976; Taylor et al., 1982). Movement of the arm produces a movement of the object, which in turn excites a transduction system or closes a switch. Thus, the movement-to-count transformation depends on the inertia of the mass, its size, shape, and elasticity, and in the case of mercury, its viscosity, surface tension, and the presence of impurities. Also involved are the dimensions and material of the containing chamber, the pathway of movement, and tendency of the mass to bounce, ricochet, or vibrate. In any event, it seems unlikely that such systems are linearly responsive to a wide range of movements, in terms of amplitude, direction, and frequency. The apparently linear calibration curves of Foster et al. (1978) hold for repetitious, unidirectional movements, so that counts are directly proportional to the number of movements; at the same time, there is a non-linear relationship to the amplitude of movements.

In our experience, mercury-switch transducers (Taylor et al., 1982) have been quite disappointing, showing little or no response to low amplitude movement (variable threshold effect), high sensitivity to vibration artifact, and spontaneous oscillation. Comparison to linear accelerometers, by mounting both on the same wrist, reveals little relationship between the count of switch closures and the RMS level of activity. In ten 60-minute repetitions, using 1-minute epochs, the correlation coefficient between Hg-switch closures and RMS activity ranged from -0.10 to +0.40. Figure 8 displays one such 60-minute record, with r = 0.00. These observations concur with those of Wong et al. (1981) and Webster et al. (1982).

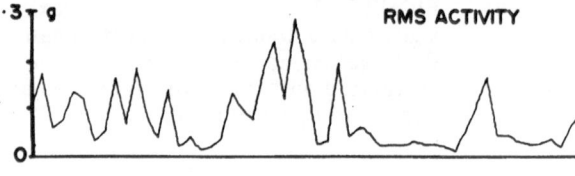

RMS ACTIVITY

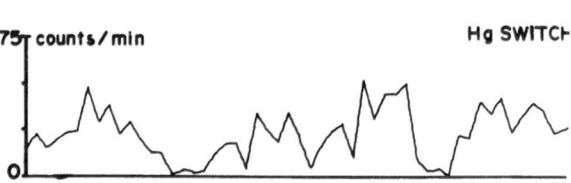

Hg SWITCH

FIGURE 8. Mercury switch transducer vs. accelerometer on same wrist. One hour's data, one minute epochs.

3.6. Analog to Digital Data Transformation

Given an activity signal which has been bandpass filtered, there are four basic methods for converting the continuous data into a form suitable for storage in digital memory. The first of these involves analog rectification and integration of the signal, with sampling and resetting the integrator's output. Drift problems, component size, and power consumption discourage this option, although it is utilized by Wong et al. (1981). The second method involves regular sampling within each epoch, with analog-to-digital conversion of the waveform, followed by computation of some summary parameter (e.g., RMS level) at the end of each epoch. The versatility offered by the choice of computational algorithms, and the linear relationship between the signal and the sampled time series, make this a desirable choice. Unfortunately, micro-power analog-to-digital converters are not yet available, and the power-drain of present circuits would sharply limit battery life.

The last two options involve the use of comparator circuits, which test the signal against some reference voltage level and provide a binary output. One choice consists of Peak Counting: counting the number of times per epoch that the signal level exceeds the reference threshold. A variant of this is Threshold Crossing Detection, which provides a count twice that of Peak Counting. The last option is similar, but by regular sampling (e.g., at 5 Hz), it counts the Time-Above-Threshold of the waveform. Figure 9 schematizes these methods of digitization.

Because of the lower current consumption, the last two methods are chosen in the present design. Given a comparator with the proper reference level, both methods are programmable; that is, the activity monitor's microprocessor can control the way the comparator output is managed (counted or sampled). The data transformation is not purely linear, since a threshold level is imposed. Furthermore, Peak Counting favors the higher frequency components of the signal, while Time-Above-Threshold favors the lower frequencies. Our design provides at option between the two, to allow further study of these signal transformations.

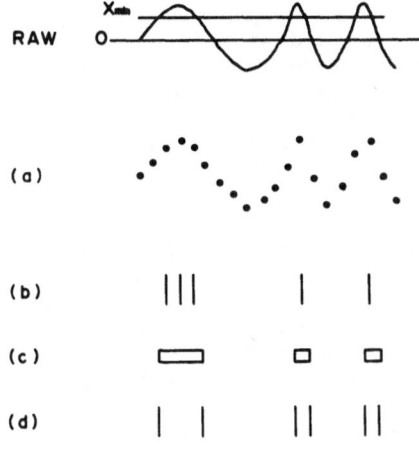

RAW

(a)

(b)

(c)

(d)

FIGURE 9. Analog to Digital transforms of signal. a) A-to-D sampling. b) Time Above Threshold. c) Peak Counting. d) Threshold Crossing.

Digitized data from the analog activity recorder were treated with algorithms which modeled Peak Counting (PC) and Time-Above-Threshold (TAT). The results for a series of 68 second epochs are plotted in Figure 10. Linear regression of each series with the original signal-RMS series produced correlation coefficients as indicated. Note that the Time-Above-Threshold count is the superior index of RMS level, which is expected since the greater power is contributed by the lower frequencies (see Fig. 4). Other data, not shown, indicate that both indices improve as the threshold rises above underlying noise levels.

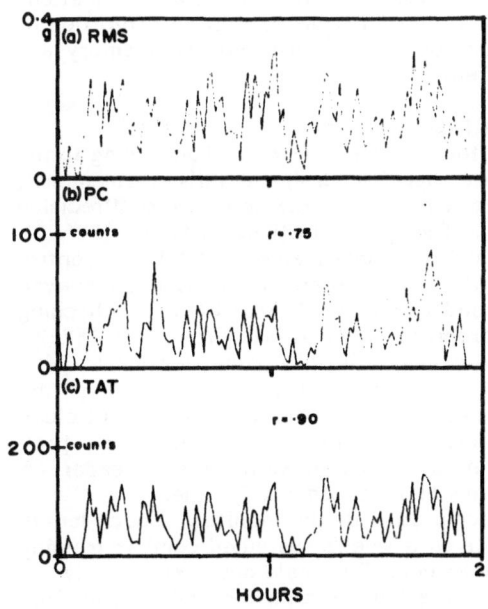

FIGURE 10. Digital Transforms and RMS Activity. a) RMS data from Fig. 1. b) Peak Counting (PC) method. c) Time Above Threshold (TAT) method.

3.7.Calibration

Calibration of the activity counter is achieved by applying known accelerations within the range of frequency and amplitude specified. Among several possibilities, the simplest is to use a pendulum with adjustable periods ranging from 2 seconds to one half-second (.5 to 2 Hz). The monitor is mounted with its sensitive axis perpendicular to the arc of the pendulum's swing. For each frequency tested, the is related to calculated values of the gravitational vector along that arc. At manufacture, the circuitry is trimmed to preset the threshold. A recording is made of counter response to pendulum excursions, and the angle of pendulum decay at which counting ceases identifies the comparator threshold setting.

3.8.Memory Capacity and Digital Dynamic Range

In older activity monitors, the count-per-epoch was limited to 255 (an eight-bit binary number). Since counts were admitted at a rate of up to ten per second, it often happened that for epochs longer than 25 seconds, counters became saturated. This in effect produced rectangular waveforms in the activity data series, which in turn created difficulties for various time series analytic methods.

In the design discussed here, the use of a microprocessor within the activity monitor permits storage of data on a bit-by-bit basis. Epochal word length, in bits, is determined by the maximum count rate and the epoch length. Since the low-pass cutoff frequency is 2 Hz, a 4 Hz Nyquist sampling frequency is imposed; as it turns out, a 10 Hz counting frequency is more conveniently derived from the system clock, so the latter is actually used. Thus, the maximum number of counts in a one minute epoch is 600 (or 10 bits), for a 10 minute epoch, 6000 (or 13 bits), and so on up to 16 bits which permits a count of 65,535 (implying an epoch of 109 minutes). Word length, in bits, and epoch length, in seconds, are separately programmable.

The total number of epochs which can be stored in the system is limited by random-access-memory (RAM) capacity, or battery life, whichever depletes first. Operating battery life is greater than 2000 Hours for the circuits used, and data collection periods of up to 720 hours, 30 days, are envisioned. The RAM capacity is 16K bytes, or 131,072 bits, so that recording time exceeds nine days for 1-minute epochs, 16 days for 2-minute epochs and so on. The relationships between word length, epoch length, and total recording time may be expressed in simple equations and stated in any computer language. An additional feature is that on saturation of memory, or with a microprocessor malfunction, all circuits but the memory are "powered down" to protect the memory contents.

4.THE WALTER REED ACTIVITY MONITORING SYSTEM

Figure 11 is a block diagram of the Monitoring System developed according to the foregoing considerations and specifications. Specific design details, refinements, software development, and production were achieved by the contractors (Precision Control Design, Inc., Ft. Walton Beach, FL). The system utilizes an MC1468705G2L (Motorola) microprocessor with self-contained read-only-memory (ROM) for control of timing, data sampling, and storage to RAM. External communication is achieved by a serial line with RS232 format, using standard MODEM/XMODEM error checking protocol implemented by the on-board microprocessor, and brought to full RS232C voltage levels by an outboard computer interface. Serial communication at 9600 baud is used to both initialize the monitor before deployment, and to "dump" the contents of RAM to a microcomputer. Initialization includes the insertion of clock time and date to the monitor's on-board clock, start/stop time and date, epoch length, data word length (in bits), counting method, and an identification header. A test of device function occurs initially and may be repeated at any time.

Figure 12 presents a 7-day time series acquired with the monitor. Epoch length was 120 seconds. The subject was a soldier on a week's sustained combat training exercise, denied sleep for three nights in mid-week. Full scale count/epoch shown is amounts to 256 movements/minute, using the threshold crossing method for counting.

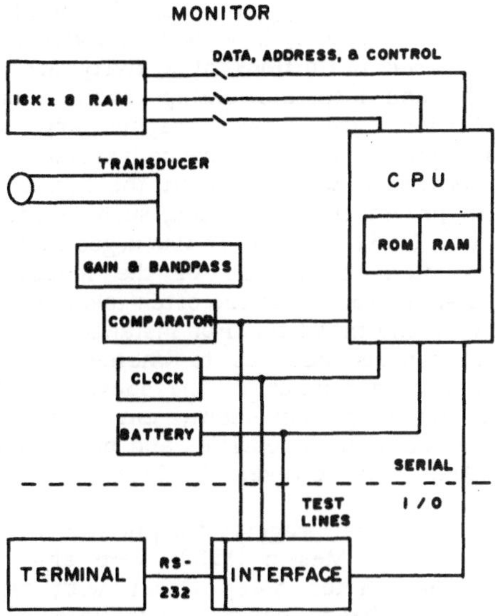

MONITOR

DATA, ADDRESS, & CONTROL

16K x 8 RAM

TRANSDUCER

C P U

ROM | RAM

GAIN & BANDPASS

COMPARATOR

CLOCK

BATTERY

SERIAL

TEST
LINES

I / O

TERMINAL

RS-
232

INTERFACE

FIGURE 11. Block diagram of new
Walter Reed Activity Monitoring
System.

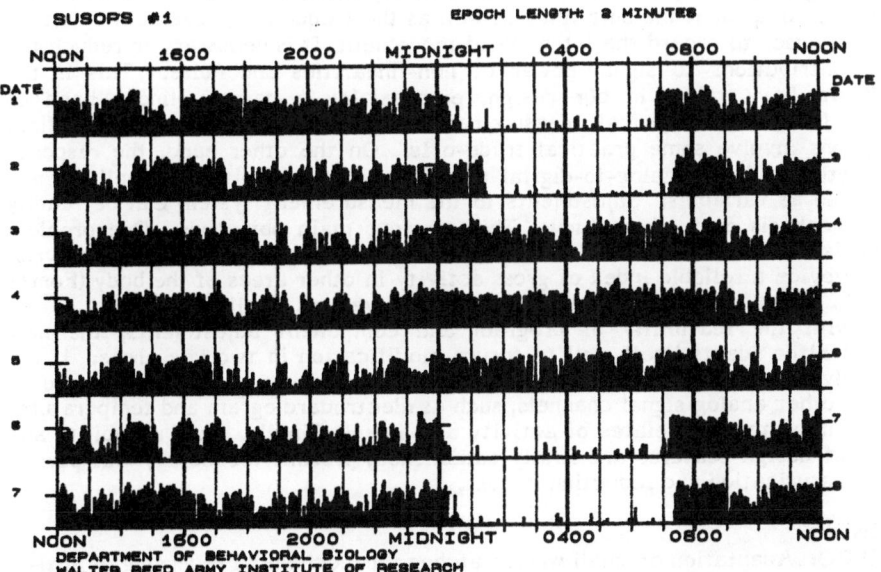

SUSOPS #1   EPOCH LENGTH: 2 MINUTES

NOON   1600   2000   MIDNIGHT   0400   0800   NOON
DATE   DATE

DEPARTMENT OF BEHAVIORAL BIOLOGY
WALTER REED ARMY INSTITUTE OF RESEARCH

FIGURE 12. Activity time series from new Monitor. Seven days of sustained
operations in young soldier, with sleep deprivation in third, fourth, and fifth nights.
Two minute epochs, with full scale = 256 movements/minute.

5.DISCUSSION

In their review of then current research on human activity, Cromwell, Baumeister, and Hawkins (1963) argued that there was a certain futility in viewing activity as a unitary, homogeneous phenomenon. Theory-based definitions of activity are as diverse as the means of measuring activity, and interrelationships even among reliable measures, or among useful theories, are weak, fragmentary, or unconfirmed. As they put it, "a precise definition of activity depends invariably on how it is measured." That point in part conveys a warning about the limits on interpretation of activity data acquired with pragmatic techniques, such as those discussed here, a caveat echoed by Webster et al. (1982, p. 744). It also urges that, if activity phenomena are to be carefully studied, definitions of the measures themselves should be precisely drawn. That is an approach not too often taken in the design of instruments for monitoring movement and motility. For instance, it is a distinction with both design and theoretical consequences as to whether human activity shall be defined simply as movement of a portion of the body, or as a complex disturbance of the environment involving movement, environmental reaction, and noise all together. In the latter case, nonlinearities and broad-band sensitivity of detectors are acceptable, even desirable; however, this intent is rarely discussed (but see Gueuning and Eugene, 1985).

It is clear that activity monitors are useful in several pragmatic applications. By comparison with EEG data, Mullaney, Kripke, and Messin (1980) were able to estimate Sleep Time, Sleep Period, and Wake After Sleep Onset with high reliability. Quantitative movement counts have been shown to correlate with residual drug effects (Crowley & Hydinger-MacDonald, 1979), serum creatine phosphokinase (Goode et al., 1979), achievement and self-image in children (Foster, McPartland & Kupfer, 1977), manic-depressive state (Wehr et al., 1982), occupational activity (LaPorte et al., 1982), and energy expenditure (LaPorte et al., 1979).

According to Wong et al. (1981), it would appear that superior correlations between oxygen consumption rate and an activity measure is achieved when the latter takes into account the amplitude as well as the frequency (movement count) of activity. In order to record the intensity of movement, it is necessary to reduce the spurious contributions to signal power of non-linearities and noise. This is the approach we have taken in our design, emphasizing a narrow, linear band of sensitivity based on empirical measurements of wrist movements. The final specifications involve some practical trade-offs. On the other hand, the response characteristics and the analog-to-digital transform of the monitor are well defined and treatable as variables: adjustments to the measurement system can be readily made on the basis of further study. This was our main objective. One problem remaining is that the choice of location is mainly one of convenience. The wrist seems to provide a reliable index of gross activity in other areas of the body (Foster et al., 1978; Webster et al., 1982), but our own observations are limited.

Along with the feasibility of program and component adjustments, the new Activity Monitor adapts itself well to future modification in two key areas: 1) the use of truly linear signal processing through analog-to-digital conversion and 2) addition of other analog signal channels, such as electrocardiogram and temperature, to monitor important correlates of activity and sleep. Finally, when reliability and relevance of design features are firmly established, present technology will permit drastic miniaturization and reduction in cost.

REFERENCES

1. Bell RQ: Adaptation of small wrist watches for mechanical recording of activity in infants and children. Journal of Experimental Child Psychology, 6:302, 1968.
2. Borbely AA, Loepfe M, Mattman P, & Tobler I: Midazolam and triazolam: hypnotic action and residual effects after a single bedtime dose. Arzneimittel Forschung - Drug Research, 33:1500, 1983.

3. Colburn TR, Smith BM, Guarini JJ, & Simmons NN: An ambulatory activity monitor with solid state memory. ISA Transactions, 15:149, 1976.
4. Cromwell RL, Baumeister A & Hawkins WF: Research in activity level. In Ellis, NR (Ed.), Handbook of Mental Deficiency. New York: McGraw-Hill, 1963.
5. Crowley TJ, & Hydinger-MacDonald M: Bedtime flurazepam and the human circadian rhythm of spontaneous motility. Psychopharmacology, 62:157,1979.
6. Foster FG, Kupfer D, Weiss G, Lipponen V, McPartland R, & Delgado J: Mobility recording and cycle research in neuropsychiatry. Journal of Interdisciplinary Cycle Research, 3:61, 1972.
7. Foster FG, McPartland RJ, & Kupfer DJ: Telemetric motor activity in children. Biotelemetry, 4:1, 1977.
8. Foster FG, McPartland RJ, & Kupfer DJ: Motion sensors in medicine, part I. A report on reliability and validity. Journal of Inter-American Medicine, 3, 1978.
9. Goode DJ, Meltzer HY, Moretti R, Kupfer DJ, & McPartland RJ: The relationship between wrist-mounted motor activity and serum CPK activity in psychiatric in-patients. British Journal of Psychiatry, 135:62, 1979.
10. Gueuning F, & Eugene C: A long-term microprocessor-based wrist-worn actimeter. Paper presented at the International Symposium on Ambulatory Monitoring, 29-31 March, 1985, Padova, Italy.
11. Kripke DF, Mullaney DJ, Messin S, & Wyborney VG: Wrist actigraphic measures of sleep and rhythms. Electroencephalography and Clinical Neurophysiology, 44:674, 1978.
12. LaPorte RE, Kuller LH, Kupfer DJ, McPartland RJ, Matthews G, & Caspersen C: An objective measure of physical activity for epidemiologic research. American Journal of Epidemiology, 109:158, 1979.
13. LaPorte RE, Cauley JA, Kinsey CM, Corbett W, Robertson R, Black-Sandler R, Kuller LH, & Falkel J: The epidemiology of physical activity in children, college students, middle-aged men, menopausal females, and monkeys. Journal of Chronic Diseases, 35:787, 1982.
14. McPartland RJ, Kupfer DJ, & Foster FG: The movement-activated recording monitor: a third-generation motor-activity monitoring system. Behavior Research Methods & Instrumentation, 8:357, 1976.
15. Mullaney DJ, Kripke DF, & Messin S: Wrist-actigraphic estimation of sleep time. Sleep, 3:83, 1980.
16. Porrino LJ, Rapoport JL, Behar D, Sceery W, Ismond DR, & Bunney WE: A naturalistic assessment of the motor activity of hyperactive boys. Archives of General Psychiatry, 40:681, 1983.
17. Taylor CB, Kraemer HC, Bragg DA, Miles LE, Rule B, Savin WM, & Debusk RF: A new system for long-term recording and processing of heart rate and physical activity in outpatients. Computers and Biomedical Research, 15:7, 1982.
18. Webster JB, Messin S, Mullaney DJ, & Kripke DF: Transducer design and placement for activity recording. Medical & Biological Engineering & Computing, 20:741, 1982.
19. Wehr TA, Sack D, Rosenthal N, Duncan W, & Gillin JC: Circadian rhythm disturbances in manic-depressive illness. Federation Proceedings, 42:2809, 1982.
20. Wong TC, Webster JG, Montoye HJ, & Washburn R: Portable accelerometer device for measuring human energy expenditure. IEEE Transactions on Biomedical Engineering, BME-28:467, 1981.

NOTE

The opinions or assertions contained herein are the private views of the authors and are not to be construed as official or as reflecting the views of the Department of the Army or the Department of Defense (AR 360-5, para 4-3).

THE SYNERGETICS OF THE EYE-MOVEMENTS OF REM SLEEP.

Petre-Quadens O., Dequae P.A.
University of Antwerp (UIA), Belgium.

1. INTRODUCTION

One of the major problems with which research on sleep has been confronted, in recent years, is the way in which the variations of the physiological parameters during sleep have been classified into different stages or states.

The use of stereotyped techniques and scoring methods has certainly provided valuable information. However, for more than a decade their popularity has prevented from more sophisticated techniques aiming at precise measurements of the quantitative variations occurring within the various physiological parameters traditionnally recorded.Owing to the state of controversy regarding the significance of the parameters involved in the recognition of Rem sleep, or paradoxical sleep, we concentrated our attention on the eye movements only. Since the discovery of the existence of the corneo-retinal potential, described by Dubois-Reymond in 1845, it has been known that the eye is a polarized system, the retinal part being negatively charged in relation to the cornea; the difference in potential is 5 to 6 μV and is independent of illumination. Electro-oculographic recordings are based upon the existence of this potential. Electrodes placed on the periphery of the eye will enable eye-movements to be recorded since the displacement of the corneo-retinal dipole changes the electric field between the electrodes. The direction of the electro-oculographic reading may indicate the direction of the eye-movement. In this case the electrodes are placed at the centre of the superior and inferior superciliary arches and at the internal angles of each eye. The first two are recording the vertical ocular movements and the other two the horizontal ocular movements.

No significant differences have been found in the normal population between the amount of horizontal and vertical eye-movements.Accordingly and for the time being, we have considered the horizontal and vertical eye-movements together. This should however not preclude the future. In the horizontal plane alone, the direction of the eye-movements towards the left or the right, may be as important during sleep as it is during wakefulness when the effects of selective learning on the Rem patterns will be tested. The left or right hemispheric dominance may be present during sleep as during wakefulness.The distinction between the vertical and the horizontal axis may also regain its actuality when sleep recordings are made in zero-G. The importance of sleep is obviously its relation to wakefulness. Rem, it is now known, is not limited to a periodical nocturnal phenomenon which is superimposed upon the sleep process. It is an ultradian function occurring both during day and night. A diurnal physiological phenomenon was therefore to be found which had the characteristics of Rem-sleep. It seems in fact, that attention is the most plausible candidate for this equivalency.

Eye-movements are typical of attention. When somebody calls after us, we turn our head and eyes towards the source of the stimulus. Also, every neurophysiologist knows of the typical EEG activation that is characteristic of the state of attention.
Just as quiet sleep and Rem-sleep alternate during the night, periods of relaxation and attention follow each other during the day.
The fundamental ultradian rhythm of rest and activity is most obvious in the young child, the kitten or the puppy. With development, attention eventually supersedes the neuromotor activity during the day.

2. FIELDS OF APPLICATION
2.1. Child development
The eye-movement frequencies higher than 1 per sec. are positively and significantly correlated with the I.Q. (p<.001) (1) (fig. 1). The higher frequency eye-movements (over 1 per sec.) already exist in the premature baby but they are still lost in long episodes of undifferentiated sleep (2).
In the full term normal neonate, they are in close connection with the quality of brain-maturation (fig. 2). The eye-movement frequencies over 1 per sec. are significantly decreased in mongoloid neonates when compared to normal neonates. This is not the case with the eye movement frequencies lower than 1 per 2 sec. (3).
These results raise the question of the meaning of the time-characteristics of the eye-movement signals recorded during sleep with respect to learning and memory processes. They stress the importance of their detection as an early diagnosis in pediatric clinics. As to the Rem-cycles, they failed to show any correlation. Moreover, the data may cast some doubt on their very existence.
During the first year of life, the eye-movement density of Rem-sleep decreased step-wise in normal infants, and became approximately stable after the age of 1 year. A parallel increase of the mean lenght of the Rem-cycles was observed (fig. 3 - 4). Past 1 year, the mean values of the Rem-cycles were similar in normal and retardates as well. The parallelism between the lengthening of the Rem-cycles and the decrease in the higher eye-movement frequencies was found to be true in normal infants only (4).
However, the data concerning the Rem-cycles call for restrictions. The standard deviations equal the mean values indicating that the Rem-cycles are a random function indeed.

2.2. Mother-child relation
During pregnancy, the woman is the temporary support of her child's brain activities. Close ties in fact link their Rem-sleep. The intensity of oculo-motor discharges increases in the pregnant woman during the second half of pregnancy, and its fluctuations over the different trimesters are identical with those observed in the premature child of corresponding gestational age (fig. 5). Similarity between the mother's and the neonate's Rem-patterns poses the problem of a common factor, responsible for it. In some cases of pathological pregnancies, for instance in placental insufficiency, the correlation between the mother's oculo-motor activity and that of the child remains true (5).When hypotrophia or dysmaturity is present in the neonate , his Rem activity is altered in the same way as it is in the mother. Yet, small-for-date neonates do not differ from mongoloid neonates in this respect, for the differences in the sleep-patterns appear only a few weeks after birth.

Physiology of Rem-sleep may be linked (as in case of immunity reactions) to a cell memory whose components, as for the antigens, cross the mother's placenta to reach the foetus and cause cell links to become established. From the anatomical standpoint, research showing an early disappearance of cell links during maturation suggests that differentiation during maturation is due to a decrease in the transmission of information between neurons, i.e. some kind of inhibition in this transmission of information which lead to the fixing of a "pattern".

It results from years of investigation on the eye-movement signals during sleep as a function of learning that the study of their combinations prevails on that of their significance. In a logical system, the signals are without semantic content and their significance is defined by the rules regulating their use only.

3. TIME-DEPENDENCY OF THE REM-PROCESS

The Rem-process can be viewed as a stochastic point process and the techniques utilized to quantify the time-dependency of such a process could be used here. Because of the existence of strong non-stationarities in the raw data the usual techniques like correlation analysis and power spectral analysis are of little value (10).

The analysis of the time-dependency of stochastic point processes requires the measurement of either the time between events (10, 13) or the number of events in an arbitrary time interval as random variable (2, 3, 4, 6, 7, 8).

These two methods are considered to be fundamentally equivalent (9).

Since a number of Rem's appear in bursts, several investigators have counted the number of Rem-bursts and their duration. But there are many definitions of Rem-bursts in the literature. Nonsequential interval histogram | plots and hazard function plots (23) indicate the distribution of the different eye-movement frequencies. The use of these methods has shown that the Rem's which appear in bursts do not fit a renewal model (exponential distribution) (11, 13).

The physical significance of time-dependency calls for precisions:time-dependency $D(m) = H(o) - H(m) /H(o)$ is a statistical measurement indeed which represents the degree of dependence of Markov processes (22, 12), where $H(o)$ and $H(m)$ are Shannon's entropy and the m-th order conditional entropy, respectively. $D(m)$ is a statistical measure representing patterns of m-th order dependence. Experimentally calculated values of $D(1)$ on rapid eye-movements shows that there is no systematic oscillation in the density of the eye-movements (11).

The structure of occurrence of Rem's quantified by transition probability matrices, corresponds to a two-state first-order semi-Markov process (14). This structure remains unchanged from one Rem period to the next one. It has also been shown that the ratio of the Rem frequencies over 1 per sec. and those lower than 1 per 2 seconds, remains relatively stable in adults over periods of several years (15) (fig. 6).

The fact that the transition probability matrices corresponding to a two-state first-order semi-Markov process remain relativily independent of Rem period rank (13, 14) suggests a dual mechanism for the Rem generation. This was already suggested by Petre-Quadens and De Lee in 1970 (1, 6, 14).

Our studies on rapid eye-movements detected by EOG-techniques during Rem-sleep have evidenced intimate connections between their pattern of occurrence and the general psychophysiological state of the human organism.

According to Holden a strictly periodic patterned activity in the nervous system would be incapable of adapting to a fluctuating irregular environment, the variability in neural activity is necessary for adapting behaviour (16).

Given the evidence that in Rem-sleep the eye-movement frequencies higher than 1 per sec. and those lower than 1 per 2 sec. have different functions, the ratio between the higher and the lower frequencies or oculo-motor index has been considered as indicating the degree of mental entropy as shown in fig. 6. It decreases as a function of age.

Results showing that the higher frequencies are related to the integration of sensori-motor information whereas the lower frequencies behave as random noise are very suggestive of the synergetic function of the brain. This function would remain unchanged whatever variations would occur in the total number of eye-movements. This hypothesis was tested in the Spacelab 1 flight where changes in gravity have induced dramatic changes in the total number of eye-movements of Rem-sleep: a 10-fold increase in early Zero-G and a drop below baseline levels after return to 1-G (17, 18). In both cases however, the oculo-motor indexes were strikingly similar (fig. 7-8).

The very complexity of the rapid eye-movement data in sleep has traditionnaly limited their evaluation to the simplest parameters and the correlates with behaviour to the broadest classifications. Mental processes are however rapid and changing. Therefore, techniques and methods have to be used that are equivalently refined and effective with epochs of data only a second or so in duration-far shorter than segments of records that are analysed with most analog computation. Such an analysis has proven fruitful in this and in other studies, where visual examination of a paper record could scarcely provide the basis for an interpretation (1, 15, 19, 20, 21). The sensitivity of the brain to environmental changes has clearly revealed changing states of activity as provocative as any other in the age-old history of the evolution of the human brain.

REFERENCES

1. Petre-Quadens O., Contribution à la phase dite paradoxale du sommeil, Acta Neurol. Belg., 69, 769-898, 1969.

2. Petre-Quadens O., De Lee C., Remy M., Eye Movement Density during sleep and brain maturation, Brain Research, 26, 49-56, 1971.

3. Petre-Quadens O., The Logic of Sleep and brain-dysfunction, Sleep, L. Popoviciu et al. (eds.) S. Karger, Basel, 126-133, 1978.

4. Petre-Quadens O., De Lee C., Eye movement frequencies and related paradoxical sleep cycles developmental changes, Chronobiologia, 1, 4, 385-355, 1974.

5. Petre-Quadens O., De Lee C., Sleep-cycle alterations during pregnancy, postpartum and the menstrual cycle, Biorhythms and human reproduction, Ferin M. et al. (eds.), Wiley and sons, New York, 335-352, 1974.

6. Petre-Quadens O., De Lee C., Eye movements during sleep: A common criterion of learning capacities and endocrine activity. Development Medicine and child neurology, 12, 6, 730-740, 1970.

7. Petre-Quadens O., De Lee C. Goffe B., Analyse stochastique des mouvements oculaires du sommeil et syndromes neurologiques. Acta Neurol. belg., 73, 20-24, 1973.

8. Dittrichova J., Paul K., Pavlikova E., Rapid Eye Movements in Paradoxical sleep in infants. Neuropaediatrics, 3, 248-257, 1972.

9. Cox D.R., Lewis P.A.W., The statistical analysis of series of events. Chapman and Hall, London, 1972.
10. Ktonas P.Y., Smith J.R., Semi-Automatic analysis of Rapid Eye movement (REM) patterns. A Software Package, Computers and Biomedical research, 9, 109-124, 1976.
11. Ktonas P.Y., Bonilla J.F., Boukadoum A.M., Quantification of Time-connectivity Patterns in Rapid Eye Movement Occurrences During Sleep, IEEE Transactions on Biomedical Engineering, BME. 28, No. 1, 31-36, 1981.
12. Ktonas P.Y., Bonilla J.F., Quantification of time-connectivity patterns in point processes, IEEE Frontiers of Engineering in Health Care, New York IEEE, 246-249, 1979.
13. Chouvet G., Structures d'occurence des activités Phasiques du sommeil paradoxal chez l'animal et chez l'homme, These d'Etat es-Sciences, Lyon, France, 1981.
14. Boukadoum A., Ktonas P.Y., Non-Random Patterns in the Occurence of Rapid Eye Movements in Human REM Sleep, Proceeding of the 4th International congress of sleep Research, Bologna, Italy, 65, 1983.
15. Petre-Quadens O., Hoffman G., Maturation of the Rem sleep patterns from child-through adulthood, Advances of Physiological Sciences: Brain and Behaviour, Adam G., Meszaros I., Banyai E.D. (Eds.), Akademiai Kiado, Pergamon Press, Budapest, 17, 55-59, 1981.
16. Holden A.V., Muhamed M.A., Chaotic activity in neural systems, Cybernetics and Systems Research, 2, R. Trappl (ed.) Elsevier Publishers B.V. (North-Holland). 245-250, 1984.
17. Petre-Quadens O., Dequae P.A., Green H.L., Stott S.F.D., Eye movements during sleep and EEG in Zero-gravity, 35th congress of the International Astronautical Federation, Lausanne, 1-5, 1984.
18. Petre-Quadens O., Green H., Eye movements during sleep in weightlessness. Science, 225, 221-222, 1984.
19. Petre-Quadens O., Sleep in Mental Retardation, Sleep and the Maturing Nervous System, Clemente C.D., Purpura D.P., Mayer F.E. (Eds.), Academic Press, New York, 383-417, 1972.
20. Chevalier B. et al., Learning effects on paradoxical sleep in man. Proceedings of the 6th European Congress on Sleep Research, Zürich 166, 1982.
21. Adey W.R., Spectral Analysis of EEG Data from Animals and Man During Alerting, Orienting and Discriminative Responses, Attention in Neurophysiology, C.R. Evans, T.B. Mulholland (Eds.), Butterworth, London, 194- 229, 1969.
22. Nakahama H., Yamamoto N., Ishii H., Aya K., Dependency as a Measure to Estimate the Order and the values of Markov Processes. Biol. Cybernetics, 25, 209-226, 1977.
23. Snyder, L.D., Random Point Processes, Wiley, New York, 1975.

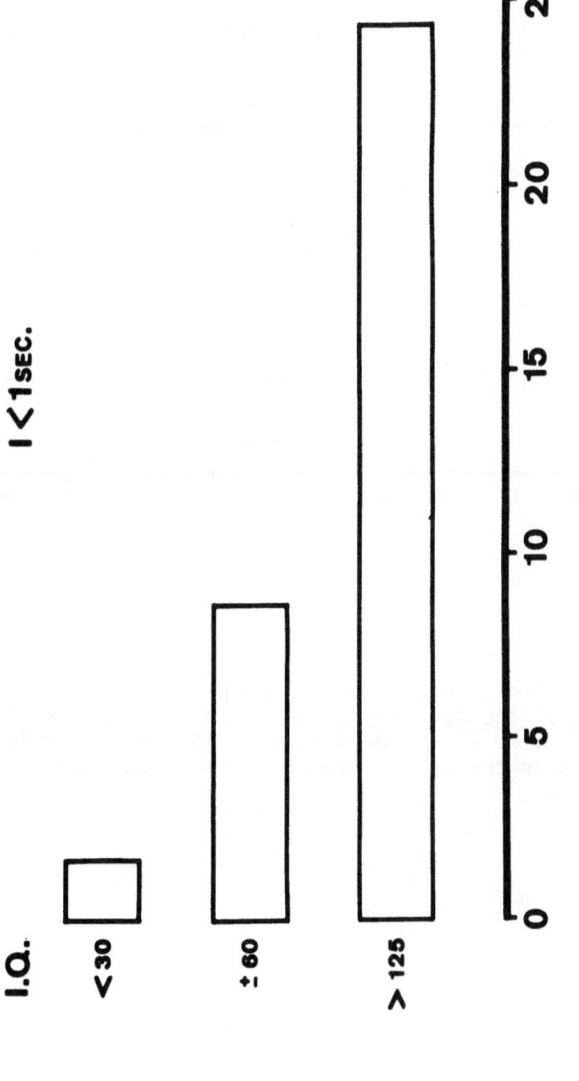

FIGURE 1. The higher eye-movement frequencies in function of I.Q. in 3 groups of children aged 6 to 8 years. In abscissa: number of the Rem-frequencies higher than 1 per second (Intervals (I)<1sec.) for 40 sec. Rem-sleep.

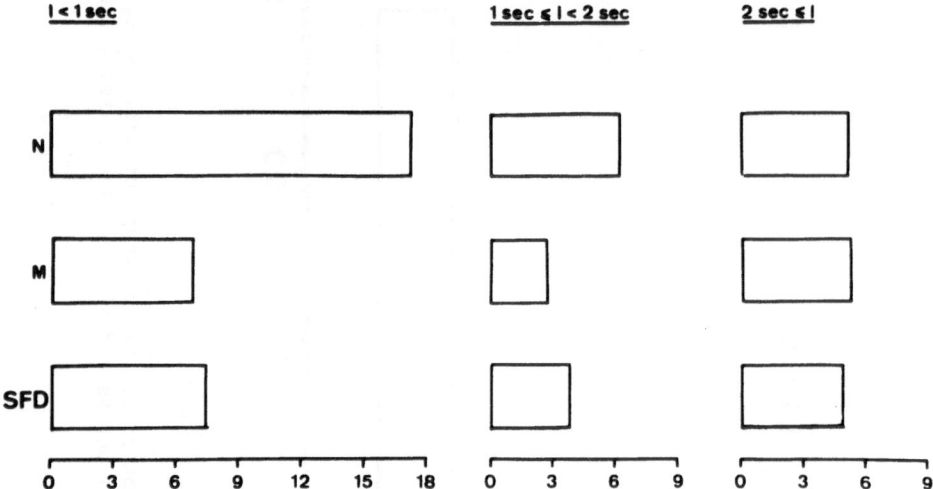

FIGURE 2. The eye-movement frequencies in normal and pathological neonates. In abscissa: number of the Rem-frequencies higher (Intervals (I)< 1 sec.) and lower than 1 per sec. (1 sec.≤I<2 sec.; I≥2 sec.) for 40 sec. Rem-sleep in full-term neonates aged 3 days, N: normal, M: mongoloid, D: small-for-date (dysmature).

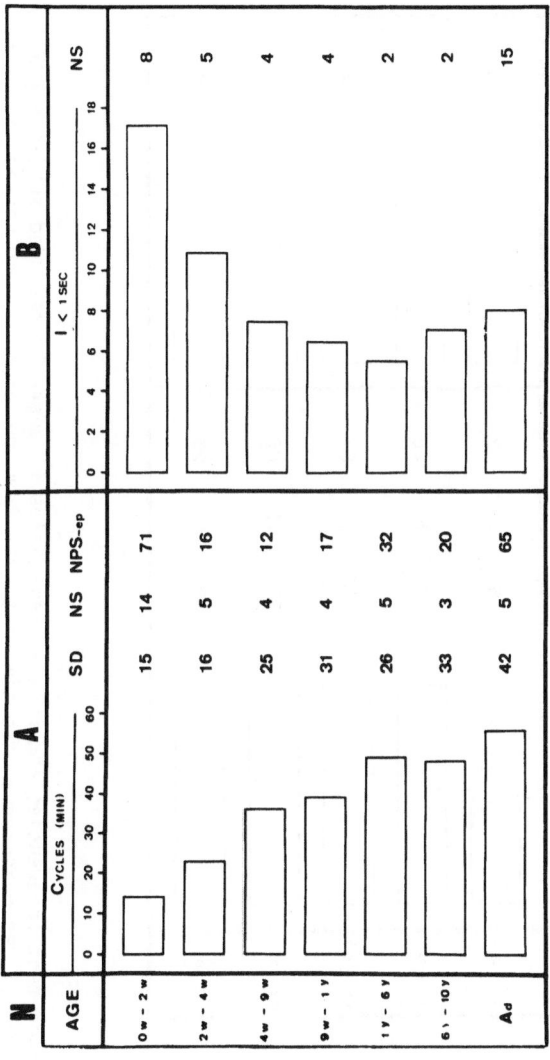

FIGURE 3. Eye-movement frequencies and related Rem-cycles in normal subjects (N). A: duration of the Rem-cycles (in min.), as measured by the time-interval from the onset of one Rem-epoch to the onset of the next one (SD= standard deviations, NS=number of subjects, NPS=number of Rem-epochs). B: number of eye-movement frequencies, higher than 1 per sec. (Interval (I)<1 sec.) per 40 sec. Rem-time. Left: age in weeks (w), years (y), adults (ad).

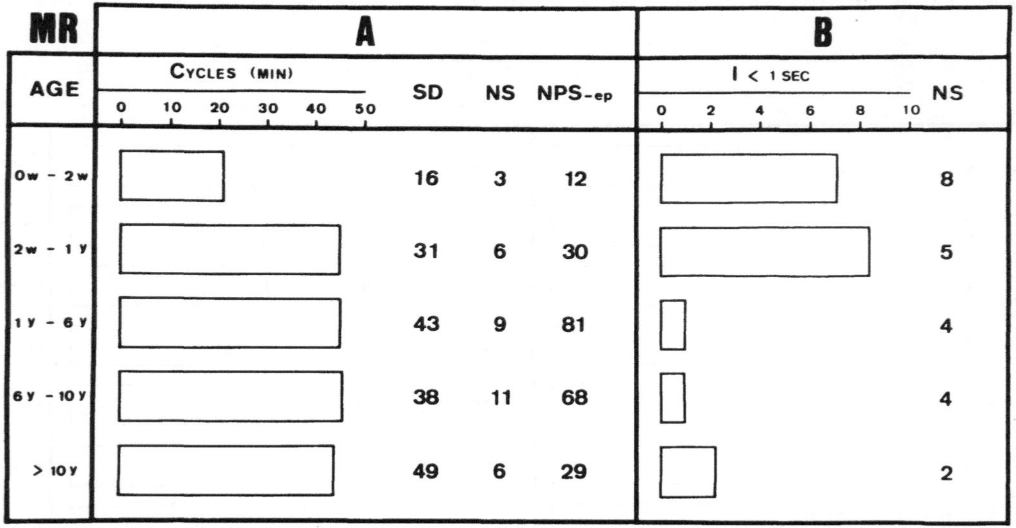

FIGURE 4. Eye-movement frequencies and related Rem-cycles in mentally retarded subjects (MR). A: duration of the Rem-cycles (in min.), as measured by the time-interval from the onset of one Rem-epoch to the onset of the next one (SD=standard deviations, NS=number of subjects, NPS=number of Rem-epochs). B: number of the eye-movement frequencies (Intervals (I)<1 sec.) per 40 sec. Rem-time. Left: age in weeks (w) and years (y).

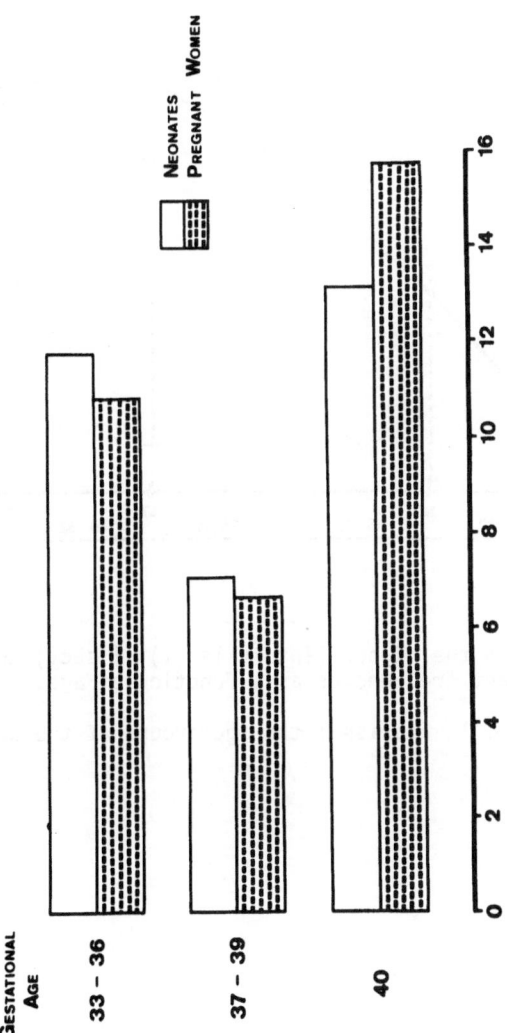

FIGURE 5. Number of eye-movement frequencies higher than 1 per sec. in pregnant women and neonates for 40 sec. Rem-sleep as a function of term (pregnancy) and gestational age (premature and neonate infants).

226

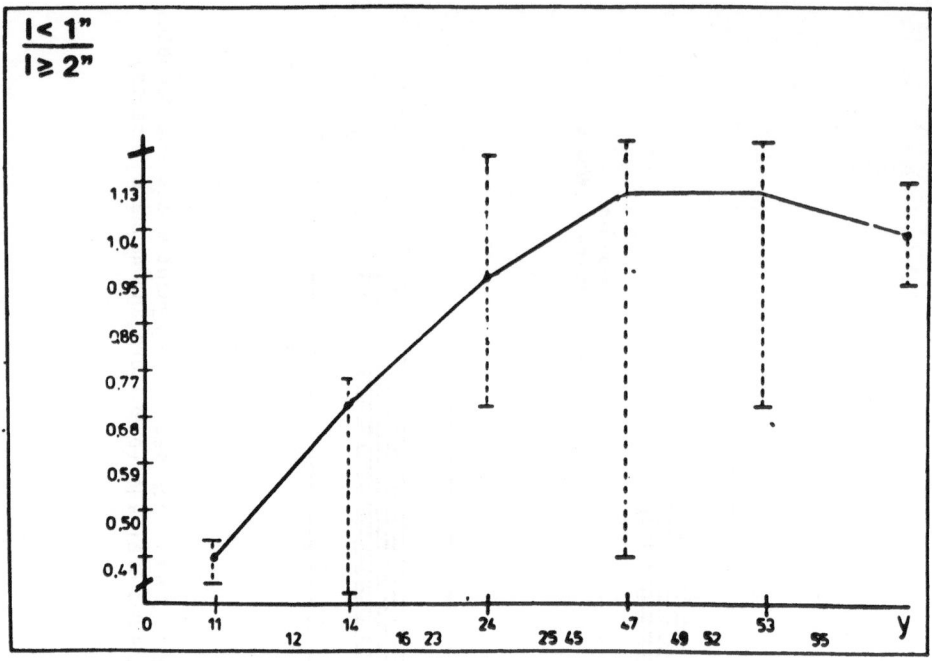

FIGURE 6. Ratio between the higher (Intervals (I) ⪦ 1 sec.) and the lower (I ⪢ 2 sec.) eye-movement frequencies as a function of age.

In ordinate: $\dfrac{I \lessdot 1 \ \text{sec.}}{I \gtrdot 2 \ \text{sec.}}$. In abscissa: the age-groups of the subjects.

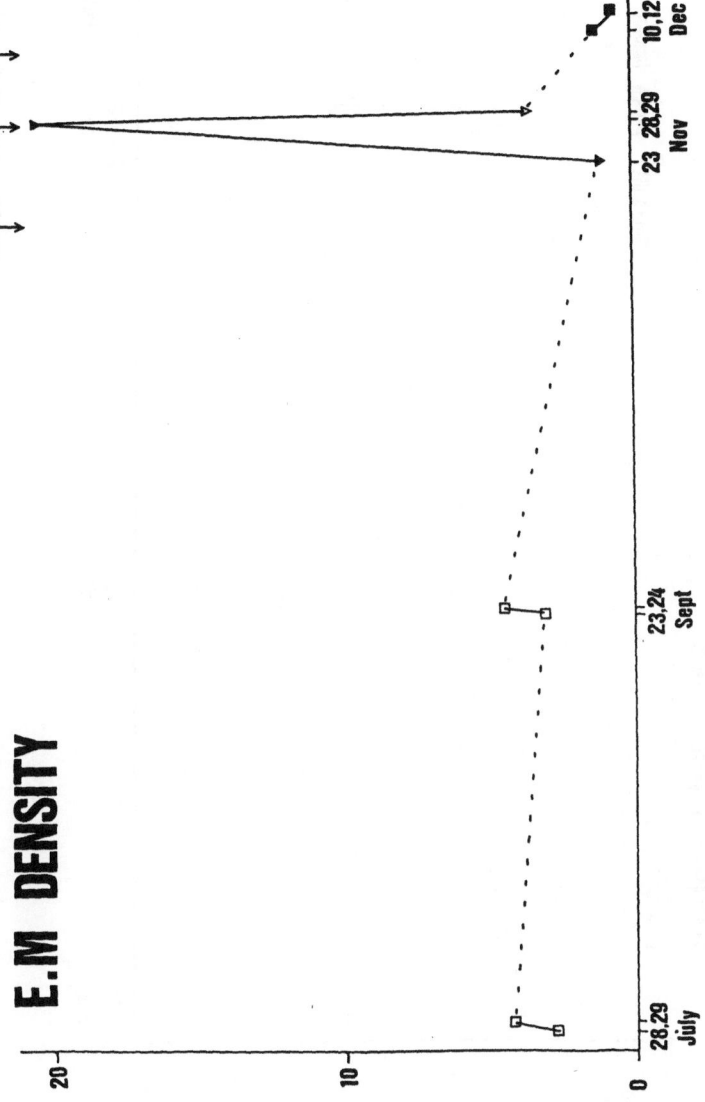

FIGURE 7. Total number of eye-movements per 40 sec. of Rem-sleep at various times before, during and after the Spacelab 1 flight.

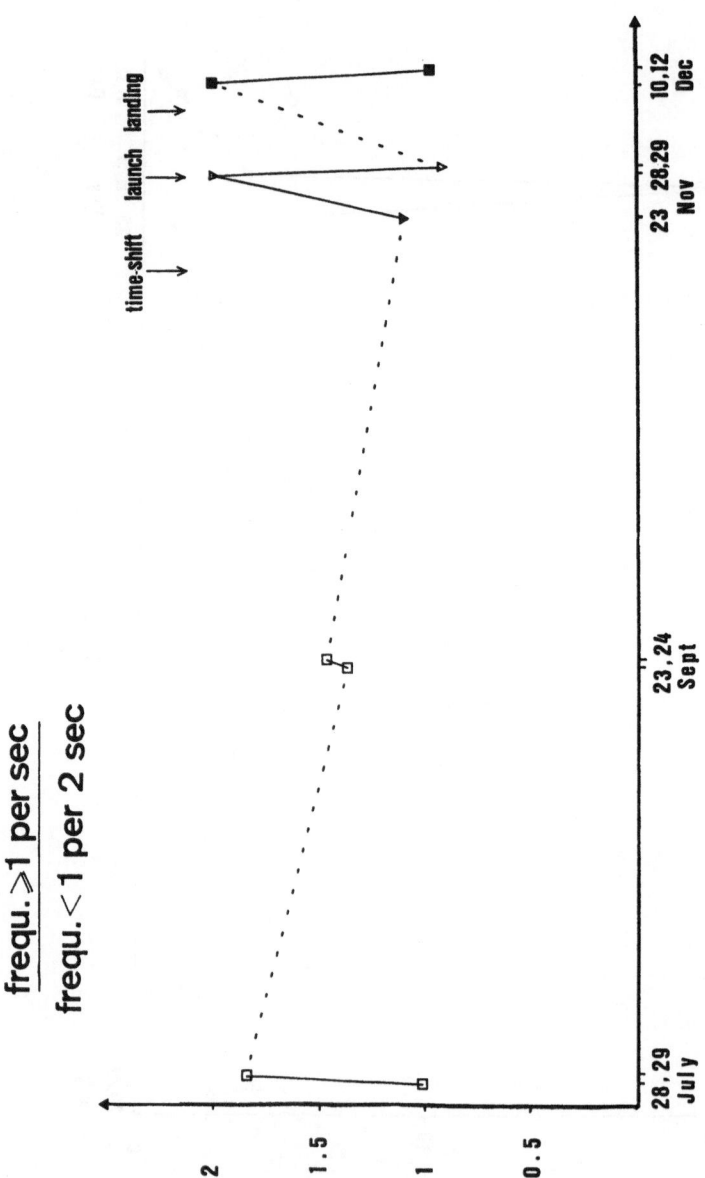

FIGURE 8. Ratio of eye-movement frequencies higher than 1 per sec. to those lower than 1 per 2 sec. at various times before, during and after the Spacelab 1 flight.

RECORDING, AUTOMATED DETECTION, AND QUANTIFICATION OF RAPID EYE
MOVEMENT (REM) PATTERNS DURING HUMAN REM SLEEP

P. Y. KTONAS AND A. M. BOUKADOUM
UNIVERSITY OF HOUSTON, HOUSTON, TEXAS, USA

1. INTRODUCTION

Rapid eye movement (REM) patterns during sleep stage 1-REM have
attracted the attention of the scientific and clinical community ever
since the re-discovery of REM sleep by Aserinsky and Kleitman in 1953.
Besides being the sign for the REM sleep stage, REM patterns have been
associated with the imagery of dreams (Dement and Kleitman 1957;
Roffwarg et al. 1962) as well as with the general psychophysiological
state of the human organism. The arrangement of REMs into bursts, and
the gradual, on the average, increase in the number of REMs and in the
number of REM bursts during the successive REM sleep periods through
the night are considered signs of normalcy, while poorly defined REM
bursts and lack of REM profusion may be indicative of a pathological
process (Barros-Ferreira and Bedoret 1972; Salzarulo et al. 1973;
Benoit et al. 1974). Sleep REM density measures (number of REMs/unit
of time) have been utilized for diagnosis and prognosis purposes. For
example, they have been used to distinguish normals from
schizophrenics (McPartland et al. 1974), as well as medical-depressive
syndromes from primary affective disorders (Foster et al. 1976), to
quantify effects of psychotropic drugs on the central nervous system
(Okuma et al. 1975), to indicate recovery of cerebral function
(Feinberg 1969), and to assess developmental changes (Petre-Quadens
and De Lee 1974).

This paper presents some critical comments and suggestions for
the recording of sleep REMs via electrooculographic (EOG)
methodologies, and for the subsequent processing of the EOG data via
automated means for the detection and quantification of REM patterns
which may possibly have chronobiological significance. Specifically,
the following will be addressed: (a) electrode montages for the EOG
recording; (b) AC vs DC coupling for the amplifying circuits; (c)
algorithms and implementations thereof for the automated REM
detection; and (d) some mathematical techniques for detailed REM
pattern quantification.

2. ELECTRODE MONTAGES FOR RECORDING REMS VIA EOG MEASUREMENTS

The EOG recording methodology is based on the fact that the
eyeball can be viewed as a dipole consisting of a positive charge in
the cornea and a negative charge in the retinal region. Eye
movements, therefore, are associated with respective movements of this
dipole which can be recorded as potential changes picked up by
periorbital surface electrodes. The most popular EOG electrode
montage for sleep REM recording is that proposed by Rechtschaffen and
Kales (1968). A two-channel montage is utilized. One electrode is
placed one centimeter above and slightly lateral to the outer canthus

of one eye, and the reference electrode is on either the contralateral ear lobe or the contralateral mastoid bone. The other channel utilizes one electrode a centimeter below and slightly lateral to the outer canthus of the other eye, having as a reference electrode the same one as for the first channel. Mostly horizontal REMs can be recorded with this montage. By moving the reference electrode to the nasion (one centimeter above the bridge of the nose), vertical as well as oblique eye movements can be recorded, provided the assumption is made (for oblique movement recording) that the eyes move in a conjugate synchronous fashion. Figure 1 gives an example of rapid eye movements recorded with this montage in the awake state (Fig. 1A) and during REM sleep (Fig. 1B).

However, for accurate eye movement recording in all directions, assuming that the movements are conjugate synchronous, three EOG channels should be utilized (Padovan and Pansini 1972). Taking into account the possible existence of disconjugate sleep REMs (Gabersek and Scherrer 1970; Gabersek 1972), a more elaborate EOG montage consisting of at least three bipolar channels per eye may be more appropriate. These channels should be able to decompose eye movements in horizontal, vertical, and oblique components (Malhotra 1984). The disadvantage of this montage is that it occupies at least six amplifier channels in the recording apparatus. Nevertheless, it is recommended if studies of detailed sleep REM dynamics are to be done. Vectooculographic methods (Uenoyama et al. 1963; Salzarulo et al. 1973; Schneider 1978a,b) could be used as well to reduce the number of channels to two per eye (one channel recording the vertical, and the other recording the horizontal component of an eye movement). Accordingly, by feeding the horizontal and vertical components of the EOG to the X and Y inputs of an oscilloscope or a plotter, one could accurately determine the direction and the amplitude of an eye movement. However, the resulting plot of REM dynamics on a two-dimensional plane may be difficult to interpret for a non-technical specialist.

3. AC VS DC COUPLING FOR RECORDING THE EOG

Due to the possible existence of low-frequency sweat artifact in the EOG records, as well as of slow changes in the resting potential of the eye throughout the night, AC-coupled amplifiers have been popular in recording sleep REMs via EOG methods. However, three important variables of interest for detailed REM studies, i.e. the amplitude and velocity of the eye movement, and the resting position of the eye after the movement, are affected by AC coupling. The latter variable is completely lost, while the other two can be distorted by as much as 90 percent depending on the time constant used (Cooper et al. 1980). In addition, if AC coupling involves second or higher-order highpass filters, resulting recovery waveforms (i.e. undershoots and overshoots) can contribute to false REM detections as shown in Figure 2 (see Ktonas and Smith (1976) for a detailed discussion of this problem).

On the other hand, DC-coupled recordings are devoid of the above problems, and are recommended if detailed studies of REM dynamics are to be done (Tursky and O'Connell 1966). In order to combat the presence of baseline drifts or of sweat artifact, a "quasi-DC" coupling is appropriate (i.e. AC coupling with a large time constant-e.g. 2 seconds or more). AC-coupled amplifiers with shorter time constants may be used where one is only interested in detecting the presence or absence of REMs (e.g. for sleep stage 1-REM detection). However, in this case, the time constant must be at least 0.3 seconds in value. Shorter time constants can lead to a more than 10 percent loss in amplitude reading when large (e.g. of 50 degrees excursion) but slow (e.g. of 50 degrees per second velocity) REMs are recorded (Cooper et al. 1980).

4. AUTOMATED REM DETECTION ALGORITHMS AND IMPLEMENTATION

Several automated REM detection systems operating on the EOG signals have been proposed (Okuma et al. 1971; Smith et al. 1971; Minard and Krausman 1971; McPartland et al. 1973; Degler et al. 1975; Whitman et al. 1975; Ktonas and Smith 1976; Kobayashi et al. 1979; Othmer et al. 1979; Martinerie et al. 1980). These systems follow a heuristic approach based on the visual detection process, whereby amplitude, slope and duration parameters of the EOG trace are measured and compared against thresholds. In some systems synchrony criteria between two EOG channels (one per eye) are utilized as well. A different approach, based on statistical detection theory, has been proposed by Yana et al. (1979), while Schneider (1978a,b) has presented a method based on the analysis of vectooculographic records in terms of slope criteria. Both hardwired and software-based implementations of the detection algorithms have been proposed. However, software-based methods are more appropriate for DC-coupled EOG data since electrographic parameters of importance in these records (e.g. amplitudes and durations) can be measured more efficiently with software programs.

A block diagram of a relatively simple analog (i.e. hardwired) automatic REM detector is presented in Figure 3. It analyzes EOG activity (recorded with a time constant of 0.1 seconds) within the frequency band (i.e. bandpass filter bandwidth) of 0.3 to 16 Hz. This band was chosen so that the system can optimally pass well-defined REM-related activity in the EOG trace of about 1-5 Hz fundamental frequency (Ktonas and Smith 1976; Boukadoum 1983) while attenuating high-frequency artifactual activity (e.g. EMG). The amplitude threshold is set at 30 μv for both channels. The AND gate ensures synchrony between the two EOG channels (Rechtschaffen and Kales montage -see section 2). After a detection, the output of the system is turned "off" for a 200-msec period in order to minimize false detections due to recovery waveforms possibly present in the AC-coupled data. The system output is also turned "off" by an artifact detector which checks for presence of muscle (EMG) artifact in one of the EOG channels. This artifact detector utilizes bandpass filtering, amplitude threshold detection, duration (defined by zero-crossings) detection, and burst-pattern detection to decide on the presence of EMG artifact (Boukadoum 1983). The system is turned "off" by this presence because usually EMG activity accompanies high-amplitude movement artifact activity which can be mistaken by the system as REM-related. Figure 4 shows an example of EMG artifact detection, while Figure 5 shows an example of system performance with EOG data from REM sleep.

REM detectors built to analyze AC-coupled EOG data detect REMs of relatively large excursions or of relatively large velocities. Some

REMs may be missed, especially if they are of small excursion and/or they occur within a REM burst. One way to alleviate this problem is to utilize large time constants (e.g. more than 2 seconds) for the EOG recording. Another way is to employ slope measurements for the EOG trace, and to indicate the possible presence of a REM when the EOG slope changes in sign abruptly. However, quasi-DC-coupled EOG recordings (e.g. time constants of more than 2 seconds) provide the opportunity for the development of much better REM detectors. These detectors should rely on amplitude, slope and duration measurements for REM detection. Nevertheless, artifact-suppression (or detection) methodologies are needed in REM detectors regardless of the mode of EOG recording. These techniques should be capable of detecting EMG and movement artifact, as well as EEG activity (mainly alpha) which may be recorded in the EOG channels via volume conduction. The presence of delta EEG activity during sleep stages III and IV can give rise to false alarms, but additional criteria built into the system (e.g. sleep staging information, muscle tone activity) can eliminate this problem (Smith 1978).

5. SOME MATHEMATICAL TECHNIQUES FOR DETAILED REM PATTERN QUANTIFICATION

Once the times of occurrence of individual REMs are defined, either visually or via automated means, several computer-based methodologies can be utilized to process the data in order to quantify patterns in these times of occurrence, of possible chronobiological significance. Accordingly, histograms of the time intervals between successive REMs (Spreng et al. 1968; Aserinsky 1971; Petre-Quadens and De Lee 1974; Chouvet 1981), definitions of "REM bursts" and counting thereof (Ktonas and Smith 1976; Boukadoum 1983), time-trend analysis of cumulative REM counts (Salzarulo 1972), as well as spectral analysis for the elucidation of periodicities in such cumulative REM count plots (Krynicki 1975; Lavie 1979; Weber et al. 1983) have been proposed. As mentioned in the beginning of this paper, REM density parameters have also been utilized by various investigators.

This section elaborates on some techniques which are appropriate for the quantification of detailed "order" in REM sequences as they evolve in time. Histograms of inter-REM intervals cannot quantify sequency patterns in REM occurrence. Although cumulative REM counts (including density measures) can provide some idea about these REM dynamics, they cannot quantify detailed patterns thereof in a satisfactory way. Similarly, spectral analysis methodologies are too crude for such an investigation. One of the proposed techniques is based on the example shown in Figure 6.

Figure 6 provides a hypothetical example of two possible REM sequences, both consisting of 12 REMs, and both occurring within the same time window, say 8 seconds. Density measures cannot separate the two sequences (since they both give rise to the same REM density measure: 12/8 = 1.5 REMs/sec). Similarly, a histogram parameter given as the ratio of the number of inter-REM intervals which correspond to a burst (underlined group of REMs) to the total number of intervals (i.e. 7/11) cannot separate the two sequences since it is the same for both cases. However, visually, the sequences are different, in that the top one is composed of a long REM burst and a few isolated REMs, while the bottom one is composed of four shorter REM bursts and one isolated REM. The proposed method, which can distinguish between the two REM sequences, is as follows: Define as "B" the "state" of inter-REM intervals within a REM burst (such intervals are defined once a burst is defined). Define as "N" the "state" of inter-REM intervals between isolated REMs as well as between isolated REMs and REM bursts. Now, compute the probabilities of transitions between states (i.e. B→B, B→N, N→B, N→N). These are listed as a state transition probability matrix (STPM) in the right part of the figure (e.g. the probability of going from the B state to the N state in the top sequence is 1/7). Obviously, the structure of these 2×2 matrices can differentiate the top REM sequence from the bottom one.

The second proposed methodology relates to the quantification of detailed REM sequence patterns within REM bursts. This methodology and the previous one are linked by the following assumptions: "The inter-REM intervals in a given REM period can be modelled as being generated by a first-order semi-Markov process with two states, B and N. The statistics of the process are summarized by the STPM corresponding to that REM period. The inter-REM intervals corresponding to the B state, however, can also be modelled as being generated by a first-order Markov process the statistics of which are summarized by another STPM (not necessarily 2×2), while the inter-REM intervals corresponding to the N state can be modelled as being generated by a renewal process". Further details on the validity of these assumptions can be found in Ktonas et al. (1981) and in Boukadoum (1983). Accordingly, state transition probability matrices can be built for the inter-REM intervals within REM bursts (the states can be defined a priori in terms of time between REMs within bursts) for each REM period of the night. The structure of these matrices (one for each REM period) should quantify the detailed REM sequence structure in REM bursts of a particular REM period. We have applied this method to REM data from young healthy adults, and preliminary results have indicated that the REM sequence structure in REM bursts may be constant from REM period to REM period regardless of the possible gradual increase in the number of REMs throughout the night (Boukadoum and Ktonas 1983).

In addition to the formation of state transition probability matrices, entropy and conditional entropy measures based on the inter-REM intervals within REM bursts can be computed, and a related REM "time-connectivity" parameter for each REM period can be formed which can quantify the degree of "order" in the REM sequences corresponding to REM bursts of that REM period (Ktonas et al. 1981). Accordingly, as mentioned above, the inter-REM intervals within a REM burst are modelled as being generated by a first-order Markov process. Furthermore, we assume this process to be realized by a stationary and ergodic Markov chain with a finite number of distinct states K and a state transition probability matrix T. Each inter-REM interval, according to its duration, is assigned to a certain process state. If, after the m-th REM, the process is in state S_j, where S_j is the state corresponding to the inter-REM interval between the m-th and the (m-1)th REM, then, after the next transition, the process will be in state S_ℓ, where S_ℓ is the state corresponding to the inter-REM interval between the (m+1)-th and the m-th REM, with conditional (transition) probability

$$\Pr[S_\ell | S_j]; \quad \ell=1,2,\ldots,K; \quad j=1,2,\ldots,K.$$

As expected, the presence of "time-connectivity" in the process under study is governed by the structure of matrix T. For example, if

$$\Pr[S_\ell | S_j] = \frac{1}{K}; \quad \forall j,\ell$$

then the process exhibits lack of "time-connectivity"; it actually exhibits the maximum amount of "disorder". Accordingly, we can quantify, on the average, the amount of "disorder" via the entropy term H_0 given by

$$H_0 = \sum_i \Pr[S_i] \times \log_2 \frac{1}{\Pr[S_i]} \ .$$

We can also quantify the amount of "disorder" in an assumed first-order Markov process (e.g. the process of inter-REM intervals within REM bursts) via the conditional entropy term H_1 given by

$$H_1 = \sum_j \sum_\ell \Pr[S_j, S_\ell] \times \log_2 \frac{1}{\Pr[S_\ell | S_j]} \ .$$

Now, we define the "time-connectivity" parameter C as

$$C = \frac{H_0 - H_1}{H_0}; \quad 0 \leq C \leq 1 \ .$$

From the above we can see that as H_1 decreases, the closer C approaches unity, and the first-order Markov process exhibits more "order". On the other hand, as H_1 approaches H_0, the more the "disorder" in the process, and the closer C approaches zero. As an example, if

$$\Pr[S_\ell | S_j] = \frac{1}{K}; \quad \forall j,\ell$$

then $H_1 = H_0$, and C = 0, i.e. there is no "time-connectivity" or "order" in the process. Sampling distributions for C, and related guidelines for its use are given in Ktonas et al. (1981).

Up to now, attention has been paid primarily to first-order statistics of the REM-generating process (e.g. number of REMs, number of REM bursts) and to their evolution throughout the night. The methodologies discussed above can serve to quantify detailed second-order properties of the process as they evolve in time during the night. Spectral analysis of cumulative REM count plots is an attempt to quantify second-order properties, but this method is too crude to unravel fine detail in these properties, and, furthermore, may give misleading results (Wong 1985). We believe that the quantification procedures described in this section are promising tools which may unravel detailed REM-generation patterns of chronobiological significance.

REFERENCES

1. Aserinsky, E., and Kleitman, N.: Regularly occurring periods of eye motility during sleep. Science, 118, 273-274, 1953.
2. Aserinsky, E.: Rapid eye movement density and pattern in the sleep of normal young adults. Psychophysiology, 8, 361-375, 1971.
3. Barros-Ferreira, M., and Bedoret J.M.: Activité oculaire et sommeil paradoxal chez le sujet normal. Rev. EEG Neurophysiol., 2, 213-220, 1972.
4. Benoit, O., Parot, S., and Garma, L.: Evolution during the night of REM sleep in man. Electroenceph. Clin. Neurophysiol., 36, 245-251, 1974.
5. Boukadoum, A.M.: Rapid Eye Movement (REM) Occurrence Patterns During Stage 1-REM Sleep in Humans: An Automated Study Using Markovian Modeling, Ph.D. Dissertation, University of Houston, 1983.
6. Boukadoum, A., and Ktonas, P.: Non-random patterns in the occurrence of rapid eye movements in human REM sleep. Sleep Research, 12, 60, 1983.
7. Chouvet, G.: Structures d'Occurence des Activités Phasiques du Sommeil Paradoxal Chez l'Animal et Chez l'Homme, Thesis, Université Claude-Bernard, Lyon (France), 1981.
8. Cooper, R., Osselton, J.W., and Shaw, J.C.: EEG Technology. Woburn, MA: Butterworth, 1980.
9. Degler, H.E., Smith, J.R., and Black, F.O.: Automatic detection and resolution of synchronous rapid eye movements. Computers and Biomedical Research, 8, 393-404, 1975.
10. Dement, W., and Kleitman, N.: The relationship of eye movements during sleep to dream imagery: An objective method for the study of dreaming. J. Exp. Psych., 53, 339-346, 1957.
11. Feinberg, I.: Sleep in organic brain conditions, in Sleep: Physiology and Pathology, Kales, A., Ed., Philadelphia, PA: Lippincott, 131-148, 1969.
12. Foster, F., Kupfer, D., Coble, P., and McPartland, R.: Rapid eye movement sleep density. An objective indicator in medical depressive syndromes. Archives of General Psychiatry, 33, 1119-1123, 1976.
13. Gabersek, V., and Scherrer, J.: Les mouvements oculaires pendant la phase paradoxale du sommeil. Acta Neurol. Latino-amer., 14, 40-50, 1970.
14. Gabersek, V.: Les mouvements oculaires au cours du sommeil. Revue d'Oto-neuro-opthalmologie, 1, 69-74, 1972.
15. Kobayashi, T., Okuno, H., and Endo, S.: Computer analysis of rapid eye movements in REM sleep periods. Jap. Society of Medical Electronics and Biological Engineering, 17, 222-229, 1979.
16. Krynicki, V.: Time trends and periodic cycles in REM sleep eye movements. Electroenceph. Clin. Neurophysiol., 39, 507-513, 1975.
17. Ktonas, P.Y., and Smith, J.R.: Automatic REM detection: Modifications on an existing system and preliminary normative data. Int. J. Bio-Medical Computing, 9, 445-464, 1976.
18. Ktonas, P.Y., Bonilla, J.R., and Boukadoum, A.M.: Quantification of time-connectivity patterns in rapid eye movement occurrences

during sleep. IEEE Transactions on Biomedical Engineering, 28, 31-36, 1981.

19. Lavie, P.: Rapid eye movements in REM sleep-more evidence for a periodic organization. Electroenceph. Clin. Neurophysiol., 46, 683-688, 1979.

20. Malhotra, J.: Electrode Montages for the Detection of Sleep Rapid Eye Movements by Electro-oculography, Master's Thesis, Electrical Engineering Department, University of Houston, Houston, Texas, 1984.

21. Martinerie, J., Joseph, J., and Naillon, M.: Computerized detection of rapid eye movements during paradoxical sleep. Int. J. Bio-Medical Computing, 11, 163-171, 1980.

22. McPartland, R.J., Kupfer, D.J., and Foster, F.G.: Rapid eye movement analyzer. Electroenceph. Clin. Neurophysiol., 34, 317-320, 1973.

23. McPartland, R.J., Weiss, B.L., and Kupfer, D.J.: An objective measure of REM activity. Physiological Psychology, 2, 441-443, 1974.

24. Minard, J.G., and Krausman, D.: Rapid eye movement definition and count: An on line detector. Electroenceph. Clin. Neurophysiol., 31, 99-102, 1971.

25. Okuma, T., Fukuma, E., and Hata, N.: "Dream detector" and automatization of REMP-awakening technique for the study of dreaming. Psychophysiology, 7, 508-515, 1971.

26. Okuma, T., Hata, N., and Fujii, S.: Differential effects of chlorpromazine, imipramine, nitrazepam, and amobarbital on REM sleep and REM density in man. Folia Psychiatrica et Neurologica Japonica, 29, 25-37, 1975.

27. Othmer, C.S., Othmer, E., Fishman, P.M., and Vannier, M.W.: Digital detection of eye movements in sleep. Sleep Research, 8, 270, 1979.

28. Padovan, I., and Pansini, M.: New possibilities of analysis in electronystagmography. Acta Otolaryng., 73, 121-125, 1972.

29. Petre-Quadens, O., and De Lee, C.: Eye movement frequencies and related paradoxical sleep cycles: Developmental changes. Chronobiologia, 1, 348-355, 1974.

30. Rechtschaffen, A., and Kales, A.: A manual of standardized terminology, techniques, and scoring system for sleep stages of human subjects. Washington, D.C.: Public Health Service, U.S. Government Printing Office, 1968.

31. Roffwarg, H.P., Dement, W.C., Muzio, J.N., and Fisher, C.: Dream imagery: Relationship to rapid eye movements of sleep. Archives of General Psychiatry, 7, 235-258, 1962.

32. Salzarulo, P.: Variations with time of the quantity of eye movements during fast sleep in man. Electroenceph. Clin. Neurophysiol., 32, 409-416, 1972.

33. Salzarulo, P., Pêcheux, M.G., and Lairy, G.C.: A vecto-oculographic approach to fast sleep eye movements in man. Electroenceph. Clin. Neurophysiol., 34, 539-542, 1973.

34. Schneider, D.: Spatiotemporal properties of rapid eye movements in human REM sleep. 1. Qualitative analysis. Waking Sleeping, 2, 63-67, 1978a.

35. Schneider, D.: Spatiotemporal properties of rapid eye movements in human REM sleep. 2. Quantitative analysis. Waking Sleeping, 2, 69-74, 1978b.

237

36. Smith, J.R., Cronin, M., and Karacan, I.: A multichannel hybrid system for rapid eye movement detection. Computers and Biomedical Research, 4, 275-290, 1971.
37. Smith, J.R.: Computers in sleep research. CRC Critical Reviews in Bioengineering, 3, 93-148, 1978.
38. Spreng, L.F., Johnson, L.C., and Lubin, A.: Autonomic correlates of eye movement bursts during stage REM sleep. Psychophysiology, 4, 311-323, 1968.
39. Tursky, B., and O'Connell, D.N.: A comparison of AC and DC eye movement recording. Psychophysiology, 3, 157-163, 1966.
40. Uenoyama, K., Uenoyama, N., and Unuma, I.: Two dimensional recording of eye movements by vector electro-oculography. Jap. J. Ophthal., 7, 155-163, 1963.
41. Weber, L.D., Muzet, A., Schieber, J.P., and Lienhard, J.P.: Characteristics of rapid eye movement production during REM sleep in man: Organization and rhythmicity. Electroenceph. Clin. Neurophysiol., 55, 151-155, 1983.
42. Whitman, R.L., Herman, J.H., and Boehling, W.A.: Processor for minicomputer analysis of "EOG's". Proceedings 28th ACEMB, New Orleans, Louisiana, 1975.
43. Wong, C.: Automated Quantification of Periodic Fluctuations in Rapid Eye Movement Density During REM Sleep in Man, Master's Thesis, Electrical Engineering Department, University of Houston, Houston, Texas, 1985.
44. Yana, K., Suzuki, Y., Tanaka, K., Saito, Y., and Kikkawa, S. Rapid eye movements as a weighted point process. Sleep Research, 8, 280, 1979.

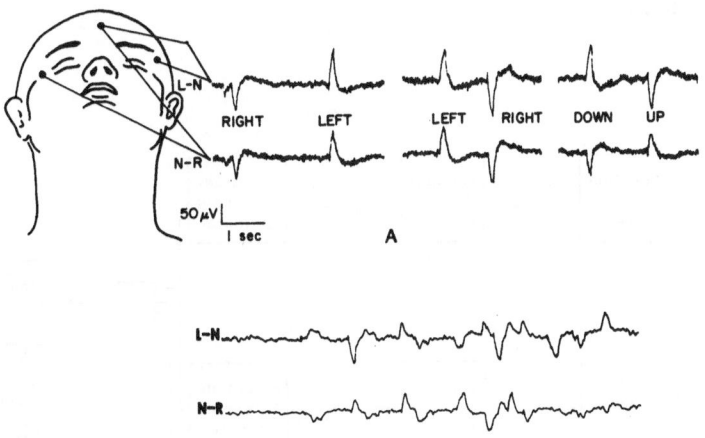

Figure 1. Rapid eye movements recorded via a common-nasion electrode montage (N: nasion, L: left eye, R: right eye). A) Voluntary eye movements in the awake state (directions indicate eye movement direction). B) Spontaneous eye movements during REM sleep. Recording time constant: 0.1 seconds.

238

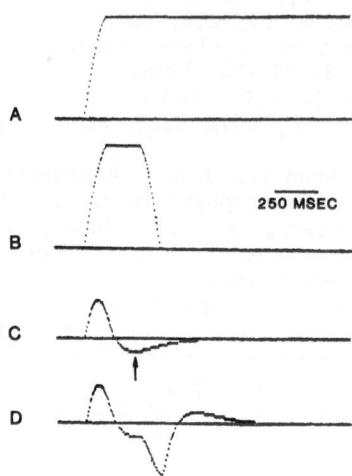

Figure 2. Recovery waveforms due to AC coupling. A) Hypothetical DC-coupled EOG waveform corresponding to a single REM excursion. B) Hypothetical DC-coupled EOG waveform corresponding to a double (to-and-fro) REM excursion. C) AC-coupled version of the EOG waveform in A (second-order highpass filter). Observe recovery waveform (arrow) which could be mistaken as corresponding to a REM. D) AC-coupled version of the EOG waveform in B.

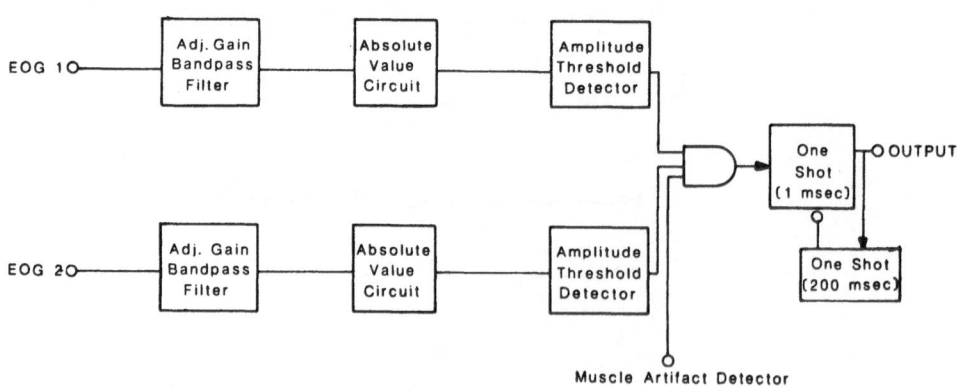

Figure 3. Block diagram of an analog automatic REM detector utilizing two EOG channels.

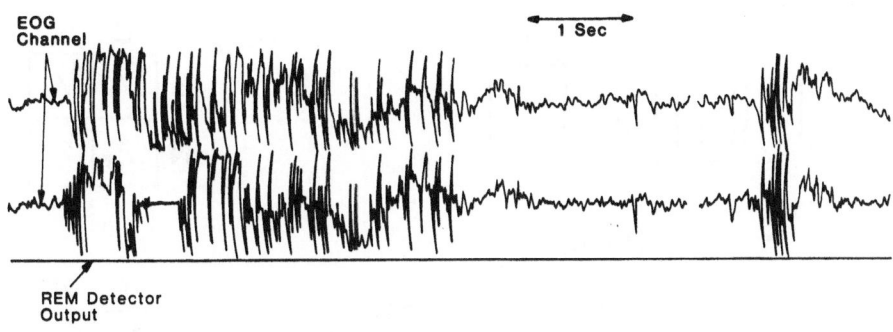

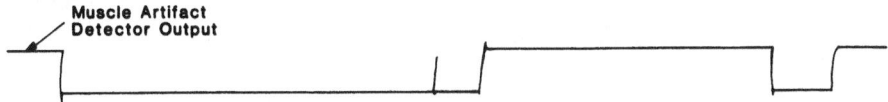

Figure 4.   Example of EMG artifact detection. A downward deflection at
the muscle artifact detector's output indicates artifact
detection.   Observe the REM-like waveforms in the EOG channels
during the presence of the artifact, and that no REM detection
occurs when the artifact is detected.

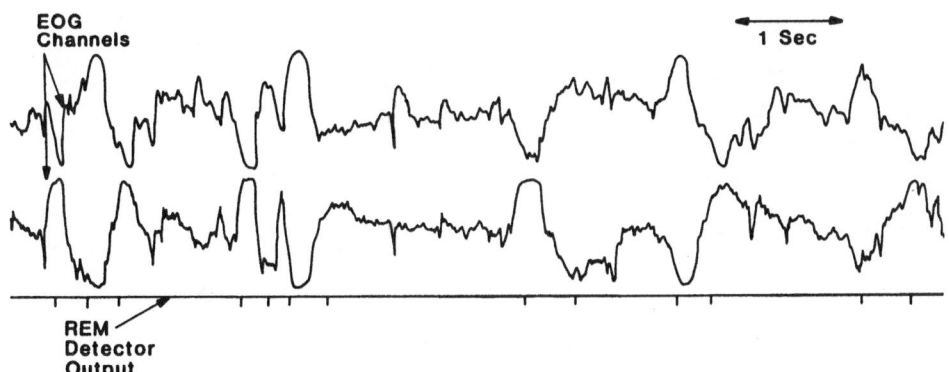

Figure 5.   Example of the automatic REM detector's performance with EOG
data from REM sleep.   The short pulses at the REM detector's
output indicate REM detections.

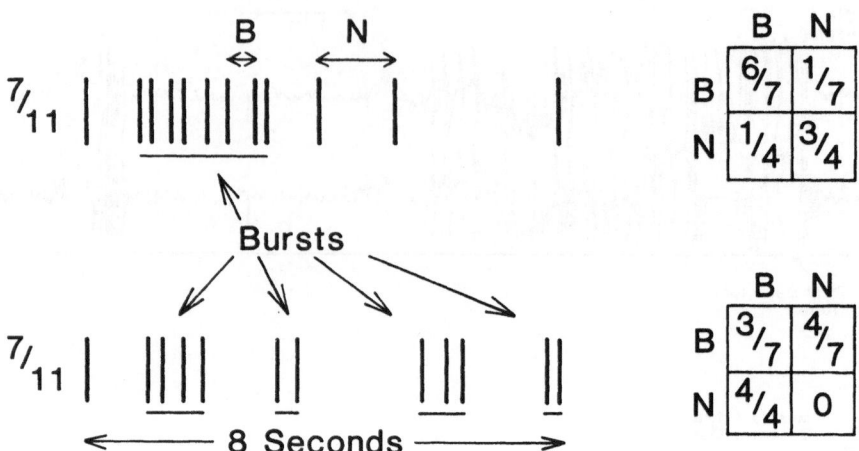

Figure 6. Two hypothetical REM sequences, differentiated by the structure of their respective state transition probability matrices on the right (see text).

INSTRUMENTATION AND DATA ANALYSIS METHODS
NEEDED FOR BLOOD PRESSURE MONITORING IN CHRONOBIOLOGY

Germaine CORNELISSEN, Chronobiology Laboratories
Univ. of Minnesota, Minneapolis, MN.

INTRODUCTION

Elevated blood pressure (BP) is a medical problem receiving much attention today, since its treatment can prevent major incapacitating diseases. A vast literature indeed indicates that a high BP constitutes an important risk factor in the development of strokes and a variety of other diseases, including those of the heart and the kidney (Australian national blood pressure study, 1980). Although the etiology of high BP remains obscure, extensive life insurance statistics document the point that early detection and treatment can prolong useful life. The remarkable "42% decrease in strokes" since 1972 emphasized by Kolata (1983a) is in the opinion of many a benefit from treating high BP. Early recognition, however, is at present unlikely because
(1) the condition is often asymptomatic and has been labeled the "silent disease";
(2) relatively few people visit a physician regularly when in apparent good health;
(3) BP is so variable that isolated measurements may be misleading;
(4) when a BP elevation is suspected or has even been clearly diagnosed, many individuals are not sufficiently educated or motivated to implement the steps necessary for a differential diagnosis and may not even be persuaded to submit to painless and often relatively inexpensive or cost-free non-drug treatment (e.g., by diet, exercise).

The variability of BP among healthy individuals is such that the identification, indeed the very definition, of high BP is highly ambiguous, mainly when relying on single time-unspecified measurements. Even when based, not on one or two (Kolata, 1983b), but on a mean of several casual rather than systematic measurements, a BP found to be "high" or "low" is often unreliable. This is due both to the large variability of BP and other body functions (see for instance Halberg and Fink, 1981), and the circumstance that unusually high or low values may occur only at certain times that may not be covered by casual sampling (Bartter, 1974).

With automatic instrumentation for indirect non-invasive BP monitoring, it becomes possible to follow the time course of BP variation around the clock in large groups (Weber and Drayer, 1984; Carandente and Halberg, 1984) to provide specifications for the measurement of BP. Automatic monitoring of

BP in healthy adults indicates that biological rhythms account, to a statistically significant extent, for predictable BP variability. The most prominent rhythms are almost invariably the circadian rhythms, with a period of about 24 hours. In men, 20 to 60 years of age (Halberg et al., 1984a), the range of change within a day averages 68.9±15.7(SD) and 56.2±14.9 mmHg for SBP and DBP, respectively, while the average pulse pressure is only 43.0±10.4(SD) mmHg. In these subjects, circadian rhythms account for a change per day of at least 24.0 mmHg for SBP and of 18.0 mmHg for DBP. In other words, on the average, a change with a predictable timing of 24 (SBP) and of 18 (DBP) mmHg can be expected to occur within 24h in any given (healthy) individual as part of the much larger total variation. More of the overall variation can be accounted for by the complementary concomitant assessment of other rhythms that also characterize BP: ultradian rhythms (or harmonics accounting for the circadian waveform) with a higher-than-circadian frequency and infradian rhythms with a lower-than-circadian frequency.

As a result of this large BP variability, in the vast majority of individuals, the highest DBP measured at one time within 24h exceeds the lowest SBP measured at another time within the same 24h. In the population referred to above, consisting of 40 men monitored on two occasions at 7.5 min intervals for 24h, the average difference (overlap) between the highest DBP and the lowest SBP is as much as 16.7±1.4(SE) mmHg. Neglect of circadian stage is thus no more warranted than the failure to distinguish systolic from diastolic BP.

Although with the advent of automatic monitoring, the large variability of BP in health and disease can no longer be disputed, any endogenous aspects of such variability remain largely ignored. Pickering et al. (1984) believe that the BP pattern of higher values during the day, intermediate values in the evening and lower values during the night, observed in the majority of people, is determined largely by factors associated with the social routine of living. A chronobiologic view is that circadian (and other) rhythms with endogenous components are synchronized by physico-chemical as well as socio-ecologic factors. The existence of an underlying intrinsic rhythmic mechanism is supported by the observation (validated statistically) that BP rises before awakening and cannot thus result only from a change in posture or activity (E Halberg et al., 1981). Halberg (1953) documented the phenomenon of an activation of both the adrenal cortex and medulla, codetermining a rise in BP prior to awakening, and postulated that the rise occurs perhaps in preparation for the start of each day's motor activities. More recently, Raftery (1984) has confirmed this finding by relying on ambulatory intra-arterial BP recording, a method of rather well-defined accuracy and precision. Studies of BP under conditions of human isolation (Halberg et al., 1984b) also support a partly endogenous (insofar as free-running), partly diversely environmental (transiently phase-trapped) BP rhythmicity.

Against this background, several questions are pertinent. First, how can BP be measured; what are the different techniques, their precision and accuracy; what is the state of the present technology? Second, how should BP be monitored; how frequently and for how long? Third, how should BP data be analyzed; what is the state-of-the-art of the available methodology? Fourth, how reliably can the effects of non-drug or drug treatment be assessed? The following sections attempt to answer these questions.

MEASUREMENT OF BLOOD PRESSURE

1. Direct measurement of blood pressure

Much progress has been made in the measurement of BP since 1733, when Stephen Hales measured the BP of an unanesthetized horse. The introduction of the mercury-filled U-tube manometer by Poiseuille and later by Ludwig was readily accepted because of the practicality of the device and the ease of its standardization. Ludwig was aware, though, that the height of the oscillations did not indicate true systolic and diastolic BP. Indeed, the BP wave reaches its peak in such a short time that the mercury manometer, because of its inertia and friction in the fluid constituting the whole system, cannot attain the maximal value. The peak-to-peak amplitude of the pressure record displayed by the mercury manometer is thus considerably less than the true pulse pressure, which is the difference between systolic and diastolic pressure. The drawback of the device (lack of a short response time) can, however, be exploited. By dampening the mercury manometer so that the amplitude of the oscillations is practically zero, and only respiratory variations in BP appear, the height of the mercury manometer represents mean pressure, i.e., the area under a single pulse wave divided by the wave length.

Attempts to develop rapidly responding systems followed. The system designed by Marey and Chauveau in 1861 reportedly exhibited a response time on the order of 5 msec and the propagation velocity of a pressure wave in 4-mm tubing used with it was 280 m/sec, thus allowing a faithful reproduction of the intracardiac pressures and the sequences in which they develop (Geddes, 1970). Since then, different techniques evolved rapidly, including mechano-optical systems, electrolytic manometers, electro-optical manometers, capacitance manometers, strain-gauge manometers, inductive manometers, mechano-electronic tube manometers, and catheter-tip manometers. These different systems are well described by Geddes (1970).

The accuracy of BP records depends directly on the response time of the transducer. A short response time requires the presence of a high natural frequency in the manometer-catheter system, that can be achieved by a high stiffness-to-mass ratio. An increase in stiffness, however, results in a decrease in sensitivity, in terms of deflection per unit of applied pressure. But the addition of levers to amplify the deflection adds mass, which, in turn, reduces the natural frequency and hence prolongs the response time. The stiffness is also inversely proportional to the volume displacement, i.e., the volume of fluid entering the transducer by applying an increase in pressure to it. It is not surprising then that the evolution of systems for reliably recording arterial BP has focused on the achievement of a high natural frequency and a low volume displacement in the transducer. BP transducers with sufficiently high natural frequencies and low volume displacements for use with catheters and small-bore cannulae or needles allowing reliable BP measurement have been available since the beginning of the 20th century. Today, BP transducers have a natural frequency in the range of 30Hz to ~10kHz, and a volume displacement of 1 to 0.01 mm^3/100mmHg (Geddes, 1970; see Figure 1-19, p45). These characteristics assure adequate BP measurement since a good reproduction of the BP wave can be achieved if the overall system frequency response extends uniformly from zero to ~10 times the cardiac frequency (20 Hz for a pulse of 120 beats/min) (Geddes, 1970).

2. Indirect measurement of blood pressure

Since direct measurement of BP is a cumbersome procedure for routine use on patients, carrying some risk of complication, its clinical application has been limited. Methods for measuring BP indirectly, i.e., non-invasively, are more attractive. It is important, however, to understand how they work and what their limitations are.

Indirect BP methods are based on the fact that if a superficial artery is palpated, a rough idea of the pressure within it can be gained by feeling the force necessary to compress it. Only since hydraulic and pneumatic artery-occluding devices were introduced, methods became available to calibrate the occluding force in terms of pressure and to relate it to the pressure within the artery. Four basic methods can be distinguished for the indirect measurement of BP, all of them relying on an externally applied artery-occluding device: (a) the palpatory; (b) the flush; (c) the oscillometric; and (d) the auscultatory method. With each, an artery is relieved of an occluding pressure and an indication of passage of the pulse wave is required. When the pulse appears, the occluding pressure is slightly below systolic pressure. With some of the methods, as the occluding pressure is reduced further, evidence is provided of its passage through diastolic pressure (Geddes, 1970).

The palpatory method is routinely used to measure systolic BP when other indirect methods fail. Accurate measurement with this method requires, however, a sensitive tactile sense. This technique was standardized by the American Heart Association in 1951, which recommended (a) the use of a cuff having a width about 0.4 times the circumference of the limb; (b) to raise the pressure of the cuff about 30 mmHg above the point at which the radial pulse disappears; (c) to reduce the pressure slowly, so that pressure in the manometer falls about 2 to 3 mmHg per beat; (d) to note the return of palpable beats at the natural rate of the heart as systolic BP. Enselberg (1961) observed the disappearance of a notch on the rising phase of the brachial artery pulse wave at diastolic BP, which may allow in some cases to use this technique to estimate diastolic BP as well.

The flush method consists of applying a suprasystolic counterpressure to a whole member, like a finger, which becomes blanched as the blood is being expelled. By slowly lowering the occluding pressure, color starts to return when the occluding pressure is just below systolic pressure. Practical use of this method in pediatric practice was introduced by Goldring and Wohltmann (1952), who called attention to the failure of the auscultatory method in newborns. In older children, these authors found that systolic BP obtained by the flush method was on the average 8 mmHg below that obtained by auscultation.

The oscillometric method relies on the detection of the first pulse as cuff-pressure falls below systolic pressure. Because cuff-pressure oscillations can be seen to accompany the appearance of the pulse, BP can be derived from cuff-pressure oscillations. As counterpressure is reduced from above sytolic to below diastolic pressure, oscillations appear, increase to a maximum and then decrease rapidly in amplitude. Systolic pressure corresponds to the appearance of oscillations. Diastolic pressure is more difficult to estimate with this method, since there is no clearly identifiable transition in the radial pulse tracing as cuff pressure passes through diastolic pressure.

The auscultatory method relies on the observation that a completely compressed artery in a normal condition does not produce any sound. Korotkoff (1905) noticed that as counterpressure drops below systolic pressure, audible sounds can be heard, that can be attributed either to phenomena pertaining to the arterial wall or to those associated with the flow of blood in the artery. Before complete disappearance of the Korotkoff sounds, murmurs are heard. Comparison with direct arterial BP measurement indicates that at the point of muffling (noted K4), the cuff pressure is slightly above DBP, while it is slightly below DBP at cessation of the sounds (noted K5), an observation that prompted the recording of both events to evaluate DBP. The auscultatory method may fail in subjects with low BP: as BP decreases, the spectrum of the Korotkoff sounds indeed shifts to the lower frequencies, beyond the sensitivity of the human ear. For the same reason, this method is sensitive to environmental noise when BP is monitored with a stethoscope. This method can be improved by using the QRS wave of the ECG to start a delay circuit which opens an electronic gate for a specified interval to enable detection of the K sounds only at a time when they are expected to occur. This is only achieved, though, at the cost of the added burden of attaching ECG electrodes to the patient.

The auscultatory and oscillometric methods are the most widely used non-invasive techniques, that have been adopted for the automatic monitoring of BP. Other promising non-invasive techniques, including Doppler methods, have been proposed but have not yet found wide acceptance (Weiss et al., 1984; p.86-87). Nelson and Egbert (1984) call attention on 16 possible sources of error in taking BP measurements:

1. Failure to use the proper size cuff.
2. Failure to apply the cuff snugly to allow for rapid and homogeneous inflation of the cuff.
3. Failure to center the cuff over the brachial artery to avoid a spuriously high reading.

4. Failure to relax arm muscles.
5. Failure to have the arm at heart level.
6. Failure to inflate the cuff rapidly to minimize the trapping of venous blood in the forearm during the time when cuff compression is between the systolic and diastolic pressures (large quantities of blood trapped distally may produce an auscultatory gap).
7. Failure to estimate systolic BP by palpation for recognizing any auscultatory gap.
8. Pressing too hard with the stethoscope endpiece.
9. Failure to use the stethoscope bell, so as to hear the low-pitched early and late Korotkoff sounds.
10. Overly rapid cuff deflation (at a deflation rate of 5 mmHg/sec and a heart rate of 60 beats/min, SBP may be underestimated by 8 mmHg).
11. Failure to record SBP at the first faint tapping sound.
12. Failure to record DBP at the point of complete disappearance of the sound (K5): recent research indicates that DBP at the muffling point is overestimated by 5 to 10 mmHg.
13. Failure to record BP in both arms at the initial visit (one study showed a 36% incidence of differential readings up to 10 mmHg in "normotensives"; "hypertensives" had a 46% rate of up to 20 mmHg).
14. Failure to record the position of the patient (there is a pressure difference between supine, sitting, and upright posture).
15. Reliance on a single BP measurement in the diagnosis of "hypertension" (ignorance of circadian rhythmicity and of large short-term variability).
16. The authors' initial point, namely the failure to have the patient in the basal state, on the assumption that ideally, BP should be recorded when the patient is free from the common stimuli that elevate it, is debatable. The alternative of studying the patient by ambulatory monitoring under the influence of habitual stimuli can also be advocated and may be more appropriately descriptive of the patient's condition.

These authors also recognize other problem areas, such as poorly audible Korotkoff sounds, the measurement of BP in "hypotensives", in the presence of arrhythmias, in obese patients, and in patients with atherosclerotic vessels (in a rigid, sclerotic vessel with double the usual wall thickness, SBP may be overestimated by as much as 32 mmHg). Finally, they call attention on instrumental errors and report results from a study wherein 31% of aneroid sphygmomanometers in several US hospitals deviated from standard by more than 3 mmHg and 18% by more than 7 mmHg, while none of the mercury-column manometers were inaccurate, although these devices are not infallible either. Observer errors are also noted.

BLOOD PRESSURE MONITORING

Several kinds of automatic devices are available to monitor BP. The need for intra-arterial invasion of monitors for the direct measurement of BP, such as the Oxford recorder, precludes their widespread use. Being interested in prevention as well as in the diagnosis and treatment of an elevated BP, focus will be placed herein on the non-invasive indirect monitoring of BP. Ideally, an automatic BP monitor should consist of a portable, miniaturized, light-weight, electronic monitor assuring reliable BP measurement and easy calibration of the instrument. In order to avoid undue costs after purchase of the monitor, the power supply should be rechargeable. Provision should be made for checking the measurements as well as the correct operation of the instrument. This implies that the option of displaying BP measurements should be made available. Some people may prefer not to have the BP values displayed if it influences their BP. Each BP measurement collected should be time-coded, a task easily achieved by incorporating a quartz clock in the instrument. Moreover, the sampling interval should be selectable. The instrument should also make adequate provisions for data storage, transfer and analysis. Data storage could be in a solid-state memory, preferably backed up with a battery so as to be non-volatile, holding enough data to cover a complete chronobiologic profile (serial BP measurements allowing the determination of BP rhythm characteristics). The instrument should offer the options of providing routine minimal analyses, along with an easily-understood summary of results, and of transfering the data to a separate computer for other analyses. A serial asynchronous communications linkage compatible with conventional personal computers should thus be provided. Data transfer is particularly important for research purposes in developing new ways to exploit the individual BP profiles on the one hand, and to derive useful new endpoints from the examination of data bases thus collected on the other hand. Monitors available today, such as those manufactured by Nippon Colin (Komaki, Japan), Squibb (Instruments for Cardiac Research, Liverpool, NY) and Del Mar Avionics (Pressurometer III, Irvine, CA) offer some of the features described above. Further efforts toward miniaturization and software capabilities for data analysis are, however, needed.

The advantages of automatic BP monitoring usually mentioned are the fact that bias due to the "white coat effect" observed in casual office BP measurements can largely be avoided, and that a 24-h mean estimates BP more accurately than one or a few isolated measurements. The possibility of measuring BP at times that would otherwise not be sampled (e.g., at night) is also acknowledged and some authors analyze day and night data separately (Reeves et al., 1984). A chronobiologic approach could further exploit features of around-the-clock BP monitoring. For instance, there is evidence to suggest that human amplitude-hypertension (elevation of the circadian amplitude in the absence of an elevation in overall mean) characterizes an early stage of BP alteration. This observation had been made earlier in the handled SHR-SP rat. In this model, a systolic amplitude-hypertension precedes a genetically-determined MESOR-hypertension (J Halberg et al., 1980). Kobrin et al. (1984) also reported that an odd-hour BP elevation during the habitual sleep span may be more harmful than one during waking.

1. Sampling rate

Not much attention has been paid to the sampling requirements of BP to obtain an adequate description of circadian BP
rhythms. One study carried out on 20 ambulatory "hypertensive" patients by di Rienzo et al. (1983) examined how well
the 24-h BP mean could be estimated with non-invasive (indirect) automatic BP monitors, using different sampling intervals. In this study, BP was monitored intra-arterially for
24h using the Oxford method. A beat-to-beat analysis of the
BP recording was provided by a computer, and the average 24-h
SBP, DBP and MAP (mean arterial pressure) values were compared
with those obtained by analyzing single BP waves of the same
recording at intervals of 5, 10, 15, 30 and 60 minutes.
Although these authors concluded that accurate assessment of a
24-h BP mean can be achieved at intervals as much as 30 or 60
min apart, their results indicate that for an adequate chronobiologic assessment of BP profiles (for studying the dynamics
of BP variability), data should be sampled at least once every
15 min.

By using the 24-h mean obtained by the continuous recording as reference, the examination of individual estimates of a
24-h BP mean from samples collected every 60 min shows a
departure as large as 15 (SBP), 8 (DBP), and 10 (MAP) mmHg.
Moreover, this study did not consider endpoints other than the
mean, pertinent to chronobiology, such as the estimation of
the extent of BP variation within 24h. Some insight into this
question can be gained by considering that the estimate of the
standard deviation of BP about the 24-h mean increases drastically for sampling intervals larger than 15 min in ~30% of the
cases studied. On this basis, a sampling rate of at least 4
samples per hour is here advocated. It has to be stressed
that this recommendation stems from the consideration of circadian rhythmicity and that much denser sampling is needed to
study changes in BP within the cardiac cycle or changes with
respiration (for instance, see de Boer et al., 1983).

On the basis of data collected at 7.5 min intervals for
24h on 40 healthy men, 20 to 60 years of age, monitored on 2
occasions with the Pressurometer III (Del Mar Avionics, Irvine, CA) (Halberg et al., 1984a), two approaches were followed to determine the characteristics of random variability
of BP and pulse. One approach examines the short-term variability in the data by computing for each 24-h profile the mean
and standard deviation (SD) of BP and pulse within each hour.
The distribution of SDs for each hour is then examined over
the 80 profiles. Table 1 summarizes the results obtained. It
can be seen that the error on SBP measurements averages ~7
mmHg, that on DBP ~6 mmHg and that on pulse ~6 beats/min.
Histograms of the within-hour SDs indicate that the distributions are highly skewed to the right (SBP: g_1=1.17; DBP:
g_1=1.46; HR: g_1=1.27, where g_1 is Fisher's coefficient of
skewness). Examination of Table 1 further reveals that the
SDs are not evenly distributed over 24h (P<0.001 by Kruskal-
Wallis test for differences of location in ranked data grouped
by single classification; Sokal and Rohlf, 1981). The
within-hour SD is larger around the time of awakening and

probably reflects the relatively rapid rise in BP and pulse associated with the transition from rest to activity. Smaller within-hour SDs are observed during the rest span for pulse. These results thus indicate that measurements taken within one hour differ on the average by 6 to 7 mmHg (BP) or ~6 beats/min (pulse). These values reflect the part of (random) variability that remains unaccounted for, even by taking circadian rhythms (with their waveform) into account.

Table 1

Within-hour variability in blood pressure (BP) and pulse, estimated by hourly standard deviations computed from samples at 7.5 min intervals over 24 h on 40 healthy men, 20-60 years of age, monitored on 2 occasions.

Time interval:	Systolic BP			Diastolic BP			Pulse		
	Mean	SD	Median	Mean	SD	Median	Mean	SD	Median
0 - 1	7.87	3.84	6.83	6.50	3.65	5.87	5.08	3.18	4.54
1 - 2	7.01	3.09	7.10	5.62	2.98	5.27	4.45	2.92	3.74
2 - 3	7.54	3.68	6.78	7.01	4.34	5.49	4.63	3.08	3.58
3 - 4	7.74	3.43	7.18	6.78	3.78	5.99	4.85	3.55	3.83
4 - 5	8.19	3.75	7.11	6.49	3.48	5.55	6.21	4.19	5.43
5 - 6	8.56	3.99	8.02	8.12	4.00	7.54	8.09	4.35	7.29
6 - 7	9.54	4.27	8.28	7.58	4.33	7.08	9.62	4.35	9.52
7 - 8	7.96	3.71	7.24	6.27	2.96	5.87	7.75	3.01	7.16
8 - 9	6.88	2.68	6.19	5.59	2.61	5.17	6.58	3.72	5.76
9 - 10	6.97	2.24	6.65	5.57	2.41	4.95	6.99	3.28	6.52
10 - 11	6.48	2.05	6.43	5.61	1.81	5.46	6.20	3.14	5.31
11 - 12	7.16	2.41	6.89	5.10	1.99	4.96	6.86	3.18	6.10
12 - 13	7.40	2.99	7.04	6.89	2.88	6.07	7.48	2.82	7.50
13 - 14	6.66	2.28	6.70	5.43	2.10	4.92	6.11	3.36	5.14
14 - 15	6.95	2.48	6.75	5.38	2.13	4.76	5.87	1.85	5.93
15 - 16	6.68	2.30	6.53	5.66	2.24	5.27	6.55	3.66	5.72
16 - 17	7.34	2.95	6.72	5.89	2.90	5.46	6.53	2.69	6.25
17 - 18	7.04	2.70	6.47	6.18	2.96	5.77	7.00	3.32	6.39
18 - 19	7.72	3.81	7.13	6.58	2.33	6.49	6.78	3.66	6.07
19 - 20	7.54	2.82	6.99	6.35	2.87	5.62	6.75	2.87	6.45
20 - 21	6.91	2.67	6.65	5.63	2.52	5.23	5.82	3.16	5.08
21 - 22	6.58	2.81	5.87	5.65	3.05	5.15	5.91	2.98	5.63
22 - 23	7.99	3.68	7.25	7.56	3.30	6.84	5.87	3.18	5.55
23 - 24	7.85	3.93	6.99	7.02	3.01	6.45	5.60	3.10	4.84
overall	7.44	3.23	6.88	6.27	3.11	5.63	6.40	3.49	5.83

Kruskal-Wallis(*)
χ^2:   58.5; P<0.001   105.7; P<0.001   221.7; P<0.001

(*) Test for differences of location in ranked data grouped by single classification (R estimator for one-way ANOVA); χ^2 test with 23 degrees of freedom (Sokal and Rohlf, 1981). This test is preferred to the one-way ANOVA in view of the skewness of the distributions (i.e., departure from normality; P<0.05).

250

Another approach consists of computing the frequency spectrum of each variable, averaged over the 80 profiles, in order to determine their noise characteristics. This approach also provides information as to the harmonic content of the circadian waveform of BP and pulse. Not only were data on SBP, DBP and HR considered, but also those on 3 other related variables: pulse pressure (PP=SBP-DBP), mean arterial pressure (MAP=SBP/3+DBPx2/3), and the rate-pressure product (SBPxHR), which provides an assessment of cardiac performance. For each variable, each 24-h profile (j=1, ..., 80) was used to determine the spectrum, characterized by an overall mean, M, and modules (A_i) and phases (ϕ_i) for periods (τ_i) ranging from the length of the observation span (24h) to the inverse of the Nyquist frequency (twice the sampling interval or ~15 min): τ_i=24h/i, where i is an integer (i=1, ..., 95). At each frequency, a population-mean cosinor (Halberg et al., 1967), summarizing the results from the 80 profiles, was applied to determine which harmonics contributed significantly to the circadian waveform. Moreover, the average power spectrum was determined by plotting $\langle A \rangle_i$ as a function of i on a log-log scale, where $\langle A \rangle_i = [\Sigma_i \Sigma_j A_{ij}^2]^{1/2}$ (i=1, ..., 95).

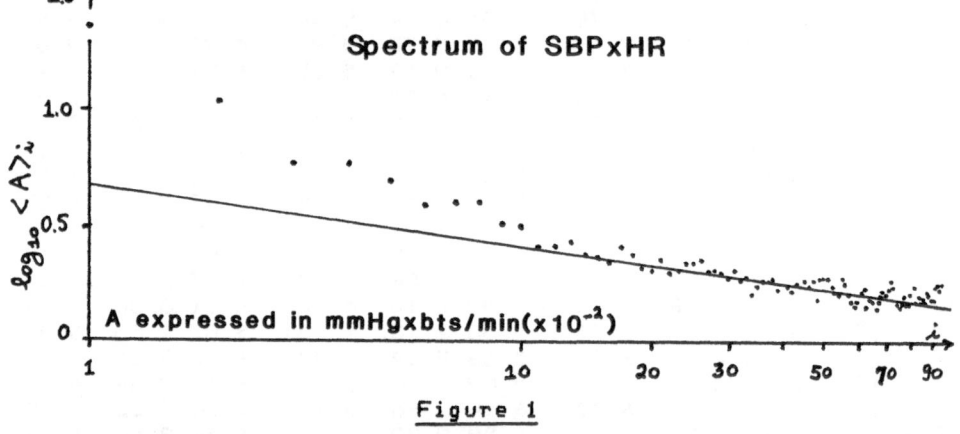

Figure 1

The population-mean cosinor results indicate that components up to the 10th harmonic may contribute to the circadian waveform (Table 2a), while higher-order harmonics were not significant. Tentatively, the rhythm may be considered to be characterized by the first 10 spectral lines and the noise by the remaining 85 spectral lines. When correlations characterize consecutive measurements errors, the spectrum is "colored" in the sense that modules (that are thought not to correspond to the deterministic signal) differ as a function of frequency. Usually, larger modules are observed at low frequencies and smaller modules at high frequencies. In such cases, it is common to represent the spectrum in a given frequency range by an expression like $\langle A \rangle_i = c/f^k$ with k usually between +1 and -1, white noise corresponding to k=0. The noise characteristics, as evaluated on the basis of the last 85 lines, are listed in Table 2b. It can be seen that the noise is correlated and that modules decrease with increasing frequency.

Table 2a

Circadian harmonic content of cardiovascular variables:
population-mean cosinor analyses.

Period (h)	SBP A	SBP ϕ	SBP P	DBP A	DBP ϕ	DBP P	HR A	HR ϕ	HR P
24.0	11.46	-223	<0.001	8.63	-206	<0.001	10.26	-209	<0.001
12.0	5.86	-257	<0.001	4.03	-244	<0.001	3.97	-263	<0.001
8.0	0.80	-303	0.005	0.37	-359	NS	1.67	-300	<0.001
6.0	1.02	-102	0.001	0.57	-179	0.037	2.31	-106	<0.001
4.8	1.27	-182	<0.001	1.17	-162	<0.001	0.58	-189	0.006
4.0	0.59	-284	0.022	0.61	-237	0.006	0.51	-258	0.017
3.4	0.27	-279	NS	0.20	-139	NS	0.59	-353	<0.001
3.0	0.98	-108	<0.001	0.52	- 26	0.010	0.75	-126	<0.001
2.7	0.44	-209	0.047	0.32	-165	NS	0.26	-290	NS
2.4	0.70	- 48	0.001	0.16	-360	NS	0.09	-142	NS

Period (h)	PP A	PP ϕ	PP P	MAP A	MAP ϕ	MAP P	SBP x HR A	SBP x HR ϕ	SBP x HR P
24.0	3.84	-261	<0.001	9.44	-213	<0.001	19.80	-215	<0.001
12.0	1.93	-281	<0.001	4.59	-249	<0.001	8.48	-260	<0.001
8.0	0.59	-265	0.006	0.43	-329	NS	2.33	-295	<0.001
6.0	1.07	- 71	<0.001	0.57	-140	0.038	3.48	-105	<0.001
4.8	0.44	-246	NS	1.20	-168	<0.001	1.50	-186	<0.001
4.0	0.41	-353	0.020	0.56	-250	0.012	0.90	-275	0.027
3.4	0.46	-285	0.029	0.11	-185	NS	0.83	-333	0.022
3.0	0.96	-138	<0.001	0.51	- 63	0.024	1.53	-122	<0.001
2.7	0.33	-251	0.047	0.33	-186	NS	0.58	-257	NS
2.4	0.61	- 67	<0.001	0.30	- 39	NS	0.61	- 65	0.045

SBP = Systolic Blood Pressure; DBP = Diastolic BP; HR = Pulse;
PP = Pulse P; MAP = Mean Arterial P; SBP, DBP, PP and MAP
expressed in mmHg, HR in beats/min, and SBPxHR in mmHgxbts/min
($\times 10^{-2}$); ϕ expressed in degrees, with $360°$ = period length, and
$0°$ = midnight; P-values not accounting for multiple testing.

Table 2b

Noise characteristics

Variable	c	k
SBP	3.85	.308
DBP	3.32	.308
HR	2.31	.205
PP	2.56	.198
MAP	3.48	.344
SBP x HR	4.76	.263

The noise spectrum in a given frequency range may be represented by an expression like: $A(f)=c/f^k$, where f is the frequency
line number and k is an exponent. White noise corresponds to
$k = 0$, while $k > 0$ indicates correlated noise.

These noise characteristics are compatible with a measurement error of ~6-7 mmHg for BP (or beats/min for pulse). The lines corresponding to the circadian rhythm can be seen to emerge from the noise, as illustrated for SBPxHR in Figure 1. For the 10th harmonic to be reliably estimated, a sampling interval of 15-30 minutes or shorter seems to be indicated, a result in agreement with that of the study by di Rienzo et al. (1983).

2. Observation span length

Because of infradian variability, circadian characteristics may change from day to day. It is thus important to determine an observation span of appropriate length for monitoring BP. Long individual recordings are valuable to answering this question. Data from a clinically healthy woman, monitored with a Nippon Colin instrument (Komaki, Japan) at ~10 min intervals, with interruptions, for 26 days (Halberg et al., 1984b), were used for this purpose. The amplitude (A) and acrophase (ϕ) of the 24-h component and the MESOR were determined for adjacent data sections covering 1, 2, 3, 4, and 5 days, in order to compare the dispersion of parameter estimates obtained over consecutive data sections as a function of interval length. A 90% prediction region for (A, ϕ) pairs from 2-day spans was derived (Nelson et al., 1983) for SBP and DBP. While all (A, ϕ) pairs from spans covering at least 2 days are inside this 2-day reference region, 33% (SBP) and 28% (DBP) of the (A, ϕ) pairs derived from one-day spans are outside this region (Cornelissen et al., 1983). The gain in predicting circadian rhythm parameters of SBP and DBP by lengthening the sampling span was gauged by the width of the 90% prediction interval for the MESOR, amplitude and acrophase, expressed as a percentage of the interval width corresponding to 1-day spans. The prediction interval width decreases by 35.4% (SE=4.7) by monitoring BP for 48h rather than 24h. Further gain is achieved by prolonging the observation span beyond 2 days (10.5% from 2 to 5 days), the total gain amounting to 45.9% (SE=6.4) for 5-day spans. These results suggest that a 24-h monitoring span may not be sufficient and that much better estimates are obtained on the basis of 48-h or longer profiles.

These same data were used to test synchronization to precisely 24h of the circadian period, by analyzing non-overlapping data sections of varying length (Bingham et al., 1984; Cornelissen et al., 1984). From the start of sampling, consecutive non-overlapping subspans ranging in length from 2 to 9 days, at 1-day intervals, were formed for separate cosinor analysis of SBP, DBP and pulse. Each variable was also analyzed over 2 adjacent 13-day subspans and over the entire observation span of 26 days. Data were averaged over 1-h intervals prior to analysis in order to reduce correlation in the residuals (difference between data and fitted cosine model) (Cornelissen et al., 1982). Regression diagnostic tests did not reject the sinusoidality assumption in most instances, but residuals were found to depart from normality in about 32% of the series. The period test was then applied to each data series in order to determine the average width of the 95% confidence interval of the circadian period as well as the average departure from 24h of the best-fitting circadian period, as a function of the length of the observation span. Results indicate that, as expected, by lengthening the duration of the observation span, a better resolution in frequency is obtained (the width of the 95% CI of the circadian period decreases), and, on the average, the best-fitting circadian period converges toward 24h. In order to see whether the circadian rhythm in BP and HR was 24-h synchronized in ordinary life, the percentage of series for which the 95% CI of the circadian period did not cover 24h was determined as a function of the subspan duration. Series on BP and HR were pooled for this computation to increase the sample size since only a limited number of series were available on any one variable for the longer observation spans. Results show that the confidence interval do not cover 24h in only a few series for either short (3- to 4-day) or long (13- and 26-day) subspans. For intermediate subspan lengths (5-9 days), as many as 35% of the confidence intervals do not include 24h (under conditions of anticipated 24-h synchronization). These results can be interpreted as follows. The period test is not sufficiently powerful to resolve the presence or absence of 24-h synchronization in short data series. Day-to-day changes in rhythm parameters and/or waveform, possibly modulated by infradian components, most likely affect series of intermediate length. As the length of the series increases, the circadian rhythmicity predominates, with its acrophase fluctuating within only a few clock-hours, thus converging to a best-fitting period of precisely 24h. These results contribute to the suggestion of monitoring BP for at least 7 days rather than for 24h, as is current practice with automatic monitors today.

The sampling requirements discussed above are concerned with the correct assessment of the dynamics of BP variation. These endpoints are particularly important for diagnostic purposes and for the proper evaluation of a patient's response to treatment (see below). For the more ambitious aim of screening large populations with a view toward prevention, the primary focus may be limited to the assessment of an overall mean and extent of predictable change within 24h. It is then cost-effective to combine automatic monitoring with self-measurements (Halberg et al., 1972), which may not be collected at a high sampling rate, but which can be taken for longer spans without requiring expensive instrumentation.

DATA ANALYSIS

It is being accepted in the medical community that pressures measured in the office or clinic are unreliable and that repeated self- and/or automatic measurements are better at predicting outcome than are single measurements. It is even being recognized that ambulatory BP measurements give better correlations than clinic readings with respect to target organ damage (Pickering et al., 1985). Moreover, the need to replace existing BP limits above which treatment should be ini-

tiated is acknowledged. If there is unquestionably more
awareness of the unreliability of casual BP measurements, investigators using automatic BP monitors have not fully exploited the capabilities offered by this new instrumentation.
Reports in the literature are primarily concerned with the assessment of a 24-h mean. In some instances (Reeves et al.,
1984; Pickering et al., 1985), data are separated between
night and day for analysis. Chronobiologic methods for data
analysis allow for a more thorough examination of the wealth
of data collected as a function of time. The inclusion of
time as a major factor in chronobiological investigations
indeed broadens the scope of methods for data analysis. In
addition to the methods of analysis of variance and covari-
ance, methods of time series analysis also become applicable.

Periodic regression has been used to model the rhythmic
behavior of biological variables. Least squares estimation
techniques of fitting relatively simple models are attractive
in view of the need to analyze non-equidistant data. Least
squares methods are, however, sensitive to outliers, in the
sense that the presence of one or a few "bad data" influences
the estimation of the parameters and their confidence intervals, and spreads the error over the entire data set. An important step in analyzing serial BP measurements thus is to
detect the presence of any outlying values (Cornelissen,
1984). The problem of detecting outliers in recordings from
ambulatory BP monitors has been addressed by Clark et al.
(1985). But the elimination of outliers, even if it is done
according to often "appropriate" criteria, may be a dangerous
procedure. Robust statistics (Rey, 1983), providing results
that are much less sensitive against small deviations from the
theoretical assumptions, may then be used with caution.

Methods of time series analysis present the advantage of
providing in addition to a more accurate estimation of the
24-h mean, estimates of rhythm parameters reflecting the
dynamics of BP variability. Test procedures are also available for comparing rhythm parameters among different populations or among several profiles from a given individual (Bingham et al., 1982). Such parameter tests allow for instance
the evaluation of a patient's response to treatment. Underlying the use of the least squares estimation techniques are
some important assumptions, including the appropriateness of
the selected model, normality of residuals, homogeneity of
variance and independence of errors. It is thus important to
verify the validity of these assumptions for a correct interpretation of the results from parameter tests.

The accumulation of data bases collected under standardized conditions on healthy individuals, in turn, makes it possible to determine reference intervals for BP measurements as
a function of (primarily circadian) rhythm stage and for
rhythm characteristics of cardiovascular variables. Such
reference values serve for an objective and positive definition of health, for the screening and diagnosis of disease,
and for gauging the subject's response to treatment. Tentative reference intervals from an as yet limited data base for
the 24-h mean (MESOR) and for the circadian amplitude of cardiovascular variables were derived as 90% prediction limits

for individuals stratified by age and sex (Halberg et al., 1984a and b). Time-specified reference limits, so-called chronodesms, can also be established for the evaluation of future single samples. Although mathematical models may in some cases be useful for constructing reference intervals (Halberg et al., 1978), the methods outlined by Nelson et al. (1983) apply to "hybrid data" (serial measurements collected from several individuals) and present the advantage of accomodating changes in variance as well as in mean as a function of rhythm stage. The latter approach involves initial pooling of data over a given time span in which changes in population characteristics can be assumed to be negligible for the purpose on hand. [Admittedly, ultradian components, e.g., reflecting changes in BP within a cardiac cycle, changes with respiration or changes in BP with periods measured in seconds or minutes, remain unassessed.] A reference interval based on the consideration of both within-subject and among-subject variability is then calculated for each time span. By computing such reference limits at increments shorter than that of the time span, displaced throughout the time series, smoothed curves are obtained. Such chronodesms were computed for several cardiovascular variables as 90% prediction limits based on measurements collected every 7.5 minutes over 24 hours by 39 presumably healthy men, 20 to 60 years of age (Halberg et al., 1984a). Any BP elevation thus can be readily checked against such reference standards and related to possible environmental influences, that should be required to be recorded in a diary as a complement to data collection.

Indices to reflect harm from an elevated BP should consider not only the 24-h mean but also the extent and the timing of BP elevation, with the likelihood that harm increases with both the magnitude and duration of BP elevation. As a first approximation, the integral over 24h of excess pressure above a critical limit can be considered (Halberg et al., 1984a and c). This index, having the units of impulse per unit area, has been denoted the hyperbaric index (HBI) and is expressed in mmHg x h. The use of such an index also requires the establishment of where the range of excess pressure begins. The upper limit of a 90% prediction chronodesm derived from data on a presumably healthy peer group monitored under standardized conditions has been proposed (Halberg and Cornelissen, submitted for publication). Such indices of BP excess can, in turn, be compared to corresponding distributions established for reference peer groups. Indeed, with ambulatory BP monitoring, isolated high BP readings can be expected to occur and it thus becomes mandatory to determine their frequency and most likely time of occurrence in reference populations.

Manufacturers of automatic BP monitors have focused on hardware problems, notably that of miniaturization. Chronobiology can add valuable software for data analysis to the existing instrumentation. The application of such methodology on a large scale would allow to correlate indices of BP excess with risk scores assessed on the basis of questionnaires, with target organ damage, and with clinical outcome. Results from such large scale surveys would, in turn, provide valuable information that could be used to improve the measure of BP ex-

cess, making provision for respite, when BP drops below-
hyperbaric-threshold, to compensate for the time spent above
threshold. There is indeed evidence indicating that the process of atherosclerosis is largely preventable and to a substantial degree even reversible (for review, see Halberg et
al., in press a).

CLINICAL APPLICATIONS

The combination of automatic BP monitoring with self-
measurements makes it possible to initiate the measurement of
BP early in life. The teaching of self-measurements has already been included in the curriculum of several schools (Halberg et al., 1984c), with the aim to bring self-help for
health care to a particularly relevant area of medicine. Continued efforts toward the introduction of self-monitoring, and
of chronobiology more generally, at an early age through the
school system, would readily allow screening for an elevated
BP on a large scale, as a step toward the prevention of major
cardiovascular diseases (Halberg et al., in press b).

Once a high BP has been detected, several options are
available. First, longer-term monitoring, preferably with automatic instrumentation, should be advocated. Second, diet
and exercise can be implemented, without any adverse effect
from taking medication when it is not needed. Third, if medication has to be administered, treatment can be optimized by
properly timing drug administration.

In evaluating a subject's response to non-drug or drug
intervention, one should be especially aware of the day-to-day
variability of a 24-h BP mean. Changes in MESOR are indeed
observed, in the absence of any intervention, between two
separate 24-h BP profiles obtained about one month apart in 22
out of 40 healthy men. A lowering of BP is found in the
second profile as compared to the first one in 14 instances
and an increase is found in the remaining 8 cases (Halberg and
Cornelissen, submitted for publication). This observation
renders the individualized assessment of a subject's response
to intervention much more difficult. Another difficulty stems
from the fact that a change in BP may occur not only as a
result of treatment, but also, at least in part, because of
unassessed factors once the environmental conditions are modified (Carandente et al., 1985; Halberg and Cornelissen, submitted for publication). Moreover, in assessing differential
treatment effects, one has to keep in mind that the regression
effect gives a misleading impression of the relationship
between treatment effect and reference measurement, the problem being that an apparent differential effect may simply reflect a regression to the mean (Berry et al., 1984).

The need to individualize the assessment of a patient's
response to treatment cannot be overemphasized (Halberg et
al., in press b). Different conclusions and interpretations
may indeed be reached whether results are summarized for the
population or for the individual. Table 3 (amplified from
Halberg et al., 1984a) provides an illustrative example,
wherein the MESOR and circadian amplitude of several cardiovascular variables derived on the basis of two 24-h BP pro-

files, obtained about one month apart, are compared. Population results indicate a very good correlation for these parameters between the two profiles, suggesting that overall a 24-h BP profile provides adequate information. A summary of individual differences between the two profiles yields a different picture, indicating that the 24-h mean differs on the average by 7 mmHg (SBP), and that in some individuals, this difference may be as much as 31 mmHg. These results clearly indicate the need to monitor BP for spans much longer than 24 hours!

Table 3

Comparison of cardiovascular rhythm characteristics derived from 2 24-h profiles, about one month apart, on 40 presumable healthy men, 20 to 60 years of age.

Endpoint		r	P	$\langle\Delta\rangle$	SD	g_1	g_2	min	Max
SBP	M	0.586	<0.001	7.13	7.09	1.410	4.694	0.18	31.09
	A	0.739	<0.001	3.16	2.66	1.267	3.956	0.08	11.16
	A+M	0.713	<0.001	7.37	7.67	1.391	4.237	0.15	31.13
DBP	M	0.652	<0.001	5.11	4.50	1.383	4.383	0.17	19.42
	A	0.742	<0.001	2.56	1.78	0.642	2.667	0.18	6.82
	A+M	0.644	<0.001	5.77	4.25	0.610	2.151	<0.01	15.15
HR	M	0.927	<0.001	3.16	2.54	0.815	2.817	<0.01	9.69
	A	0.768	<0.001	2.61	2.24	1.097	3.524	0.34	8.66
	A+M	0.897	<0.001	4.51	3.65	1.178	3.759	0.12	14.56
PP	M	0.482	0.002	8.74	6.02	0.546	2.570	0.06	23.22
	A	0.270	0.089	3.16	2.96	1.821	6.635	0.17	13.88
	A+M	0.544	<0.001	9.20	7.16	1.130	3.280	0.81	28.09
MAP	M	0.690	<0.001	4.63	4.22	1.367	4.771	0.22	19.40
	A	0.793	<0.001	2.36	1.57	0.246	2.069	0.01	5.83
	A+M	0.734	<0.001	5.03	4.05	0.726	2.628	0.03	15.98
SxHR	M	0.850	<0.001	7.38	6.56	1.892	7.116	0.37	32.00
	A	0.826	<0.001	4.00	3.39	1.181	3.786	0.36	13.76
	A+M	0.879	<0.001	9.09	7.89	1.752	6.712	0.01	39.38

SBP = Systolic Blood Pressure; DBP = Diastolic BP; HR = Heart Rate; PP = Pulse P; MAP = Mean Arterial P; SxHR = SBP x HR; SBP, DBP, PP, MAP expressed in mmHg, SxHR expressed in mmHgxbts/min($\times 10^{-2}$); M = MESOR; A = Amplitude of 24-h component; r = correlation coefficient; P= associated P-value; $\langle\Delta\rangle$ = average absolute difference between the 2 profiles; SD = standard deviation of $\langle\Delta\rangle$; g_1=coefficient of skewness; g_2=coefficient of kurtosis.

Against this background, considerations for intervention studies regarding a change in BP should include:
1. The use of a randomized experimental design wherein subjects receive all planned treatments in a random sequence, so as to assess the effect of treatment individually;

2. The use of capsules for dietary or drug intervention so as to be able to compare the agent under study with a placebo in a double-blind approach, for both individual and group comparisons;
3. The inclusion of untreated controls in the study design;
4. Reliance on several clinical endpoints and on several statistical approaches to interpret results preferably for the individual.

CONCLUSIONS

Current instrumentation for automatic indirect BP measurement has its unquestionable merits and has served as a basis for the specification herein of sampling requirements (sampling rate and length of observation span). The pioneering investment of industry has already yielded invaluable results that allow today the accumulation of data bases from which more realistic reference standards can be derived. Software development for the assessment of rhythm characteristics and of indices of pressure excess should gauge the need for and the effects of therapy. The short-comings of currently available automatic monitors, also discussed herein, should prompt further developments of instruments that are lighter and cheaper, so as to allow their more widespread use, and to make feasible the long-term assessment of BP for the determination of a given individual's personalized BP characteristics.

ACKNOWLEDGMENTS

The advice and support of Franz Halberg are gratefully acknowledged, as is the cooperation of Erna Halberg. Mr Masayuki Shinoda (President, Nippon Colin Ltd., Komaki, Japan) provided invaluable automatic instrumentation for this research and for the acquisition of reference data bases.

REFERENCES

1. Australian National Blood Pressure Study. Lancet i, 1261, 1980.
2. Bartter FC: Periodicity and medicine. In: Chronobiology. LE Scheving, F Halberg, JE Pauly (eds). Igaku Shoin Ltd, Tokyo, 6-13, 1974.
3. Berry DA, ML Eaton, BP Ekholm, TL Fox: Assessing differential drug effect. Biometrics 40: 1109-1115, 1984.
4. Bingham C, B Arbogast, G Cornelissen, JK Lee, F Halberg: Inferential statistical methods for estimating and comparing cosinor parameters. Chronobiologia 9: 397-439, 1982.
5. Bingham C, G Cornelissen, E Halberg, F Halberg: Testing period for single cosinor: extent of human 24-h cardiovascular "synchronization" on ordinary routine. Chronobiologia 11: 263-274, 1984.
6. Carandente F, G Ferrario, VF Ferrario, P Giani, L Vizzotto, F Halberg, W März, G Cornelissen, EM Schaffer: Infradian, mostly circaseptan profiles for the diagnosis and treatment of blood pressure elevation. Abstract, 2nd Eur. Mtg. on Hyperten-

sion, Milan, Italy, June 9-12, 1985.
7. Carandente F, F Halberg (eds): Chronobiology of blood pressure in 1985. Chronobiologia 11 (3), 1984, 152pp.
8. Clark LA, L Denby, D Pregibon, GA Harshfield, TG Pickering, S Blank, JH Laragh: A data based method for bivariate outlier detection: application to automatic blood pressure recording devices. Presentation at the NIH Workshop on 24-hour monitoring of blood pressure, Bethesda, Maryland, June 20-21, 1985.
9. Cornelissen G: Automatic detection of multiple outliers in physiologic time series, notably temperature. In: Annual review of chronopharmacology. Proc. 1st Montreux Conf. on biological rhythms and medications, A Reinberg, M Smolensky, G Labrecque (eds). Pergamon Press, Oxford, 157-160, 1984.
10. Cornelissen G, E Halberg, F Halberg: Circadian cardiovascular rhythms in ordinary life. Minn. Acad. Sci. 49: 18, 1984.
11. Cornelissen G, F Halberg, R Fanning, EL Kanabrocki, LE Scheving, DP Redmond, F Carandente: Differences in internal and external timing of circadian rhythms in human rectal temperature and motor activity. In: Biomedical Thermology, M Gautherie, E Albert (eds). Alan R Liss Inc., 167-184, 1982.
12. Cornelissen G, W Nelson, E Halberg, F Halberg: Individualized reference region for circadian rhythm parameters of systolic and diastolic blood pressure and heart rate. Minn. Acad. Sci. 51: 9-10, 1983.
13. de Boer RW, JM Karemaker, J Strackee: Beat-to-beat variability of heart interval and blood pressure. Automedica 4: 217-222, 1983.
14. di Rienzo M, G Grassi, A Pedotti, G Mancia: Continuous vs intermittent blood pressure measurements in estimating 24-hour average blood pressure. Hypertension 5: 264-269, 1983.
15. Enselberg CD: Measurement of distolic pressure by palpation. New England J Med. 265: 272-274, 1961.
16. Geddes LA: The direct and indirect measurement of blood pressure. Year Book Medical Publ. Inc., Chicago, 1970, 196pp.
17. Goldring D, H Wohltmann: Flush method for blood pressure determinations in newborn infants. J. Pediat. 40: 285-289, 1952.
18. Halberg E, F Halberg, K Shankaraiah: Plexo-serial linear nonlinear rhythmometry of blood pressure, pulse and motor activity by a couple in their sixties. Chronobiologia 8: 351-366, 1981.
19. Halberg F: Some physiological and clinical aspects of 24-hour periodicity. J Lancet 73: 20-32, 1953.
20. Halberg F, A Ahlgren, E Haus: Circadian systolic and diastolic hyperbaric indices of high school and college students. Chronobiologia 11: 299-309, 1984c.
21. Halberg F, G Cornelissen: "Personalized" blood pressure, salt and rhythms. Submitted for publication.
22. Halberg F, JIM Drayer, G Cornelissen, MA Weber: Cardiovascular reference data base for recognizing circadian mesor- and amplitude-hypertension in apparently healthy men. Chronobiologia 11: 275-298, 1984a.
23. Halberg F, H Fink: Juvenile human blood pressure: need for a chronobiologic approach. In: Hypertension in children and adolescents. G Giovannelli, M New, S Gorini (eds). Raven Press, New York, 45-73, 1981.

24. Halberg F, E Halberg, F Carandente, G Cornelissen, W März, J Halberg, JIM Drayer, MA Weber, E Schaffer, P Scarpelli, B Tarquini, M Cagnoni, N Tuna: Dynamic indices from blood pressure monitoring for prevention, diagnosis and therapy. In: Proc. Int. Symp. Ambulatory Monitoring, Padua, March 29-30, 1985, in press b.

25. Halberg F, E Haus, E Halberg, G Cornelissen, P Scarpelli, B Tarquini, M Cagnoni, D Wilson, K Griffiths, H Simpson, L Reale: Chronobiologic challenges in social medicine: illustrative tasks in cardiology and oncology. Proc. 2nd Int. Conf. Medico-social aspects of chronobiology, Florence, Oct. 2, 1984, in press a.

26. Halberg F, EA Johnson, W Nelson, W Runge, RB Sothern: Autorhythmometry -- procedures for physiologic self-measurements and their analysis. Phys. Teacher 1: 1-11, 1972.

27. Halberg F, JK Lee, W Nelson: Time-qualified reference intervals -- chronodesms. Experientia (Basel) 34: 713-716, 1978.

28. Halberg F, LE Scheving, E Lucas, G Cornelissen, RB Sothern, E Halberg, J Halberg, F Halberg, J Carter, KD Straub, DP Redmond: Chronobiology of human blood pressure in the light of static (room-restricted) automatic monitoring. Chronobiologia 11: 217-247, 1984b.

29. Halberg F, YL Tong, EA Johnson: Circadian system phase: an aspect of temporal morphology; procedures and illustrative examples. Proc. Int. Congress of Anatomists. In: The cellular aspects of biorhythms, Symp. on biorhythms, Springer-Verlag, 20-48, 1967.

30. Halberg J, E Halberg, DK Hayes, RD Smith, F Halberg, CS Delea, RS Danielson, FC Bartter, E Haus: Schedule shifts, life quality and quantity -- modeled by murine blood pressure elevation and arthropod life-span. Int. J. Chronobiology 7: 17-64, 1980.

31. Hales S: Statical Essays, vol. 2: Haemostaticks. London, W Innys and R Manby, 1733.

32. Kobrin I, W Oigman, A Kumar, HO Ventura, FH Messerli, ED Frohlich, FG Dunn: Diurnal variation of blood pressure in elderly patients with essential hypertension. J. Am. Geriatr. Soc. 32: 896-899, 1984.

33. Kolata G: Incidence of strokes declines. Science 220: 591, 1983a.

34. Kolata G: Heart research briefing: what is the meaning of childhood hypertension? Science 220: 833, 1983b.

35. Korotkoff NS: On the subject of methods of measuring blood pressure. Bull. Imp. Military Med. Acad. St Petersburg 11: 365-367, 1905.

36. Ludwig C: Beiträge zur Kenntnis des Einflusses der Respirations bewegungen auf den Blutlauf im Aortensysteme, Müller's Arch. Anat.: 240-302, 1847.

37. Nelson W, G Cornelissen, D Hinkley, C Bingham, F Halberg: Construction of rhythm-specified reference intervals and regions, with emphasis on "hybrid" data, illustrated for plasma cortisol. Chronobiologia 10: 179-193, 1983.

38. Nelson WP, AM Egbert: How to measure blood pressure accurately. Primary Cardiology: 14-26, Sept. 1984.

39. Pickering TG, GA Harshfield, RB Devereux: Ambulatory moni-

toring of blood pressure: the importance of blood pressure during work. In: Ambulatory blood pressure monitoring. MA Weber, JIM Drayer (eds). Springer-Verlag, New York, 193-197, 1984.

40. Pickering TG, GA Harshfield, RB Devereux, JH Laragh: What is the role of ambulatory blood pressure monitoring in the management of hypertensive patients? Hypertension 7 (2): 171-177, 1985.

41. Raftery EB: Understanding hypertension. The contribution of direct ambulatory blood pressure monitoring. ·In: Ambulatory blood pressure monitoring. MA Weber, JIM Drayer (eds). Springer-Verlag, New York, 105-116, 1984.

42. Reeves RA, AM Johnson, AP Shapiro, YM Traub, R Jacob: Ambulatory blood pressure monitoring: methods to assess severity of hypertension, variability and sleep changes. In: Ambulatory blood pressure monitoring, MA Weber, JIM Drayer (eds). Springer-Verlag, New York, 27-34, 1984.

43. Rey WJJ: Introduction to robust and quasi-robust statistical methods. Springer-Verlag, 1983.

44. Sokal RR, FJ Rohlf: Biometry, Freeman and Co, 2nd ed., 1981.

45. Weber MA, JIM Drayer (eds): Ambulatory blood pressure monitoring, Springer-Verlag, New York, 1984, 249pp.

46. Weiss SM, KA Matthews, T Detre, JA Graeff (eds): Stress, reactivity, and cardiovascular disease. Proc. of the Working Conference, NIH Publ. No 84-2698, 1984, 253pp.

NONINVASIVE CHRONOBIOLOGICAL BLOOD PRESSURE MEASUREMENTS' CLINICAL VALUE
AND PERSPECTIVE

V. R. McCALL[*] AND W.C. McCALL[**] Product Applications Research, Del Mar
Avionics, Irvine, CA[*] and Anaheim Memorial Hospital, Anaheim, CA [**]

INTRODUCTION

Hypertensive cardiovascular disease is the most common illness treated
by primary care physicians. It is an insidious process with well-
recognized morbidity and mortality. The sequelae of hypertension can be
reduced by drug therapy, but antihypertensive medications are costly and
have adverse side effects. The safe and cost-effective use of these
medications requires the accurate assessment of each patient's individual
need for therapeutic intervention.

The World Health Organization recommends that the patient's blood
pressure (BP) must be measured on at least two occasions over a four-week
period prior to establishing the existence of mild hypertension[1] (defined
as a diastolic BP between 90 and 104 mmHg). Traditionally, patients have
been evaluated using the average of three separate readings taken at
three different times. Using these criteria, patients studied with
uncomplicated diastolic hypertension of 100 mmHg or less have not
revealed support for the premise that therapeutic intervention is
routinely necessary.[2-6]

Previously, it has been felt that the BP measured in an office
represented the mean pressure over each 24-h span. Therapeutic
intervention was predicated on this assumption. Several years ago,
patients were encouraged to take their own BP at home. Confusion and
doubts arose when the reported home measurements varied widely from those
measured by the physician. Such recordings demonstrated that large
variations are quite common and that BP recorded in the medical
environment may not represent that in the patient's milieu. The
discrepancies in measurements, coupled with epidemiological observations
that many patients with office elevations did not develop target organ
damage over prolonged time spans, resulted in a reluctance on the part of
many in the medical community to label and actively stimulate patient
compliance in a lifelong therapeutic regimen.

Thus, high BP assessment has been limited primarily to random
measurements of BP in the physician's office. The inadequacy of these
measurements is self-apparent since only a minimal sampling of
measurements can be obtained in an environment which is not consistent
with the patient's usual daily loads and activities.

To address the problem of borderline hypertension, a number of
intervention approaches have been recommended and debated, ranging from
"do nothing--wait and observe"[7] to treating patients aggressively with
sustained diastolic BP of more than 90 mmHg.[8] The term "sustained" has

also been thrown open to debate when considering either a 24-h monitoring span or intermittent random (or average) measurements.[9]

We believe now that casual BP readings are unreliable when determining the magnitude or severity of hypertensive disease. If the objective of therapeutic intervention is to lower or control the patient's BP (throughout his usual 24-h day), then a new measurement method that can assess the cardiovascular strain (load) over time (24 h) should be able to distinguish those patients who will benefit the most from drug treatment. Thus, to evaluate the elevated BP of patients suspected of having sustained hypertension, we used a fully automated device for one circadian period in an attempt to establish the patient's designation as hypertensive and his need for therapeutic intervention.

The use of fully automated devices has bridged the gap between casual and home BP measurements, demonstrating the variability of blood pressure and revealing the existence of identifiable pattern subgroups.[10,11] These patterns in both normotensive and untreated hypertensive subjects appear to establish the daily duration of cardiovascular load,[12] thus leading directly to identifying those patients who will or will not develop cardiovascular complications. Although this premise has not as yet been widely validated, this prognostic correlation has recently been observed and reported by Perloff,[13] Carrageta,[14] Garrett,[11] Devereux,[15] and others.

Previous findings have demonstrated circadian variation in both normal and hypertensive populations utilizing both direct and indirect measurements. Recent publications have attested to the (a) reliability,[16] (b) accuracy,[17,18] (c) reproducibility,[19] (d) long-term validity,[20] and (e) potential usefulness of fully automated, environmental, indirect BP measurements.[18,21]

The clinical usefulness of the indirect method has been mentioned by other authors but only two previous papers have been published covering the diagnostic use in medical practice of the 24-h pattern.[10,11] Equally, there is the widely held belief that hypertensive disease is a routinely progressive disease, implying that progressive severity should be both time-and age-related.

To investigate this premise, along with our efforts to evaluate patients suspected of having sustained hypertension, we used a fully automated BP measuring device for one circadian period. We also attempted to establish the patient's need for the diagnosis of hypertension and his need for therapeutic intervention.

PATIENTS AND METHODS

One hundred fifty-two sequential office patients who revealed mean elevations greater than or equal to 140 systolic or 90 diastolic BP on three successive office visits were then tested with a battery-operated, fully automated, ambulatory indirect BP monitoring and memory storage device (Del Mar Avionics Model 1978 Pressurometer) over one complete 24-h span. Blood pressure and heart rate samples were automatically taken at 7.5-min intervals[20] with the patient awake or asleep. Additional samples, documented by diary entry, were initiated by the patient whenever specific tasks were undertaken. Each sample time, ECG-heart rate, systolic and diastolic BP were instantaneously stored in an incorporated battery-operated, solid-state memory.

Following both initial applications and return of the patient to the office, the device was simultaneously compared to the auscultatory technique. Measurements with an error difference of less than 5 mmHg were encountered routinely. These findings correspond to those previously reported.[16,17,19]

Following return of the patient, the application of the system was inspected to assure that it had not been dislodged during use. The BP monitoring device (Model 1978) was then connected to an electrostatic printing system (Del Mar Avionics 1979 Pressurometer Charter) containing interface electronics and solid-state memory circuits designed to transfer, store and process the environmentally recorded data. The charter system automatically edited obvious artifactual data and although manual line editing was available, this added feature was rarely required. Our results have been similar to others,[16] demonstrating greater than 95% valid readings throughout the recording span.

RESULTS

The 152 patients in this study ranged in age from 20 to 82. No attempt has been made to divide the patients by ethnicity or sex. All patients were classified into groups by 24-h pattern utilizing the following classification table (Table 1).

Following classification into groups by 24-h pattern, the study population was divided into 10-year age groups (Table 2).

TABLE 1. Definition of Patient Groups

Measurements Group Type	Definition	% of 24-Hour Greater Than 140/90*
I	Elevated only in the medical environment (pseudohypertensive)	Less than 10%
II	Labile or ultradian variability	10-30%
III	Blood pressure elevated during day: normotensive at night	30-75%
IV	Sustained blood pressure (elevations awake and asleep) (infradian)	75-100%

*Estimated percent of elevated BP readings that are above 140 systolic or 90 diastolic during the 24-h recording span.

TABLE 2. Study Population by 10-Year Age Groups

GROUP	AGE GROUPS 20-30	31-40	41-50	51-60	61-70	71-80	81-90	TOTAL
I	6	8	7	23	11	4	0	59
II	1	4	8	11	8	0	0	32
III	3	5	12	18	5	1	0	44
IV	2	1	1	5	3	4	1	17
TOTAL	12	18	28	57	27	9	1	152

The total number of patients with elevated BP increases with age; the percentages in the population of the groups I, II, and III hypertensives do not appear to change much with age. Group IV (sustained) hypertensives (small in number in this study population) appear to be much less prevalent than previously suspected.

Only 11.2% of all patients (regardless of age or sex) were shown to be sustained hypertensives.

Following classification into age groups by 24-h pattern, the data were divided into under 50-year (mean age 38) and over 50-year (mean age 61) age groups to determine whether the subgroup patterns change with age (Table 3).

TABLE 3. Classification by Age and Groups

	Total All Patients by Group Types				Percent
Total Patients	I	II	III	IV	of Total
Under 50 Years (55) Mean 38	21 (38.2%)	11 (20%)	19 (34.6%)	4 (7.2%)	36%
50 Years and Over (97) Mean 61	38 (39.2%)	21 (21.6%)	25 (25.8%)	13 (13.4%)	64%
Total (152)	59 (39%)	32 (21%)	44 (29%)	17 (11%)	100%

DISCUSSION

The findings in this series of patients substantiated the fact that randomly taken BP measurements in a primary care environment could not be relied upon when deciding whether all patients would truly benefit from antihypertensive therapy. Casual BP readings are unreliable for determining the magnitude or severity of hypertensive disease.

We do not know whether Groups I, II, and III are unique types of hypertension or are part of the natural progression of the disease process. Tables 2 and 3 show no obvious difference in the frequency distribution within the groups according to age. In many cases, the labile pattern variations shown in Groups I and II (along with simultaneous heart rate information) have been found to be due to physical activity, alcohol, pain, excitement, hyperkinesis, or emotional factors rather than systemic hypertension. This makes selected cases amenable to therapeutic modalities other than traditional hypotensive step-care agents.

Group III appears to be either unique or an extension of Groups I and II. Also, this group may fall into the category of circadian amplitude hypertension[9]. Our findings also revealed that it was impossible to differentiate between Groups III and IV solely utilizing daytime, random or office BP readings.

In our predominantly white, middle-class practice, we found that 38% of patients with presenting BP of 140/90 or above do not fall into the category of hypertension in need of treatment. These findings agree with those reported by Pickering[22] who found that one-third of those patients with diastolic BP between 90 and 104 did not need treatment, and Carrageta who reported 28% in 148 patients.[14] This conclusion is especially true if the objective of therapeutic intervention is to control the patients' BP during their average daily activities.

In patients assumed to have borderline hypertension, the percentage of readings found elevated during the recording period has been observed by Horan.[23] In his study, the borderline patient population was monitored over a 24-h span. Elevated readings ranged from a minimum of 7.9% to a maximum of 81%. We[10] reported a 17.7% incidence of patients who had no BP elevations during the test but did have random office elevations in a primary care setting, along with an additional 14.5% with typical Group I patterns.

In the 11% of the patient population classified in this study as Group IV, we found nearly 100% of their BP measurements to be elevated. In our opinion the sustained elevations found in Group IV hypertensives indicate a high risk and a need for a thorough systemic hypertensive workup followed by aggressive therapeutic intervention. This observation has recently been substantiated by Kobrin et al[24] who reported that patients with hypertension during sleep suffer more generally from cardiovascular complications.

INFERENCES
1. Four chronobiological patterns are empirically evident in the suspected hypertensive patient population.
2. Fully sustained hypertension appears to be less prevalent than previously suspected.

PERSPECTIVE
Both diagnosis and treatment of high BP require instrumental extension of the human senses for proper assessment of the patient. Peak spans of elevation or depression of systolic and diastolic BP associated with environmental situations or conditions (load effects on the cardiovascular system) are manifest. There are several clinical indications for fully automatic, indirect ambulatory BP monitoring, including: 1. Borderline hypertension; 2. Labile (essential) hypertension; 3. Malignant hypertension as caused by: pheochromocytoma; renal artery stenosis or aneurysm; adrenal hyperplasia or adenoma; or Cushing syndrome; 4. Cerebrovascular accident.

When a patient is found to be hypertensive in the office (usually identified by three consecutive elevated readings on three consecutive office visits) the physician is faced with a decision; should the patient be sent home with a sphygmomanometer and have someone take and record serial readings throughout the 24-h span or start him immediately on anti-hypertensive drug therapy. Up to now, the former decision was usually made, but home BP readings were generally reported to be significantly different than the office readings. The physician was again faced with a decision; were the lower home readings a result of untrained personnel taking the BP or was the patient truly normotensive at home and only hypertensive in the office? It is this type of decision which makes automatic, indirect ambulatory blood pressure monitoring such an advance for the medical profession. If the patient's test results reflect the need for medication to control the hypertension, pharmaceutical intervention is begun. During this therapeutic phase, the patient will undergo 24-h ambulatory BP tests to evaluate: 1. Regulation of drug dosage - establishing the optimal drug dosage time and span to insure control; 2. Effectiveness of medication - establishing the minimal drug dosage required for maintenance over an entire 24-h span and proving that the drug works; 3. Periodic evaluation of patient status - has the status of the patient's condition altered enough to warrant an alteration in the strength or frequency of the drug being taken?

Several physicians were recently polled as to why they made fully automated, indirect, ambulatory BP monitoring an integral part of their differential diagnosis of hypertensive patients. The reasons for utilizing ambulatory BP monitoring were generally stimulated by problem cases within the practice. They cited the following problems with present and traditional office diagnostic methods and findings. 1. Poor correlation with target organ involvement; 2. Degree of variability unrecognized (lability); 3. Circadian variations not assessed; 4. Nocturnal elevation not assessed; 5. Decisions based on random (few) measurements, yet: a. Patient committed to a lifetime of drug therapy; b. Social impacts of the label "hypertensive". Questions the physician may now explore for a given patient include:
1. What is the relationship of the patient's office readings, or home readings to an average BP taken over 24-hours?
2. Are readings more than 140/90 frequent or rare?
3. What percentage of BP in normal subjects exceed these limits?
4. Can hypertension itself and its risks to an individual be defined better by 24-h recordings as compared to casual measurements?
5. Will medication once or twice a day maintain goal pressures all day?
6. Will the high pressure and heart rate fall too low in the patient with coronary or cerebrovascular disease?
7. Are myocardial and cerebral infarctions precipitated by hypertension during the preceding minutes or hours?
8. Is there a basic circadian rhythm to BP irrespective of sleep, body position, activity or emotion? How does it vary in health and disease? These, and many other questions, can be answered with the results of a 24-h ambulatory BP. These answers can make any curious physician ready to cope more effectively with the hypertensive patient and the realities of BP variations.

Surveyed physicians include the following criteria for a totally automated ambulatory blood pressure monitoring device: 1. Noninvasive application; 2. Accuracy of systolic and diastolic BP measurement equal to the standard cuff method; 3. Simultaneous heart-rate monitoring capability; 4. Totally automatic time-documented cycling, awake and asleep, with demand cycling capability; 5. Portability approximately comparable to ambulatory ECG recorders; 6. Mechanical and electronic ruggedness and reliability. 7. Easy serviceability; 8. Easy method of cross-checking data with standard auscultatory techniques; 9. Compliance with national AAMI standards. 10. Patient acceptability with minimal time per sample and lowest squeezing pressure compatible with accuracy. The data reduction and report presentation requirements as stated by the physician are: 1. Simple numerical presentations of systolic, diastolic BP and mean pressures; 2. Simultaneous heart-rate data; 3. Simultaneous time-course documentation; 4. Simple graphic presentations for clinical assessment; 5. Automatic and manual editing of artifactual data; 6. Statistical analysis and percentage of hypertensive readings' capability; 7. One-page summary report generation; 8. Double-product presentation to assess cardiovascular load over time.

REFERENCES
1. Buhler, FR, AE Doyle, FH Epstein et al. Guidelines for the Treatment of Mild Hypertension: Memorandum from a WHO/ISH Meeting. Bull WHO 61:53-56, 1983.
2. Hypertension Detection and Follow-Up Program Cooperative Group: Five- Year Findings of the Hypertension Detection and Follow-Up Program: I. Reduction in Mortality of Persons with High Blood Pressure, Including Mild Hypertension. JAMA 242:2562-2571, 1979.
3. Management Committee of the American Therapeutic Trial in Mild Hypertension: Untreated Mild Hypertension. Lancet 1:185-191, 1982.
4. Management Committee: Initial Results of the Australian Therapeutic Trial in Mild Hypertension. Clin Sci 57 (Suppl 5):449S-452S, 1979.
5. Smith, WM. Treatment of Mild Hypertension: Results of a Ten-Year Intervention Trial. Circ Res 40 (Suppl 1):I-98--I-105, 1977.
6. Helgeland, A. Treatment of Mild Hypertension: A Five Year Controlled Drug Trial: The Oslo Study. Am J Med 69:725-732, 1980.
7. Kaplan, NM. Therapy for Mild Hypertension: Toward a More Balanced View. JAMA 249:365-367, 1983.
8. Moser, M. "Less Severe" Hypertension: Should It Be Treated? Am Heart J 101:465-472, 1982.
9. Halberg, F, E Halberg, J. Halberg, Francine Halberg. Chronobiologic Assessment of Human Blood Pressure Variations in Health and Disease. Ambulatory Blood Pressure Monitoring, 137-156, 1983.
10. McCall, WC, VR McCall. Diagnostic Use of Ambulatory Blood Pressure Monitoring in Medical Practice. J of Fam Prac 13:25-30, 1981.
11. Garrett, BN. The Role of Ambulatory Blood Pressure Monitoring in the Evaluation of Hypertension. Dateline Hypertension, Volume I, No. 5:1 & 7, Aug/Sept., 1983.
12. Mallion, JM, R DeGaudemaris, JL Debru et al. Mesure de la Pression Arterielle en Ambulatorire par Methode Automatique. Arch Mal Coeur 73:95-101, 1979.
13. Perloff, D, M Sokolow, R Cowan. The Prognostic Value of Ambulatory Blood Pressure. JAMA 249:2792-2798, 1983.
14. Carrageta, MO, R Soares, A Martins. Twenty-Four Hour Assessment of Once-Daily Beta-Blocker Antihypertensive Effects. Presented at the International Symposium on Blood Pressure-Variability, Vienna, Austria, January 28, 1983.
15. Devereux, RB, TG Pickering, GA Harshfield, HD Kleinert et al. Left Ventricular Hypertrophy in Patients with Hypertension: Importance of Blood Pressure Response to Regularly Recurring Stress. Circ 68:3, 470-476, 1983.
16. Kennedy, HL, NE Padgett, MJ Horan. Performance Reliability of the Del Mar Avionics Non-Invasive Ambulatory Blood Pressure System. Ambul Electrocardiol 4:13-17, 1979.
17. Harshfield, GA, TG Pickering, JH Laragh. A Validation Study of the Del Mar Avionics Ambulatory Blood Pressure System. Ambul Electroardiol 4:7-12, 1979.
18. Sheps, SG. Evaluation of Pendolol Dosage on Hypertension by Automatic Indirect Blood Pressure Monitoring. Archives of IM 145:54-57, January, 1985.

269

19. Weber, M, JIM Drayer, Nakamura, F Wyle. The Circadian Blood Pressure Pattern in Ambulatory Normal Subjects. Am J Cardiol 54:115-119, 1984.
20. DiRienzo, Grassi, Pedott, Mancia. Continuous Versus Intermittent Blood Pressure Measurements in Estimating 24-Hour Average Blood Pressure. Hypertension 5:264-269, 1983.
21. Prisant, LM, R Trincher, AA Carr. Ambulatory Blood Pressure Monitoring. J of Med Ass'n of GA 73:784-786, November, 1984.
22. Pickering, TG, GA Harshfield, HD Kleinert et al. Blood Pressure During Normal Daily Activities, Sleep, and Exercise. Comparison of Values in Normal and Hypertensive Subjects. JAMA 247:992-996, 1982.
23. Horan, MJ, HL Kennedy, NE Padgett. Do Borderline Hypertensive Patients Have Labile Blood Pressure? Ann of Intern Med 94:466-468, 1981.
24. Kobrin, I, W Oigman, A Kumar, HO Ventura, FH Messerli, FG Dunn. Diurnal Variation of Blood Pressure in Elderly Patients with Essential Hypertension. J Am Ger So 32(12):896-899, December, 1984.

REPETITIVE BLOOD PRESSURE MEASUREMENTS: CLINICAL ISSUES, TECHNIQUES, AND DATA ANALYSIS

M. A. WEBER, J. I. M. DRAYER, D. D. BREWER, Hypertension Center, Veteran Administration Medical Center, Long Beach, CA.

INTRODUCTION

The major impetus for an interest in blood pressure readings, obtained either conventionally or by automated equipment, has been a need to better understand and to more accurately diagnose clinical high blood pressure states. Hypertension is a common chronic condition that may affect up to 25% of the adult population. The major importance of this condition is that it is a risk factor for premature cardiovascular disease, especially strokes and heart attacks (1). It has been demonstrated that treatment of high blood pressure by pharmacologic methods decreases the incidence of these major complications and probably prolongs life (2). Thus, there has been a strong incentive to identify individuals with high blood pressure and to provide them with appropriate therapy.

Particular attention has focused on mild hypertension, which is clearly the most common form of hypertension. A group of experts, the Joint National Committee on Detection, Evaluation, and Treatment of High Blood Pressure (3), has recommended that diastolic hypertension be diagnosed at values of 90 mm Hg or above. Indeed, actuarial data suggests that diastolic blood pressures in excess of 83 mm Hg are associated with a greater than average risk of death, and the Committee has designated diastolic pressures in the range 85 to 89 mm Hg as high-normal. Individuals in this range should be followed fairly closely to determine any trends in their blood pressures. Obviously, when dealing with blood pressures in this range it can be difficult, and potentially fallacious, to discriminate between the relatively small differences that determine normalcy or hypertension. This problem is particularly important when therapeutic implications are involved.

This issue has been highlighted by some interesting studies. In the Australian Therapeutic Trial on Mild Hypertension (4) it was found that over a quarter of the patients with mild hypertension treated with a placebo for three years actually had normal blood pressure by the end of the study. It is noteworthy that the patients were admitted to that study after only two conventional measurements of their blood pressures had been in the hypertensive range. Moreover, most of these placebo responders became apparent within the first few weeks of the study. These findings imply that a large proportion of individuals exhibiting a normalization of blood pressure during placebo therapy were, in all likelihood, normotensive individuals in whom an erroneous diagnosis of hypertension had been made. Our own experience with therapeutic trials on a smaller scale has also tended to support this conclusion (5). In another study it was recently shown that blood pressure in patients whose antihypertensive therapy was discontinued often stayed low (6). In fact, it was found that over half the patients were still not in need of reinstitution of treatment during periods of up to four years following discontinuation of their original therapy, again raising the question as to whether these individuals were ever truly hypertensive.

It is evident that blood pressure can vary markedly from minute to minute, and it is thus not surprising that there is a potential for erroneous diagnoses to be made. There is a need for methods of assessment that can take into account the variations in blood pressure and thereby improve the accuracy of diagnosis and provide better information concerning hypertension. Unfortunately, there is as yet no clear agreement as to how best to evaluate blood pressure. Equipment and methods that can obtain multiple and long-term measurements of blood pressure have been available for only the past few years, and there are still some technical problems to be solved. Additionally, methods for treating and analyzing the data produced by these techniques have not yet been standardized. A major problem will be to link data obtained by these methods to long-term clinical prognosis.

AVAILABLE EQUIPMENT

Techniques for automated monitoring of blood pressure have been available for several years, especially in intensive care units or in cardiac catheterization laboratories. However, most recent attention has focused on devices that are portable, less invasive, and less expensive. Some of the currently used techniques are summarized in Table 1. We have focused on three major characteristics of these methods: whether they are automated, have the capacity to measure ambulatory blood pressure, and can provide data for full 24-hour periods.

TABLE 1. Types of equipment used for obtaining blood pressure data. Further descriptions are given in the text.

	Automatic	Ambulatory	Full 24-Hour Duration
Multiple conventional manual readings (self or observer)	No	Partly	No
Remler equipment[a]	Semi	Yes	No
Dinamap[b]/Arteriosonde[c]	Yes	No	Yes
Pressurometer III[d]/ICR[e]	Yes	Yes	Yes
"Oxford System" intra-arterial[f]	Yes	Yes	Yes

(a)Remler Co., Brisbane CA; (b) Applied Medical Research, FL; (c) Roche Medical Electronics, Cranbury, NJ; (d) Del Mar Avionics, Irvine, CA; (e) Spacelabs, Bellevue, WA; (f) not commercially available.

Before considering advanced equipment, it is appropriate to evaluate methods based on the conventional approach for measuring blood pressure. Many individuals have acquired conventional mercury or aneroid sphygmomanometers, and measure their own blood pressures at home or at other sites. Industrial nurses or other health personnel routinely measure blood pressure and can provide multiple readings at different times of the day or over periods of weeks or months. A lack of standardization for these types of measurements can make interpretation difficult, although the recent availability of small and inexpensive electronic devices for home blood pressure measurements may add some consistency to the results obtained. Unfortunately, the quality of these newer devices is unpredictable, and pressures measured by them are often different from those obtained concurrently with conventional sphygmomanometers. Difficulties of interpretation, especially in reconciling blood pressures at the work site with those obtained either in the physician's office or at home also make it difficult to reach clinically helpful conclusions. At present, therefore, self-measured blood pressures cannot be used with confidence as an aid to diagnosis.

Data obtained from studies with the Remler equipment (7) has been used in a number of hypertension studies. This semiautomatic device requires the patient to manually inflate the conventional blood pressure cuff used in this system, but the rest of the measurement, specifically the perception of the Korotkoff sounds, is performed by the device. Moreover, this equipment is able to store all measurements taken during a period of several hours. It is small and light enough to allow the patient to be ambulatory, and it has the additional virtue of reliability and accuracy. Its principal drawback is that it requires the physical participation of the patient in obtaining the blood pressure measurement, and thus cannot provide readings during sleep.

An alternative approach is to use completely automatic but non-portable devices such as Dinamap or Arteriosonde (8). As with the Remler equipment, the Dinamap uses a conventional blood pressure cuff which it automatically inflates at selected intervals of from 1 to 15 minutes. It uses oscillometric perception rather than the Korotkoff sounds, a method which appears to be satisfactory. Because of its large size this equipment is not portable but is useful for measuring blood pressure in patients who can spend extended periods of time in one area. It has been possible to get good 24-hour data in hospitalized patients using this device, and it has a good record of reliability (8,9). It is reasonably inexpensive and provides a continually updated hard copy printout of all blood pressures achieved during the monitoring period.

Devices such as the Pressurometer III (Del Mar Avionics) or the Instruments for Cardiac Research model (Spacelabs) have similar attributes to the Dinamap, but additionally are portable. Thus, they are able to provide full 24-hour data in ambulatory subjects. At the conclusion of the monitoring period, these devices are linked to microcomputers that then give full printouts of all data obtained. They are able to measure blood pressure, again using the conventional arm cuff, at intervals varying from 1 minute to 1 hour during the full day. Because of the high developmental costs in producing devices of this compactness, they are still relatively expensive and perhaps beyond the means of many practicing clinicians. There have also been some questions of reliability and accuracy during the early developmental phases of this equipment, but these problems are fast being solved. Although used far more in Europe than in the United States, continuous blood pressure monitoring through an intra-arterial catheter, usually placed in the brachial artery, probably provides the greatest quantity and detail of data. In fact, because of its truly continuous nature, this form of monitoring provides a blood pressure measurement with every heart beat. This approach has been regarded as the standard against which other methods should be judged. The negative aspects of intra-arterial monitoring obviously are related to the discomfort of having an intra-arterial device inserted and safety concerns such as bleeding or the loss of blood supply to the distal arm and hand. Although misadventures with this equipment have been few, apprehension about its use in the fully ambulatory patient, especially outside the hospital, has limited its use in the United States.

USING THE TECHNOLOGY

Perhaps the biggest problem with blood pressure monitoring has been the premature use of automated or semiautomated equipment without first establishing standardized protocols for its use. Presumably there are two influences on blood pressure in any individual subject: the intrinsic and circadian characteristics of the blood pressure itself, and the added impact of environmental and other external factors on that blood pressure pattern. Most monitoring studies have attempted to evaluate the intrinsic and extrinsic characteristics of the blood pressure at the same time, thereby making interpretation of the data excessively complex. Because of this concern, some of our early studies were performed (using the Dinamap equipment) in patients maintained in a comparatively restful and standardized setting within a comfortable hospital room (8,9).

Recently, however, we have more frequently used ambulatory monitoirng equipment (either the Pressurometer III or the ICR) in subjects going about their usual daily routines at work and at home (10,11). Although the data achieved by this method has been useful and interesting, it has not really allowed us to make qualitative assessments as to the impact of varying stimuli and circumstances on blood pressure. It is also necessary to question whether subjects undergoing monitoring, even when they appear to follow a standard pattern, are truly having a typical day. They are conscious of wearing the equipment and naturally tend to alter their activities to facilitate the frequent measurements of blood pressure. For example, it is known that measurements obtained while driving a car tend to be inaccurate, and patients may alter this aspect of their activity accordingly. Similarly, certain types of manual work cannot be readily carried out while wearing this equipment. Patients become very much aware of every minor incident throughout the day that might have an impact on blood pressure, and perhaps focus excessively and with too much subjectivity on each event. There has also been some concern as to whether patients can sleep as well as usual while wearing a monitor, although interestingly most subjects undergoing the procedure appear to rest reasonably well and to exhibit the typical circadian decreases in blood pressure that occur during the nighttime hours.

VALIDATING THE METHODS
One of the first tasks to be undertaken with the whole-day blood pressure monitoring technique was to show that it is reproducible from day to day. This evaluation was carried out in 56 normal volunteers who each underwent the entire procedure on two separate occasions approximately six weeks apart (10). The values for their blood pressures are shown in Figure 1. For simplicity, the 24-hour day was divided into 12 consecutive 2-hour segments, and the data in the figure show for all patients together the averages of the blood pressure values during each of the 2-hour periods throughout the whole day. For the patients as a whole, the blood pressure measurements on the two monitoring days correspond closely. To test the reproducibility of the circadian pattern of the blood pressure, we also analyzed data in which the two hour periods throughout the day within each patient were ranked in increasing order of blood pressure values. Again, there was close correspondence between the two days, suggesting that the pattern of the blood pressure as well as its actual values is reproducible (10).

Despite these encouraging results for the group as a whole, comparison within individual subjects showed that for at least one-third of them there were some clear differences between the two days of monitoring (10). Of course, we could not determine whether these differences, when they did occur, reflected true variations in the basic circadian pattern of blood pressure, or whether the discrepancies simply reflected differences in work routine or in other events on one day as compared with the other. Importantly, since the averages for the subjects as a whole were so reproducible, this technique can be used to assess antihypertensive therapy (as discussed below), for differences between data obtained on two separate days can be attributed to treatment effects rather than to chance variations in the blood pressure.

The usefulness of whole-day blood pressure monitoring has also been established in studying characteristics of various types of patients. For example, a comparison of younger and older hypertensive patients was able to document that older patients, as might be expected from other physiologic considerations, have a clearly greater

274

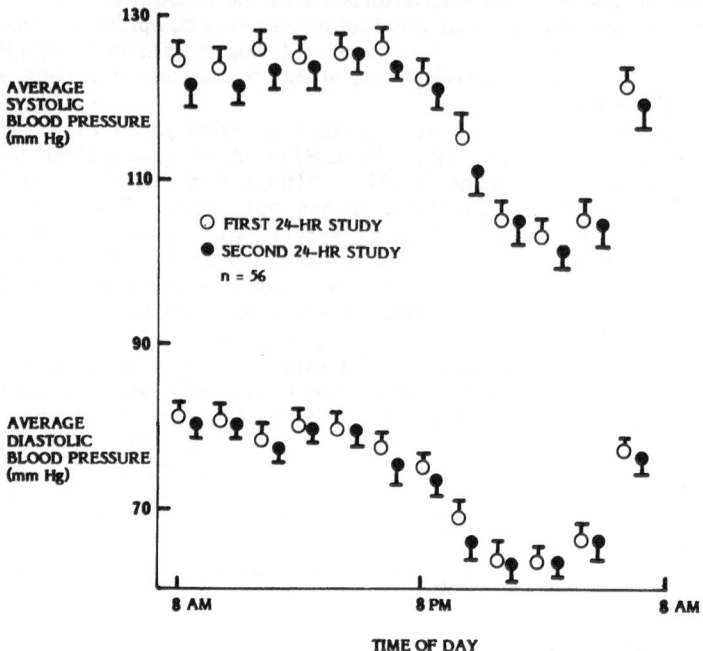

Figure 1: Systolic and diastolic blood pressure values during two separate 24-hour ambulatory monitoring periods in each of 56 normal volunteers. Values shown are the averages for 12 two-hour periods during the day.

variability in their blood pressure throughout the day (12). The whole-day monitoring technique was also found to be of particular value in studies of cardiac left ventricular hypertrophy in hypertensive patients. Although it had been predicted that blood pressure should be related to the thickness of the left ventricle, conventional casual readings of blood pressure correlated only poorly (13). However, if longer term blood pressure monitoring averages were used rather than the conventional readings we were able to document a close correlation, indicating the superiority of long-term values in explaining physiologic phenomena. Thus, despite some of the early concerns with this new technique, these findings support the idea that long-term blood pressure monitoring is the most appropriate and relevant method for evaluating blood pressure and its relationships.

DIAGNOSTIC IMPLICATIONS

Actuarial and epidemiological blood pressure data used to establish the likelihood of cardiovascular complications have been based on casual (conventional) clinical measurements. Accordingly, this type of data has been the basis for recommendations such as those given by the Joint National Committee on Detection, Evaluation, and Treatment of High Blood Pressure (3) concerning the diagnosis and management of hypertension. The prognostic value of casual blood pressure readings has been clearly defined in large-scale studies due to the high number of subjects evaluated, but the variability of casual values within individuals makes this type of measurement less valuable when making a clinical decision in a single patient.

Unfortunately, there are no data linking cardiovascular prognosis and blood pressure values obtained from long-term monitoring techniques. Thus, despite the reliability and reproducibility of the long-term methods, considerable care and judgment will be required if they are to be used as the basis of diagnostic and therapeutic assessments.

At this early stage of experience with blood pressure monitoring the methodologies for analyzing data are still preliminary. Indeed, no standard methods have been established for presenting and evaluating data and for determining prognosis. The most simple approach is to use the average of all blood pressures measured throughout the 24-hour period as being the representative value for the day. This approach is simple and reproducible (10). In a preliminary evaluation of this method, we have found that when patients previously diagnosed as being hypertensive (by conventional means) are compared with normal controls there is a great deal of overlap (11). Indeed, approximately 25% of hypertensive patients when assessed in this fashion actually fell within the range defined by the normal volunteers. Because it is sometimes inconvenient to perform whole-day monitoring, we have assessed the usefulness of a shorter two-hour monitoring period and have shown that it will, in fact, serve a similar purpose to the whole-day average in helping to discriminate hypertensive individuals (unpublished data).

A drawback to these approaches of using blood pressure averages obtained during differing periods of time, is that the variability of blood pressure is not taken into account. Is it possible that qualitative differences between patients, even when their averages are similar, might indicate differing prognosis. Unfortunately, as discussed earlier, prognostic data linked to these techniques is not available. Another approach, however, is to study the incidence of abnormal readings (arbitrarily greater than 90 mm Hg diastolic blood pressure or greater than 140 mm Hg systolic blood pressure) during the day (14). As with the average blood pressure method, however, this method also indicates that approximately a quarter of hypertensive patients may actually be in the normal range. Interestingly, even normal individuals have a proportion of readings within the elevated range, and again it will be necessary to study prognosis so as to determine what frequency of abnormal readings is acceptable and part of a normal pattern.

A possible solution to the problem of analyzing long-term monitoring data is to use classical chronobiologic methods. We have shown previously that blood pressure data is highly susceptible to this type of treatment (15). Although there are various approaches that could be used, Figure 2 indicates two comparatively simple concepts that might be of diagnostic value. The PTE shown in this figure represents the percentage of time that blood pressure is elevated, whereas HBI denotes the hyperbaric impact. In essence, this computed parameter totals the "areas" above the curve of blood pressures felt to be higher than an arbitrarily determined critical value. An attraction of these approaches is that they are able to reduce the multiple values obtained during the whole-day of monitoring activity into simple values. Potentially, as our research progresses, we might be able to make a straightforward determination of whether a patient is hypertensive or within a normal range.

BLOOD PRESSURE MONITORING IN THERAPY

An important consideration in the treatment of hypertension is not only the decrease in blood pressure but also the duration of this antihypertensive effect. From a practical standpoint, it is sometimes helpful to be able to use pharmacologic anti-hypertensive therapy on a once-daily basis. Ambulatory whole-day blood pressure monitoring reliably provides a means for determining whether this goal is being achieved. Results obtained with this method have already been published (16), and represent at the present time the most practical and frequent use of this new technology. Many newer antihypertensive agents are now undergoing clinical trials using whole-day blood pressure monitoring methods for evaluation. One potential benefit of this method is that it might eliminate the so-called placebo responder from

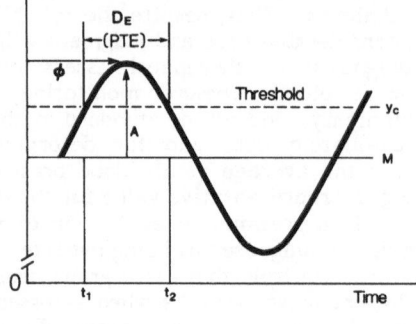

Duration of Elevation, D_E
Percent Time Elevation, PTE
timespan (D_E) during which variable is elevated above given threshold, expressed as a percentage of 24 h, unless otherwise specified.

$$D_E = (t_2 - t_1)$$

$$PTE = \frac{D_E}{24} \times 100$$

$$\left.\begin{matrix} t_1 \\ t_2 \end{matrix}\right\} = \frac{24}{2\pi}\left[\arccos\left(\frac{y_c - M}{A}\right) - \phi\right]$$

Hyperbaric Impact, HBI
measure of excess load exerted upon the arterial walls, i.e., the area of blood pressures above a given threshold.

$$HBI = \int_{t_1}^{t_2}\left[M + A\cos\left(\frac{2\pi}{24}t + \phi\right) - y_c\right]dt$$

Figure 2: A fitted cosine curve derived from a 24-hour blood pressure monitoring period. PTE=precent time elevation; HBI=hyperbaric index. Fuller descriptions are given in the text.

drug studies. Obviously this would provide far greater sensitivity in clinical trials, but again this claim has yet to be fully tested.

PRESENT DEVELOPMENTS
    The main problem being experienced at present is in linking data obtained during long-term blood pressure monitoring to physiological and pathophysiological mechanisms and events. Because the onset of hypertensive cardiovascular complications may sometimes take years to unfold, it seems likely that many of these answers will not be immediately forthcoming. This critical information will become available only as a result of large-scale multicenter efforts to accumulate the large data base necessary to study the relationships between blood pressure monitoring data and cardiovascular prognosis. Technical problems with the blood pressure monitoring equipment have now, to a large extent, been solved. Although unsuccessful monitoring procedures still can occur, investigators and clinicians can now use this technique with a high level of confidence that they will generate usable data.

REFERENCES

1. Kannel WB, Castelli WP, McNamara PM, Sorlie P: Some factors affecting morbidity and mortality in hypertension. The Framingham Study. Milbank Mem Fund Q, 47:116-142, 1969.

2. Hypertension Detection and Follow-Up Program Cooperative Group. Five-year findings of the hypertension detection and follow-up program. I. Reduction of mortality in persons with high blood pressure, including mild hypertension. JAMA 242:2562-2571, 1979.

3. Joint National Committee on Detection, Evaluation, and Treatment of High Blood Pressure. Arch Intern Med 144:1045-1057, 1984.

4. Report by the Management Committee. The Australian therapeutic trial in mild hypertension. Lancet 1:1261-1267, 1980.

5. Drayer JIM, Weber MA: Monotherapy of essential hypertension with a converting enzyme inhibitor. Hypertension 5:108-113, 1983.

6. Finnerty FA, Jr.: Step-down treatment of mild systemic hypertension. Am J Cardiol 53:1304-1307, 1984.

7. Gould BA, Hornung RS, Kieso HA, Altman DG, Cashman PMM, Raftery EB: Evaluation of the Remler M2000 blood pressure recorder. Comparison with intra-arterial blood pressure recordings both at hospital and at home. Hypertension 6:209, 1984.

8. Weber MA, Drayer JIM, Wyle FA, DeYoung JL: Reproducibility of the whole-day blood pressure pattern in essential hypertension. Clin Exp Hypertension A4:1377-1390, 1982.

9. Weber MA, Drayer JIM, Wyle FA, Brewer DD: A representative value for the whole-day blood pressure. JAMA 248:1626-1628, 1982.

10. Weber MA, Drayer JIM, Nakamure DK, Wyle FA: The circadian blood pressure pattern in ambulatory normal subjects. Am J Cardiol 54:115-119, 1984.

11. Drayer JIM, Weber MA, Nakamura DK: Automated ambulatory blood pressure monitoring: a study in age-matched normotensive and hypertensive men. Am Heart J 109:1334-1338, 1985.

12. Drayer JIM, Weber MA, DeYoung JL, Wyle FA: Circadian blood pressure patterns in ambulatory hypertensive patients. Am J Med 73:493-499, 1982.

13. Drayer JIM, Weber MA, DeYoung JL: Blood pressure as a determinant of cardiac left ventricular muscle mass. Archives Int Med 143:90-92, 1982.

14. Drayer JIM, Weber MA: Definition of normalcy in whole-day ambulatory blood pressure monitoring. A7:195-204, 1985.

15. Halberg F, Drayer JIM, Cornelissen G, Weber MA: Cardiovascular reference data base for recognizing circadian mesor- and amplitude-hypertension in apparently healthy men. Chronobiologia 11:275-341, 1984.

16. Drayer JIM, Weber MA, DeYoung JL, Brewer DD: Long-term blood pressure monitoring in the evaluation of antihypertensive therapy. Archives Int Med 143:898-901, 1983.

Michael A. Weber, M.D.
VA Medical Center (W130)
5901 East Seventh Street
Long Beach, CA 90822
(213)494-5746

HYPERBARIC IMPACT GAUGES EXCESS BLOOD PRESSURE DURING PREGNANCY

PAUL J. MEIS, FRANZ HALBERG[*] AND FRANCES BOYETTE-KOURI, Bowman Gray
School of Medicine, Winston-Salem, NC and The University of Minnesota,
School of Medicine, Minneapolis, MN[*]

INTRODUCTION

Although several investigators[1,8,12] have described alterations of
blood pressure (BP) over the course of human pregnancy, and ample evidence exists that circadian rhythms of BP are demonstrable during pregnancy,[1,6,9,10,11] no longitudinal data exist of 24-hour BP patterns over
the course of gestation in healthy women, nor does information exist
about BP rhythm changes over the course of pregnancy in "hypertensive"
women. We have described circadian rhythms of systolic and diastolic BP
of three clinically healthy and two "hypertensive" pregnant women, with
sequential measurement over the course of gestation in one healthy and
one diabetic hypertensive patient. Further, the systolic and diastolic
BP excess for each study is quantified by use of the hyperbaric index
technique.[5]

PROCEDURE

Materials and Methods

Systolic and diastolic BP were recorded using noninvasive BP
recording apparatus (Vita-Stat 900S) at 10-minute intervals during waking
and 60-minute intervals during sleeping times over a 24-hour time span.
The subjects were three clinically healthy pregnant women, one pregnant
woman with sickle cell anemia and preeclampsia, and one pregnant woman
with diabetic nephropathy and retinopathy. The latter, along with one
clinically healthy subject, was studied sequentially throughout pregnancy. The clinically healthy subjects were studied in their homes, and
the "hypertensive" subjects were studied in hospital. All subjects were
permitted to ambulate or sit in a chair. Food and liquid intake were
allowed as desired.

Separately, for systolic and diastolic BP, a single 24-hour cosine
fit was used to derive rhythm parameters: the rhythm-adjusted mean or
mesor, the circadian amplitude, and the acrophase. Indices of BP excess
were also computed in relation to a time-specified variable threshold,
so-called chronodesmic limits[5] according to Halberg et al.[3,5]

These indices are the percent time of elevation and the duration of
elevation, i.e. the time span in hours during which the BP exceeds the
upper limit of the chronodesm for adult women, a 24-hour hyperbaric
impact (24-h HBI) and a 10-year HBI as a projection of cumulative excess.

RESULTS

Measures of BP excess are shown in Table 1. Systolic and diastolic
BP deficit were also sought, but none was found in the five subjects
investigated. Two of the clinically healthy subjects had no systolic BP
excess and all three had no diastolic BP excess during the weeks of
pregnancy indicated in Table 1, as assessed by the 24-h HBI. The third
healthy person (who was studied sequentially through gestation), during
the 18th week of pregnancy had a mean systolic BP excess of only 5 mm Hg,

associated with a 10-year HBI projection of slightly more than 100,000 mm Hg x h. The small HBI of this subject was reduced to near zero during the 25th week and to zero during the 37th week of pregnancy, in keeping with the BP-lowering effect of pregnancy as such. A BP-lowering effect was also seen with advanced pregnancy in a patient with diabetic nephropathy whose diastolic 24-h HBI in the 16th week of pregnancy was 277 mm Hg x h only to drop to 3 and then to 84 mm Hg x h during the 28th and 31st weeks of pregnancy. Postpartum the HBI was again at 353 mm Hg x h corresponding to a 10-year projection of over 1,288,000 mm Hg x h. In the same patient, however, the systolic 24-h HBI was not lowered by pregnancy, but showed the reverse course. The systolic 24-h HBI during the 16th week of pregnancy was 649 mm Hg x h, corresponding to a linear 10-year projection of excess of over 2,000,000 mm Hg x h. This 24-h HBI increased by the 28th week of pregnancy to 661 and rose further to 937 mm Hg x h by the 31st week. After delivery, the systolic hyperbaric impact of this woman dropped to 472 mm Hg, corresponding in this case to a 10-year projection of just over 1.7 million mm Hg x h. Table 1 shows that patient 4, with sickle cell anemia and preeclampsia, had a substantially elevated 24-h HBI for both systolic BP (106 mm Hg x h) and diastolic BP (121 mm Hg x h) corresponding to a 10-year projection of 386,000 and 442,000 mm Hg x h respectively.

DISCUSSION

Comparative differences of the effects of gestation on systolic and diastolic BP have been shown in previous studies[2,12] with diastolic BP exhibiting a larger decrease than systolic in mid-pregnancy, though both tend to reach pre-pregnant values (or higher) at term. Subject number five, whose pregnancy was complicated by diabetic nephropathy, shows a similar trend, with diastolic BP decreasing during pregnancy while systolic actually increased.

The importance of considering the circadian rhythms of BP in examining deviations from usual standards was pointed out in a recent publication by Scarpelli et al[11] who show that an arbitrary dividing line (mean arterial BP of 85 mm Hg) as an indication of fetal risk is misleading when applied to individual patients unless rhythm-adjusted guidelines are considered. Also of importance, however, is the consideration of gestational age adjusted BP guidelines as the same authors, perhaps unwillingly, demonstrate. The authors quoted by Scarpelli (Page and Christianson)[8] derived their data from, and intended their reference guideline (a mean arterial pressure of 90 mm Hg rather than the 85 mm Hg quoted) for women in the second trimester of pregnancy only. This guideline was applied, perhaps inappropriately, by Scarpelli et al to BP data from third trimester pregnant patients.

The results of this study demonstrate the practicality of measuring circadian rhythms of BP in pregnant women using noninvasive techniques in either the home or hospital locale. Blood pressure patterns over at least 2 and preferably 7 days can then be analyzed using chronodesmic reference standards for single samples and rhythm parameters to distinguish health from mesor-or amplitude-hypertension.

In order to extend the application of the hyperbaric index and other techniques of chronobiologic assessment, several requirements must be met. These include (1) reasonably priced equipment for automatic or continuous monitoring of the physiologic parameter over at least a 48-to 72-hour time span; (2) automatic storage of the data with sufficient capacity to permit a reasonably dense data base (i.e. for blood pressure, measurements every 10 minutes for 72 hours); (3) easy loading of the

280

stored data into mini- or microcomputer using a program which will
generate the chronobiologic parameters desired and make comparisons with
appropriate 24-hour reference limits. These requirements are well within
the limits of current technology but are not as yet developed.

The results here recorded and, in particular, the circumstance that
no subject showed a BP deficit, that is, no subject showed a BP below the
chronodesmic limits used, are, however, qualified by the nature of the
reference standard used. Our reference standard was determined for a
group of 15 clinically healthy menstrually cycling women 27-37 years of
age who each provided at ˜10-minute intervals for one to four 24-hour
spans automatically recorded BP series throughout the course of a year.
As an urgent task, the circadian BP patterns of clinically healthy should
be established for separate gestational stages from women with an uncomplicated pregnancy. Such a body of data will permit a better use of
chronobiologic methods in order to identify and quantify BP deviations
suggestive of disease states. Only until such a reference standard
becomes available can our inappropriately applied chronodesm from non-
pregnant women be used.

REFERENCES
1. Beilin L.J., Deacon J., Michael C.A., Vandongen R., Lalor C.M.,
    Barden A.E., Davidson L.: Circadian rhythms of blood pressure and
    pressor hormones in normal and hypertensive pregnancy - Clin. Exp.
    Pharmacol. Physiol. 9, 321-326, 1982.
2. MacGillivray I., Rose G.A., Rowe B.: Blood pressure survey in
    pregnancy - Clin. Sci. 37, 395-407, 1969.
3. Halberg F.: Quo vadis basic and clinical chronobiology: promise
    for health maintenance. Am. J. Anat. 168:543-594, 1983.
4. Halberg F., Carandente F., Cornelissen G., Katinas G.S.: Glossary
    of chronobiology. Chronobiologia 4, Suppl. 1, 1974, 189 pp.
5. Halberg F., Drayer J.I.M., Cornelissen G., Weber M.A.: Cardio-
    vascular reference data base for recognizing circadian mesor-and
    amplitude-hypertension in apparently healthy men. Chronobiologia
    11:275-278, 1984.
6. Meis P.J., Halberg F., Buster J.E., Marshall J.R.: Circadian
    rhythms in blood pressure, breast surface temperature, and blood
    dehydroepiandrosterone sulfate in human pregnancy. Potential
    chronotherapeutic markers - Chronopharmacology and Chrono-
    therapeutics. Florida A & M University Foundation, Tallahassee,
    Florida, USA, 1981; pp. 159-175.
7. Nelson W., Cornelissen G., Hinkley D., Bingham C., Halberg F.:
    Construction of rhythm-specified reference intervals and regions,
    with emphasis on 'hybrid' data, illustrated for plasma cortisol -
    Chronobiologia 10, 179-192, 1983.
8. Page E.W., Christianson R.: The impact of mean arterial pressure in
    the middle trimester upon the outcome of pregnancy - Am. J. Obstet.
    Gynecol. 125, 740-746, 1976.
9. Redman C.W.G., Beilin L.J., Bonnar J.: Variability of blood
    pressure in normal and abnormal pregnancy. In: Lindheimer, Katz,
    and Zuspan (Eds): Hypertension in Pregnancy. Wiley, New York,
    1976; pp. 53-60.
10. Sawyer M.M., Lipshitz J., Anderson G.D., Dilts P.V., Halperin L.:
    Diurnal and short-term variation of blood pressure: Comparison of
    preeclamptic, chronic hypertensive, and normotensive patients -
    Obstet. Gynecol. 58, 291-296, 1981.

11. Scarpelli P.T., Fersini C., Sensi G., Corti C., Croppi E., Romano S., Tarquini B.: The maternal 24-h blood pressure (BP) profile as a predictor of fetal distress - Chronobiologia 11, 141-145, 1984.
12. Schwarz R.: Das Verhalten des Kreislaufs in der normalen Schwangerschaft - Archiv. fur Gynakologie. 199, 549-570, 1964.

TABLE 1

Check for Blood Pressure Excess in Pregnant Women
Circadian Rhythm Parameters and Indices of Excess
Derived from Fit of 24-h Cosine*

Subj. ID & Diagnosis¶	Week of Preg.	Mesor	Amplitude	Acrophase (360°≡ 24h)	PTE (%)	Timespan BP>y_c Hours	24-h HBI	10-yr HBI**
		(mm Hg)					(mm Hg x h)	
				SYSTOLIC				
1E-h	12	100.4	8.9	-269°	0	0	0	0
2H-h	22	109.1	9.8	-247°	0	0	0	0
3S-h	18	117.0	16.9	-228°	23	5.5 (around 15^{24})	27	100,152
	25	114.1	12.0	-211°	2	0.6 (around 14^{17})	<1	1,169
	37	118.5	5.8	-215°	0	0	0	0
4P-s	34	126.8	5.9	-291°	72	17.2 (around 23^{21})	106	386,252
5G-d	16	150.6	4.0	-220°	100	24 (around 02^{33})	649	2,369,559
	28	151.1	2.6	-158°	100	24 (around 04^{13})	661	2,414,266
	31	162.6	4.4	-224°	100	24 (around 10^{58})	937	3,421,479
	post-p	143.2	5.5	-195°	100	24 (around 06^{57})	472	1,723,505
				DIASTOLIC				
1E-h	12	59.8	6.2	-264°	0	0	0	0
2H-h	22	64.4	5.4	-231°	0	0	0	0
3S-h	18	57.7	2.9	-254°	0	0	0	0
	25	59.7	6.8	-210°	0	0	0	0
	37	63.3	1.8	-72°	0	0	0	0
4P-s	34	86.7	2.3	-345°	88	21 (around 02^{00})	121	442,427
5G-d	16	93.3	2.2	-211°	100	24 (around 04^{41})	277	1,011,816
	28	79.8	3.4	-246°	16	4 (around 01^{08})	3	12,309
	31	80.9	8.8	-20°	45	10 (around 02^{00})	84	308,125
	post-p	96.5	3.3	-164°	100	24 (around 06^{24})	353	1,288,821

*Vs. chronodesmic limits (y_c) for non-pregnant, menstrually cycling women.
¶h = health; d = diabetes; s̄ = sickle-cell anemia and preeclampsia.
PTE = percent time elevation; HBI = hyperbaric impact
**10-year HBI = HBI projected over next 10 years.

THE NON-INVASIVE AUTOMATIC 24-H MONITORING OF BLOOD PRESSURE GAINS UNIVERSATILITY BY THE IMPLEMENTATION OF DATA ANALYSIS SYSTEMS DEVELOPED BY CHRONOBIOLOGY

P. CUGINI[+], P. LUCIA[+], G. MURANO[+], C. LETIZIA[+], D. SCAVO[+], R. ROMANO[++], A. GASPARETTO[++], G. LEONE[+++]

[+]I Patologia Medica, [++]Istituto di Anestesiologia e Rianimazione [+++]Istituto di Terapia Medica Sistematica, "La Sapienza" University of Rome, Rome, Italy

1. INTRODUCTION

Basically, the automatic equipments designed for the temporal BP non-invasive monitoring can be divided in two main groups. The quasi-portable devices allow a real-time control of BP. The fully-portable pressurometers document on a delayed basis the pressor values previously recorded on a mass memory.

Until now, bioengineering developed a technology essentially oriented toward the common requirements of medical practice. The quasi-portable pressurometers, with their visual monitors, audible alarms, readible print-out, are ideal for use in surgery and emergency room. The fully-ambulatory recorders, with their remote reading, are of choice for non-time vital situations such as the definition of borderline disorders in BP. Because of such clinical finalities, data analysis systems have been fundamentally dedicated to give a numerical and/or graphical representation of raw values versus time. Such a type of data handling appears to be dramatically poor in comparison with the informative potentiality of the 24-h BP monitoring. Aim of the present paper is to document that some mathematical statistical procedures developed by chronobiology may be highly recommended for optimizing the universality of pressurometers already available. Therefore, our research group will present some paradigmatic investigations concerning the 24-h BP monitoring in both the basic and clinical fields of medical science. It must be stressed that our experience mainly deals with quasi-portable devices manufactured by Invivo Research Laboratories (Tulsa, Oklahoma, USA, model Omega 1000), and by Nippon Colin (Komaki City, Japan, model BP-203 X). Such devices display systolic (S) and diastolic (D) BP, mean arterial pressure (MAP) and heart rate (HR).

2. ILLUSTRATIVE INVESTIGATIONS OF OUR LABORATORY

Figure 1 shows an example of integration between the 24-h BP monitoring and the chronobiologic procedure of cosinor (1,2) for investigating a basic problem of clinical physiology con-

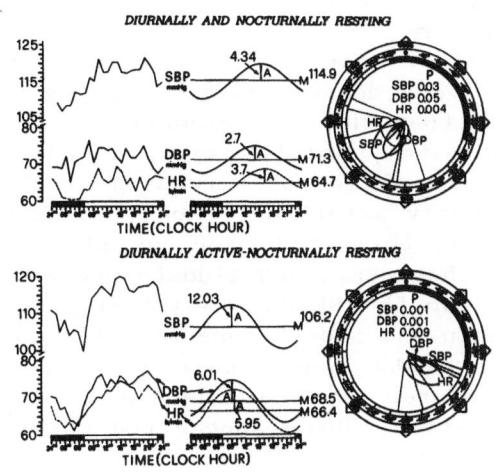

Figure 1. Effects of motor-rest activity on the 24-h patterns of blood pressure shown by chronograms and cosinor-derived best fitting cosine curves and polar plots.

cerning the effects of motor-rest schedule on hemodynamic function.

The conventional repre_sentation (left panel) is complemented with the cosinor-derived rhythmometry (other panels) which documents several additional findings, i.e., SBP, DBP and HR:1. are characterized by a well-defined circadian rhythm (CR) in subjects either diurnally-nocturnally recumbent or diurnally active-nocturnally resting, as demonstrated by P values; 2. show an increase and an advance, respectively in circadian variability and fluctuation in subjects active by day and resting by night, as illustrated by amplitude and acrophase values. It is apparent the gain of information which can be achieved by handling data by means of cosinor procedure even in the basic field of clinical physiology, since one can speculatively suggest that a routine of diurnal activity causes in the hemodynamic function to globally reset its chronoorganization.

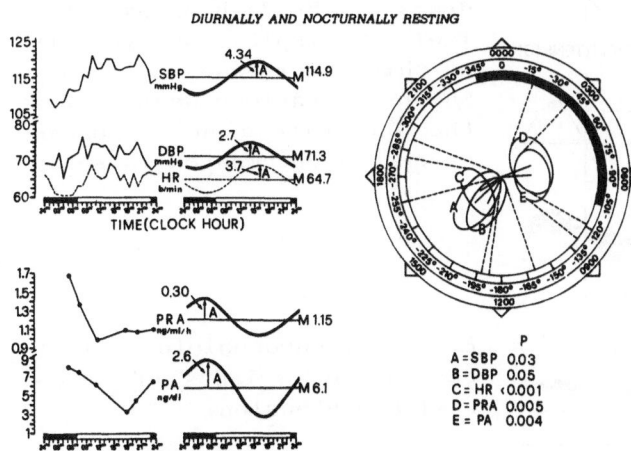

Figure 2 shows an example emphasizing the importance of information, compacted to four main

Figure 2. Cosinor-derived circadian rhythmometry for the rhythm of blood pres_sure as compared with the cyclicity of plasma renin and aldosterone.

284

parameters (waveform, mesor, amplitude, acrophase) by the cosinor procedure, as a rapid and suitable tool for comparing
the 24-h BP patterns with other biorhythmic variables, which
cannot be investigated with very dense serial sampling along
the time scale. It is clear that the circadian phase for the
biohumoral variables investigated, namely renin and aldosterone, occurs in early morning, while the circadian crest for
SBP and DBP is located in early afternoon. Such a difference
in time is highly significant (P<0.001). Because of such an
asynchronism, one can argue that renin and aldosterone are not
the immediate determinants for the BP CR. To investigate the
temporal relationship of renin and aldosterone with BP via the
conventional statistics, raw data should have been analyzed
by means of particular procedures, such as the cross correlation or the lead-lag correlation, which appear too much specific for optimizing the universatility of pressurometers.

Figure 3 illustrates in its left panel the chronobiologic variants of arterial hypertension which can be documented by applying the cosinor procedure to the 24-h patterns of DBP (3).
By assuming the occurrence of high BP values at odd hours (4),
and considering essential hypertension as characterized by the
usual timing in circadian BP acrophase (idiophasic hypertension), our research group hypothesized the existence of the
"heterophasic hypertension" whose "acrophase shifted", or "reverse", or "desynchronized" variants could be per se diagnostic for etiopathogenetically secondary types (5). Accordingly,
the cosinor procedure has
been applied to investigate
the hypertensive states affecting human beings and the
effects of antihypertensive
drugs on the 24-h BP patterns.
Table I displays a synopsis
of this investigation.

Shifts of various degrees for
the DBP circadian acrophase
have been documented in sever

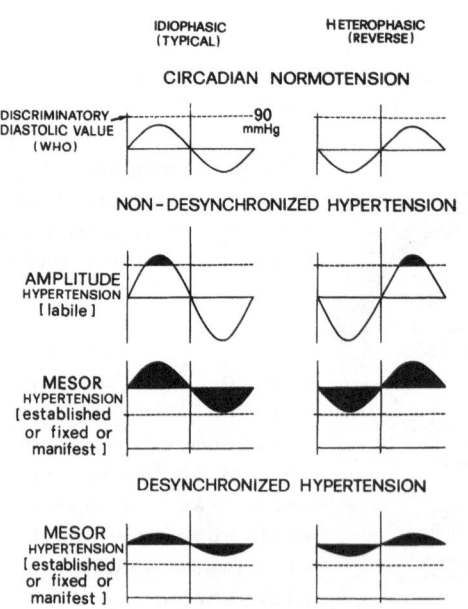

Figure 3. Chronobiologically-
recognized variants of arterial hypertension.

285

TABLE I-Etiopathogenetic classification of hypertensive states by means of the cosinor procedure applied to the 24-h patterns of blood pressure (diastolic behavior)

Clinical types of hypertension	Hypertension			
	Idiophasic	Heterophasic		
		shifted acrophase	reverse	desynchronized
Essential	+			
Renovascular	+			
Renal transplantation	+	+	+	+
11-β Hydroxylase deficiency		+		
Conn's syndrome			+	
Cushing's syndrome		+		
Iatrogenic corticoid excess		+		
Pheochromocytoma		+		
Licorice syndrome	+			
Conventional therapy with:				
-Propranolol			+	
-Atenolol			+	
-Penbutolol	+			
-Metoprolol		+		
-Labetalol		+		
-Clonidine	+	+		
-Nifedipine	+			
-Captopril	+			
-Hydrochlorothiazide			+	

al types of secondary hypertension and in relation to some antihypertensive conventional therapies, suggesting that the cosinor-derived rhythmometry of the 24-h monitoring may be used not only for the screening and clinical follow-up but also for the differential diagnosis of hypertension.

Figure 4 displays the combination of the 24-h BP monitoring with an analysis system for handling hemodynamic data in clinical conditions devoided of a CR for BP and/or HR. In this specific example, SBP and DBP values have been statistically evaluated by the bivariate analysis of gaussian distribution which has been tridimentionally plotted. The first diagram relates to clinically healthy subjects.

BIVARIATE GAUSSIAN DISTRIBUTION FOR SYSTOLIC (S) AND DIASTOLIC (D) BLOOD PRESSURE (BP)
(mmHg)

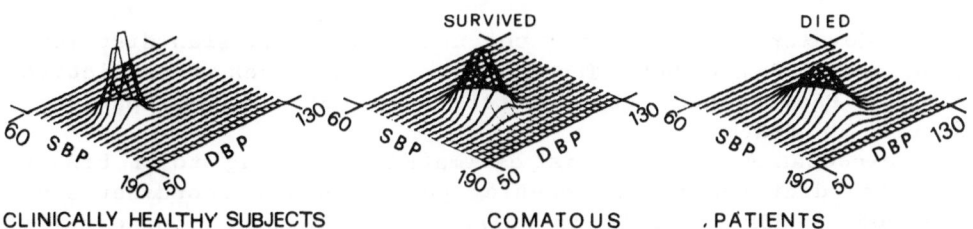

Figure 4. Bivariate gaussian analysis applied to 24-h patterns of systolic (SBP) and diastolic (DBP) blood pressure for discriminating long-term comatous patients, who survived or died, by taking into account the normal distribution.

The area covered by the curve can be, thus, regarded as the bivariate reference region which includes the 99% of distribution for both SBP and DBP values. The other two diagrams relate to patients surviving or dying from a long-term coma non-dépassè (stage II-III) due to cerebral apoplexia or acute in-

286

toxication by sedatives.

The regions of distribution clearly indicate that SBP and DBP
have a particular distributive frequency in comatous patients.
The bivariate discriminant analysis found that the 24-h BP pat
terns significantly discriminate (D=15.1; F=106; P<0.001) the
patients without or with a letal prognosis. This implies that

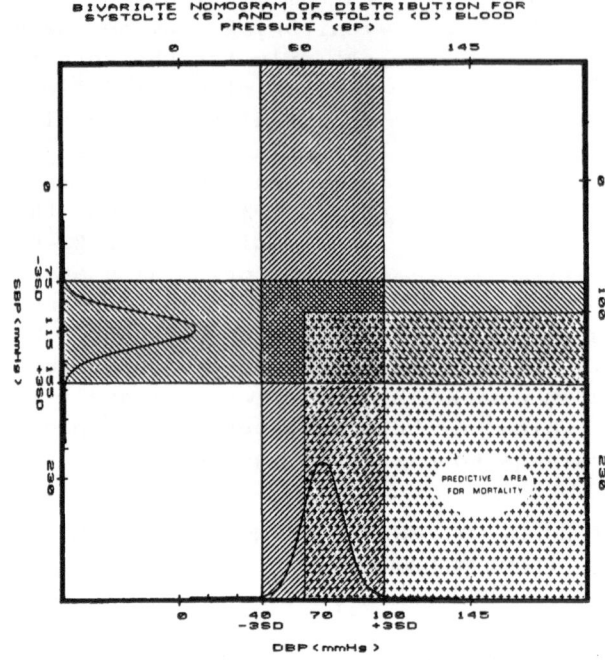

Figure 5. Planegraph
for predicting the
mortality in patien-
ts with a long term
coma non dépassè due
to vascular accident
or acute intoxica-
tion by sedatives,
via the 24-h monitor
ing of blood pres-
sure.

time-qualified BP da
ta can be reliably
used for assessing
the risk of mortali-
ty in such a specif-
ic area of pathology,
via the statistical
analysis in the fre-
quency domain. A
planegraph has been,
thus, developed by plotting the univariate gaussian distribution for SBP and DBP. The figure 5 shows such a predictive
diagram facilitating the identification of comatous patients
at risk of death.

The expectancy of life is estimated according to a binary
decision dictated by the meeting point for the coordinates of
the median SBP and DBP, in relation to the region predictive
of mortality.

CONCLUSIONS AND RECOMMENDATIONS

Two conclusions are stressed by this presentation. The 24-h
BP monitoring is fundamental not only for clinical but also
for basic medicine. At the present, data analysis systems implemented are too inappropriate for allowing the pressurometers to show all their investigative potentiality, data hand
ling being mainly descriptive and statistical algorithms es-
sentiality conventional. A larger universality is, thus, recom
mended.

With respect to this, the present paper documented that the

24-h BP monitoring may gain versatility, flexibility and practicability by adding some specific chronobiologic procedures
to data analysis systems.
The cosinor procedure is of crucial importance since the tempo
ral BP variability can be statistically validated in its rhythmicity. Furthermore, the information compacted to four parameters (waveform, mesor, amplitude, acrophase) is highly
useful for a possible correlation of BP with other time-dependent variables, avoiding the additional implementation of unusual procedures for cross-section analysis. Lastly, the cosinor-derived rhythmometry and best-fitting curve are basic for
estimating behaviors (idiophasic or heterophasic hypertension,
amplitude-or mesor-hypertension) and updated indices (hyperbaric impact, percent time elevation, overall mean pressure
excess, mean pressure excess, etc.) via the 24-h monitoring
(6, 7).
As documented, the statistical analysis of frequency distribution associated with the plot of univariate and bivariate gaus
sian curves can optimize the capability of pressurometers to
investigate the 24-h hemodynamic patterns devoided of rhythmicity. The statistical analysis in the frequency domain, thus,
complements the inferential statistics of cosinor. In addition, the bivariate gaussian analysis allows the SBP and DBP
to be evaluated as a "unum". Physiologic and pathologic states can be, thus, estimated in this biunivocal correspondence
and differentiated by the bivariate discriminant analysis. The
procedure can be used for correlating MAP with HR as well.
Lastly, it must be stressed that the median pressure and/or
pulse may have a practical importance as a predictor in some
clinical conditions at risk of death.
Technologically, any innovation will cause modifications invol
ving hardware and/or software. Changes should be, thus, considered under the cost-effectiveness viewpoint. Our recommendations appear to be not utopian considering that the software
to be implemented has been already developed.

REFERENCES

1. Halberg F., Tong Y.L., Johnson E.A.: Circadian system pha-
   se-an aspect of temporal morphology; procedure and illustra
   tive examples. In "The cellular aspects of biorhythms".
   Springer-Verlag, Berlin, 1967, pp. 20-48.
2. Halberg F., Johnson E.A., Nelson W., Runge W., Sothern R.:
   Autorhythmometry: procedures for physiologic self-measurements and their analysis. Physiology Teacher 1,1-11, 1972.
3. Halberg F., Lauro R., Carandente F.: Autoritmometria. Dal
   singolo dato di laboratorio allo studio delle serie tempo-
   rali per la diagnosi di malattia. La Ricerca Clin. Lab. 6

(suppl. 2), 1-45, 1976.
4. Halberg F., Scheving L.E., Lucas E., Cornelissen G., Sothern R.B., Halberg E., Halberg F., Carter J., Straub K.D.,
Redmond D.P.: Chronobiology of human pressure in the light
of static (room-restricted) automatic monitoring. Chronobiologia 11, 217-247, 1984.
5. Cugini P., Lucia P., Murano G., Letizia C., Scavo D., Verna
R.: On determinants of circadian variability for blood pres
sure. In: Proceedings of the II Meeting "Blood pressure ambulatory monitoring in the study of pathophysiology of hypertension and the evaluation of the effect of the treatments" Roma, April 16, 1984.
6. Halberg F., Drayer J.I.M., Cornelissen G., Weber M.A.: Cardiovascular reference data base for recognizing circadian
mesor-and amplitude-hypertension in apparently healthy men.
Chronobiologia 11, 275-298, 1984.
7. Halberg F., Ahlgren A., Haus E.: Circadian systolic and
diastolic hyperbaric indices of high school and college
students. Chronobiologia 11, 299-309, 1984.

Chronobioengineering for human blood pressure*

Erna Halberg@, Franca Carandente¶, Robert B. Sothern@ and Franz Halberg@†
University of Minnesota, Minneapolis, MN 55455, USA
University of Milan, Milan, Italy

*Dedicated to the memory of Howard Levine, academic pioneer of blood pressure chronobiology, who at a time when ambulatory instrumentation for blood pressure measurement was not available practiced self-measurement for over a decade, including the terminal span (even the last hours) prior to death from amyotrophic lateral sclerosis.
†Support: U.S. National Institute of General Medical Sciences (GM-13981); Minnesota Mining and Manufacturing Inc., St. Paul, MN; Medtronic Inc., Minneapolis, MN; Fondazione Hoechst, Milan, Italy. Mr. Masayuki Shinoda, President, Nippon Colin Ltd., Komaki, Japan, provided invaluable automatic instrumentation for this research and for the acquisition of several special reference data bases.

In terms of the number of people involved who could benefit from proper instrumentation, the challenge to engineers in both academy and industry that is posed by the need for a chronobiologic approach to blood pressure is second to none. The result of proper monitoring and introduction of preventive measures could lead to a reduction in suffering from cardiovascular disease, one of the major diseases of modern civilization. In addition, industry would gain a huge market for blood pressure and related instrumentation. Scrutiny is therefore warranted of what is currently available in terms of such instrumentation, bad as well as good, useful as well as useless.

Machines in public places, i.e., airports and shopping centers, may compute 'good days' and 'bad days' once a birthday is indicated and some money inserted. These machines are obvious put-ons; even a contemporary principal proponent of birthday-determined 'biorhythms' admits that they have no basis in scientific fact. Other machines, often in the same public places, measure a single blood pressure (BP) or heart rate (HR). The time has come to recognize that both kinds of machines are worthless. The one yielding a single BP or HR is the greater put-on if it serves as the sole basis for decisions regarding health. BP in health can indeed vary by as much as 30-70 mm Hg in 24 hrs, Figure 1.

Leading health professionals may not realize this point. The president of the American Heart Association undertook a study with two BP measurements (Kolata, 1983). Others advocate a BP measurement on three different occasions (Rosner and Polk, 1979). An authority recognized worldwide in the field advocates 10 such casual measurements as a practical basis for diagnosis and treatment (Tobian, 1968). As a cost-effective alternative, everybody can learn—preferably early in childhood schooling—how to self-measure BP

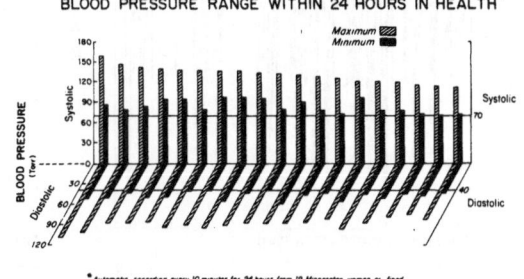

BLOOD PRESSURE RANGE WITHIN 24 HOURS IN HEALTH*

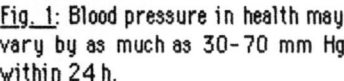

Fig. 1: Blood pressure in health may vary by as much as 30-70 mm Hg within 24 h.

290

Fig. 2: Time plots of BP variability in clinically healthy woman, monitored longitudinally from May 8 to July 9 and from August 9–21, 1984. The horizontal line drawn at 140 mm Hg corresponds to the upper limit for SBP by the World Health Organization. Note that this woman, in presumed cardiovascular health, exhibits many values above 140 mm Hg.

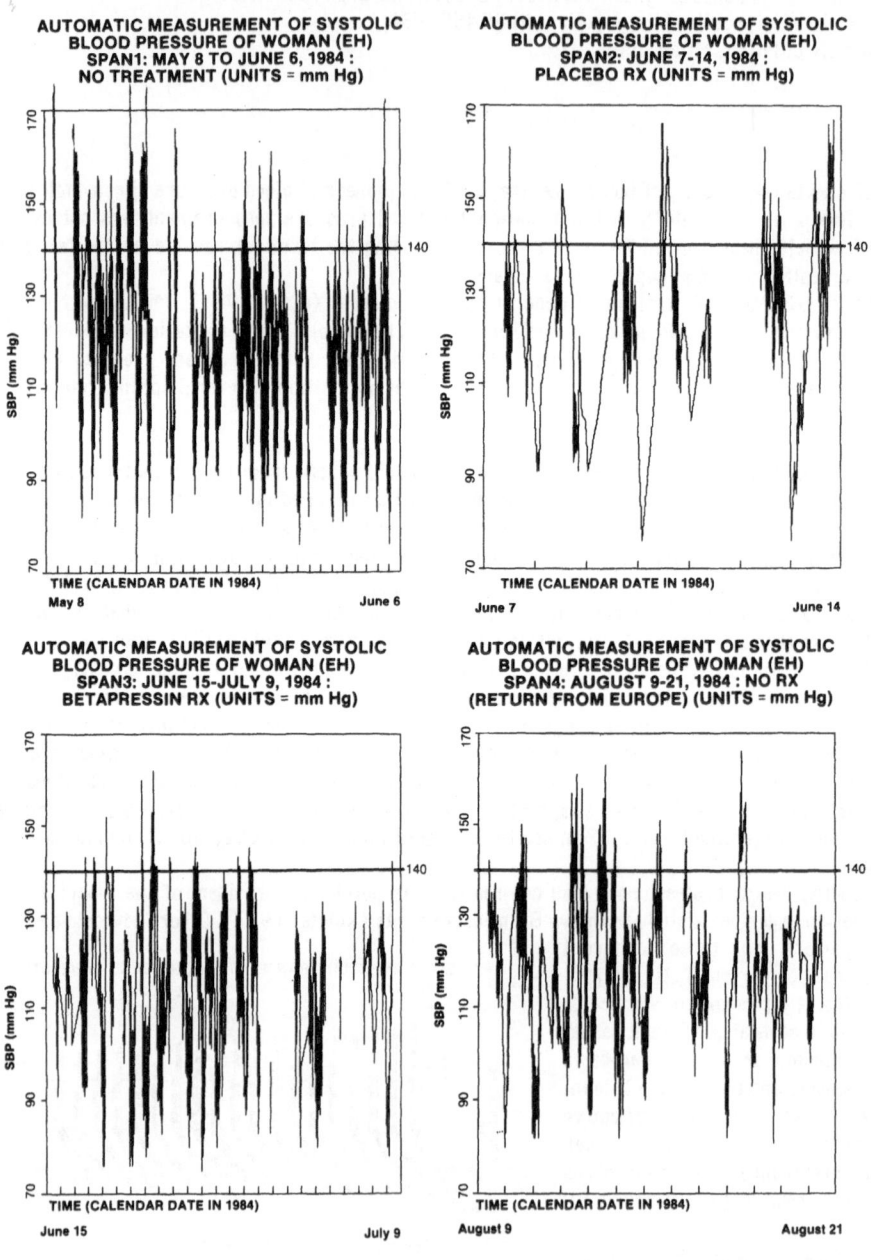

several times throughout the day and night and to derive a set of statistics from these data. Automatically, BP series are more readily obtained by night as well as by day, with currently available instrumentation.

Government, academy and industry all have an interest in the automatic monitoring of human BP, notably when it is excessive, since cumulative excess leads to major diseases. Health is everybody's concern. In addition, government has to manage (and contain the cost of) health care. There is no better way than prevention to achieve this goal. Ethical industry realizes that in the long run, a good health product is most rewarding. Government, industry and academy will eventually realize that good bioengineering should be equated with chronobiologic engineering (Halberg, F., 1983) for three reasons: 1) rhythms—algorithmically-formulatable phenomena, validated by inferential statistical means—are omnipresent in biology; 2) they are of critical importance, predictably tipping the scale between life and death in a number of responses to various agents, including potentially noxious ones such as drugs; 3) information on rhythms is useful since it can be exploited by modern engineering methods, provided appropriate hardware and software can be matched with satisfactory data bases and interpreted in the light of dynamic concepts. Rhythm assessment can then serve the primary and secondary prevention of major cardio-cerebro-reno-vascular diseases as well as their diagnosis and therapy, cost-effectively in the home.

The assessment of changes in human BP then becomes a task for everyone, regardless of sex, age, ethnicity or social standing. The detection of a high BP and its lowering help to prevent heart and kidney disease and stroke. Human BP varies greatly, not only from the contraction of the heart (systole) to the heart's relaxation (diastole), but also during 24 hours, a week and much longer bioperiodicities (Sothern and Halberg, in press). At a given time of day, the diastolic (D) BP (heart relaxed) can be 18 mm Hg higher than the systolic (S) BP (heart contracted) at another time of day, while the D or SBP can vary an average of 40 mm Hg within the same 24 hours. Figures 2 and 3 show this great variability of human BP in a clinically healthy woman monitored with the instrument manufactured by Instruments for Cardiac Research (ICR, Liverpool, New York). Part of this variability can be quantified by algorithms implemented in a set of computer programs. Algorithms are rules for getting a specific output from a specific input. Each step of an algorithm must be precisely defined so that it can be translated into language compatible with a computer or pocket calculator, the tools of the chronobiologist.

One task of this symposium with respect to BP is to emphasize the need for a so-called microscopic chronobiologic approach, to distinguish it from (macroscopic) data inspection in tabulations or graphs.

The task of home monitoring is already greatly facilitated by available automatic instruments, even if all of them are expensive and the fully ambulatory ones all too weighty. Nonetheless, for those of us (Halberg et al., 1983; Levine et al., 1980; Sothern and Halberg, in press) who self-measured manually for many years, these automatically measuring instruments, their limitations notwithstanding, are extremely welcome. Verlin McCall's records by the Pressurometer III (Del Mar Avionics, Irvine, CA), even if we look at them with the unaided eye (by macroscopy), provide important information on the extent of change. When properly analyzed (Halberg et al., 1984a, 1985), fully automatic and room-restricted monitoring are complementary. Our room-restricted data stem from a very sturdy, reliable, portable though not wearable automatic monitor, manufactured by Nippon Colin Ltd. (Komaki, Japan; NC), and the pioneering Arteriosonde (Hoffman-LaRoche, Cranbury, New Jersey, USA) (E. Halberg et al., 1981).

Figures 2-3 present data obtained with the lightest among the fully ambulatory instruments available (ICR), but one which is costly to maintain apart from initial acquisition costs, since batteries must be replaced daily. Early in its use, we had equipment failures, apparent as gaps in Figure 2. It must be realized that dense monitoring with this instrument, as it is now built, cannot be continued, say at 10-minute intervals for longer than 24 hours. Eventually, however, the shortcomings of this instrument and similar ones will have to be overcome; clearly, records such as those in Figures 2-3 are not readily obtained by self-measurement. Another shortcoming of this instrument is that it exhibits digit preference, especially in the measurement of DBP (Figure 4). It

<u>Fig. 3</u>: Circadian pattern of BP data shown in Fig. 2.

**AUTOMATIC MEASUREMENT OF SYSTOLIC
BLOOD PRESSURE OF WOMAN (EH,AGE 64)
SPAN1: MAY 8 TO JUNE 6, 1984 : NO TREATMENT
HOURLY MEANS AND STANDARD ERRORS**

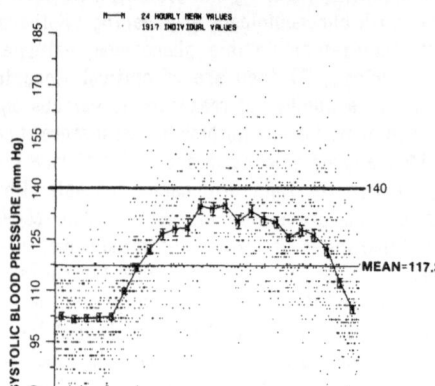

**AUTOMATIC MEASUREMENT OF SYSTOLIC
BLOOD PRESSURE OF WOMAN (EH,AGE 64)
SPAN2: JUNE 7 TO JUNE 14, 1984 : PLACEBO RX
HOURLY MEANS AND STANDARD ERRORS**

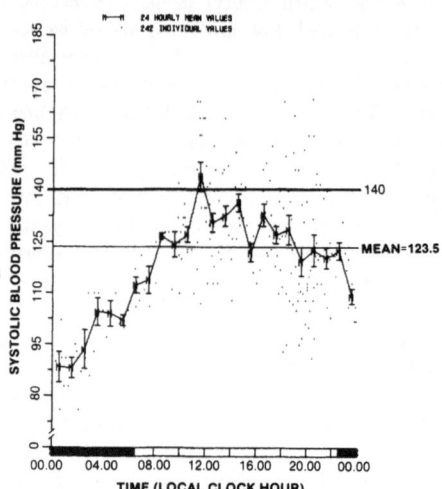
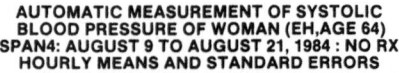

**AUTOMATIC MEASUREMENT OF SYSTOLIC
BLOOD PRESSURE OF WOMAN (EH,AGE 64)
SPAN3: JUNE 15 TO JULY 9, 1984 : BETAPRESSIN RX
HOURLY MEANS AND STANDARD ERRORS**

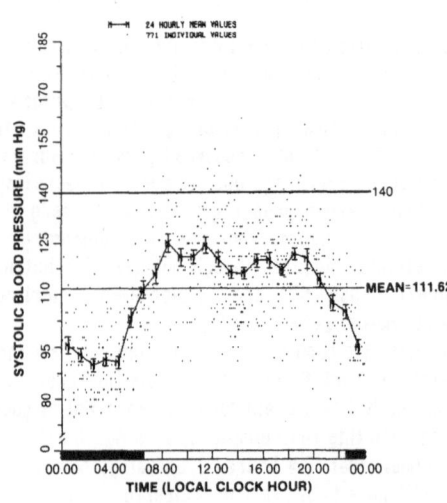

**AUTOMATIC MEASUREMENT OF SYSTOLIC
BLOOD PRESSURE OF WOMAN (EH,AGE 64)
SPAN4: AUGUST 9 TO AUGUST 21, 1984 : NO RX
HOURLY MEANS AND STANDARD ERRORS**

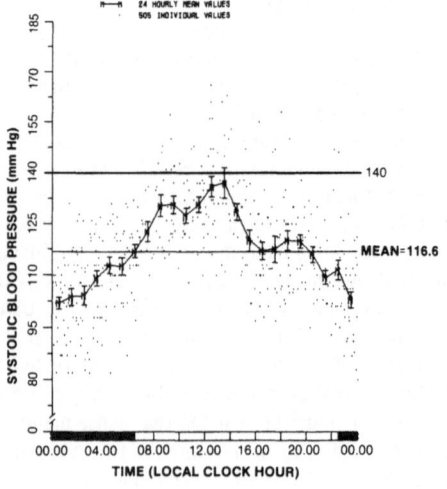

4a: DBP

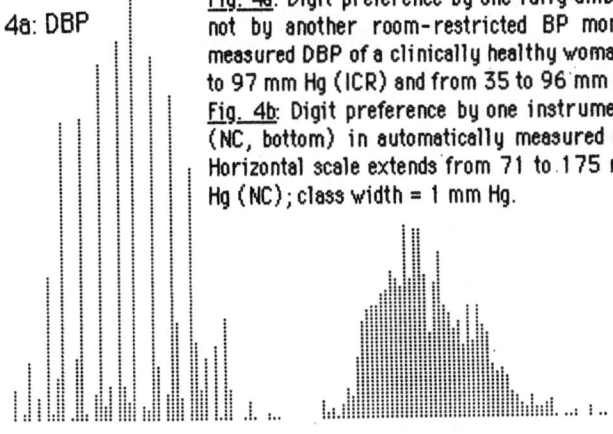

Fig. 4a: Digit preference by one fully ambulatory BP monitor (ICR, left), but not by another room-restricted BP monitor (NC, right) in automatically measured DBP of a clinically healthy woman. Horizontal scale extends from 42 to 97 mm Hg (ICR) and from 35 to 96 mm Hg (NC); class width = 1 mm Hg.

Fig. 4b: Digit preference by one instrument (ICR, top), but not another one (NC, bottom) in automatically measured SBP of a clinically healthy woman. Horizontal scale extends from 71 to 175 mm Hg (ICR) and for 81 to 170 mm Hg (NC); class width = 1 mm Hg.

can be readily seen that there are many dots corresponding to certain numbers but not to certain other numbers. As opposed to human digit preference, which may favor numbers ending in 0 or 5 and even numbers over odd, the machine may 'prefer' certain other numbers.

4b: SBP

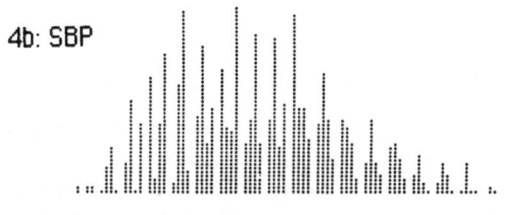

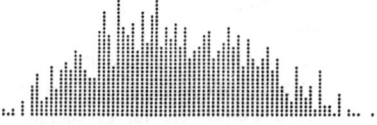

This shortcoming, the undue weight and the need to buy expensive batteries for each day's recording and even the inability to record densely for spans longer than 24 hours are certainly outweighed by the fact that electrodes need not be used with this instrument. The product-moment correlation with a sphygmomanometer reading is certainly not the 'gold standard' and the pressure measured by an internal line may serve as such in the want of a more objective standardized artificial arm. In any event, with the ICR, one can obtain reasonable data under fully-ambulatory conditions with relatively little nuisance for considerable spans, as can be seen from Figures 2 and 3. Data over such spans and longer ones may be needed in order to optimize treatment of certain patients. A new generation of instruments will have to overcome the costs of initial acquisition, the new batteries every 24 hours, the undue weight and the digit preference, while safeguarding the great merit of the ICR: recording without electrodes.

Use of the current instrumentation is nonetheless very much worthwhile, as emphasized by Figures 2 and 3. Data during the first span constitute a reference for the second span, during which a placebo was taken daily. A fleeting comparison by the naked eye of the data in May with those in August when no treatment was administered may suggest that in August, the values are much lower, notably since there appear to be fewer values above the 140 mm Hg line. Further analysis shows that this result is a mistaken impression by the naked eye, which views data along different time scales. The overall means, Figure 3, are nearly identical in the 2 no-treatment spans, where the data are stacked along the scale of single idealized days, as instruments for home monitoring should do. In other words, future instruments may have an update each day and, if need be, at any given moment of the entire accumulated series, folded into a single idealized day or any other appropriately chosen time span. Nearly 2,000 individual values, for the span from May 8 to June 6, are shown with their means and standard errors for consecutive 1-h intervals. It can be seen that one of the hourly mean values during the placebo span is above the 140 mm Hg line. If one happened to sample only in this window, one may well interpret the result to indicate the need for treatment.

294

Fig. 5: Illustration of circadian rhythm characteristics of SBP in a clinically healthy woman.

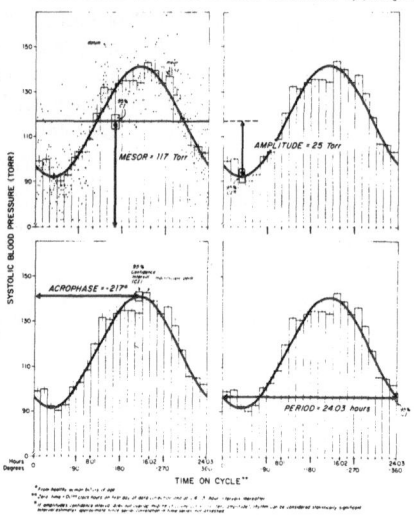

HYPOTHESIS TESTING* AND *ESTIMATION* OF
CIRCADIAN PARAMETERS OF SYSTOLIC BLOOD PRESSURE
ESTIMATED BY NON-LINEAR LEAST-SQUARES FIT
OF COSINE CURVE TO 7 DAYS OF DATA* (summarized by plexogram)

In the context of the entire curve, it becomes apparent that we are dealing with an individual in apparently good cardiovascular health and that the vast majority of the values, including many other hourly means, are much lower than 140 mm Hg.

Cumulative displays over a desired span serve to characterize the results first, but added features should also be provided by future instruments. Available software should yield more than just a 24-h mean. Chronobiologic parameters can be useful. These are shown in Figure 5, illustrating the characteristics of a circadian rhythm for the same woman during an earlier span. We can focus first on the midline-estimating statistic of rhythm, the MESOR, M, which may differ slightly from the 24-h mean when the BP data are not equidistant or do not cover an integral number of periods. In this figure, we find, again for the original data, a very great variability during just 7 days. In this case of a woman living on a 24-h social routine, as anticipated, the period is extremely close to 24 hours (actually of 24.03 hours). Figure 5 also shows the amplitude, a measure of predictable extent of change and the acrophase, a measure of timing of overall high values. Data storage for long recording spans can be facilitated if an algorithm computes and stores averages for consecutive hours or even longer spans, perhaps with any prominent ultradian characteristics. Actually, the ultradian components may determine the span for averaging, such as 1.7-hour spans or even changing spans, when frequency multiplications and divisions of the ultradian component do occur.

From the viewpoint of focus upon the circadian component, the averaging serves to reduce the effect of correlations in the data. Thus, averaging provides a more appropriate set of circadian characteristics while also reducing the numbers to be stored. Moreover, for circadian estimates, that are not concerned with an evaluation of ultradians, it is a great technical advantage to measure only at longer intervals, thereby reducing the energy necessary for cuff inflation. The saving in power may then be converted into a reduction in weight and size of the instrument. Parameter tests (Bingham et al., 1982) can also be carried out on the results of home and work monitoring. To turn back to Figures 2 and 3, such tests do not reveal a difference between span 1 and span 2 for SBP, but there is a significant difference (P<.001) between the MESOR in spans of placebo and betapressin (penbutolol, a beta-blocker) administration. There is also a statistically significant difference between the span with the beta-blocker and the subsequent no-treatment span. Ultradian and circadian BP rhythm characteristics and measures of BP excess (Halberg et al., 1984a) may be stored and used for any infradian analyses.

A reduction in size is required if the instrument is to be used routinely to assess the extent and timing of excess pressure, to be considered for the timing of treatment and for gauging its efficacy. To document this point, we refer to the records of 28 patients of Yerlin and Willifred McCall (McCall Y.R. and McCall W.C., this volume; Halberg et al., 1985). These patients were suspected of a high blood pressure on the basis of values above 140/90 SBP/DBP on three occasions, in a physician's office. Data were obtained at 7.5-minute intervals for 24 hours. All series cover a very wide range of values, yet 3 of them are described by an amplitude compatible with the diagnosis of amplitude-hypertension. An amplitude of 35.6 (double amplitude 71.2) mm Hg in a 43-year-old woman is clearly outside the reference limits for the circadian amplitude (Halberg et al., 1984a,b).

In considering the amplitude and acrophase as a parameter pair, written (A,ø), a new level of

Fig. 6: Cosinor display of circadian rhythm in blood pressure and heart rate of a clinically healthy woman.

Circadian Cardiovascular Rhythms
Automatically Monitored in a 60-year old Woman*

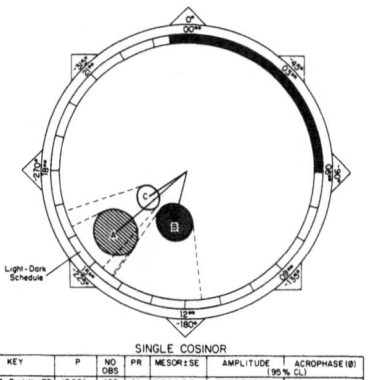

SINGLE COSINOR						
KEY	P	NO OBS	PR	MESOR±SE	AMPLITUDE	ACROPHASE (θ) (95% CL)
A Systolic BP	<0.001	422	21	109±1.05	76(58, 93)	-229°(-215,-244)
B Diastolic BP	<0.001	420	11	62.7±0.4	4.2(2.7, 5.7)	-193°(-173,-215)
C Pulse	<0.001	440	19	68.1±0.3	3.8(2.9, 4.7)	-236°(-221,-251)

P= probability of hypothesis amplitude=0, No obs = number of observations, PR = Percent rhythm, 95% CL=
95 % confidence limits derived from cosinor ellipse

*Mesor and amplitude of systolic and diastolic blood pressure (BP), expressed in torr, pulse mesor and amplitude expressed in beats/min, acrophases in degrees, with 360° = 24 hrs, 0° = local midnight

information is gained, concerning both the timing and the extent of BP change. This combined index is shown in the polar cosinor plot with a circular scale, in which midnight is shown on top, noon at the bottom, 06^{00} on the right and 18^{00} on the left, Figure 6. This display also provides the uncertainty of each characteristic, i.e., of amplitude and acrophase not only separately, by the intersects of the joint confidence region with the vector and its prolongation for A and by tangents to the confidence region for ø, but also as a joint confidence region for (A,ø) displayed as an added feature. The tabulation below the cosinor numerically indicates results from the least-squares fit of a 24-hour cosine curve to the data.

What we wish to know in determining BP includes, beyond a description of the rhythm, an assessment of any excess characterizing the BP of the given person, the so-called hyperbaric index (HBI). This excess can be esti-mated as the product of the extent and the duration of values exceeding a peer-group reference limit (Halberg et al., 1984a). Of necessity, when the preferable personalized chronodesmic reference standard is still lacking, the upper chronodesmic limit of a peer group can be used. Indices of BP excess are useful to optimize the timing of any treatment, if needed. It seems logical indeed that, in any one patient, the current palliative anti-hypertensive treatment modes should be so timed as to remove the BP-excess, when it actually occurs. A major question to be asked next in this context is whether the pattern of excess is a random one and, if not, to what extent timing of excess may be quantifiable by the fit of a single cosine curve. The excess pressure can be computed as fractionated 3-hourly HBI's, to which the single cosinor can be applied. Specification of the timing of the BP excess is then indicated by the acrophase, which in turn can be used to time treatment. Clearly, a mere indication of when excess recurs reproducibly, whatever its form may be, is needed and is best individualized in terms of a reference standard obtained on several occasions in health, starting as early in life as possible, in school if not at birth. Ideally, of course, the proper reference standard for a given individual is that individual's pressure behavior before the onset of amplitude-hypertension. With the teaching of chronobiologic computer and health literacy in schools, for preventive measures, this goal of providing a personalized chronodesm for every school child is not out of reach. It would serve best if preventive measures are instituted as soon as there is a change in (A,ø) pair, which change may well precede the change in MESOR (Halberg et al., 1984b). The reference to the physiologic change in a peer group is a second choice; the excess is quantified not in terms of when the BP as such is high, but rather on the basis of when BP deviates from the time course of BP in peers.

With respect to the 28 patients of Verlin and Willifred McCall, they were classified into 4 groups of patients, all monitored because of a suspicion of high BP, Table 1. A first set of 8 records stems from patients diagnosed as office-hypertensives or, as Verlin McCall called them, pseudo-hypertensives, or perhaps 'white-coat' hypertensives. These patients have an HBI below 50 mm Hg x h, which is compatible with HBIs found for clinically healthy individuals. In the second group, labeled (by macroscopic inspection) as non-circadian labile hypertension, one patient (subject 09 in Table 1) accumulates, within the first 6 hours of the night, an HBI of 140 mm Hg x h, while the HBI is low for the remainder of the day. One may worry, of course, about the possibility that high HBIs by night and relatively low ones by day are simply the result of the choice of reference limits, since we are not dealing with a fixed threshold (e.g., at 140 mm Hg), but rather with a wavy reference standard, which is much lower by night than by day. This line of thought is

Table 1: Circadian rhythm characteristics of BP excess (HBI) in 28 patients suspected of high BP*

			Systolic BP			Diastolic BP		
Age	Sex	M	A	ø		M	A	ø
Group I: office hypertension								
01	45	F	0.03	0.05	-157°	0		
02	45	F	3.50	4.12	-39°	0.03	0.04	-225°
03	45	M	0			0		
04	58	F	2.53	2.12	-157°	16.97	9.61	-183°
05	54	M	0.39	0.34	-28°	0.79	1.56	-113°
06	46	M	0.14	0.24	-15°	0		
07	57	M	4.54	4.28	-172°	0.26	0.36	-202°
08	39	M	3.98	5.01	-71°	0.10	0.02	-100°
Group II: labile hypertension								
09	30	M	23.29	27.94	-35°	14.94	19.77†	-97°
10	34	F	6.71	7.64†	-289°	4.87	5.19	-234°
11	66	M	24.68	35.69†	-192°	0.53	0.95	-201°
12	83	M	14.23	17.72	-193°	0.10	0.10	-147°
13	60	M	23.63	25.67	-96°	3.38	3.28	-66°
14	52	M	2.48	3.01	-163°	7.23	6.58	-172°
15	74	F	32.51	19.41	-116°	9.37	5.24	-150°
16	38	F	13.03	3.80	-104°	17.51	8.42	-161°
Group III: daytime hypertension								
17	55	M	44.99	38.24	-181°	8.08	12.97†	-195°
18	48	M	19.41	19.60†	-160°	0.43	0.37	-187°
19	63	M	21.11	16.04†	-140°	4.88	1.12	-314°
20	19	M	10.76	10.61	-346°	0.22	0.42	-15°
21	43	F	16.24	18.94†	-132°	9.70	13.97†	-168°
22	42	M	62.37	4.46	-48°	16.13	12.03	-167°
Group IV: sustained hypertension								
23	62	F	68.58	42.19	-35°	14.65	17.62	-24°
24	61	M	31.52	38.10	-40°	3.12	5.51	-36°
25	30	M	33.83	8.83	-62°	0.08	0.15	-91°
26	31	M	30.62	34.17†	-53°	0.13	0.25	-67°
27	59	M	58.12	40.32†	-85°	0.91	1.21†	-76°
28	72	M	44.26	26.85	-71°	1.06	1.90	-49°

*M=MESOR, A=Amplitude; M and A expressed in mm Hg x h (HBI computed over consecutive 3-hour intervals); ø=Acrophase (360°≡24 hours; 0°=00^{00}); overfit results from the constraint that HBI is ≥0 by definition.
†P<0.05 in testing H_0: A=0.

not generally applicable, however. Clearly, in another patient in the second group, the highest HBIs occur between noon and 15^{00} (subject 11 in Table 1). In two other patients of this group, the highest HBIs occur between 09^{00} and 12^{00} (subjects 12 and 15 in Table 1). In a third group, with BP elevated during day and labeled as normotensive at night, one finds exceptions to this statement by macroscopic criteria. Patients with sustained high BP, in group IV, have their BP elevated while awake or asleep, macroscopically. In this case, chronobiologic analysis reveals periodicity in HBI with the excess occurring by night in all cases, Table 1.

In looking at DBP, at first glance, it is readily apparent that there is much less excess in this variable in the 28 cases examined. In the first group, though, in which no systolic excess was found, there is a diastolic MESOR-hypertensive (subject 04 in Table 1) among the office hypertensives, with a total HBI for DBP exceeding 120 mm Hg x h, with the excess occurring mostly by day rather than by night. An excess occurring primarily by night rather than by day is seen for patients in group IY, described as exhibiting sustained high BP by day and by night.

The minimum that should be done (even if one ignores the timing of excess) is to assess first, say for 3 consecutive days or preferably for 7 days, the excess for systolic BP each day, the excess for diastolic BP each day, and any tachycardia. In addition, rhythm parameters should be given as an indication of whether the amplitude and acrophase are within or outside their prediction limits. At this early stage of chronobiologic information, such summaries should convey to physician and lay person alike not only what a MESOR, amplitude and acrophase indicate, but also whether or not the amplitude, acrophase or MESOR are within or outside their reference limits.

To turn back to the hyperbaric index, it has been introduced thus far as derived from original data. If instrumentation for dense automatic measurement is not available, a reasonably fair approximation of the HBI can be derived from a cosine curve which can be fitted to data that are much less dense than those obtained with the sampling rates now possible with automatic instrumentation. For the instrumentation of the future, it is mandatory that cross-calibrated instruments for self- and automatic measurement be available, as repeatedly emphasized in this session. The ideal hardware which we wish to have may still be years away. A self-measurement device which allows for data coding in an instrument (such as an autochronor [Del Pozo et al., 1983]) may be the item of most general use for every primary care physician.

Such instrumentation would allow every person to determine salt-sensitivity. Non-drug treatment should and must be tried before drugs are prescribed for a high BP. Again, an autochronor for self-measurement and self-coding, and preferably self-analysis of the data, may be the most urgent item to be procured and the most readily obtained. This item could indeed serve every school child and every adult and would allow the recording of the data as one goes, notably of BP, but also some other pertinent performance variables, and it would provide a ready analysis of the characteristics of BP as well as of other variables which should be readily understood worldwide.

References

1. Bingham C., Arbogast B., Cornélissen Guillaume G., Lee J.K., Halberg F. (1982): Inferential statistical methods for estimating and comparing cosinor parameters. Chronobiologia 9: 397-439.
2. Del Pozo F., Perez Subias M., Halberg F., Burillo Y., Hermida Dominguez R.C. (1983): Microprocessor-based system for self-measurement applications. Proc. 5th Ann. Conf. IEEE Engineering in Medicine and Biology Society, Columbus, OH, September 10-12, 1983, pp. 413-418.
3. Halberg E., Halberg F., Shankaraiah K. (1981): Plexo-serial linear-nonlinear rhythmometry of blood pressure, pulse and motor activity by a couple in their sixties. Chronobiologia 8: 351-366.
4. Halberg F. (1983): Quo vadis basic and clinical chronobiology: promise for health maintenance. Am. J. Anat. 168: 543-594.
5. Halberg F., Drayer J.I.M, Cornélissen G., Weber M.A. (1984a): Cardiovascular reference data base for recognizing circadian mesor- and amplitude-hypertension in apparently healthy men. Chronobiologia 11: 275-298.
6. Halberg F., Halberg E., Hermida Dominguez R.C., Halberg J., Cornélissen G., McCall W.C., McCall Y.R., März W., del Pozo Guerrero F. (1985): Chronobiologic blood pressure (BP) and heart rate (HR) self-monitoring at home, workplace, school and elsewhere. IEEE/7th Ann. Conf. Engineering in Medicine and Biology Society, Chicago, September 27-30, 1985, pp. 660-664.
7. Halberg F., Lagoguey M., Reinberg A. (1983): Human circannual rhythms over a broad spectrum of physiological processes. Int. J. Chronobiol. 8: 225-268.
8. Halberg F., Scheving L.E., Lucas E., Cornélissen G., Sothern R.B., Halberg E., Halberg J., Halberg Francine, Carter J., Straub K.D., Redmond D.P. (1984b): Chronobiology of human blood pressure in the light of static (room-restricted) automatic monitoring. Chronobiologia 11:

217-247.

9. Kolata G. (1983): Heart Research Briefing: What is the meaning of childhood hypertension? Science 220: 833.

10. Levine H., Cornélissen G., Halberg F., Bingham C. (1980): Self-measurement, automatic rhythmometry, transmeridian flights and aging. In: Chronobiology: Principles and Applications to Shifts in Schedules, L.E. Scheving, F. Halberg, eds., Sijthoff and Noordhoff, Alphen aan den Rijn, The Netherlands, pp. 371-392.

11. McCall V.R., McCall W.C. (this volume): Noninvasive chronobiological blood pressure measurements: clinical value and perspective.

12. Rosner B., Polk B.F. (1979): The implications of blood pressure variability for clinical and screening purposes. J. Chron. Dis. 32: 451-461.

13. Sothern R.B., Halberg F. (in press): Circadian and infradian blood pressure rhythms of a man 20-37 years of age. Proc. 2nd Int. Conf. Medico-Social Aspects of Chronobiology, Florence, Oct. 2, 1984.

14. Tobian L.M. (1968): Practical therapeutics: how to treat benign essential hypertension. GP 37: 124-132.

Blood pressure self-measurement in schools for chronobiologic discriminant analysis between two groups of children with and without family history of hypertension

Salvatore Romano*, Paolo Tommaso Scarpelli# and Franz Halberg†
Institutes of Medical Physics (*) and Medical Clinics (#), University of Florence, Italy; Chronobiology Laboratories, University of Minnesota (†)

Introduction

The purpose of this study is to verify the possibility and to quantify the degree of discrimination between two groups of primary school children, one of which is at risk of developing a high blood pressure (BP) as far as family history of hypertension is concerned. A self-measurement approach was considered of more practical use for an epidemiologic study as compared to the more reliable but more cumbersome automatic invasive or even indirect monitoring with currently available heavy instrumentation in 9-year-olds.

The second approach may in turn be used to ambulatorily follow those children who had been identified as "hypertensive" (or as having abnormally high BP) at the first screening.

Some precautions are needed to verify the reliability of the self-measurements. The criteria of self-consistency adopted in this study may be indirectly related to the compliance of the subjects to properly follow the protocol suggested.

Subjects and methods

The subjects studied are part of the 510 9-year-old students engaged in the first experiment made in Florentine schools in 1983 with the assistance and financial support of Provveditorato agli Studi of Florence and Regione Toscana. Measurements are available for systolic (S) BP, diastolic (D) BP and heart rate (HR) for one day at 2-h intervals from 07^{00} to 03^{00}. As a criterion of reliability and admittance to the study, the following conditions had to be met:

1) No missing data in any of the three variables measured.

2) Less than 9 equal measurements in each of the 3 time series collected.

According to an anamnestic questionnaire, 179 reference children (with no hypertensive and/or diabetic family history) and 130 children with pure hypertensive family history were included in the study.

The following statistical analyses were employed:

1) Each variable of the two groups was analyzed for circadian rhythm detection by the population mean-cosinor method (1) in order to check the significance of that cyclic component. The same analysis was performed on SBP x HR, DBP x HR, (SBP+DBP) x HR and (SBP-DBP) x HR. The last two should be related to some extent to the amount of work performed by the heart.

2) The two groups were compared by multivariate analysis of variance (2) taking as statistical variates the raw data themselves and the cartesian components of the amplitude-acrophase vector representing the individual circadian rhythm as it is detected by single cosinor (3).

3) A discriminant analysis was applied, using the method of Penrose reduction (4) of variates into two parameters defined as "size" and "shape". This reduction consists of 3 steps:

a) All data were normalized dividing each of them by the pooled within-group standard deviation at each timepoint.

b) The size is roughly the mean value between timepoints of all individual normalized data. It has some correspondence with the circadian MESOR.

c) The shape was computed as a linear combination of the individual normalized data with weighting coefficients

$$w_i = D_i/D - 1$$

where D_i is the mean difference of normalized data between two groups at time t_i and D is the overall mean. It has some correspondence with the time pattern (say the circadian component).

As source variates for discriminant analysis, the raw data of SBP, DBP and the pool were considered together with the cartesian components of the corresponding amplitude-acrophase vector.

Results

The results of the mean cosinor analysis are reported in Table 1. A statistically highly significant circadian rhythm is documented in both groups for all the variables analyzed, the only exception being DBP in the group at risk.

Table 1: Population-mean cosinor results: children without (N) or with (H) a family history of high BP

Variable	Group	MESOR (SD)	Amplitude (95% CL)	Acrophase (CL) (hr^{min})
SBP	N	105.2 (0.60)	1.79 (1.44, 2.13)	13^{23} (11^{43}, 15^{06})
(mm Hg)	H	105.0 (0.73)	2.97 (2.70, 3.23)	12^{14} (11^{04}, 13^{16})
DBP	N	67.5 (0.61)	0.12 ( )	12^{48} ( )
(mm Hg)	H	67.0 (0.78)	1.48 (0.47, 2.49)	13^{38} (10^{39}, 16^{05})
HR	N	74.4 (0.68)	4.65 (3.75, 5.55)	16^{31} (15^{49}, 17^{13})
(beats/min)	H	73.4 (1.83)	3.28 (1.01, 5.56)	15^{47} (13^{23}, 18^{27})
SBP x HR	N	130.6 (1.45)	9.69 (7.82, 11.6)	15^{55} (15^{11}, 16^{38})
(mm Hg/s)	H	129.4 (1.49)	11.7 (9.05, 14.1)	15^{48} (15^{08}, 16^{28})
DBP x HR	N	83.8 (1.09)	5.27 (3.72, 6.82)	16^{27} (15^{27}, 17^{30})
(mm Hg/s)	H	82.9 (1.32)	7.65 (5.60, 9.69)	16^{20} (15^{32}, 17^{07})
(SBP+DBP)xHR	N	214.4 (2.41)	14.9 (11.7, 18.2)	16^{06} (15^{20}, 16^{53})
(mm Hg/s)	H	212.3 (2.61)	19.2 (14.8, 23.5)	16^{01} (15^{21}, 16^{40})
(SBP-DBP)xHR	N	46.8 (0.88)	4.53 (3.35, 5.70)	15^{18} (14^{18}, 16^{21})
(mm Hg/s)	H	46.6 (1.05)	4.13 (2.67, 5.59)	14^{49} (13^{30}, 16^{17})

The results of the multivariate analysis of variance are reported in Table 2. The two groups are statistically significantly different with regard to both the raw BP data and the amplitude-acrophase vector. No difference was found for the remaining variables. According to the promising results obtained for BP, discriminant analyses should give good results as well.

Table 2: Multivariate analysis of variance

Variable	Raw data (11 d.f.) x^2	P	Single cosinor (2 d.f.) x^2	P
SBP	22.784*	<0.025	8.367*	<0.025
DBP	19.155	(0.1)	6.048	<0.05
HR	6.110	n.s.	4.517	n.s.
SBPxHR	8.116	n.s.	2.375	n.s.
DBPxHR	11.786	n.s.	5.385	(0.1)
(SBP+DBP)xHR	8.932	n.s.	3.933	n.s.
(SBP-DBP)xHR	9.057	n.s.	0.908	n.s.

Table 3 reports the levels of significance of the discriminating function and the proportions of the two groups, with respect to the overall median, for all the reduced variates considered.

The best, though still poor, discrimination is observed when the raw data of SBP and DBP are pooled, obtaining 22 variates before performing the Penrose reduction. In Figure 1, the corresponding cartesian plot of each individual point, in shape and size coordinates, is shown as well as the discriminating straight line. It is apparent that the size parameter is almost ineffective in the discrimination. This result is in keeping with the fact that the two populations do not differ with

Table 3: Statistical significance of discriminant function and distribution matrix (%)

Var.	P-value	Raw data Distribution matrix Family history of high BP No	Yes	P-value	(A,ø) from single cosinor analysis Distribution matrix Family history of high BP No	Yes
SBP	<.0002	75 (41.9)	80 (61.5)	<.02	83 (46.4)	72 (55.4)
		104 (58.1)	50 (38.5)		96 (53.6)	58 (44.6)
DBP	<.0003	78 (43.6)	77 (59.2)	<.05	78 (43.6)	77 (59.2)
		101 (56.4)	53 (40.8)		101 (56.4)	53 (40.8)
SBP & DBP	<.0001	74 (41.6)	81 (62.3)	<.004	76 (42.5)	79 (60.8)
		105 (58.7)	49 (37.7)		103 (57.5)	51 (39.2)

statistical significance when the circadian MESORs are compared. By contrast, the multivariate analysis of variance shows a statistically significant difference in the circadian rhythm, a result in keeping with the discrimination power of the shape parameter.

Figure 1: Discriminant analysis: Penrose variates reduction (shape and size). Systolic and diastolic BP (raw data) of children without (•) and with (*) family history of hypertension. Above: Gaussian distribution of discriminant functions; below: bivariate distributions of shape and size.

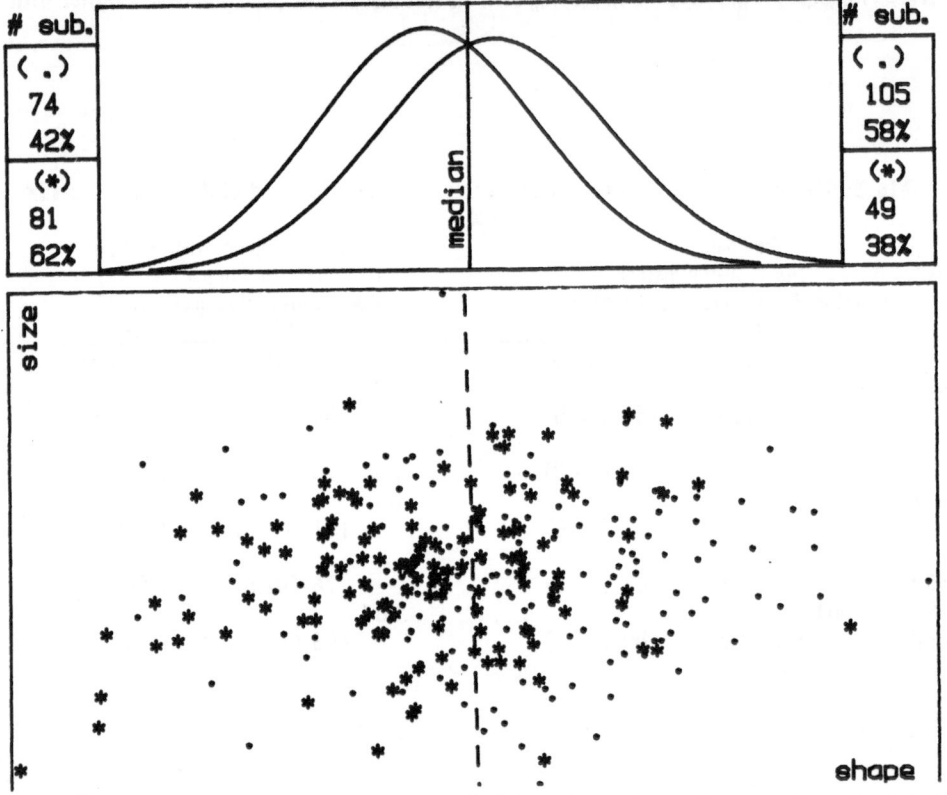

Conclusion

Some interesting results are found from the chronobiological point of view in the assessment of risk of developing hypertension on the basis of autometric measurements only, in that the two groups are shown to be different as far as the circadian rhythm is concerned, particularly the amplitude.

The discriminant analysis showed the highest significance of the discriminating function after pooling the SBP and DBP raw data. The least significance was found when using as variates the cartesian coordinates describing individual circadian rhythms. This result suggests that some information is lost in fitting the cosine function to the collected data.

The poor percentage of discrimination of the subjects in the two groups indicates that more sophisticated automatic measurements may be needed as a complement to autometry.

The use of several combinations of BP and HR failed to improve the discrimination. The product of BP x HR is a measure of the rate of the baric loading of arterial wall (systolic, diastolic or differential). As far as the circadian rhythm is concerned, the daily baric overloading (DBO) may be calculated, as exceeding area, by integration over the time span within which the rate is greater than a reference value (say the acrometron of the reference group). This new index is complementary to the hyperbaric index earlier proposed by Halberg et al. (5), which does not take heart rate into account.

The results concerning the distribution of DBO in the two groups studied are not presented in this paper because of the lack of significance as a discriminant parameter.

Independently of any discrimination between children with or without a family history of high BP, and despite the limitations of self-measurements in assessing the dynamics of BP variability, the value of teaching autorhythmometry at an early age has to be stressed. From an educative point of view, students gain a better understanding of the role of BP and the risk of developing cardiovascular diseases later in life. They also learn how to take BP and HR measurements, and thus acquire the necessary skills to monitor themselves and to detect any change in their BP, which may prompt earlier intervention. Autorhythmometry may thus lead the way toward primary prevention.

References

1. Halberg F., Tong Y.L., Johnson E.A.: Circadian system phase—an aspect of temporal morphology; procedures and illustrative examples. Proc. Int. Cong. Anatomists. In: The Cellular Aspects of Biorhythms, Symposium on Biorhythms, Springer-Verlag, 1967, pp. 20-48.
2. Radhakrishna Rao C.: Advanced Statistical Methods in Biometric Research. John Wiley and Sons, Inc., New York, 1952.
3. Halberg F., Halberg F., Johnson E.A., Nelson W., Runge W., Sothern R.: Autorhythmometry procedures for physiologic self-measurements and their analysis. Physiol. Tchr. 1: 1-11, 1972.
4. Penrose S.L.: Some notes on discrimination. Ann. Eugenics 13: 228-237, 1947.
5. Halberg F., Ahlgren A., Haus E.: Circadian systolic and diastolic hyperbaric indices of high school and college students. Chronobiologia 11: 299-309, 1984.

INSTRUMENTATION FOR HUMAN BLOOD PRESSURE RHYTHM ASSESSMENT BY SELF-MEASUREMENT

P.T. Scarpelli*, S. Romano*, R. Livi*, L. Scarpelli*, G. Cornélissen¶, M. Cagnoni*, F. Halberg¶

*Istituto di Clinica Medica Generale e Terapia Medica II, Florence, Italy
¶Chronobiology Laboratories, University of Minnesota, Minneapolis, MN, USA

Introduction

Herein, we wish to document the need for instrumentation for autorhythmometry, notably of blood pressure (BP). Autorhythmometry has been introduced by us in schools, in the home and in the clinic. Despite obvious limitations of the existing instrumentation, the merits of autorhythmometry pertain to (early) diagnosis, (optimal) treatment and, first and foremost, to prevention, as illustrated by the following results.

Autorhythmometry in schools: a step toward prevention of high blood pressure

We have taught 9-year-old students in Florence how to self-measure their systolic (S) and diastolic (D) BP. An Erkameter, a mercury sphygmomanometer, manufactured in Bad Tölz, Germany, was used to that effect. In this endeavor, students learned how to take their BP and became aware of the importance of measuring their BP around the clock in view of the existence of rhythms in several important body functions. Moreover, they gained insight into the risks associated with an elevated BP. At a very early age, these children thus were introduced to self-help for health care.

From an epidemiologic viewpoint, family histories of these children, regarding cardio-cerebro-reno-vascular disease risk, were obtained by asking them to answer questionnaires. This aspect of the study aimed at obtaining information concerning any correlate of BP values and BP rhythm characteristics with the epidemiologically assessed risk of developing cardiovascular diseases.

Results indicated that in the absence of any difference in overall mean (rhythm-adjusted mean or MESOR), the circadian amplitude (A) and acrophase (ø) of SBP differed in children with or without a family history of high BP. This difference primarily came about because of a higher amplitude in children with a family history of high BP (Scarpelli et al., in press). This result is interesting in view of previous evidence pointing to an elevation of the circadian BP amplitude preceding an elevation of overall BP mean. The first evidence for an increase in circadian amplitude prior to an increase in overall BP mean was observed in the handled stroke-prone SHR-SP rat (J. Halberg et al., 1980). A higher circadian amplitude of diastolic BP was observed in black children as compared to matched Caucasian children (Ramlow et al., 1985). This result is to be aligned with the high risk of developing diseases associated with a high BP in black populations. On the basis of automatic instrumentation for BP monitoring, the circadian amplitude was found to first respond to intervention, before observing a response in the overall BP mean. One example concerns the circadian rhythm of systolic BP following salt restriction in a MESOR-hypertensive man (Lee et al., 1982). An increase in the circadian amplitude of BP may also occur in response to cessation of treatment (switch from a ß-blocker to a placebo) (Scarpelli et al., 1978a and b). Similarly, circadian amplitude-hypertension may signal an incomplete therapeutic effect (Halberg et al., in press a).

The results of our study in 9-year-olds, discussed in more detail elsewhere (Romano et al., this volume; Scarpelli et al., in press), prompted the following recommendations:

1. Digital sphygmomanometers should be preferred to avoid problems in hearing the Korotkoff sounds and to avoid digit preference in BP readings.

2. Samples by night are important for the correct evaluation of the circadian amplitude.

Awaiting cheaper automatic instrumentation, self-monitoring within a family may be preferable, where another family member takes the measurements by night to avoid interference of the BP recording with the awakening of the subject.

3. Preference for a 48-h or longer recording span over a 24-h profile. Day-to-day variation in BP MESOR is indeed not uncommon, even under standardized conditions such as hospitalization (Carandente et al., in press).

Once the discipline and know-how of self-measurements are acquired, low-cost equipment with data storage capability is most useful. Del Pozo et al. (1983) describe a microprocessor-based system for self-measurement applications, called the autochronor. Ideally, such a system should offer capabilities for 1) multivariate data acquisition and 2) the implementation of a sampling sequence that can be automatically programmed from a local time routine serving the multiple purposes of a) programming the sampling sequence, with eventually a varying sampling rate; b) calling attention of the subject to prompt the start of the measuring routine; c) time-coding of measurements; d) time-keeping of special events (diary); and e) assessing the time elapsed to complete performance tasks.

With such equipment on hand, it should become possible to establish individualized reference values that serve for the prevention of cardiovascular complications later in life, before disease sets in. Once a heightened risk is recognized, blood pressure monitoring by automatic ambulatory instrumentation is advocated.

Autorhythmometry in the home and clinic

Daily self-measurements of BP at regular intervals for an appropriate length of time has proved to be an easy and well-accepted procedure by our patients (Scarpelli et al., 1978b). Several kinds of information can be obtained from the data so collected. First, the reliability of the diagnosis is improved and the efficacy of the treatment can be monitored more closely. Second, patients themselves can immediately determine the results of treatment. Therefore, it is usually accepted with true enthusiasm.

Autorhythmometry also serves the purpose of assessing the individual responsiveness to therapy. Using a chronobiologic protocol based on five-times-a-day autometric data gathering and weekly processing by computerized methods, the recurrent monitoring of individual responsiveness under habitual life conditions and the accomplishment of a personalized dose adjustment were reached in one renovascular and four primary hypertension patients treated with prazosin (Romano et al., 1981). The response to treatment of the renovascular patient is noteworthy in that the BP average decrease was accompanied by a nearly threefold augmentation of the circadian BP amplitude.

Around-the-clock monitoring of BP is also helpful in properly timing treatment. Treatment was adjusted in chronobiologic fashion in a 61-year-old patient with established MESOR-hypertension (Halberg et al., in press b). In this particular case, BP, monitored automatically, was found to be elevated in relation to a time-specified reference interval. An index of BP excess, defined as the hyperbaric index (HBI), representing the excess BP above the critical threshold, integrated over 24 hours (Halberg et al., 1984), was computed for each 24-h profile, as were 3-hourly fractionated HBIs, showing that the excess BP occurred primarily at night. Hence, this elevation escaped notice in check-ups at noon. Once recognized, the treatment was optimized by timing medication (Schaffer et al., 1985). The timing of BP elevation may be important since Kobrin et al. (1984) reported that the prevalence of clinical cardiovascular complications was 43% (6/14) in those elderly patients with essential hypertension who had a decrease by night and 100% (7/7) in those patients with a nocturnal increase in pressure.

The following two sections illustrate the usefulness of autometry accompanied by the derivation of chronobiologic indices in the clinic. |One example pertains to the monitoring of patients with malignant hypertension, the other describes a case of iatrogenous reversible MESOR-hypertension.

1. Monitoring of patients with malignant hypertension

Ten patients with malignant hypertension self-measured their BP and heart rate (HR) several times a day for several days. Table 1 provides the clinical information concerning these patients.

Table 1: Clinical data of male patients with malignant hypertension

ID	Family history of high BP	Age at diagnosis	Age at start of Rx	Treatment (Rx) (dose/day)	Comment
CB01	no	44	49	900 μg Clonidine 75 mg Hydralazine	left ventricular hypertrophy
GU02	yes	20	42	1200 μg Clonidine 4 mg Prazosin 20 mg Frusemide	Rx modifications discontinuation of self-measurement; died at age 47 of cerebral hemorrhage
GF03	no	47	48	450 μg Clonidine 32.5 mg Hydralazine	Rx modification Left ventricular hypertrophy
MR04	-	35	35	600 μg Clonidine 100 mg Hydralazine	Rx modification; died at age 36 of cerebral hemorrhage
CG05	-	43	43 56*	Clortalidone 600 μg Clonidine	signs of heart failure at age 56; discontinuation of self-measurement
PS06	-	46	46	1200 μg Clonidine 100 mg Hydralazine	discontinuation of self-measurement
PA07	-	17	17	450 μg Clonidine 100 mg Hydralazine	bilateral vesico-ureteric reflux found at age 8
TA08	yes	45	50	Propranolol & Hydralazine	myocardial infarction at age 52; Rx modification; discontinuation of self-measurement
GA09	yes	43	44	1200 μg Clonidine 200 mg Hydralazine 4 mg Prazosin 60 mg Frusemide	left ventricular hyper-trophy; died at age 46 of myocardial infarction
MG10	no	20	24*	600 μg Clonidine 100 mg Hydralazine	ventricular hypertrophy low compliance died at age 25 of cerebral hemorrhage

*Age of patient at first observation accompanied by self-measurement.

The self-measured BP and HR data were analyzed by the single cosinor method (Halberg et al., 1977), to derive estimates of MESOR (overall 24-h mean), amplitude (measure of predictable extent of change around the MESOR) and acrophase (measure of timing of overall high values), Table 2. These rhythm parameters served to compute the HBI against peer-group time-specified reference limits (Halberg et al., 1984). The MESOR, amplitude and HBI were further compared between those patients who died from cardiovascular complications (n=4) and those who are still alive (n=6).

As can be seen from Table 2, the circadian amplitude tends to be higher in the patients who died from cardiovascular diseases than in those who are still alive. A statistically significant difference in the circadian amplitude is observed for DBP ($P=.017$), while for SBP, the difference is of borderline statistical significance ($P=.103$).

A population-mean cosinor (Halberg et al., 1977), Table 3, indicates that HR is practically out of phase with SBP and DBP. The fact that BP excess peaks at night and that SBP and DBP both have their acrophase by night, although a population rhythm cannot be established for SBP and DBP in the ten patients with malignant hypertension, is noteworthy.

Table 2: Circadian blood pressure characteristics of patients with malignant hypertension*

	Systolic BP				Diastolic BP			
	M	A	ø	HBI	M	A	ø	HBI
Patients who are still alive (group 1)								
CB 01	236.6	2.13	-19°	2303	131.5	1.35	-75°	921
GF 03	200.6	4.26	-151°	1439	131.4	1.82	-199°	920
CG 05	213.3	1.45	-9°	1745	119.8	1.84	-332°	641
PS 06	220.7	4.05	-40°	1923	124.7	5.24	-89°	758
PA 07	210.2	5.23	-234°	1670	124.6	1.42	-185°	757
TA 08	210.1	4.58	-25°	1668	123.3	1.12	-323°	725
Patients who died from cardiovascular complications (group 2)								
GU 02	229.9	8.27	-20°	2144	148.7	6.12	-356°	1336
MR04	218.9	5.64	-57°	1879	148.9	3.26	-25°	1339
GA 09	193.5	6.45	-185°	1269	111.0	6.62	-183°	430
MG 10	181.9	2.78	-301°	991	127.2	4.46	-276°	818

Comparison of circadian blood pressure characteristics between the two groups **

	Systolic BP			Diastolic BP		
	$(\bar{Y}_2 - \bar{Y}_1)$	t	P	$(\bar{Y}_2 - \bar{Y}_1)$	t	P
MESOR (mm Hg)	-9.2	0.85	0.418	8.1	1.05	0.323
Amplitude (mm Hg)	2.17	1.84	0.103	2.98	2.99	0.017
HBI (mm Hg x h)	-221	0.85	0.418	193	1.05	0.323

*M=MESOR; A=Amplitude; ø=Acrophase (360°=24 h; 0°=local midnight); M and A expressed in mm Hg; HBI=24h hyperbaric index expressed in mm Hg x h.
** $(\bar{Y}_2 - \bar{Y}_1)$ =Difference in mean between group 1 $(\bar{Y}_1)$ and group 2 $(\bar{Y}_2)$; t = Student t statistic.

Table 3: Population-mean cosinor of cardiovascular variables in ten patients with malignant hypertension*

Variable	PR	P	M ± SE	A (95% CI)		ø (95% CI)	
SBP	5	0.664	211.6 ± 5.2	1.26	( )	-39°	( )
DBP	6	0.969	129.1 ± 3.8	0.28	( )	-10°	( )
HR	14	0.006	73.7 ± 3.0	2.89	(0.78; 5.62)	-237°	(-212°; -313°)
HBI:SBP	73	<.001	213. ±16.	36.5	(24.8; 48.7)	-52°	(-40; -68)
HBI:DBP	70	.001	108. ±11.	17.7	(8.8; 26.8)	-33°	(-10; -64)

*PR=Percent Rhythm; M=MESOR; A=Amplitude; ø=Acrophase (360°=24 h; 0°=local midnight); SE=standard error; CI=confidence interval; M and A are expressed in mm Hg (SBP and DBP), in beats/min (HR) and in mm Hg x h (HBI); rhythm parameters for HBI determined by fitting a 24-h cosine curve to 3-hourly fractionated HBIs; the fact that the HBI was computed against time-specified reference limits may have contributed in part to the statistical significance of its circadian rhythm; results of population-mean cosinor are of ordering value only, in view of the difference in amplitude found between patients who died and those who are still alive, and who were pooled for the purpose of this analysis focusing on the timing of overall high values.

2. Iatrogenous reversible 'MESOR-hypertension'

On January 18, 1985, a 20-year-old man was admitted to the Hospital of the University of Florence for "hypertension" without any relevant family history. A high BP had been discovered four months earlier, when treatment was started with a daily dose of 25 mg of a diuretic (Clortalidone), taken after getting up. The patient had suffered from rhinitis since May 1984. In June 1984, he started to inhale, 2-4 times per day, a decongestant (Biorinil) containing fluoroprednisolone and a vasoconstrictor, as well as an antihistamine and an antibiotic. The patient showed hypokalemia with an increased urinary potassium excretion. The inhalant was continued during the first 6 days in the hospital and discontinued thereafter. Autorhythmometry was started on the day of hospitalization, with 5 BP measurements per day, at 08^{00}, 12^{00}, 16^{00}, 20^{00} and 00^{00}. A 24-h urine aldosterone determination was also obtained daily. Aldosterone was highest while the patient was on the drug (11.63 nM/L) and dropped to 7.8 nM/L after 15 days off the drug (usual value range: 0.19-0.97). Plasma potassium rose and urinary potassium declined following treatment removal ($P<.05$). Chronobiologic serial sections (Halberg et al., 1977), carried out to follow the time course of SBP, DBP and HR, showed decreasing trends in MESOR, Table 4.

Table 4: Decrease in blood pressure and heart rate after discontinuance of an inhalant decongestant

Variable	Decrease (per day)	Correlation r	P	Estimated MESOR Last day before discontinuance of treatment	After 19 days off treatment
SBP (mm Hg)	2.04	.973	<.001	152	111
DBP (mm Hg)	1.37	.947	<.001	100	73
HR (beats/min)	0.58	.558	<.01	88	76*

*HR tended to increase again toward the end of the monitoring span.

The HBI computed with reference to peer-group reference limits showed decreasing trends: before discontinuance of Rx, the HBIs were 269 (SBP) and 160 (DBP) mm Hg x h, while no BP excess was found for the last 4 days of the monitoring span (Scarpelli et al., 1985).

Conclusions

Chronobiology offers tools for an individualized objective and positive quantification of health by the inferential statistical estimation of rhythm characteristics. The clinical data discussed herein illustrate the need to monitor BP around-the-clock for several days or weeks to assess the response to intervention on an individualized basis. Moreover, evidence is presented of the need for automatic monitoring to recognize BP elevation at odd hours. The question remains in this era of automatic ambulatory monitoring whether recorders operating over long spans may not be more appropriate than those currently available providing 24-hour records. A combination of automatic monitoring and autorhythmometry may serve as a compromise while awaiting cheaper and lighter instrumentation. The wealth of data collected with automatic monitors should also be exploited by wedding appropriate software for their analysis to the existing hardware. Chronobiologic indices accounting for the rhythmic behavior of BP indeed allows focus not only on a 24-h (static) mean, but also on the dynamics of BP variability. Since rhythm alteration may indeed precede an overall elevation of BP mean, early clues as to a heightened risk of cardiovascular complications may thus be provided. Moreover, once disease has set in, chronobiology also provides means to optimize treatment timing and to gauge response to treatment of the individual patient. Instrumentation of the future, allowing for strategic BP sampling over long spans, light enough not to hinder the patient, but with the capability of recording, storing, analyzing and summarizing the data as one goes, according to a chronobiologic design to examine the spectral structure of the data and determine any BP excess with respect to time-specified reference limits, could thus serve the multiple purposes of early diagnosis, treatment optimization and prevention.

References

1. Carandente F., Ferrario G., Ferrario V.F., Giani P., Vizzotto L., Halberg F., März W., Cornélissen G., Schaffer E.M. (in press): Infradian, mostly circaseptan profiles for the diagnosis and treatment of blood pressure elevation. 2nd Eur. Meeting on Hypertension, Milan, Italy, June 9-12, 1985.
2. Del Pozo F., Perez Subias M., Halberg F., Burillo V., Hermida Dominguez R.C. (1983):

Microprocessor-based system for self-measurement applications. Proc. 5th Ann. Conf. IEEE Engineering in Medicine and Biology Society, Columbus, OH, September 10-12, 1983, pp. 413-418.

3. Halberg F., Carandente F., Cornélissen G., Katinas G.S. (1977): Glossary of chronobiology. Chronobiologia 4, Suppl. 1, 189 pp.

4. Halberg F., Drayer J.I.M., Cornélissen G., Weber M.A. (1984): Cardiovascular reference data base for recognizing circadian mesor- and amplitude-hypertension in apparently healthy men. Chronobiologia 11: 275-298.

5. Halberg F., Halberg E., Carandente F., Cornélissen G., März W., Halberg J., Drayer J., Weber M., Schaffer E., Scarpelli P., Tarquini B., Cagnoni M., Tuna N. (in press b): Dynamic indices from blood pressure monitoring for prevention, diagnosis and therapy. In: Proc. Int. Symp. Ambulatory Monitoring, Padua, March 29-30, 1985.

6. Halberg F., McCall Y., McCall W., Sothern R.B. (in press a): Circadian amplitude-hypertension signals incomplete therapeutic MESOR reduction and need for timing beta-blockers. Proc. Int. Soc. Chronobiol., Little Rock, Ark., USA, Nov. 3-6, 1985. Chronobiologia.

7. Halberg J., Halberg E., Hayes D.K., Smith R.D., Halberg F., Delea C.S., Danielson R.S., Bartter F.C. (1980): Schedule shifts, life quality and quantity—modeled by murine blood pressure elevation and arthropod lifespan. Int. J. Chronobiol. 7: 17-64.

8. Kobrin I., Dunn F.G., Oigman W., Kumar A., Ventura H.O., Messerli F.H., Frohlich E.D. (1984): Essential hypertension in the elderly: circadian variation of arterial pressure. In: Ambulatory Blood Pressure Monitoring, M.A. Weber, J.I.M. Drayer, eds., Springer-Verlag, New York, pp. 181-185.

9. Lee J.Y., Gillum R.F., Cornélissen G., Koga Y., Halberg F. (1982): Individualized assessment of circadian rhythm characteristics of human blood pressure and pulse after moderate salt and weight restriction. In: Toward Chronopharmacology, Proc. 8th IUPHAR Cong. and Sat. Symposia, Nagasaki, July 27-28, 1981, R. Takahashi, F. Halberg and C. Walker, eds., Pergamon Press, Oxford/New York, pp. 375-390.

10. Ramlow J., Halberg F., Prineas R., Mandel J. (1985): Automatic circadian 24-h profiles of systolic & diastolic pressure and radial pulse in black & white boys. Chronobiologia 12:76-77.

11. Romano S., Gizdulich P., Scarpelli P.T. (1981): Use of an autorhythmometric experimental design to achieve individual adjustment of antihypertensive treatment. Meth. and Find. Exp. Clin. Pharmacol. 3: 223-231.

12. Romano S., Scarpelli P.T., Halberg F. (this volume): Blood pressure self-measurement in schools for chronobiologic discriminant analysis between two groups of children with and without family history of hypertension.

13. Scarpelli P.T., Livi R., Scarpelli L., Cagnoni M., Romano S., Cornélissen G., Halberg F. (1985): Decongestant-associated aldosteronism and high blood pressure (BP) described and quantified by autorhythmometry. Proc. Int. Soc. Chronobiol., Little Rock, Ark., USA, Nov. 3-6, 1985. Chronobiologia 12: 271.

14. Scarpelli P.T., Romano S., Buricchi L., Corti C., Menniti P., Gizdulich P. (1978a): Controllo dell'effetto antiipertensive del prazosin mediante autoritmometria della pressione arteriosa. In: Problemi e Prospettive dell'Ipertensione Arteriosa, C. Bartorelli, A. Bertelli, A. Giotti, U. Teodori, eds., ESAM, Rome, pp. 173-190.

15. Scarpelli P.T., Romano S., Lamanna S., Buricchi L., Cai M.G. (1978b): Autorhythmometry in hypertension: some methodological aspects and clinical implications. Chronobiologia 5: 407-424.

16. Scarpelli P.T., Romano S., Cagnoni M., Livi R., Scarpelli L., Croppi E., Regioni F., März W., Halberg F. (in press): Blood pressure self-measurement as part of instruction in the Regione Toscana. Proc. 2nd Int. Conf. Medico-Social Aspects of Chronobiology, Florence, Oct. 2, 1984.

17. Schaffer E.M., Cornélissen G., Halberg F. (1985): Chronobiologic indices for treatment of MESOR-hypertension. Proc. Int. Soc. Chronobiol., Little Rock, Ark., Nov. 3-6, 1985. Chronobiologia 12: 272.

CHRONOBIOLOGIC ELECTROCARDIOGRAPHIC MONITORING
IMPLICATIONS TO SCREENING AND TREATMENT IN THE CORONARY
ARTERY DISEASE

U.MANZOLI,   M. LUCENTE, A.G. REBUZZI
Cardiology Department-Catholic University "S.Coure" Roma-Italy

The Holter system of ECG monitoring plays an important role in the screening, diagnosis and treatment of coronary heart disease (CHD).

In the majority of cases, the diagnosis of angina pectoris is clinical: description of characteristic features of the pain (quality, localization, and propagation, short duration time) is usually sufficient for diagnosis. However, to confirm the suspicion of angina requires objective evidence of ischemic attacks. For this purpose, ECG is the most practical method.

Of course, since ischemic attacks are transient and consequently cause transient electrical changes, the ECG to be positive, must be made during the ischemic event. This can be achieved in clinical practice by recording the ECG after induction of an ischemic attack by means of a provocative test, or by prolonging the ECG until the ischemic event spontaneously occurs. This has become possible since the introduction of dynamic ECG monitoring. The Holter system allows us to recognize that the majority of ischemic attacks occur without any symptoms ("silent angina"); on this account only prolonged ECG recording allows us to record full documentary evidence. Besides this, Holter ECG allows us to characterize the attack (type of signal, time and value of ECG changes), to observe its trend in time, to evaluate the occurence of ischemic attacks during the stresses of daily life and to note the effects of medical treatment.

Continuous ECG monitoring emphasizes the extreme variability of ECG signals to which the spontaneous ischemic attack may give rise.

Although transient ST-segment elevation, described by Prinzmetal as typical of the "variant form", is the ECG feature most frequently observed (in about 70% of events), spontaneous ischemic attacks may also manifest transient ST-segment depression, or transient T-wave changes (voltage increasing, flattening, inversion, "normalization" of abnormal T-wave in the basic ECG tracing). All these different morphologic aspects may also appear in the same patient, or on the other hand it is possible that one patient may manifest all attacks with the same ECG feature.

Myocardial perfusion imaging studies (by means of ionic tracers such as thallium 201) have shown that attacks with ST-segment elevation, T wave pseudo-normalization or increased T-wave voltage , are always related to a massive,transmural reduction of myocardial perfusion. In these cases, there is good correlation between the ECG localization of the ischemic signal and localization of the perfusion imaging defect. Ischemic attacks characterized by ST segment depression appear to be related to smaller perfusion defects, remaining presumably restricted to subendocardium. In this case, it is common to observe a dissociation between localization of the ECG changes and site of the perfusion defect.

As to the other signals to which an ischemic attack may be related, such as T-wave flattening and/or inversion, their pathophysiologic significance is not yet clearly known, but probably is also a matter of subendocardial ischemia.

The different distribution of myocardial ischemia-transmural or subendocardial- and consequent ECG features of the ischemic attack, are correlated with the severity and localization of obstruction, with the basic conditions of coronary circulation, and with the presence or absence of collaterals.

Ischemic attacks with ST-segment elevation, T wave pseudo-normalization or T-wave voltage increasing are generally correlated with severe spasm of one main coronary vessel. Those with ST segment depression may be due to a less severe spasm of one main coronary artery, or to an occlusive or subocclusive spasm of one minor guage artery, or to occulusive spasm of one main vessel, when this happens in a coronary tree with fixed obstruction and well-developed collaterals, which partially counterbalance the reduction of the flow produced by spasm.

We have applied the principles of chronobiology to computerized dynamic ECG monitoring, in order to "microscopically" identify the phenomena of ischemia of the heart. The aim of the study was to evaluate whether frequency of ischemic attacks might have any identifiable distribution during 24 hour period, and if ventricular premature beats might have any circadian variation. Whether circadian variation is present in some or in all ischemic patients has diagnostic and therapeutic implications, and may be useful in planning cardiovascular therapy.

MATERIALS AND METHODS

The study population consisted of 65 patients hospitalized with ischemic heart disease (43 patients with primary angina, 10 with effort angina and 12 patients with acute myocardial infarction (AMI)).

All the subjects were synchronized to the hospital routine, adhering to a common schedule. In all patients (except in subjects with acute myocardial infarction) the Holter ECG recorder was applied the day before the beginning of the experiment in order to avoid stress.

In 39 patients with primary angina, Holter ECG monitoring was applied for 24 hours. In four patients monitoring was prolonged for 168 hours and in one patient for 360 hours. In all patients the diagnosis of primary angina was confirmed by angiographic studies.

312

For effort angina, 10 patients were studied with bicycle stress tests twice a day (in the morning and in the afternoon) and after they performed a 24 hour Holter ECG monitoring.

For myocardial infarction 12 patients, aged 51-66 years, performed Holter ECG monitoring in the 1st-7th-14th and 21st day after AMI, to evaluate frequency, periodicity and characteristics of VPB's.

Three patients, that needed lidocaine therapy, were excluded from the first recording and 1 subject, that needed mexilitine therapy from the 17th day after AMI, was excluded from the last recording.

RESULTS

PRIMARY ANGINA

24 hour ECG D: 315 ischemic attacks (120 asymptomatic) were observed in 39 patients; there were ST-segment depressions in 198 recordings and ST-segment elevation in 32. T waves were inverted in 85 recordings (Fig. 1.). Chronobiologic analysis documented circadian rhythm of all ischemic attacks with Acrophase at -101.5 degrees, Mesor of 6.47 and Amplitude of 7.5. No circadian periodicity of symptomatic attacks (about 30%) was shown. Blood pressure and heart rate also showed circadian rhythms.

168 hour ECG D (Fig. 2.): The ECG monitoring was prolonged for one week in 4 of 39 patients and 218 ischemic attacks were observed (153 asymptomatic and 65 symptomatic). These attacks were accompanied by ST-depression 120 times and with a ST-elevation 139 times. In one patient there was an inverted T-wave. Circadian periodicity was documented only in 1 patient.

360 hour ECG D: In a single patient with 15 days Holter ECG monitoring, 60 ischemic attacks were documented (36 with ST elevation and 24 with ST depression) (Fig.3.) Cosinor analysis revealed a periodic variation of HR of QRS and of SVT.

EFFORT ANGINA

The stress test ST segment depression was greater in the morning trial session than in the afternoon (2.3 mm versus 1.7 mm). The pressure-rate product on exercise was higher in the afternoon than in the morning. The workload was also higher in the afternoon. After treatment with molsidomine the ST-segment displacement on stress test ECG was significantly reduced, without significant differences between the morning and the afternoon. The pressure-rate product was decreased in the morning as in the afternoon. Holter ECG monitoring showed in all the patients a circadian rhythm of ST displacement with an acrophase of the group at -105 degrees, a mesor of 7.4 and an amplitude of 1.04. After treatment, this circadian rhythm disappeared.

MYOCARDIAL INFARCTION

The mean HR and VPB frequency on the 1st-7th-14th and 21st day after AMI are reported in table 1 and table 2. There was a positive significant correlation between mean HR and mean PVBs frequency on the second, third, and fourth recording. No correlation was found in the first recording. (Fig.4.).

The chronobiological analysis of the data showed, on the 7th day after AMI, a circadian rhythm of HR with acrophase at -242.37 degrees, mesor of 68.9 and amplitude of 48.2. VPBs showed a circadian rhythm only in 8 patients with acrophase at -253.77 degrees, mesor of 60.13 and amplitude of 36.74.   On the 14th and 21st day after AMI all the patients presented circadian rhythm of HR while it was demonstrated for VPBs in 9 and 10 patients respectively.

No circadian rhythm was shown on the first day.

DISCUSSION

Angina pectoris is caused by an acute and transient imbalanace between coronary blood flow and myocardial O_2 demand.

The first description of this clinical picture, which represents one of the clinical forms of ischemic heart disease, was by Heberden in 1768. This kind of angina, triggered by exercise or other conditions to increase the O_2 myocardial demand, is the classical "effort angina". Today this is called "secondary angina", since the attack is secondary to an increasing myocardial O_2 demand not matched by a proportional increasing of flow because the presence of critical coronary stenosis.

More recently, another form of angina has been documented, characterized by chest pain attacks without apparent relation to increased myocardial O_2 demand. This kind of angina has been called ("spontaneous reduction of flow without increasing of myocardial O_2 demand).

First in 1959 Prinzmetal described the characteristic features of this other kind of angina, which was called "variant angina", as opposed to classical Heberden's effort angina. In the Prinzmetal's picture, the "variant" form is characterized by pain at rest, or during activites which do not significantly increase myocardial O_2 demand. The ECG shows transient ST-segment elevation, i.e. on opposed signal in front of the usual ST-segment depression of the "effort angina". Prinzmetal believed that the "variant form" of angina was due to coronary spasm. In recent years, several studies have better established the clinical and ECG features of spontaneous angina, and they show it's extreme variablity.

PRIMARY ANGINA

In Japan where primary angina is present in approximately 25% of all patients with angina (1), a pattern of circadian variation with most attacks occuring in the early morning hours, has been described both for spontaneous and provoked attacks (6-12).

In our experience we have found a circadian rhythm of spontaneous attacks in 39 patients with primary angina with acrophase in the early morning hours, has been described both for spontaneous and provoked attacks (6-12).

In our subjects, blood pressure and HR have different acrophases and this result suggests that there are different mechanisms underlying these different periodicities.

Jansen and co-workers have demonstrated that there is a circadian variation of the tone of the large coronary arteries in patients with Prinzmetal's "variant angina". The tone of vascular smooth muscle (including that a coronary artery) depends on the presence of calcium ions which are required for activation of miofibrillar ATPase. Physiologically, a highly potent CA^{++} – antagonistic action is exerted by H^+ In the early morning, metabolism decreases and H^+, which are produced by metabolism, also decrease, wheras in the afternoon metabolism increases and H^+ increase. This may be related to circadian variation in the tone of large coronary arteries. There are many other factors that might play a role in the genesis of circadian variation of arterial tone. Several hormones and minerals undergo a daily variation of their concentration and particularly Ca^{++} reaches a peak in the morning. Involvement of autonomic nervous system has been postulated as a pathophysiologic mechanism. The importance of "intrinsic rhythms" of myocardial cells has been demonstrated by Kraft and by Solensky and our results in patients with angina support this.

EFFORT ANGINA

Our study confirms the presence of a circadian variation in exercise capacity and in ST-segment displacement with a higher exercise tolerance in the afternoon when compared to the morning. These data are in agreement with the acrophases of myocardial ischemia founded at 7:00 a.m. by 24 hour Holter monitoring.

Because sympathetic discharge occurs in response to exercise and stimulation of alpha adrenergic receptors is known to result in coronary spasm, it is possible that vasoconstriction also plays an important role in the pathogenesis of effort angina.

Pharmacologic treatment produces a significant increase in exercise tolerance with reduction of the ST-segment depression and suppresses the difference between responses to exercise in the morning and the afternoon.

The effect of treatment with Molsidomine may be due to the drug effect on the prolonged elevation of CGMP levels. A part of the action of the drug could be also related to an improvement in the prostacycline/TXA2 equilibrium provoked by Molsidomine.

MYOCARDIAL INFARCTION

Our study shows a remarkable correlation between PVB frequency and underlying HR. This correlation is present in only two patients in the first day after AMI, but is seen in an increasing number of subjects on subsequent days. Our observations do not permit statements about the mechanism of the observed relationship, but one may speculate.

There might be increased ischemia at faster HRs with increasing conduction delay, which could cause reentrant VPBs. On the other hand the higher sympathetic drive, associated with higher HR, might accentuate phase 4 diastolic depolarization and might permit the emergence of VPBs due to enhanced automaticity.

Chronobiologic data obtained for HR show no difference from those reported in healthy or cardiopathic patients. Only

on the first day did we   not observe circadian variation of
HR. It is   possible that the absence of synchronisation plays
an important role.

The literature has been conflicting with respect to VPB
frequency. Three studies focused on patients with recent
myocardial infarction and found ventricular ectopy increased
or unchanged during the day. The mechanisim responsible for
this diurnal variation in ventricular irritability have not
been elucidated, but probably are mainly related to
sympathetic withdrawal and lessening of higher central nervous
system activity occuring during the sleep. These effects may
result in an elevation of the ventricular stimulation
threshold.

Our observation of a diurnal pattern of VPBs in
increasing number of patients from the first to the last
monitoring may be due to the possibility that particular
active disease states may produce ventricular irritation which
over-rides the general effect of the sleeping state. As for
the HR, the circadian variability is "normalized" during the
following days when the patient's rhythms return to normal
pattern.

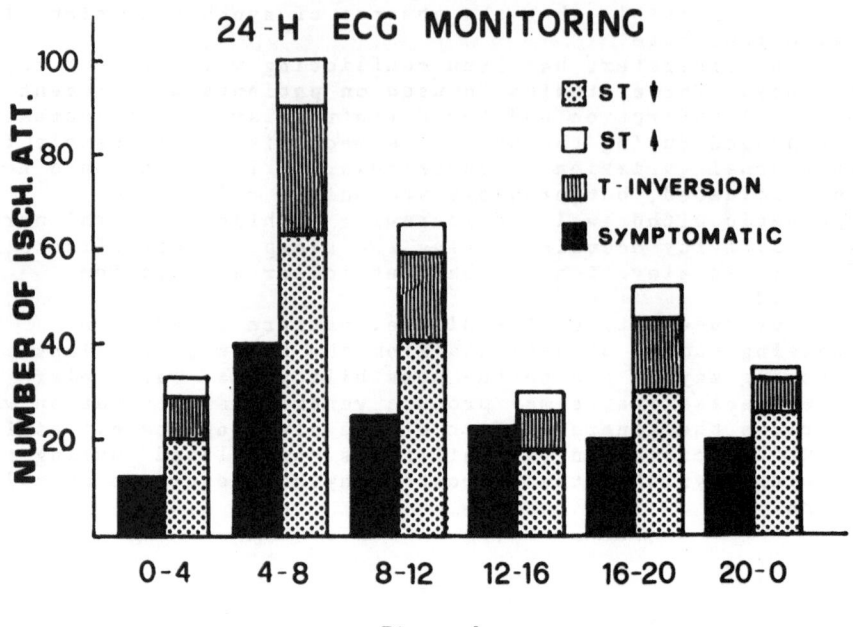

Figure 1

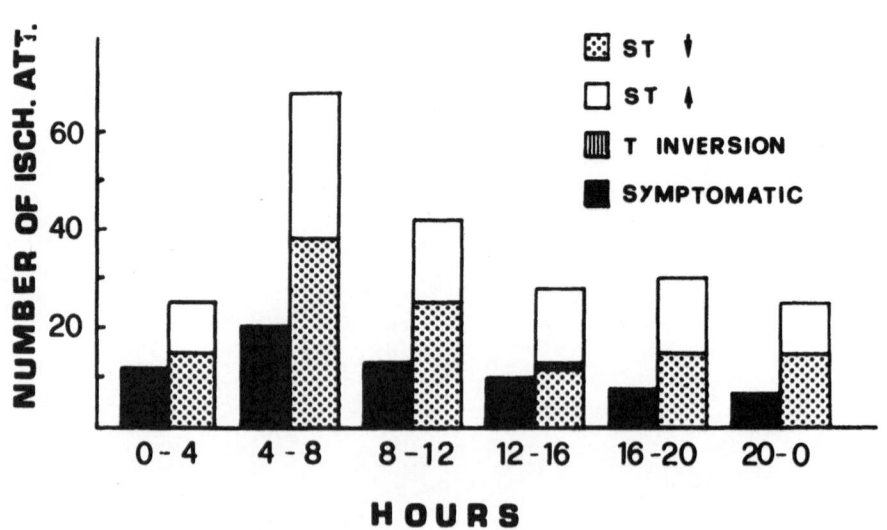

Figure 2

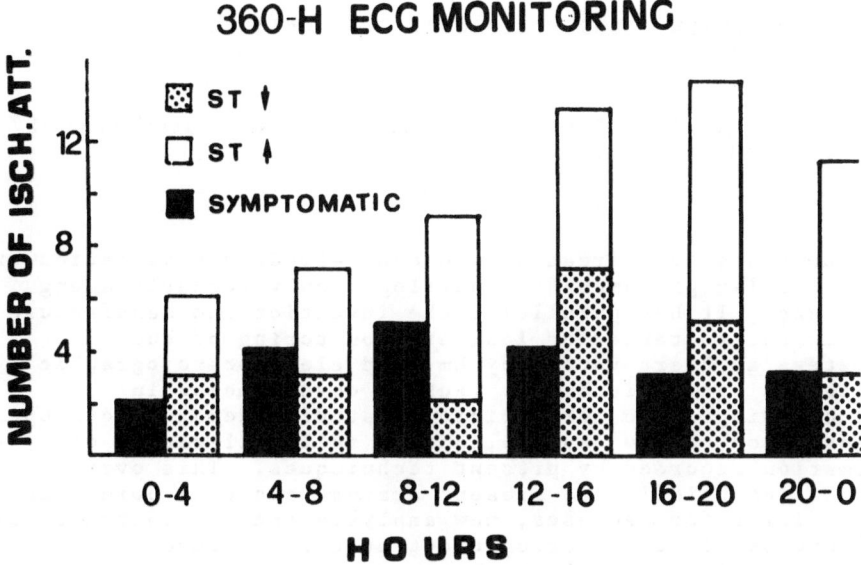

Figure 3

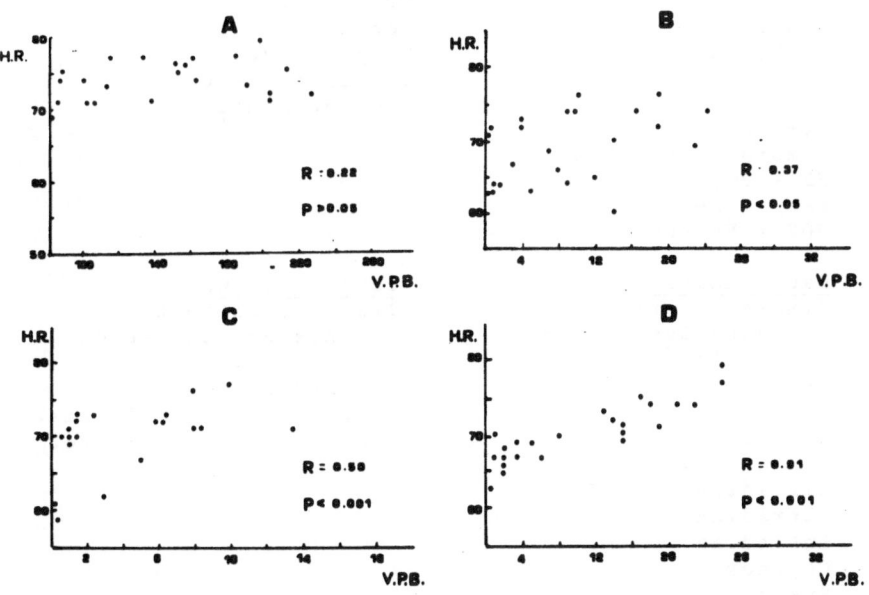

Figure 4

OVERVIEW: CHRONOBIOLOGIC ECG MONITORING

CHARLES N. LEACH, JR., Department of Cardiology, New Britain General Hospital, New Britain, CT.

Awareness of circadian and other-frequency variation of cardiovascular phenomena has developed only recently among clinicians. It has paralleled the invention and manufacture of equipment suitable for longterm monitoring of such parameters as heart rate, rhythm, and electrocardiographic changes indicating ischemia. Future developments in electrocardiographic chronobiologic studies depends both upon the invention of new devices, and on full utilization of information recorded by present technicques. This overview will outline briefly the present status, and will point out possibilities for new uses, new analysis and new instruments- with emphasis on those brought out at this conference.

The following table presents a much-condensed outline of present day ECG monitoring:

Phenomena	Data Acquisition
Heart Rate	Holter Monitor
Arrhythmias	Event Recorder
Atrial	Trans -Telephonic
Ventricular	Scheduled
Ischemia	Symptom-Cued
AV Block	Implanted Recorder
Pacing	Bedside Monitor
Symptoms	
Combinations -E.G.	
BP + Pulse	
Resp + Pulse	
PO2 + Rhythm	

Data Analysis	Interventions
Simple Counting	Instruct Patient
Evaluate Complexity	Administer Medication
Relate To	Adjust Device
Symptoms	Pacemaker Function
Activities	Anti-Tachycardia Pacemaker
Medication	Implanted Defibrillator
Chronobiologic	
Circadian	
Ultradian	
Infradian	
Cosinor	
Spectral	
Chronodesm	

Not all modalities listed are in common use at present
by clinicians or in the research setting. Furthermore, the
utility of even the simplset measurement,(heart rate for
example) has not been fully explored.

HEART RATE
Circadian fluctuations of pulse rate have been known for
many years, although little diagnostic use has been made of
the phenomenon. Its absence has long been recongnized as
suggesting a hypermetabolic (usually hyperthyroid) state.
More recently, Mann (1) has pointed out the absence of
circadian rate fluctuation in autonomic dysfunction.
Diminished circadian (and ultradian) heart rate fluctuation
accompanies extreme old age; and exaggerated variations occur
in anxiety states and neurasthenia. An intriguing recent
report (2) relates the loss of circadian heart rate variation
to the occurrence of autonomic neuropathy in diabetes
mellitus. Thus, the chronobiologic characteristics of the
heart rate most likely reflect severity and prognosis in
diabetics. One is tempted to speculate that heart rate
abnormalities also predict arrhythmias and sudden death. Loss
of heart rate variability after myocardial infarction has been
noted by Manzoli (3), and Kleiger (4) reports that this
phenomenon also predicts mortality. He suggests on the basis
of studies in dogs that there is reduced vagal baroreceptor
cardiac responsiveness.
In addition to its diagnostic and prognostic value, the
chronobiologic assesment of heart rate appears to be of value
in controlling the cardioltoxicity of chemotherapeutic agent
adriamycin. Hruschesky (5) has pointed out the value of
circadian timing in cancer chemotherapy. At this conference,
he has described a device for measuring respiratory sinus
arrhythmia. By its use (6), he has moved the control of
adriamycin toxity from the circadian to the ultradian domain.
Understanding and application of chronobiologic pulse
monitoring is close to fruition, but more clincial
investigation is needed. Inexpensive and easily-applied new
chronobiologic monitors (of which Hruschesky's is a good
example) are essential for this purpose. Furthermore,
physicians must be made aware of the chronobiologic data
present in Holter monitor studies, and they must be assisted
in its application by user-friendly equipment design.
Automated or semi-automated monitoring devices are presently
on the market. Exemplified by the Avionics Trendsetter and
the Pegasys respectively, their algorithms are not yet equal
to analysis of atrial or complex arrhythmias. However, data
such as pulse rate, upon which chronobiologic interpretations
may be based, are neither complex nor difficult to recogonize
from templates. Thus, presently-available automated
monitoring equipment could easily be adapted to analyze for
circadian and other frequency rhythms.
VENTRICULAR ARRHYTHMIAS
Ventricular arrhythmias furnish a second example of the
importance of chronobiologic ECG monitoring. Lown (7) first

320

called attention to the striking decline of VPC frequency
during sleep. Orth-Gomer (8), Sensi (9), Leach (10) and
Rebuzzi at this conference have investigated circadian and
infradian variation in ventricular ectopic activity (VEA).
Orth-Gomer (8) has applied chronobiologic analysis of VPC
frequency in a population with coronary disease to predict
mortality when simple measurement of VPC frequency was
insufficient.

Attempts to relate diagnosis prognosis and VEA
chronobiology is smaller series (9,10,11,12) have not as yet
proved successful. To date, investigations of VEA have been
largely descriptive, without testing interventions and without
elucidating the mechanisms by which VEA frequency varies—
though such variation is often attributed to varying vagal and
sympathetic tone. Knowledge of the chronobiology of VEA in
individual patients offers a basis for a chronobiologic
approach to their management. The author has thereby suceeded
in improving dosing intervals and optimizing dosage of
anti-arrhythmic medications. This allows improved efficacy,
reduced side effects, and avoids interuption of sleep by
reducing nocturnal dosing when VEA is often minimal.
Unfortunately, the utility and eminent practicality of this
chronobiologic approach to VEA therapy has not yet become
common knowledge among physicians, and rigid dosing schedules
persist.

At the Nato conference, the author presented an
investigation of the chronbiology of VEA carried out with Drs.
Halberg and Ruskin in an unmedicated hospitalized population
with various diagnoses. (10). We documented striking
individual circadian VEA rhythms which were independent of
etiology. Group mean cosinor analysis did not reveal a
significant group rhythm. (Fig.1.). This study demonstrated
the importance of individualizing chronobiologic data, and by
inference the need for inexpensive and user-friendly
monitoring devices for individual use.

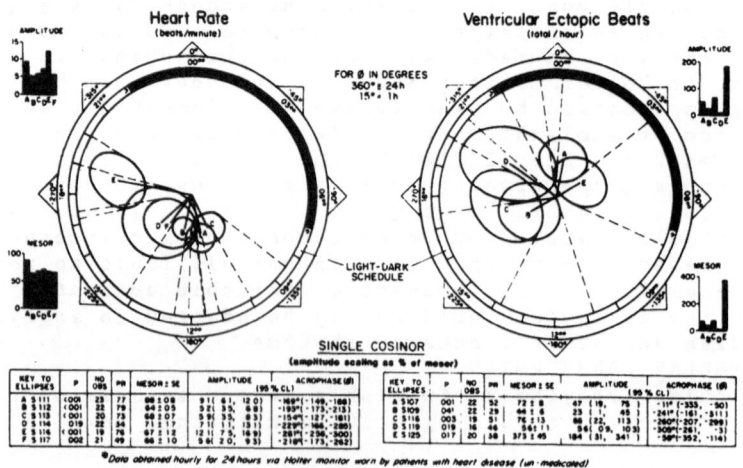

Figure 1.

Monitoring must also at times be extended into the infradian domain. As an example was cited out study (13) of a comatose patient with high-grade VEA following failed coronary bypass surger. In this investigation, we documented infradian variation of VPC and ventricular tachycardia frequency, and of the length of episodes of ventricular tachycardia. Of particular interest was the non-congruence of these frequency and duration rhythms. (Fig. 2). This suggests the possibility of different mechanisms, and indicates the need to monitor not only the quantity of ECG phenomena, but also their complexity and their interrelationships, in order to obtain full chronobiologic data. In this connection, tha author is presently analyzing a very large database in search of circannual variation in VEA and of the factors which may determine it.

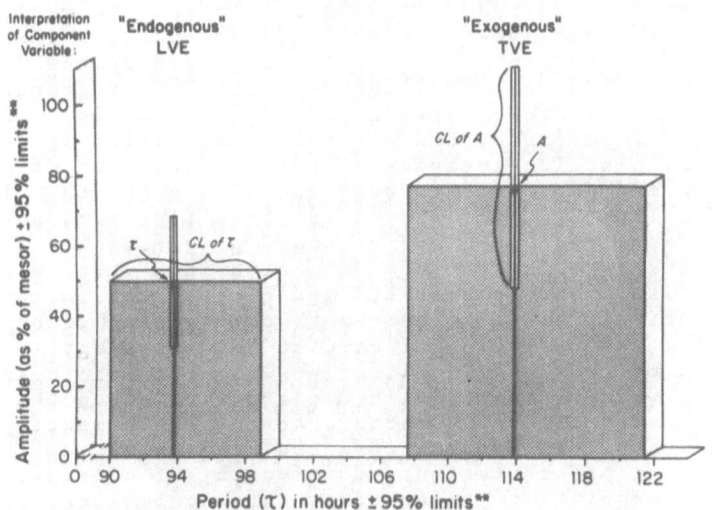

Infradian Components of Differing Period (τ) Characterize Hourly Total Ventricular Ectopies (TVE) and Longest Runs of VE (LVE) in a Patient Comatose after Coronary Bypass Surgery*

* EKG of a 66-year-old white man (MT) with past history of myocardial infarction monitored continuously for 10 days until death from ventricular fibrillation.

** Confidence limits obtained from plexo-serial linear-nonlinear least squares analyses (CL).

Figure 2

ECG Evidence Of Myocardial Ischemia

Cardiac chronobiology will also be useful in the characterization and therapy of myocardial ischemia. With the advent of high-fidelity FM ambulatory ECG recorders skepticism

(14) has given way to awareness that ST segment shifts in fact
often reflect ischemia (15). Particularly convincing are the
studies of Schang (16) and Biagini (17), who reduced the
frequency and degree of asymptomatic ST segment abnormalities
by administering nitroglycerin. Furthermore, Biagini
documented their coronary-spastic etiology by angiography
(17). The chronobiology of ST segment abnormalities and
ischemia has been investigated by Yasue (18). In patients
with Prinzmetal angina (due to coronary vasospasm), he
documented striking circadian variation of both symptomatic
and asymptomatic episodes as reflected by ST abnormalities
and ventricular arrhythmias. Further work by the same author
has documented circadian fluctuation of exercise-induced
coronary spasm with preponderance in the morning hours (19).
Awareness of the frequency and significance of asymptomatic ST
segment shifts and their circadian variation will in time lead
the clincian to a new, chronobiologically adapted endpoint of
therapy (15). It will also expand the population of patients
requiring treatment for Myocardial Ischemia. The demand for
precise, low-cost and chronobiologically adapted ambulatory
monitoring equipment will increase - both for diagnosis and
for assesment of therapy. Biological rhythms in myocardial
ischemia are operative in other frequency domains than the
circadian. Infradian variation is suggested by the
observation of Grunzig (20) that episodes of crescendo angina
(intermediate syndrome) have a periodic character. This has
therapeutic importance, and may relect variation in coronary
vasomotion, platelet activity or both. Variation of platelet
activation and adhesion has been shown to occur the ultradian
scale by Folts (21), who showed rhythmic fluctuation of
platelet deposition in a dog coronary preparation. This
suggests that a combined form of monitoring, which might
include measurement of both ECG and clotting parameters might
most effectively bring to bear both our evening technology and
our growing understanding of cardiac chronobiology.
     Each of the three applications of chronobiologic ECG
monitoring which I have outlined was discussed on the basis of
their own research by the authors at this NATO meeting. In
each area, important recent advances have been made, but each
is still in rapid evolution and is worthy of consideration
from the viewpoints represented at this conference: technical,
chronobiologic and clinical. An important goal for our
participants was to project the future of ECG monitoring in
this regard, the contribution of Drs. Rebuzzi and Manzoli
confirms the circadian periodicity of cardiac ischemia- both
"primary" and "secondary"; and that of ventricular ectopic
activity. Implicit in their elegant presentation is the need
to monitor and stress test for ischemia and VEA in full
awareness of their temporal distribution. They also
demonstrate the need for chronobiolgic analysis of ECG data in
the infradian domain.
     Dr. Hruschesky's presentation stressed the importance
and clinical utility of analysing for ultradian periodicity in
ECG data, especially heart rate. Plenary discussion included
the presentations of Drs. Ivan Bourgeois and Philip

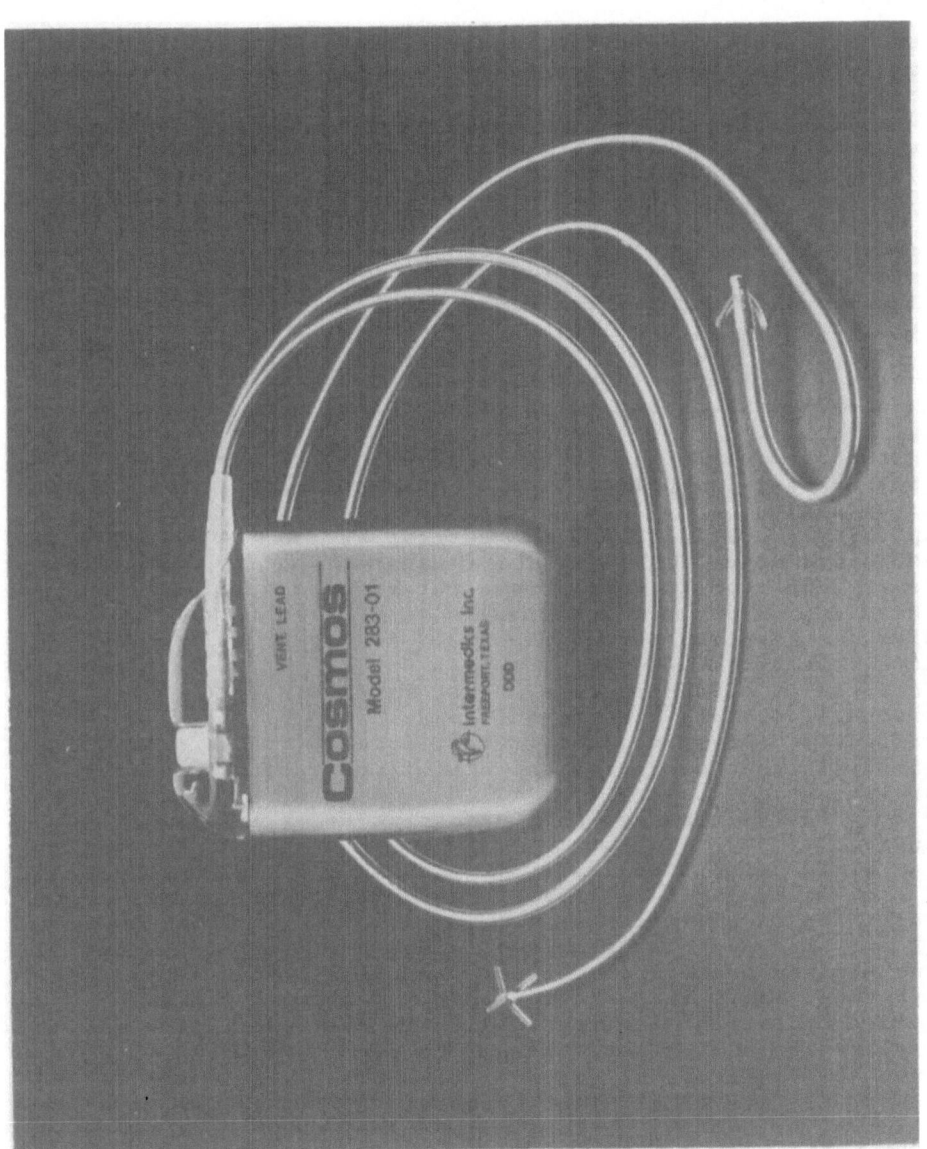

(Fig 3.) An Implanted Monitor of ventricular Ectopic
          Activity: The COSMOS Dual Chamber Pacemaker

Schoenfeld, which appear elsewhere in this volume. They
joined the above authors in a subgroup to develop consensus as
to which aspects of ECG monitoring appear promising for
technical improvement and chronbiologic applications. These
comprise a "dream sheet" which expresses the group's idealized
concept of improved ECG monitoring:

1. ECG data should be sufficiently dense and extensive to
allow analysis of infradian and ultradian rhythms as well as
circadian.
2. This will require sensors (such as electrodes, cuffs,
microphones, etc.) which are durable and comfortable for the
subject.
3. Extended monitoring will also require cost reduction. This
may be obtained by reduced cost of instruments (which is
already well underway), by greater ease of application, or by
less costly data reduction (as can be achieved by automation).
4. Automated data reduction needs greater reliablity. The
best of present instrumentation is seriously deficient in the
recognition of complex arrhythmias, ventricular fusion beats,
and atrial activity. Automation also needs to be extended to
the recognition and reporting of chronobiologic features of
data.
5. Extended monitoring can be improved by the use of implanted
units for certain applications. These will require
miniturization, and improved (perhaps rechargeable) power
supplies. A hybrid example in current use is the Intermedics
COSMOS pacemaker (fig.3), which tabulates ventricular ectopic
activity and reports totals when interrogated. (22).
6. Handling of data on individuals must be improved.
Individual baseline Chronodesms (23) can be established for
future reference, and periodic lifelong sampling of such
parameters as blood pressure, heart rate, VEA, and pulse
characteristics may then reveal departures (or more
importantly, threatened departures) from health.
7. Several other technical aspects of monitoring require
improvements:
    a. Analysis and graphic presentation of heart rate
phenomena.
    b. ST segment analysis. (24).
    c. Analysis of artificial pacemaker function and
recognition of pacemaker signals.
8. There is a need for easily-obtained combined monitoring of
phenommena such as blood pressure and heart rate; VEA and
heart rate, heart rate and ischemia. Combined data are
recorded by present equipment, but are not effectively
correlated by analysis techniques or report formats.
Clinicians require such easily-accessible correlations to
allow definition of clinical syndromes and their proper
therapy.
9. Chronopharmacology will require adjustment of cardiac
therapies to phenomena such as heart rate and arrhythmias, or
to the presence of silent evidence of myocardial ischemia.
Clinical decisions as to adequacy of beta blockade depend more
upon heart rate than drug levels, and this simply measured

325

parameter might easily be incoporated in a feedback system for
control of an implanted drug administration device.
Similarly, VEA could control automated anti-arrhythmic drug
delivery and ST segment shifts could cue administration of
coronary vasodilators. The group also favored development of
equipment to utilize cardiovascular cues for administration of
non-cardiac medications such as Adriamycin. Awareness of the
chronobiology of cardiovascular phenomena will improve the
precision with which these feedback controls are used.
10.Chronobiologic cardiac pacing offers another focus for
clinician and engineer. The work of Manzoli documented
circadian variation of pacing thresholds, R wave amplitutde,
AV delay, QT interval and other phenomena. Measurement of
these factors by the pacemaker may allow feedback adjustment
of pacer output and sensing; and the AV delay and refractory
periods of dual chamber devices. Similar feedback controls
may be applied to anti-tachycardia pacemakers.
11. Finally, the group recognized the importance of increased
and widespread awareness of the utility of chronobiology among
those who employ cardiac monitoring to help patients.
Instruments and displays must be adapted to analyze for and
express findings in time-qualified terms. And the vocabulary
of chronobiology must be introduced to daily use in the clinic
and developmental laboratory to facilitate efficient
applicaton of its principles.

BIBLIOGRAPHY

1. Circadian variation of blood pressure in autonomic failure,
Mann, S., Altman, D., Raferty, B., Bannister, D.M., Circ 68:
477,1983
2. Abnormalities of Ambulatory 24 hour Heart Rate in Diabetes
Mallitus. Ewing J, Borsey D Q, Travis P, Bellavere F, Neilson
J and Clarke B. Diabetes 32:101 Feb.1983.
3. Manzoli: Chronobiologic Electrocardiographic Monitoring:
Nato Conference.
4. Heart rate and mortality following M.I, Kleiger, Pace 3:
547 1984
5. Circadian timing of cancer chemotherapy. Hrushesky, W.
Science 228:73 1985
6. The respiratory sinus arrhythmia measure of cardiac age.
Hrushesky, W, Fader D, Schmitt O & Gilbertsen V. Science
224:1001 1984
7. Sleep and Ventricular Premature Beats. Lown B, Tykocinski
M, Garfein A, & Brooks P. Circ 48:691 1973
8. The Circadian Rhythm of Ventricular Arrhythmias. Orth-Gomer
K, Halberg F, Sothern R, Akerstedt T, Theorell T, Cornelissen
G. Toward Chronopharmacology 1981, Takahashi, 1982.
9. Circadian Rhythm of Ventricular Ectopy. Sensi S, Manzoli
U, Capani F, Domenicelli B, Lucente M, Schiavoni G, Coppola E,
Chest 77:580 1980 (Letter)
10. Circadian Variation of Frequent Human Ventricular Ectopy.
Leach C, Ruskin J, Halberg F. Federation Proceedings,40:1981
11. Arythmies Ventriculaire du Prolapsus Valvulaire Mitral.
Miane B, Laurent M, Revillon L, Almange C, Leborgne P. Sem.
Hop Paris 19-20:954,1981

12. Arrhythmias in Patients with Mitral Valve Prolapse.
Winkle R, Lopes M. Fitzgerald J. Goodman D,. Schroeder J,
Harrison D. Circ. 52:73, 1975
13. Infradian Variablity in Total (TE) and Longest Runs (LE)
of Cardiac Ectopies, Heart Rate, Blood Pressure and
Temperature of a Comatose Man. Leach C, Ruskin J, Halberg F, &
Sothren R. Chronobiologia 10:138 1983
14. Frequency response characteristics of ambulatory ECG
monitoring systems and their implications for ST segment
analysis. Bragg-Remschel D, Anderson C, Winkle R, Am. Heart
J. 103:20,1982.
15.New Approach to Managemnet of Patients with both
symptomatic and asymptomatic episodes of myocardial ischemia,
Cohn, P.F., Am J Card 12/84 P 1358
16. Transient Asymptomatic ST Segment Depression During Daily
Activity. Schang S, Pepine C. Am J Cardiol 39:396,1977
17. Vasospastic Ischemic Mechanism of Frequent Asymptomatic
Transient ST-T Changes During Continuous Electrocardiographic
Monitoring in Selected Unstable Angina Patients. Biagini A,
Mazzei M, Carpeggiani C, Testa R, Antonelli R, Michelassi C,
L"Abbate A, Maseri A. Am Heart J 103:13, 1982.
18. Coronary Arterial Spasm in Ischemic Heart Disease and its
Pathogenesis. Yasue H, Omote S, Takizawa A, Nagao M, Circ Rsch
(Suppl I) 52:147,1983.
19. Circadian Variation of Exercise Capacity in Patients with
Prinzmetal's Variant Angina: Role of Exercise-Induced Coronary
Arterial Spasm. Yasue H, Omote S, Takizawa A, Nagao M, Miwa K,
Tanaka S, Circ 59:938,1979.
20."Percutaneous Transluminal Coronary Angioplasty" Harvard
Medical Post Grad Course Cardiac Angiography 1982, Gruentzig,
A.
21. Blood Flow Reductions in Stenosed Canine Coronary
Arteries: Vasospasm or Platelet Aggregations? Folts J,
Gallager J, Rowe G. Circ 65:248, 1982.
22.Sanders R, Martin R, Frumin H, Goldberg M J, Data storage
and retrieval by implantable pacemakers for diagnostic
purposes, Pace 1984 Nov, P1228-33
23.Quo Vadis Basic and Clinical Chronobiology: Promise For
Health Maintenance. Halberg F, Am J. Anat 168: 543-594,1983
24.International Symposium on Ambulatory Monitoring.
(Padua,3/29-30 1985- Semi Automated ST segment Analysis:
Validation Results, Problems and Lessons Learned. Cashman P,
Kohli R, Khurmi N, Bowles M, Raftery, E. (Abst).

A CASE FOR CLINICAL CONCENTRATION UPON THE ULTRADIAN
FREQUENCY DOMAIN

WILLIAM J. M. HRUSHESKY, Mayo Memorial Bldg., University of Minnesota,
School of Medicine, Minneapolis, MN

Most currently available chronobiological monitoring
devices have been designed for evaluation of physiologic
rhythms in the circadian and infradian domains. Discrete
(e.g. respiration or pulse) or continous (e.g. blood pressure,
temperature) physiologic parameters occur with high density
within these circadian and infradian rhythms. Both the
relative density of these data and the length of the measured
span necessary for accurate evaluation of such rhythms cause
severe theoretical and practical problems for those interested
in quantifying them. An important culprit on the theoretical
side, is the same villain who is at the root of all
homeostatic science, non-rhythm qualified data averaging. The
inferred defense for this practice is the untested and
unwarranted assumption that the circadian and infradian rhythm
characteristics are more pertinent or meaningful than is the
predictable variability within the ultradian frequency domain.
Non (circadian stage) rhythm qualified data averaging cannot
be justified in order to estimate a suboptimally broad "normal
range", and it cannot be justified when handling long dense
data series used to estimate circadian and infradian rhythm
characteristics. The practical limitations on collection of
long dense data series are the absence of comfortable,
reliable sensors and durable "intelligent" data analyzers
which can be effectively applied to the clinical realities of
outpatient or inpatient medical practice.
    The amount of information thrown away when the commonly
applied data averaging techniques are employed can be
illustrated by a consideration of pulse. 1,2,3,4,
There is every reason to suspect that the fundamental heart
beat frequency, its ultradian rhythms and their harmonics
might be as revealing and useful as circadian or infradian
pulse patterns. There is also every reason to expect that
averaging pulse data without regard to their position within
the respiratory cycle, the well described high amlitude 10-20
second pulse rhythms, or the many other ultradian rhythms,[5]
might be less than optimal.
    Both these theoretical and the practical consideration
of physiologic data gathering and analysis have stimulated my
interest in the analysis of continuos non-averaged biologic
data.

The respiratory modulation of pulse was chosen for study because 10 to 20 complete cycles can be evaluated within a couple of minutes. The of use highly reliable sensors for determining pulse and respiration, and the interface of these excellent quality signals with a microcomputer, allow internal synchronization of the pulse within the breathing cycle. This phase locks the two systems and diminishes noise, which would otherwise occur as the respiratory and pulse phase drift back and forth across one another. This instrument (Fig.1) then analyzes the quality of these data, eliminating poorly phase locked cycles (error greater than 1/N where N equals the number of beats per respiratory cycle) and fitting a cosine model by least squares analysis to the relationship of pulse and breathing of each cycle. The inspiratory error (distance from breathing signal and actual initiation of inspiration) in each cycle may then be subtracted from the acrophase of that cycle, and the cycles can be combined using the population mean cosiner rhythm averaging technique.[1]

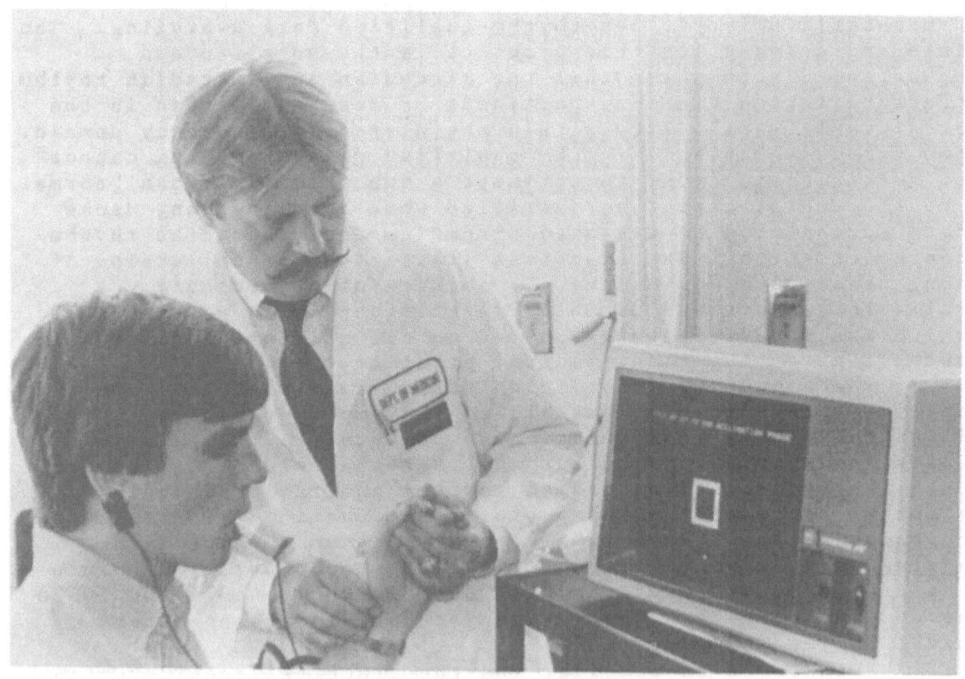

Figure 1

This quantitative evaluation of the respiratory sinus arrhythmia occurs on-line within two minutes. Every pulse datum is evaluated; no data are averaged; data are analyzed and stored in analyzed and raw forms and are easily interfaced with any microcomputer or mainframe.

In order to be most revealing, the pulses sampled for circadian analysis should be qualified as to where in these ultradian rhythms the samples originate. In childern and young adults, for example, the amplitude of pulse variation associated with respiration is usually much greater than the amplitude of the (averaged) circadian rhythm in pulse. There may also be a great deal of information defined by the ratios of the amplitude of various ultradian pulse rhythms to one another and to that of the circadian rhythm. In any event, this information must not be discarded by arbitrary data averaging which disregards these powerful ultradian rhythms.

Pulse data obtained in this way have allowed quantitative evaluation of cardiovascular physiologic aging, cardiovascular aerobic training, ischemic cardiomyopathy, and doxorubicin induced cardiomyopathy. This system has also been used on a limited scale to investigate other ultradian pulse rhythm and the interaction of these ultradian rhythms with one another and with the overlying circadian rhythms of pulse 6

In summary: As a practicing physician-scientist-chronobiologist who wishes to monitor ultradian, circadian and infradian rhythms in the physiologic function of patients and research subjects, it is my opinion that while non-invasive sensors, data recording, handling and analysis instrumentation are adequate for handling continous ultradian data, they are not up to the task of dealing with long spans of continuos data. Furthermore, currently available systems are not comfortable or convenient enough for routine use by ill patients. Additionally, current data averaging techniques commonly used for circadian data collection disregard ultradian rhythms in human physiology which may be more profound and at least as interesting and informative as circadian and infradian rhythms.

I conclude that ultradian physiologic rhythms contain a great deal of medically useful information which is easily extractable from data series given present technology. Circadian and infradian physiologic monitoring and data-averaging must consider this in order not to mislead. I also believe that implanted radio-sensor technology combined with much more powerful limited or single purpose dedicated micropressor-based instuments, using on-line analysis and universal interface systems, are an absolute necessity for evaluating longer period biologic rhythms. These insruments must ultimately be the size and convenience of a wristwatch. Finally, there may well be much more exciting and relevant biological information in the quantitative relationship of various ultradian rhythms with one another and with circadian and infradian rhythms than there is in any single rhythm or domain.

References

1. Hrushesky, W.J. M., Fader. D., Schmitt, O. and Gilbertson, V.: The respiratory sinus arrhythmia: A measure of cardiac age. Science 224: 1001-1004,1984.

2. Smith, Joseph M. and Cohen, Richard J.,: Simple finite-element model accounts for wide range of cardiac dysrhythmias. Proc. Natl. Acad. Sci. 81: 223-237,1984.

3. Adam, Dan R., Smith, Joseph M., Akselrod, Solange, et al.: Fluctuations in T-wave morphology and susceptibility to ventricular fibrillation. J. Electrocardiology 17 (3),1984,pp 209-218.

4. Gordon, D., Cohen Richard J., Kelly, D., Akselrod, Solange, et al.: Sudden infant death syndrome: Abnormalities in short term fluctuations in heart rate and respiratory activity. Pediatric Research 18 (10),1984,pp. 921-926.

5. Akselrod, S., Gorden, D., Ubel, Andrew F., et al.: Power spectrum analysis of heart rate fluctuation: A quantitative probe of beat to beat cardiovascular control. Science 213: 220-222.1981.

6. Hrushesky, W. J. M.: The Sine-o-graph pulse monitor: A potential quantifier of cardiovascular wellness. In A. Reinberg, M. Smolensky, G. Labrecque, eds., Vol. T. Annual Review of Chronopharmacology. New York: Pergamon Press, pp 325-328,1984.

REQUIREMENTS FOR CHRONOBIOTECHNOLOGY AND CHRONOBIOLOGIC
ENGINEERING IN LABORATORY MEDICINE

ERHARD HAUS, St. Paul-Ramsey Medical Center and Ramsey Clinic, St. Paul, MN

I. THE PROBLEM:

The requirements for chronobiotechnology and chronobiologic engineering in laboratory medicine are determined by the nature of the biologic system to be explored and by the kind of data needed to apply chronobiology in a meaningful quantitative manner to clinical medicine, i.e, to the problems of individual patients.

Time dependent, regularly recurring, rhythmic and thus predictable changes in several frequency ranges characterize the living mammalian organism in its metabolism, its cell proliferation and function. The rhythmic changes, which take place whether we want to study them or not, lead to reproducible and sometimes high amplitude variations in most clinical and laboratory parameters (1-11). Information on the clinical importance of the human time structure for clinical medicine has been accumulating during the last two decades (1,12-16). The frequencies of interest in human biologic systems range from milliseconds to seasonal variations and probably even to rhythms with periods of several years duration superimposed upon aging trends.

Whatever measurements are taken to study these rhythmic variations, they have to be adequate in sampling density and in the length of the sampling span to allow a quantitative inferential statistical description of the rhythms and of their parameters with variance estimate for each. Only if the requirements for sampling and analysis can be met in individual subjects will chronobiology exert its full impact on physiology, work hygiene, and medicine.

The past and present limitations of the application of chronobiology to clinical medicine has been due to a considerable degree to the difficulty of obtaining statistically meaningful and rhythmometrically quantifiable information on rhythmic functions and their parameters from single subjects under socially acceptable conditions and at an acceptable cost. It is one of the present challenges to laboratory medicine to provide such data on individual patients to allow the time dimension to assume its critical role in physiology and medicine.

Most information on rhythmic variations of laboratory functions, thusfar available has been obtained from groups of subjects sampled over one or over a few of the periods to be studied. Comparison of single or of a few values obtained from an individual subject, with the rhythm adjusted usual range (chronodesm) derived from an appropriate peer group, may give some useful information if high amplitude rhythms are concerned. In the many rhythmic functions with low amplitudes, however, the chronodesm will be so broad as to offer little advantage over the use of time unqualified 'usual values'. It would be desirable

to compare the rhythm parameters of laboratory functions between
individual subjects, and to study the phase relation of different
laboratory functions to each other within the same subject. Statistical
methods for the comparison of rhythm parameters and the calculation of
so called 'parameterdesms' have recently been described (17). However,
to do this in a meaningful manner and to avoid the often useless and
risky speculation inherent in chronobiologic statements based on
inadequate data, a sufficient amount of information has to be collected
to allow a quantitative, statistical evaluation. In the past, this has
been done for a number of laboratory functions in a few selected
subjects, which were studied either intensively by frequent (e.g.,
every 20 minute) sampling over single 24-hour spans with
hospitalization and relative immobilization by intravenous catheters,
removal from his or her customary surrounding, etc. Alternatively
single or a few individuals were followed for prolonged time spans
with, e.g., urinary collections (18-20) which for the general every day
use in patients is neither technically feasible nor socially
acceptable, and would not necessarily be always correct if the
collections are performed during conditions of daily life and by
untrained personnel.

The considerable volume of data accumulated over the last two
decades allows to define and to delineate areas in which chronobiologic
methods are essential to obtain meaningful results in the study of
laboratory parameters. In addition, there are numerous areas in which
chronobiologic study designs, and analyses may open new avenues in the
exploration of disease states, their diagnosis and their treatment. The
investigation of the present role and of the potential application of
chronobiology to laboratory medicine leads to a number of observations
and conclusions.

1) Almost all laboratory parameters studied are periodic in one
or more often in several frequency ranges (1). Rhythmic variations with
large amplitudes may be detectable in single individuals with
relatively few appropriately timed measurements. Rhythms with small
amplitude and/or high variability, however, may require extensive
sampling in order to allow their description and quantification by
inferential statistical methods in a single subject, or such rhythms
may become manifest only as group phenomenon.

The length of the observation span and the sampling intervals
required for statistical rhythm detection depend on the spectral region
and on the characteristics of the rhythm to be studied. An estimate of
the number of periods needed for rhythm detection in an individual or
of the number of subjects needed for the detection of a rhythm as a
group phenomenon is possible only after the characteristics of the
rhythm have been established, and the interference by superimposed
higher frequencies and the amount of noise to be expected are
approximately known. The sampling requirements will be considerably
greater for demonstrating a rhythm of unknown period, especially if it
is unexpected.

In many but not in all functions of clinical interest, the
circadian frequency component seems to have the highest amplitude. This
is not the case, e.g., for hormones related to reproduction which in
women during the reproductive years have a higher circatrigintan
(menstrual) rhythm amplitude and apparently also not for certain
immunologic functions, which manifest themselves among others in

transplantation biology where a prominent circaseptan periodicity seems to be operational in determining in part the response of the host's immune system to an allograft (21). In some functions, like e.g., in plasma DHEA-S, the circannual variation may be larger in extent than the circadian amplitude (22).

The circadian rhythms are modulated by ultradian rhythms with a higher frequency and are themselves superimposed upon rhythms with lower frequencies, i.e., in the circaseptan, circatrigintan and circannual frequency range. The higher frequencies may lead to spurious results and to aliasing in (infrequent) spotchecks of individuals studied for their circadian rhythm (see below Figure 4). The lower frequencies may alter mesor, amplitude and acrophase of a circadian rhythm and/or may imitate trends in some of these functions. The multifrequency mammalian time structure has to be kept in mind in experimental designs as well as in clinical studies.

2) There is a limited number of laboratory functions showing high amplitude circadian rhythms (1). These are predominantly found in endocrinology and in hematology with a few also in clinical chemistry (Figures 1-3). Rhythms of relatively large amplitude require time qualified reference intervals [chronodesms (23)] for the interpretation of individual measurements. In these parameters, the determination of reference limits irrespective of time, may be too broad and hence not discriminating. High amplitude rhythms of different frequencies which characterize some variables of vital interest in biology and medicine may contribute a large fraction of the variability seen in clinical data. Sampling at time points chosen (on the basis of previous chronobiologic information) by pertinence rather than only by convenience is essential to obtain meaningful and comparable results in such parameters. In some laboratory functions, the same value when checked against an appropriate chronodesm, may in fact be too low at one time, quite normal at another and even too high at yet another time (19,24-26).

For some parameters which show marked interindividual variations, even the time qualified reference ranges obtained from well selected and apparently appropriate peer groups may be quite large. In such cases, it is essential for the evaluation of a laboratory test in a given clinical situation to keep in mind the rhythm parameters of rhythm adjusted level (mesor), the usual timing (acrophase), and the extent of the rhythm as characterized either by its amplitude and/or by the range of the recurring change encountered (the latter i.e. in the case of non-sinusoidal variations). Consecutive measurements of a given individual have then to be evaluated against this background.

Time qualified reference ranges (chronodesms) are desirable for high amplitude rhythms, not only in the circadian but in all frequency ranges. The choice of the method chosen for establishing these reference ranges will depend on the shape of the rhythmic variation, the distribution of the measurements and the number of measurements available. The non-Gaussian distribution of the values found in many laboratory functions often requires the use of nonparametric statistics (i.e. percentiles) to delineate the usual range in a chronodesm.

3) Many circadian (and other) rhythms encountered are of low amplitude and do not pose a diagnostic problem in today's clinical practice. They may, however, gain in importance if the sampling requirements for a statistically valid evaluation of low amplitude

rhythms can be met (ideally by frequent noninvasive sampling by
socially acceptable procedures over a prolonged time span by automatic
miniaturized instrumentation preferably interfaced with a data
processor or computer). The low amplitude rhythms indicate the usual
sequence of many metabolic events and by phase and/or amplitude
alterations may indicate early pathology. Temporal abnormalities in
some low amplitude circadian rhythm parameters have in some instances
been found to precede the relatively coarse abnormalities presently
regarded as clinically important in time unqualified spot checks. The
circadian rhythm in serum bilirubin, for example, has too small an
amplitude to present a problem for the diagnosis of jaundice. However,
it may be of considerable biological interest since changes in the
circadian rhythm of serum bilirubin have been reported as one of the
earliest signs of liver damage (27). Rhythm alterations may indicate
early pathology by revealing temporal changes of laboratory values
which, by a conventional approach, would be regarded as within the
'usual range'.

4) Rhythm parameters like the rhythm adjusted mean (mesor), the
extent of the rhythm (amplitude) and its timing (acrophase) have become
new end points in physiology and pathology. The usual ranges of these
parameters [parameterdesms (17)] have to be established in individuals
and in appropriate peer populations and deviations from these usual
values have to be recognized in a statistically meaningful manner.

5) The circadian rhythms in most laboratory functions can be
detected in diurnally active, clinically healthy ambulatory subjects
following their habitual daily routine. For most functions
standardization beyond that used for blood drawing in the laboratory
did not appear essential for rhythm detection (some exceptions, e.g,
plasma catecholamines, plasma renin, etc. are obvious).

6) Time dependent changes in drug kinetics have recently been
reviewed by Reinberg (28), and will have to be applied to the
evaluation of clinical drug level studies.

7) It has to be emphasized that a given clock hour is not
necessarily representative of the biologic time of an organism.
Circadian periodic changes must not be misinterpreted as time of day
effects. The same time of day may have an entirely different meaning
for two individuals on two different living schedules. Phase shifts,
phase drift, and within group desynchronization have to be kept in mind
in the interpretation of experimental or laboratory results. Such
rhythm disturbances may occur during an ongoing study or during a
course of treatment of a patient. Thus, in the study of human subjects
or populations, chronobiologic sampling should be accomplished against
the background of the subject's rest-activity and sleep-wakefulness
patterns, working schedules, and dietary habits--including the times of
the main meals. Inquiry into some or all of these simple biologic
reference functions provides information on the subject's
synchronization and may be critical if sampling has to be limited to a
single or to a few time points. Many other periodic variables can serve
as potential reference functions. Potential reference functions or
marker rhythms in the circadian domain are among others body
temperature, urinary volume, some urinary and salivary functions,
notably electrolytes and corticosteroids (29-31); sweat electrolytes,
etc. The pertinence of a reference function for the rhythm under study,
however, will have to be explored and documented in each instance.

The detection and characterization of pertinent reference functions, which can serve for monitoring the biologic timing of patients in general, and of certain vital functions (e.g. the time of maximal cell proliferation in the hematopoietic cells in the bone marrow) specifically may often be essential for the choice of the right time for treatment to obtain optimal results. Timing of drug administration may also be used to protect the patient during treatment with agents showing undesirable side effects, e.g., many of the agents used in cancer chemotherapy. The problem in this area is to determine which functions may be pertinent as phase reference for the susceptibility resistance cycles to a certain agent. A reference function (e.g., for the susceptibility cycle to a chemotherapeutic agent) has to be not only periodic in the same frequency and easily measurable but has to maintain in the disease state to be treated and during the treatment a fixed phase relation to the susceptibility cycle to be monitored. After a potential reference rhythm has been found to be pertinent, one will have to establish the sampling requirements to obtain statistically valid results on the parameters of this rhythm in a single subject in an ongoing and timely manner.

Preferably, a reference function should be longitudinally measurable at frequent intervals by noninvasive methods. Variables measurable by physical or physico-chemical end points that do not involve expensive and/or lengthy chemical analyses, and which can be recorded automatically in a computer compatible form are particularly attractive.

Automatic measurement and recording and possibly even telemetering of some biochemical or physical reference functions will be of crucial importance and will, in the long run, greatly reduce the cost of chronobiologic studies. Automated monitoring of reference functions will allow the determination of the biological time of a subject, and will make it possible to limit sample collection for invasive (e.g., blood) and costly procedures (e.g., for chemical hormone analysis) to few but well defined time points chosen for their pertinence for the parameter under study.

The practical application of human chronobiology to environmental and work physiology and to clinical medicine will depend critically on the availability of automated instrumentation for the study of low amplitude and of marker rhythms.

II. CHRONOBIOLOGIC INFORMATION ON LABORATORY DATA OBTAINED BY CONVENTIONAL SAMPLING TECHNIQUES:

In order to apply the study of biological rhythms of laboratory functions to medical practice, we first have to define the sampling requirements to obtain statistically meaningful results in single subjects and will have to see if and how these sampling requirements can be met. But even if sampling can be obtained over an adequate time span, with appropriate sampling intervals, the cost, e.g., of the chemical determinations of a given metabolite or hormone may be prohibitive for routine application.

Of importance for the 'detection' of rhythms in the invariably 'noisy' biological time series and for the rhythmometric analysis of data of single subjects, is the extent of the rhythmic variation which has to be expected. The information available on the extent of circadian variations of laboratory data are derived almost exclusively from groups of subjects studied over one or over a few 24-hour spans.

The extent of the circadian variation as found by cosinor analysis in a number of hematologic, biochemical and endocrine variables in groups of healthy young adult subjects studied at St. Paul-Ramsey Medical Center, St. Paul, Minnesota, are shown in Figures 1-3. All subjects followed a diurnal activity pattern with rest at night. They ate three regular meals habitually and followed the same schedule on the day of the study. They were synchronized to some extent through their activities as medical technologists, clerical workers and physicians at St. Paul-Ramsey Medical Center, and students at the University of Minnesota. The day of the study, the subjects spent at St. Paul-Ramsey Medical Center. They were ambulatory and followed an activity pattern not too different from their daily activities. Heavy exercise and alcoholic beverages were avoided. Blood was drawn six times over a 24-hour span, beginning at noon of one day and ending at 0800 of the following day. All chemical determinations were done in the clinical chemistry and special chemistry laboratories of St. Paul-Ramsey Medical Center. Each subjects' data were analyzed by single cosinor and those of the entire group by population mean cosinor. In Figures 1, 2, and 3, the extent of the circadian variation is presented as the peak-trough difference of the cosine curve best fitting to the data (the double amplitude) expressed in percent of the mesor of each function (Figures 1, 2, 3).

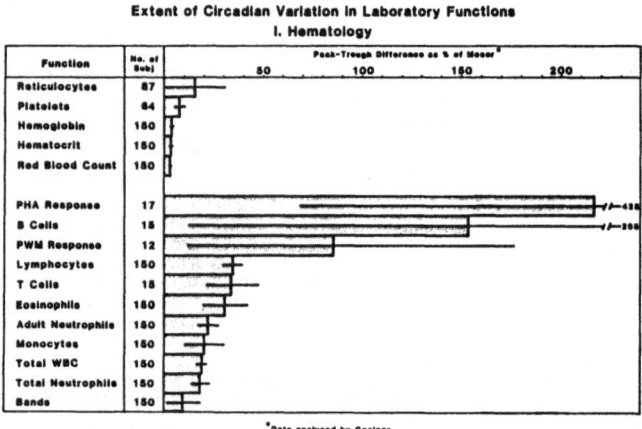

Figure 1: Extent of circadian variations in hematologic parameters. The peak-trough difference of the cosine curve best fitting to the data (double amplitude) is shown expressed as percent of mesor.

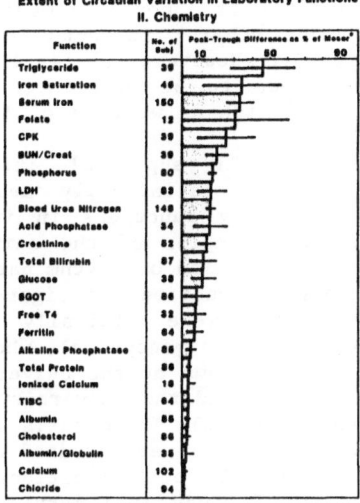

Extent of Circadian Variation in Laboratory Functions
II. Chemistry

Figure 2: Extent of circadian variation of various serum constituents in clinically healthy young adult and adult subjects. The peak-trough difference of the cosine curve best fitting to the data (double amplitude) is shown expressed as percent of mesor.

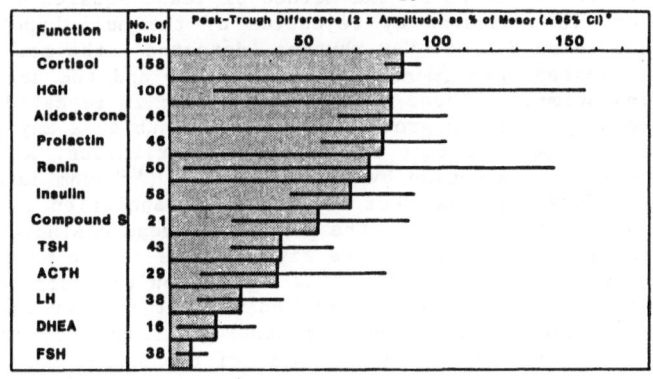

Extent of Circadian Variation in Laboratory Functions
III. Endocrinology

*Data analyzed by Cosinor

Figure 3: Extent of circadian variation in serum hormone concentrations in clinically healthy young adult and adult subjects of both sexes. The peak-trough difference of the cosine curve best fitting to the data (double amplitude) is expressed as percent of the mesor.

It is obvious that only a limited number of circadian periodic functions have large enough amplitudes to pose a diagnostic problem in todays state of the science of laboratory medicine. Such high amplitude rhythms are found, among others, in hematology (Figure 1) and in endocrinology (Figure 3). However, since differences in rhythm parameters have been shown to be associated with disease (1,26) rhythmometric analyses of high as well as of low amplitude rhythms will have to be accomplished.

Only very little generally applicable information on the sampling requirements for obtaining statistically meaningful rhythmometric results for common laboratory functions in individual subjects are thusfar available. A few examples of the sampling requirements for obtaining quantitative information on rhythm parameters by cosinor analysis is shown for some endocrine functions in Figures 5-9. The subjects from whom these data were obtained were clinically healthy women of different ages ranging from young adult to menopausal, who were studied under as far as feasible comparable conditions at the University of Minnesota, U.S.A. (two-thirds of the subjects) and the University of Kyushu, Fukuoka City, Japan (one-third of the subjects). The details of this study were published elsewhere (32). The same subjects were studied up to four times, each time during a different season. In both locations, the subjects were hospitalized for the day of study, and carried an indwelling catheter through which 2 ml of blood were sampled every 20 minutes for the determination of cortisol and prolactin and 15 ml every 100 minutes for the determination of these and of 13 other hormonal variables as shown in Figure 5. Also here, the chemical analyses were done in the special chemistry laboratories of St. Paul-Ramsey Medical Center, St. Paul, Minnesota. The data obtained from the Americans and Japanese women were very similar, although not identical (32), and were pooled for the purpose of this presentation. The rhythmometric analysis of the data was done by single, and for groups of subjects by population mean cosinor as indicated in the legends to the figures. In the single cosinor procedure, a cosine curve is fitted by the method of least squares to the data. 'Rhythm detection' is indicated by rejection of the null hypothesis for zero amplitude in an F-test. For rhythms 'detected', the method then yields the rhythm adjusted mean (mesor), the amplitude and the acrophase with their variance estimates. These values as obtained in repeated sampling spans of the same subject or in groups of different subjects may serve as input for a population mean cosinor for further quantitation. A rejection of the zero-amplitude assumption by single cosinor ('rhythm detection') refers to the given data set, and does not allow extrapolation to a population as a whole. As the name implies, the population-mean cosinor, by comparison aims at extrapolation far beyond the given sample to the population as a whole. Use of one or the other test hence depends on the purpose of a given study. If the sample is to be characterized without further inferences to others in the population, the single cosinor is much more efficient; when inference is to be drawn on the basis of the sample for the population as a whole, the population-mean cosinor is indicated (23).

The cosinor analysis requires that the data obtained can be reasonably well represented by a cosine curve and nonsinusoidality limits the applicability of the method. Unfortunately, few biologic rhythms of laboratory functions are ideally sinusoidal. More often, there are ultradian frequencies superimposed on the circadian rhythms which themselves are superimposed on infradian cycles like the circatrigintan or menstrual cycle, circannual cycles, etc. The latter,

if the data are collected over a limited time span, may present
themselves as trends rather than as rhythms. The higher frequencies on
the other hand may lead to a considerable degree of aliasing, an
example of which is shown in a patient in whom measurements of plasma
cortisol obtained at 20 minute intervals were available (Figure 4).

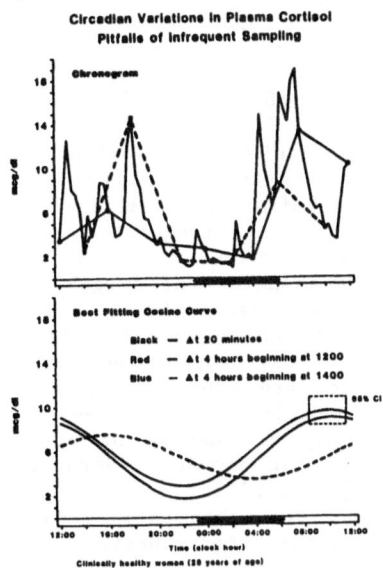

Figure 4:   'Aliasing' of circadian rhythm in plasma cortisol (sampled
             every 20 minutes) if sampling is limited to 4 hour
             intervals. Note apparent difference in acrophase if
             sampling at 4 hour intervals would have begun at 1400
             instead of 1200. Inadequate sampling density may lead to
             erroneous results.

As shown in the figure, if instead of the samples obtained at 20 minute
intervals, only the samples collected at 4 hour intervals were studied (as
it has been often the case in chronobiologic investigations), the apparent
circadian variation as suggested by its best fitting cosine curve will
appear to be quite different if sampling would have been started at 1200
and continued at 4 hour intervals, or if sampling would have been started
at 1400. The sampling at different clock hours would have introduced an
artifact by aliasing due to the high amplitude 'episodic variations' (which
most likely are the expression of ultradian cycles) of cortisol secretion
which are superimposed upon the circadian rhythm. No synchronization
between the two frequencies is known which would allow to predict other
than with a certain degree of probability, the occurrence of ultradian
peaks or troughs at a given clock hour.
      The superimposed ultradian variations or episodic secretions make
for many functions 'single point' measurements at circadian stages
defined on the basis of information obtained from peer groups or even
from the subject itself rather difficult to interpret if not useless
since samples taken only a few minutes earlier or later may show

substantially different values. In functions showing high amplitude
ultradian or 'episodic' variations, a more meaningful 'single sample'
can be derived from prolonged continuous blood aspiration (e.g. with a
withdrawal pump) or from several collections over a certain time span
(e.g. 4 samples obtained at 15 minute intervals), which can be pooled
for the chemical determination of some analyte. The time span and/or the
sampling interval for such an 'integrated' sample would depend upon the
function to be studied, and i.e, upon the half life time in circulation of
the substance to be measured. Preferable would be, of course, continuous or
frequent short interval monitoring, preferably with a non-invasive or only
minimally invasive sensor which minimizes the interference of the
investigator with the subject.

For the laboratory evaluation of the higher frequencies the need
for extremely short sampling intervals may represent a problem and
sometimes a limitation. A limitation is also the amount of material
(e.g. blood) that can be removed throughout a sampling span (e.g. 24
hours) without interfering with the system to be measured, and is
especially in the lower frequencies the length of the sampling span
required to obtain statistically meaningful quantitative end points.

Rhythmometric procedures can be used to 'detect' rhythms in noisy
time series of laboratory values brought about by superimposed rhythms
of several frequencies which are continuously adjusted, modulated and
altered by regularly or randomly recurring environmental stimuli (24).
Rhythm 'detection' especially of unknown or unexpected frequencies,
however, requires a considerable amount of data collected over numerous
periods of the rhythm in question. Frequently unsatisfactory results of
rhythmometric procedures may come about simply due to the inadequacy of
the data available to obtain representative and statistically
meaningful results (which, of course, is not the fault of the
procedure). Nevertheless, the cosinor and related rhythmometric
procedures have provided some statistical end points for the
measurement and the quantitation and comparison of rhythms, and their
parameters and with all qualifications in mind allow a rhythm
comparison between subjects, different populations and different
functions. If quite empirically, 'rhythm detection' by cosinor is taken
as end point, a hierarchy of circadian rhythms identifiable by this
procedure in clinically healthy subjects comes to the fore. Figure 5 shows
the percentage of subjects in whom 'rhythm detection by cosinor analysis
could be obtained at different levels of statistical significance in a
number of endocrine functions of clinically healthy women.

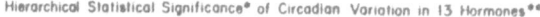

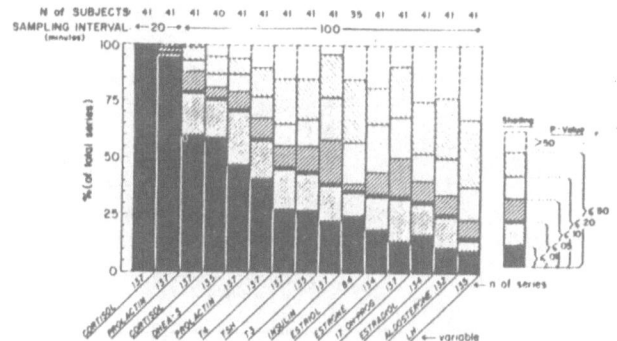

Figure 5:   Hierarchy of statistical significance of circadian variation
             in 13 hormones in plasma of clinically healthy women sampled
             at 20 minute and/or 100 minute intervals during 24-hours for
             individualized rhythm assessment. Analyses ('single cosinor')
             are based on least squares fit of 24-hour cosine function.
             The p value is dervied from an F test of the zero amplitude
             hypothesis. Forty-one subjects (for estriol 35) were sampled
             over 132-137 (84 for estriol) 24-hour spans. Cortisol and
             prolactin are shown at left sampled at 20 minute intervals
             and are shown again evaluated in samples obtained at 100
             minute intervals together with the other parameters.

At the far left, prolactin and cortisol are shown with sampling obtained at
20 minute intervals. In almost all instances, rhythm detection can be
achieved with this sampling schedule by cosinor analysis in these two
functions in a single subject studied over a single 24-hour span. The same
parameters are shown again farther to the right of the figure together with
the other functions, which were studied at 100 minute intervals only. If
the sampling frequency for cortisol and prolactin is reduced to 100 minute
intervals, still a large percentage but not all subjects show 'rhythm
detection' for cortisol and even fewer for prolactin. The decrease in
sampling density from 20 to 100 minutes leads to a certain, but not
dramatic loss of information. The comparison of the 13 hormonal functions
sampled at 100 minute intervals over one 24 hour span shows that there are
considerable differences in the number of individuals in whom 'rhythm
detection' was signaled by the cosinor analysis of each subject's data.
Apart from cortisol and prolactin, a large percentage of subjects
showed a circadian rhythm detectable by cosinor analysis under the
conditions of this study in aldosterone, while FSH, a predominantly
menstrually cycling variable, was found to be at the very low end of the
circadian spectrum.

The effect of increase or decrease of sampling density in the same subjects on 'rhythm detection' by cosinor is shown for plasma cortisol and prolactin in Figure 6a and b.

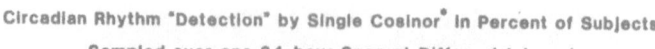

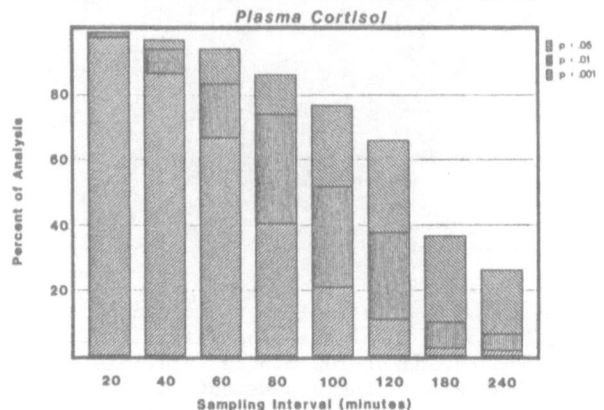

Figure 6a: Circadian rhythm in plasma cortisol concentration detected by single cosinor (p < 0.05) in percent of subjects sampled over one 24-hour span. Sampling occurred at 20 minute intervals. Samples obtained at different intervals were chosen for analysis. Number of profiles 140. Individual rhythm detection and quantification by single cosinor in 90 percent of subjects could be obtained by sampling at 60 minute intervals.

In the case of plasma cortisol (Figure 6a), a decrease of sampling density from 20 minutes to a 60 minute sampling interval will still give in over 90 percent of cases 'rhythm detection' by single cosinor within one 24 hour span. If the sampling interval is further increased to 120 minutes, 'rhythm detection' will still be obtained in over 65 percent of the subjects examined.

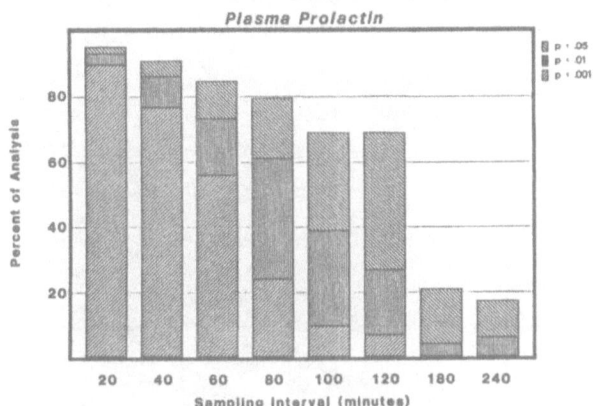

Circadian Rhythm "Detection" by Single Cosinor[*] in Percent of Subjects
Sampled over one 24-hour Span at Different Intervals

Plasma Prolactin

[*]Rejection of the no-rhythm (zero-amplitude assumption) in F-test

Figure 6b: Circadian rhythm in plasma prolactin concentration detected
by single cosinor (p < 0.05) in percent of subjects sampled
over one 24-hour span. Sampling occurred at 20 minute
intervals. Samples obtained at different intervals were
chosen for analysis. Number of profiles 140. Individual
rhythm 'detection' and quantification in prolactin in over 90
percent of subjects studied required sampling at 40 minute
intervals.

In prolactin (Figure 6b), which apparently represents a somewhat less
regular function, 'rhythm detection' in 90 percent of the subjects examined
required sampling at 40 minute intervals or less. At 120 minutes sampling
interval, however, the 'rhythm detection' rate was also around 65 percent.
     A rejection of the no-rhythm (zero-amplitude) assumption, however,
does not necessarily imply an agreement of the rhythm characteristics
in the original and decimated samples. A given sample size may be
sufficient to describe a rhythm, but (as shown in Figure 4) may lead to
parameter estimates that are widely divergent from those based upon all
data. By the same token, for the analyses in these figures, the shape
and the frequent non-sinusoidality of the waveform are ignored. The fit
of harmonics for a description of the waveform also has to be
considered in making a decision as to sample size, as described
elsewhere (32). Further work will have to ascertain, with harmonics,
the extent of deviation of the rhythm characteristics from a standard.
Thus, if a given acrophase is to be estimated within a certain number
of degrees, one will have to analyze all series now available to state
the number of samples required for the extent of conformity desired
with the characteristic based upon the complete sample.
     The study of blood or plasma parameters in chronobiology is
presently limited by the need for invasive sampling procedures and the
amount of blood which can be removed by frequent and/or prolonged

344

sampling. With measurements obtained at 4 hour intervals over a single 24 hour span, as it is frequently done in clinical studies, only a small percentage of subjects will show 'rhythm detection' by the cosinor procedure even in high amplitude circadian rhythms such as plasma cortisol or prolactin (Figure 7a and b).

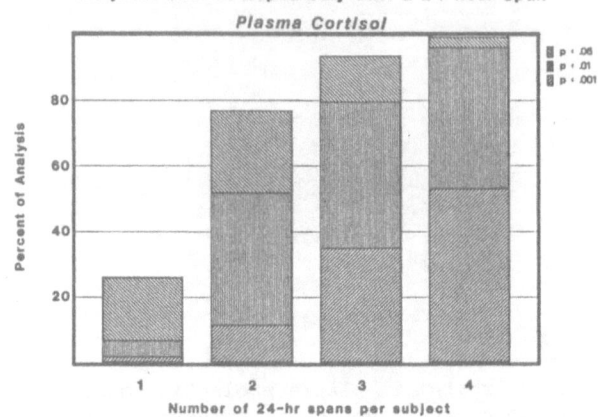

Figure 7a: Circadian rhythm 'detection' in plasma cortisol as indicated by single cosinor in 1,2,3 or 4 24-hour profiles (6 samples obtained at 4-hour intervals) obtained from the same 30 subjects sampled once during each season. In the central two columns, 100 groups of 2 or 3 profiles of the same subjects were examined (formed by random allocation from the four sets of data available from each subject).

Four 24-hour profiles (24 samples) allowed rhythm 'detection' and quantification by single cosinor in all subjects.

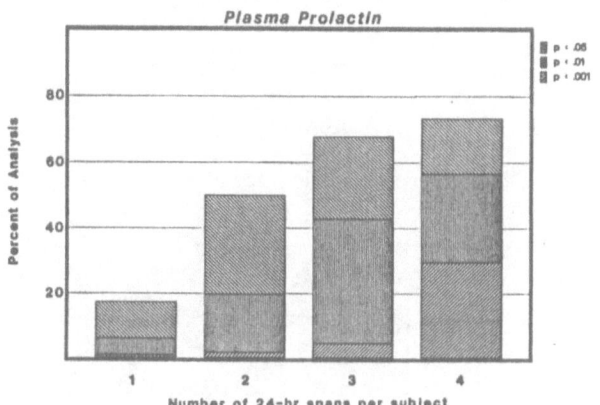

Circadian Rhythm "Detection" by Single Cosinor[*] In Percent of (Same)
Subjects Studied Repeatedly over a 24-hour Span
Plasma Prolactin

[*]Rejection of the no-rhythm (zero-amplitude assumption) in F-test

Figure 7b: Circadian rhythm in plasma prolactin as described by single
cosinor with rejection of the null-hypothesis for amplitude
in an F-test with a $p < 0.05$ in 1, 2, 3 or 4 24-hour
profiles (6 samples obtained at 4-hour intervals). The
profiles were obtained from the same 30 subjects sampled once
during each season. In the central two columns, 100 groups of
2 or 3 profiles of the same subject were examined (formed by
random allocation from the four sets of data available from
each subject).

Four 24-hour profiles (24 samples) yield indication of
statistical significance ($p < 0.05$) in about 75 percent of
subjects.

Improvement in 'rhythm detection' in individual subjects can be achieved by
increasing the data base by studying the same subject several times. The
subjects shown in Figure 7a and b were studied four times over a single
24-hour span each during different seasons (six samples were taken during
each 24-hour span at 4 hour intervals). In the premenopausal women this was
done by necessity during different stages of the menstrual cycle. The
24-hour profiles, although from the same subjects, thus were not
obtained during consecutive 24-hour spans.
    In the study of populations, the group size can be increased in
order to obtain statistically meaningful results. The gain in 'rhythm
detection' by single cosinor analysis by increasing the group size is
shown in Figure 8a & b.

346

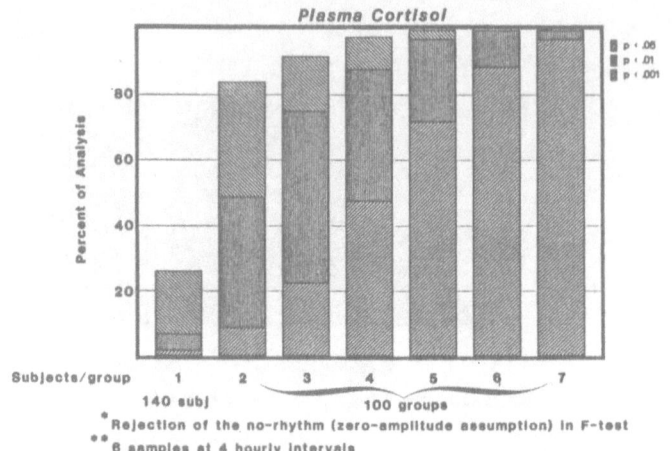

Circadian Rhythm "Detection" by Single Cosinor in 140 Single Subjects
and in 100 Randomly Chosen Groups of 2 to 7 Different Subjects
Studied over one 24-hour Span Each[**]

*Rejection of the no-rhythm (zero-amplitude assumption) in F-test
[**] 6 samples at 4 hourly intervals

Figure 8a: Circadian rhythm 'detection' in plasma cortisol as indicated
by single cosinor in 100 individual subjects and in 100
randomly allocated groups of 2 to 7 different subjects
sampled over a single 24-hour span each (6 samples obtained
at 4 hour intervals).

Groups of 5 subjects allowed rhythm 'detection' by single
cosinor in all instances.

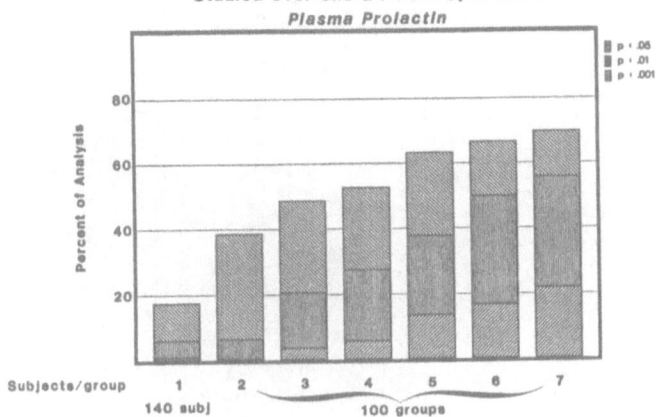

Figure 8b: Circadian rhythm 'detection' in plasma prolactin as indicated
by single cosinor in individual subjects and in randomly
allocated groups of 2 to 7 different subjects sampled over a
single 24-hour span each (6 samples obtained at 4 hour
intervals).

Groups of 4 subjects yield statistical significance by single
cosinor ($p < 0.05$) in slightly more than 50 percent, and
groups of 7 in slightly over 70 percent of the groups
examined.

These figures show the percentage of single cosinor analyses indicating
'rhythm detection' in individual subjects and in 100 groups of 2 - 7
different subjects chosen from the same pool at random. In cortisol, groups
of 4 to 5 different subjects of the population studied will in almost all
instances allow 'detection' and description of a circadian rhythm by single
cosinor. This result is similar to that obtained by repeated sampling of
the same subject (Figure 7a). In prolactin, however, groups of randomly
matched different subjects of the same pool show 'rhythm detection' by
single cosinor only in about 55 percent if groups of 4 are investigated (or
compared to 73% if four series of the same subject are examined), 63
percent in groups of 5 and slightly above 70 percent in groups of 7. In
prolactin, individual differences thus seem to be more pronounced than in
cortisol.

If extrapolation from the data set examined to the population as a
whole is desired, the population mean cosinor is the appropriate method

348

for analysis.

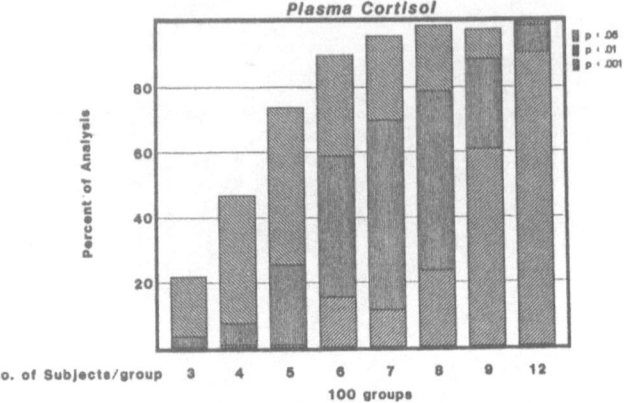

Circadian Rhythm "Detection" by Population Mean Cosinor
in 100 Groups of 3 to 12 Randomly Chosen Different
Subjects Studied over one 24-hour Span Each

Figure   9a: Circadian rhythm 'detection' in plasma cortisol by population
mean cosinor for randomly allocated groups of 3 to 12
different subjects studied over one 24-hour span each (6
samples obtained at 4 hour intervals).

With this technique of analysis, statistical significance of
the circadian rhythm as group phenomenon is indicated in
95-100% of groups of 7 to 8 subjects.

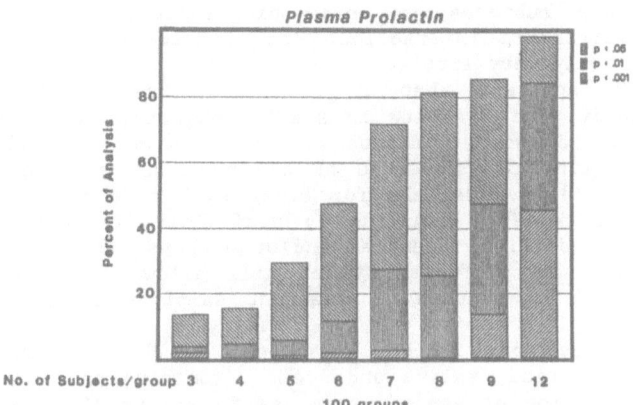

Circadian Rhythm "Detection" by Population Mean Cosinor*

in 100 Groups of 3 to 12 Randomly Chosen Different

Subjects Studied over one 24-hour Span Each

*Rejection of the no-rhythm (zero-amplitude assumption) in F-test

Figure 9b: Circadian rhythm in plasma prolactin as described by
population mean cosinor for randomly allocated groups of 3 to
12 subjects studied over one 24-hour span each (6 samples
obtained at 4 hour intervals).

With this technique of analysis, statistical significance at
the p < 0.05 level of the circadian rhythm as group
phenomenon is indicated in over 70 percent of groups of 7
subjects and in almost all instances in groups of 12
subjects.

For the analysis of the data presented in Figures 9a and 9b, the time
series of each subject were analyzed by single cosinor and the rhythm
parameters obtained by single cosinor served as input for the population
mean cosinor analysis of randomly allocated groups of subjects. As seen in
the figures, the population mean cosinor requires a larger group size to
allow extrapolation beyond the given data set. In plasma cortisol, analysis
by single cosinor indicated 'rhythm detection' in 85 and 93 percent of
groups of 2 and 3 subjects respectively, while the population mean cosinor
required groups of 6 and 7 subjects to achieve the same percentage (Figures
8a and 9a). In plasma prolactin, the single cosinor indicated 'rhythm
detection' in a data set of two subjects in almost 40 percent, and three
subjects in 50 percent, while the population mean cosinor required groups
of six subjects to obtain an indication of 'rhythm detection'. In larger
groups (e.g., 7 subjects), this difference disappears and the population
mean cosinor becomes equally effective. The comparison of cortisol (Figures
7a,8a,9a) and prolactin (Figures 7b,8b,9b) indicates differences in
sampling requirements for the two variables with less regularity and
possibly more individual features of the rhythm characteristics to be found
in prolactin.

It appears that in plasma prolactin 'rhythm detection' by cosinor analysis is achieved more easily in data of the same subject, even if sampled months apart than from the combination of the same number of profiles from different subjects. Each of the subjects may have a slightly different usual activity-rest pattern, which may have prevailed in spite of the uniform conditions on the day of sampling or each of the subjects may have his individual curve shape, ultradian-circadian interaction, etc., factors about which we today still know only very little.

It is apparent that in order to obtain meaningful and statistically valid results in single subjects, the sampling frequency in the study of most functions will have to be substantially increased over that clinically feasible at the present time. For this purpose techniques and/or materials for study will have to be sought, which provide for reliable sampling by noninvasive or minimally invasive methods. In addition, chemical and/or biophysical procedures will have to be found and perfected, which will allow the analysis of the parameters to be studied by frequent sampling in a cost-effective manner.

Among the body fluids, which can be obtained by noninvasive methods, are urine, saliva and sweat. Promising and well documented is the determination of steroid hormones in saliva (26). Alternatively of interest are measurements which can be obtained through the intact skin or a mucosal surface (e.g., the partial pressure of oxygen). Electrochemical or optical sensors applied on or implanted under the skin or even built into a contact lens may allow for the monitoring of analytes by frequent measurements over a prolonged time span with relatively non-invasive methodology. Approaches and instrumentation for relatively non-invasive chronobiologic studies in the gastrointestinal tract are presented by Dr. Kirt Vener in this volume.

III. BIOTECHNOLOGIC APPLICATIONS OF POTENTIAL USE IN CHRONOBIOLOGY-
     OPPORTUNITIES AND AVENUES FOR CHRONOBIOLOGIC ENGINEERING

For the application of chronobiology to clinical medicine, longitudinal monitoring of rhythmic body functions in single subjects is essential. Technology will have to be provided which allows the measurement of rhythmic functions in high, medium, and low frequency ranges in a cost effective, and as far as feasible, non-invasive manner.

High-technology chronobiologic monitoring of certain body functions will have a place in intensive care units or for patients undergoing potentially traumatic procedures (e.g., the induction treatment of acute leukemias, and other forms of cancer chemotherapy). Such applications are very expensive and will be applicable only to a limited number of patients in critical condition. Apart from applications in critical care, the current trend for cost containment has shifted patient care away from the hospital into the outpatient setting and from the treatment of existing disease to health maintenance. Home monitoring of body functions by the patient has become commonplace for blood pressure, body temperature, blood sugar, ketones, and some other blood and urine parameters (33). In chronobiology, autorhythmometry with simple inexpensive instrumentation has provided much information on some rhythmic functions especially in the circadian and lower frequency ranges. In the past, the number of parameters, which could be studied by these methods was limited, and so was the possibility for a timely rhythmometric evaluation of the data.

Recent developments in clinical chemistry, electronics and microprocessor technology, however, have led to the development of a new generation of instruments which measure a wide variety of laboratory parameters, and which in the 'low-tech approach' are either simple enough to allow the use by the patient at home or by other minimally trained people in the patients' surrounding, or which in the 'high-tech approach' consist of a biosensor and a recording device applied to or even implanted into the patient. Either approach can provide prolonged series of measurements as a function of time suitable for the study of rhythms in a cost effective manner.

(1) Dry Multilayer Film Chemical Analyses

One of the most active areas of innovative technology which is expected to have considerable opportunities for chronobiology is that of dry 'slide' or multilayer film chemistries in combination with reflectance, fluorescence and potentiometric analyses (34,35). There are a number of commercially available small, dry chemical analyzers suitable for home measurements of some parameters like blood glucose and ketones, which are relatively inexpensive and which require very little technical skill to operate. All that must be done to start an assay is to apply a small amount of sample to the slide. This is presently done by an office nurse or a technician in the physician's office and can be taught without much difficulty to many if not most patients. The performance of the dry reagent chemistries have been shown to be in most instances comparable to the more established procedures (34,35). Several of the instruments which are presently commercially available have been reviewed in a number of recent articles (34,36-38).

In dry chemistry procedures, the complete chemistries are miniaturized into a disposable dry format. Each reagent carrier contains all the chemical constituents required for a specific analysis applied on a support material, usually a thin rigid plastic or plastic-like material which may be transparent or reflective. The reflective zone in the carrier reflects to a detecting system any light not absorbed by the chemistry of the carrier. The reagent zone assembly on the carrier is often quite complex, and may include separation membranes, masking layers or trapping layers. All steps of the procedure required by the analyses are integrated into the analytical element. Separation steps mays be included into the carrier, e.g., plasma is separated from red blood cells by the carrier matrix as the red blood cells are removed by washing or wiping. Different reagent layers may be separated by semipermeable membranes. The conventional multiple step procedures are reduced to one single step. No prior reconstitution of reagents is required and the manipulations necessary consist of simply applying the sample. The amount of material required varies between 10 and 50 µliters, and if needed, the procedures could often be subjected to further miniaturization. An analysis is complete in one to seven minutes.

The chemical reactions occurring on dry reagent carriers usually are monitored by diffuse reflectance spectroscopy (39) and sometimes by fluorescence (40). In these procedures, the diffuse reflection from a matte surface is of interest which is the result of light interacting with the various chemical and physical factors in the reaction volume of the carrier including the absorption, transmission and scattering properties of the illuminated material. During the reaction on the carrier, a chromophore is either generated or degraded and is illuminated at a suitable wavelength. The amount of diffuse light recovered with the aid of the reflective layer is a measure of the progress of the reaction. The intensity of light reflected by the reaction media at one or several time points is determined relative to a known reflectance standard. As with transmittance, reflectance is not linear with concentration and require a data processor with the appropriate algorithms (41). The reactions resulting in the appearance or disappearance of fluorescence are monitored by front phase analysis in which irradiation and fluorescence are from the same surface of the carrier (42).

The technology of making dry reagent chemistries is sufficiently advanced that carriers can be developed for almost any chemical analysis. The waste of reconstituted but unused solutions is eliminated providing for more cost effectiveness in the use of the reagents. Since the reagents are stored dry until use, their shelf life is prolonged beyond that of reconstituted conventional chemistries.

Dry reagent chemistries are presently commercially available for nearly all the commonly tested blood metabolites (Table 1).

Table 1:   Examples of Dry Reagent Chemistries Presently Available
For Routine Clinical Use

Blood Metabolites

Glucose
Blood Urea Nitrogen
Uric Acid
Cholesterol
Triglycerides
Creatinine
Bilirubin
Ammonia
Calcium

Enzymes

Creatinine kinase
Lactate dehydrogenase
Aspartate transaminase
Alamine transaminase
α -amylase
γ -glutamyltransferase
Alkaline phosphatase

Therapeutic Drugs

Theophylline
Antibiotics Gentamycin
  Amikacin
  Tobramycin
Anticonvulsants
  Carbamazepine
  Phenytoin
  Pimidione

Electrolytes

K^+
Na^+
Cl^-
CO_2

The dry reagent chemistries, which were developed for electrolyte analysis are based on ion selective membranes using either electrochemical or spectroscopic analysis. In some respects, the principles used are very close to those which apply for the construction of ion selective electrodes. Also, the ionophores used in some drug chemistry carriers are similar to those used in electrodes. Enzyme determinations frequently require coupled multiple step procedures and may involve several enzyme systems and co-factors.

Dry chemistry procedures also lend themselves for competitive protein binding assays. This type of assay is widely used in drug level determinations. An example for this is the determination of the blood concentrations of the antiasthmatic drug theophylline (34). The competitive protein binding assay used for this purpose is based on a substrate-labeled fluorescence immunoassay (43). Upon placing the sample on the carrier, a competition for antibody binding sites is established between the theophylline present in the serum and a theophylline conjugate. The unbound conjugate remaining is proportional to the theophylline in the samples and is monitored by fluorescence. Following a similar competitive binding principle, dry chemistry carriers have been described for the detection of antibiotics like gentamicin, amikacin and tobramicin, and for the anticonvulsant drugs carbamazepine, phenytoin and primidone.

Instrumentation for dry reagent carriers presently available ranges in size from hand held devices designed for a single analyte to multi-parameter instruments. The instruments are microprocessor controlled allowing to store calibration curves and to time the chemical reaction on the carrier. Numerous small instruments are presently used in the determination of glucose in whole blood, e.g., the Glucometer (Ames Division, Miles Lab, NIC), the Accu-chek bG (Boehringer Mannheim Corp), the Easy Test (Australia Bio-transducers) and the Hypo-count IIB (hypoguard LTT).

Larger manual and automated instruments are available for the handling of a wide variety of chemistries. These include, among others, the Seralyzer reflectance photometer (Ames Division, Miles Lab Inc.) and the Ektachem and its variants by Eastman-Kodak. In these instruments, each test has a specific module that contains part of the computer memory for the test, i.e., the algorithm and the optical interference filter. Analysis time may range from 30 seconds to four minutes depending on the nature of the chemistry. The instrument's microprocessor maintains control of several operations including temperature, timing of reactions, calculations and display of clinical results. In addition, the system alerts the user to malfunctions and operator errors. The Seralyzer represents a manual instrument which requires that each chemistry and sample be introduced individually on the instruments table by the operator. Fully automated instrumentation is also available for use in larger laboratories as exemplified by the Ektachem 400 Analyzer (Eastman-Kodak). In this instrument, the operator need only provide the samples and select the desired tests. The instrument automatically selects the reagent carrier from a cassette, calibrates the selected chemistry, applies the sample and reports the results. It is capable of more than 500 tests per hour and can hold 1,600 dry reagent chemistries. This instrument can be programmed to run any of 16 currently available tests, and can be updated to run additional tests as they become available. The system reports malfunctions, diagnoses problems and tells how the operator can correct them.

For the use in clinical chronobiology, it would be very easy to develop small instruments with limited scope (one, two or three types of measurements only) for autorhythmometric studies using, e.g., saliva constituents as noninvasive end points. Such an instrument could be complemented by a data processor or microcomputer which may be as small as a programmable pocket calculator. Rhythmometric programs for instruments of that size are already available (44). These instruments could be directly linked to the chemical analyzer or, if separate, the patient would only have to enter the measured data with the type of rhythmometric analysis to be performed predetermined by the investigator. The information obtained could either be stored in the calculator/microcomputer and be evaluated by the medical investigator at the occasion of the patient's next visit, or in certain instances immediate feedback could be provided to the patient. The technology of measurement in clinical chemistry and the computational capability are both available, but have not yet been brought together for the specialized use in chronobiologic applications.

Because of their stability and discrete formats, dry reagent chemistries allow cost effective, low volume testing. In conjunction with the relatively low cost of small single or multi-purpose instruments, chronobiologic monitoring in physicians' offices and for some functions autorhythmometry of biochemical parameters in the patient's home may become feasible. This may open the door for the study of low frequency rhythms (e.g., in the circaseptan range). Applied to chronopharmacology, the capability to follow reference functions in different frequency ranges as well as to perform time qualified drug level determinations, may in some instances, allow patients to monitor and control the timing and the dose of their own medication.

(2) Biosensors

Recent progress in automation, miniaturization, and in the development of new techniques of measurement has lead to the development of instrumentation, which can give information about a large number of biochemical analytes in diverse body fluids by electrochemical or biochemical-optical probes which can be used inside or outside the human body. A high tech approach to measurements and data processing eliminates some of the uncertainties and potential errors which may occur in autorhythmometry by the patient. Such methods of measurement would especially be applicable in situations where the patient, due to the environmental conditions or due to his disease state or other circumstances, is not in a position to execute his own measurements and data entry or transfer.

Electronic instruments have changed medical practice in the hospital and more recently, even in the home. The monitoring of body functions has become an integral part of patient care in intensive care units, in neonatology, post-surgical and post-traumatic care and has become indispensable in the management of coronary heart disease and in numerous other disease states. Monitoring of the physical and/or chemical composition of the blood is widely used in anesthesia, i.e., in the form of continuous measurement of blood oxygenation and of the concentration of anesthetics in respiratory air and/or in blood.

Medical instrumentation has benefited from the information explosion in electronics. Today, self-contained medical instruments can carry out complex signal processing that only recently required a separate computer. The highly sophisticated processing capabilities of laboratory instruments, however, require high quality signals from sensors that serve as interphase between the biologic function to be measured and the electronic data processing system.

Chemical and biochemical sensors can deal with a wide range of species including gases, ions and a great variety of biologic compounds including hormones, enzymes and even whole cells. Within the last decade, there has been a rapid development of biophysical and biochemical sensing devices and the number of printed articles appearing in this field has skyrocketed to over 2,000 per year. The following overview is merely intended to outline for chronobiologists the present trends and the scope of some recent developments in the field, and to provide a limited number of key references of more specialized articles on some areas and some types of instrumentation with potential chronobiologic applications (45-49).

The majority of the sensors currently used in biomedical science are electrochemical in nature and in operational mode. Conductivity, amperometric, and potentiometric measurements can be obtained by the way of ion selective electrodes. Some of these electrochemical sensors have found practical application in the clinical laboratory and after a transition period of about 15 years, have now largely replaced the flame photometer in the determination of sodium, potassium, and calcium. In addition, however, by incorporation of appropriate biocatalysts such as enzymes in the membranes, much more complex biochemical and medical sensors can be constructed.

The combination of electrodes measuring simple end points like a change in hydrogen ion concentrations, CO_2 or ammonia with a more elaborate system leading over one or several steps of reactions to this end point provides for a wide variety of analytical possibilities. Enzymes and enzyme combinations can be used. Immune electrodes (responding either to antigen or antibody present in the material to be examined) and affinity sensors have been developed which use the principles of competitive binding analysis and provide an optical or electrochemical end point recognizable by a biosensor.

Most recently, the development of solid state technology has lead to the development of chemically sensitive field effect transistors (CHEMFETS) and their variants like ion specific field effect transistors (ISFETS). Some of these devices are amenable to miniaturization and mass production and can be produced at relatively low cost. Similar in some respects to the electrochemical applications, are optical probes ('optrodes') in which a change in color or fluorescence is measured spectrophotometrically or fluorometrically through a light conducting probe with an indicator, or an enzyme system in contact with the analyte to be measured or with the probe extending into a reaction chamber in which, e.g., a competitive binding process may take place.

(3) Ion selective electrodes:

The development of ion selective electrodes goes back to 1906 when Cremer described a probe for measuring pH. This glass electrode used together with a reference electrode and a potentiometer forms a useful analytical technique which has revolutionized the field of chemical analysis both of cations as well as anions (45,50-52). The electrodes sense the free activity of the ion species not the total concentration. The analytical useful range of ion specific electrodes is usually about 10^{-1} to 10^{-5} mole and the response time depending upon the type of electrode between a fraction of a second up to 1 minute. The response is logarithmic with the precision of the measurement constant over the dynamic range. These electrodes are widely used in clinical and environmental chemistry where a large number of samples must be assayed with a need for a rapid and inexpensive method of analysis.

Ion selective membranes may be designed for specific applications (Ion selective electrodes, ISE) (52-55).

Table 2: Ion-Selective Membrane Electrodes

Electrode Type	Measured Species
Glass membrane	$H^+,Na^+,Ag^+,Li^+,Cs^+,Rb^+,NH_4^+,TI^+$
Liquid Membrane ion exchanger	$Cu^{2+},CI^-,Mg^{2+},Ca^{2+},NO_3^{2-},CIO_4^-,UO_2^{2+}$, organic cations and anions, some drugs
Neutral carrier	$K^+,Li^+,H^+,Ca^{2+},Na^+,NH_4^+,Sr^{2+},Ba^{2+},Cd^{2+}$
Crystal membrane Single crystal	F^-
Polycrystalline	$S^{2-},Ag^+,Hg^{2+},CI^-,Br^-$
Mixed crystal	$CI^-,Br^-,I^-,CN^-,SCN^-,Cd^{2+},Pb^{2+},Cu^{2+}$
Gas sensors using ion electrodes as elements	CO_2,NH_3,H_2S,SO_2,HCN

After:Rechnitz, 1982 (61)

Table 2 summarizes the main classes of ion selective membrane electrodes, and some of the analytes for which they are presently being used. Recent advances in membrane technology and the combination of the sensor devices with a microprocessor have made in vivo monitoring possible, e.g., the continuous measurement of sodium and potassium in undiluted urine of catheterized patients. This type of system is found in intensive care units and is used during open heart surgery. At the present, adequate solvent polymeric membranes for clinically relevant measurements are available among others for sodium, potassium, calcium in blood serum and whole blood, and for sodium and potassium in undiluted urine. Also liquid membrane microelectrodes useful for intracellular studies of sodium, potassium, calcium, magnesium and hydroxyl ion have been described (54,55). Runs of over 24-hours can be performed with these devices without deterioration of performance (56).

The potential of such electrodes alone or incorporated into more complex biosensors is virtually unlimited. The selectivity of these systems may be tailored to a certain degree and they allow the construction of cell assemblies in a wide variety of shapes and sizes. The membranes to be used have to provide selectivity, stability of the measured cell potential difference, a reasonably short response time and an adequately long life time. In view of these goals, highly lipophilic membrane components (e.g. plastizers) have been incorporated in ISE membranes. Most electrodes are relatively stable and provide measurements with a clinically relevant precision for several hours or more without need for intermediate calibration. The life time of the membranes is expected to be several months (57). The speed of response under field conditions is for many electrodes adequate for the measurement of higher frequency rhythms extending to the range of the cardiac and respiratory cycles in small animals (58).

(4) Bioselective chemical sensors - bioselective electrodes:

Bioselective chemical sensors are designed to respond selectively and sensitively to a specific analyte. They depend on a matrix bound bioactive substance for molecular recognition and on an electronic device for signal transduction. The molecular recognition of the analyte to be determined is responsible for the selectivity of a biosensor. A variety of bioactive substances like enzymes, binding proteins, lectins, hormone receptors and antibodies have been used for molecular recognition in matrix bound forms. These substances determine the specificity, and to a large degree also the sensitivity of the sensor. Their characteristics and their binding concepts with the analyte to be measured have to be taken in account in the design of the molecular recognition site of a biosensor. Various ways of immobilization of these substances in the matrix or on the surface of an electrochemical device can be followed (53,55,59).

Bioselective electrodes can be constructed by combining ion or gas sensing membrane electrodes with a substance or phase that converts the compound to be measured over one or several steps of reactions to a species sensed by the electrodes (53,54,60-62). By using this approach, the measurement capabilities of membrane electrodes can be extended to many classes of biological compounds, and chemical or immunochemical amplification can be used in a multiple step procedure to greatly enhance the sensitivity of the method. A variety of materials can be employed as biocatalysts extending in different systems from isolated enzymes to whole cells, and to plant and animal tissue sections.

An enzyme electrode consists of a thin layer of enzyme immobilized on or incorporated in the surface of the membrane of an electrochemical sensor (53-55,61). The enzyme reacts with the substance to be determined consuming a co-reactant or generating an electroactive product, which can be monitored electrochemically. Both potentiometric and amperometric indicating electrodes have been used in enzyme based sensors. Bioselective enzyme-electrodes have been developed for a wide variety of biologically and clinically important substances (Table 3). These devices have the advantage to be simple and inexpensive and require a minimum of treatment. The detection limits reached are quite favorable. Enzyme based electrodes have a long life expectancy and a fast response time. Multienzyme electrodes have been developed which allow the determination of a wide variety of compounds.

Automated potentiometric gas sensing systems are ideally suited for use as detectors in enzyme-immunoassay arrangements. Enzyme-immunosensors depend on the molecular recognition of the analyte by an antibody for selectivity and on the chemical amplification of an enzyme for sensitivity. In such a sensor, an antibody bound to the membrane, and e.g., an ammonia sensor device can be assembled with considerable gain in sensitivity over conventional techniques. The ammonia liberating enzyme adenosine deaminase can be used as a label and can be covalently coupled to protein antigens. The activity of the enzyme in the reaction mixture can be monitored with a variety of sensing systems which measure the rate of ammonia production. By using enzyme and immunologic agents in conjunction with gas sensing

Table 3: Examples of Substances Analyzed with Bioselective Enzyme Based Electrodes

Substance	Enzyme	Sensor	Concentration Range mM/L
Acetic Formic Acid	Alcohol Oxidase	Pt (O_2)	0.1–100
Alcohols	Alcohol Oxidase	Pt (O_2)	0.5–100 mg%
		Pt (H_2O_2)	0.5–100 mg%
Amygdalin	β–Glucosidase	CN^-	0.01–10
Cholesterol	Cholesterol Oxidase	Pt (H_2O_2)	0.1–10
D–Amino Acids	D–AA Oxidase	Cation	0.05–10
Glucose	Glucose Oxidase	pH	1–100
		Pt (H_2O_2)	0.1–20
		Pt (O_2)	0.01–100
	Glucose Oxidase & Catalase	Gas (O_2)	0.1–20
L–amino Acids	L–AA Oxidase	Pt (H_2O_2)	0.01–1
		Pt (O_2)	0.1–10
		Gas (O_2)	0.1–10
		NH_4^+	0.1–10
L–asparagine	Asparaginase	Cation	0.05–10
L–glutamic Acid	Glutamate Dehydrogenase	Cation	0.1–100
L–glutamine	Glutaminase	Cation	0.1–100
L–Tyrosine	L–Tyrosine Decarboxylase	Gas (CO_2)	0.1–100
Lactic Acid	Lactate Dehydrogenase	$Pt[Fe(CN)_6^{4-}]$	0.1–2
Nitrate	Nitrate Reductase/ Nitrite Reductase	NH_4^+	0.1–10
Nitrite	Nitrite Reductase	NH_3 (Gas)	0.1–50
Penicillin	Penicillinase	pH	0.1–10
Phosphate	Phosphatase/ Glucose Oxidase	Pt (O_2)	0.1–10
Succinic Acid	Succinate Dehydrogenase	Pt (O_2)	0.1–10
Sulfate	Aryl–Sulfatase	Pt	0.1–100
Urea	Urease	Cation	0.05–10
		(Gas) NH_3	0.05–50
		(Gas) CO_2	0.0–10
Uric Acid	Uricase	Pt (O_2)	0.1–10

After: Guilbault 1982 (53)

detectors, methodologies for measuring a host of clinically important substances have been developed.

In microbial sensors, matrix bound microbial cells and an electrochemical device are assembled in a similar fashion as in enzyme sensors. The respiratory activity of the microbial cells can be measured with a Clark type oxygen electrode, or metabolites of the matrix bound microbial cells can be detected by an appropriate electrochemical system (63). Organelle and tissue sensors incorporate the multienzyme systems of subcellular organelles and animal tissues confined in a proper matrix for molecular recognition similar to those used in enzyme and microbial devices (64).

Bacterial cells or tissue sections may, in some cases, offer advantages over enzyme electrodes in terms of higher biocatalytic activity and may improve the life time of the probe, and eliminate the need for added cofactors or activators. Such devices may extend the range of use for biocatalytic membrane electrodes to biochemical constituents not readily measured with conventional electrodes. In addition, bacterial electrode selectivity and sensitivity may be improved by bacterial induction and/or by genetic manipulation techniques (63).

Membrane electrodes have been developed among others for the determination of a variety of drugs (65) and recently also of hormones using enzyme immunoassays (66).

Potential problems with bioselective potentiometric membrane electrodes are the need for frequent calibration, a relatively slow dynamic response time which may fall into the 2–7 minute range, and the time required to recondition the electrode between measurements, which may be as long as 20 minutes. A major limiting factor is also the sensitivity of potentiometric membrane electrodes. Also, there may be interference from other volatile and nonvolatile acids or bases that may be present in the sample. A limitation of glass electrode based gas sensors is the technical difficulty encountered when trying to miniaturize such devices. The latter problems have been improved to some degree by the development of polymer membrane type ion selective electrodes as sensing elements.

(5) Chemically Sensitive Field Effect Transistors (CHEMFET)

Semiconductor technology has been successfully applied to the development and fabrication of miniature chemical and biochemical sensors (67,68). Some of these are derived from the same technology as used in the microelectronics industry, namely microfabrication and microlithography. There are numerous advantages to the application of semiconductor technology to chemical sensors. Modern techniques using optical mask exposure can mass produce devices with two micron geometrics. Todays x-ray and electron beam lithography systems routinely produce devices with 0.5 micron geometrics. Microlithographic techniques have been applied, not only in the production of sensors and detectors, but also in the design of numerous other miniaturized instrument components in instrumentation of potential importance for the monitoring of biologic functions by portable or even implantable devices.

First reported by Bergveld, 1970, (69) the Chemically Sensitive Field Effect Transistor (CHEMFET) is essentially a conventional insulated-gate field effect transistor which has its metallic gate contact replaced by a chemically sensitive coating and a reference electrode (67,70) (Fig. 10). A current is made to flow by the

360

application of a voltage across the source and the drain contacts.
Interactions of the ions in solution with the membrane result in a
change of the interfacial potential. The variations in the electric
field in the gate region located between source and drain produce
corresponding variations in the observed drain current. In these
devices, the surface field effect due to the absorption and
disassociation of surface sites on the gate insulator is the desirable
potential generating mechanism. It is usually associated with rapid
response and long term stability.

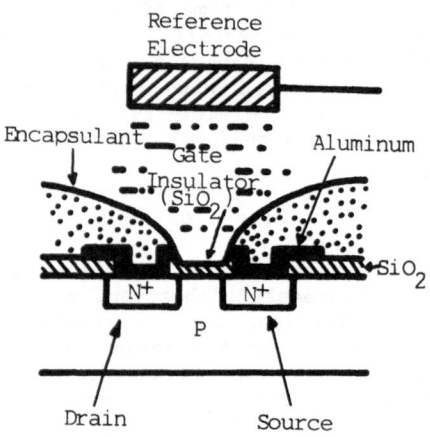

Figure 10: Structure of a simple silicon dioxide gate ion sensitive
field-effect-transistor (ISFET). This ISFET is rendered pH
sensitive by exposing the bare silicon dioxide gate insulator
to the sample solution ('bare gate' ISFET). Alternatively,
chemically sensitive membranes can be applied on top of the
gate insulator to create more complex sensors.

Four types of CHEMFETS with biomedical applications have been
described, which are of considerable promise also for chronobiologic
applications. These are gas sensitive, ion sensitive, enzyme sensitive
and immunosensitive CHEMFETS (67,68,71)
The leading challenge in the construction of chemical microsensors
is to develop reproducible coatings that are compatible with the device
and selective to the chemical species of interest. The ultimate
performance of chemical microsensors will be determined by the coating
chemistry.
The ion sensing CHEMFET (or ISFET as it is often called) has
advantages in its small size (e.g., less than 1 mm square area) and low
output impedance which makes it ideal for in vivo monitoring and/or for
the analysis of small sample volumes. The small size allows the design

of multiple ion sensor assemblies. In addition to detecting ions in solution (72-75) and reducing gases,(72,76) CHEMFETS offer a tremendous potential for immunological and enzymatic assays (67,70). Several mechanisms of interaction are possible between the immobilized enzyme or antibody coating and the CHEMFET. Because selectivity may be degraded by the complex medium to be analyzed (e.g., blood or urine), the use of multiple microsensors together with pattern recognition techniques will be essential. For this purpose, an array of sensors may be used, which respond in a reproducible, but probably non-linear way to the target molecule and to known interferences. This approach will require suitable algorithms to provide qualitative and quantitative analytical information. The ever diminishing costs of computation power, however, will make such an approach feasible in the future.

CHEMFETS can easily and inexpensively be mass produced and their small sizes are particularly attractive if expensive enzymes or antibodies are to be used in a disposable device. The main technological problem which has prevented the wide scale use of CHEMFETS is related to the encapsulation of the devices. No traces of moisture or ion contaminants can be allowed to penetrate beyond the ion selective coating or instability results. Packaging them is an area that will require a major commitment before mass produced sensors will be available.

(6) Bioaffinity sensors:

The principle of detection by affinity sensors is based on the competitive binding of the analyte to be measured and a labeled analogue with receptor sites, which are specific for the analyte and the competing labeled ligand. The end points to be measured with these devices can be electrochemical, optical or heat production or consumption.

If the ligand and the reagent are larger molecules than the analyte, they can be confined by a dialysis membrane that allows the analyte to transfer freely between the phases. An essential feature of the ligand is that its electrical thermal or optical properties change in a measurable way upon binding to the reagent. The detected parameters may be based on the property of the ligand alone or on the combination of ligand with reagent. The response of the system depends on the relative affinity of the ligand and the analyte for the immobilized reagent. The transducer, depending upon the end point measured can be an electrode, a CHEMFET, a thermistor or an optrode (77,78).

The use of antibodies as a specific reagents in such a system does allow the design of many possible sensors. However, since in such rather complex systems more processes and larger molecules are involved, the response times may be relatively slow. The sensitivity of these probes is adequate for the range of clinical interest as applied to numerous substances in blood and other body fluids. The glucose sensor described by Schultz, et al (1982) (79,80) reaches a sensitivity in the 10^{-3} range. Sensitization of the procedure can be attained by enzyme amplification techniques as was shown by Ikariyama et al (1982)(78) for thyroxine in the concentration range from 10^{-8} to 10^{-6} gm/mL and for biotin in the concentration range from 10^{-9} to 10^{7} gm/mL (81).

(7) Thermobioanalyzers:

Most enzymatic reactions are accompanied by considerable heat evolution in the range of 5-100 kJ/mole. Some of the possibilities and advantages of analytical devices using immobilized enzymes can,

362

therefore, be applied to a combination of the immobilized enzyme with a thermometric probe (82).

A wide variety of different substances can be determined by this approach (Table 4).

Table 4: Examples of Substances Analyzed with the Enzyme Thermistor and Related Thermal Bioanalyzers

Substance	Immobilized Biocatalyst	Conc. Range (mM/L)
Clinical Analysis		
Ascorbic Acid	Ascorbic Acid Oxidase	0.05-0.6
ATP	Apyrase or Hexokinase	1-8
Cholesterol	Cholesterol Oxidase	0.03-0.15
Cholesterol Esters	Cholesterol Esterase + Cholesterol Oxidase	0.03-0.15
Creatinine	Creatinine Iminohydrolase	0.01-10
Glucose	Glucose Oxidase/Catalase	0.002-0.8
Glucose	Hexokinase	0.5-25
Lactate	Lactate 2-monoxygenase	0.01-1
Oxalic Acid	Oxalate Oxidase	0.005-0.5
Oxalic Acid	Oxalate Decarboxylase	0.1-3
Triglycerides	Lipase, Lipoprotein	0.1-5
Urea	Urease	0.01-500
Uric Acid	Uricase	0.5-4
Soluble Enzyme Analysis		
Urea	Urease (soluble)	0.1-100 U/ml
H_2O_2	Catalase (soluble)	0.1-100 U/ml
Immunological Analysis (TELISA)		
Albumin (antigen)	Immobilized Antibodies + Enzyme-Linked Antigen	10^{-13} mol/L (detection limit)
Gentamicin (antigen)	''	0.1 ug/mL (detection limit)
Insulin (antigen)	''	0.1-1.0 U/mL (detection limit)

After: Mosbach and Danielsson, 1981 (89)

In principle, the chances are excellent for finding a suitable candidate for a particular biochemical substrate to be analyzed among the more than 2100 different enzymes that have so far been characterized and allotted a specific number. The concentration of numerous compounds of clinical interest lies well within the detection range. The same measuring device can also be applied with slight modifications to the growing area of immunochemical analyses, i.e., antigen-antibody determinations. This type of procedure has been described as 'thermometric enzyme link immunosolvent assay (TELISA) (77). Excellent sensitivity down to 10^{-13} mole/liter has been found with the Telisa technique, which may serve for the automated determination of hormonal variables, enzymes, etc., in flow systems and other applications outside the patient's or animal's body where interference from other sources of heat production can be eliminated.

The methods provided by this technique depend for their specificity on the enzyme or other reaction systems used in the measurement device. The detection of a change in heat production (either increase or decrease) is entirely nonspecific and is applicable to an almost unlimited array of chemical systems. The sensitivity of this approach, however, is somewhat limited (10^{-5}) except when used in the Telisa technique.

(8) Chemical sensors based on fiber optics:

The devices developed in this category involve a reagent phase on the end of a fiber optic. In operation, the interaction of the reagent phase with the analyte leads to a change in the optical properties of the reagent phase which is probed and detected through the fiber optic (83). Depending on the particular device, the optical property measured can be absorbance, reflectance, luminescence, fluorescence or something else. An example of such a device would be a pH sensor based on an immobilized dye whose color or fluorescence properties vary with pH (84,85). Optical sensors are in their design either reversible or non-reversible. A sensor is reversible if the reagent phase is not consumed by its interaction with the analytes. If the reagent phase is consumed, then the sensor is non-reversible. For such a device to be useful for sensing over a prolonged time span, the relative consumption of reagent phase must be small, or there must be provisions for renewing the reagent.

The term optrode is used to describe such devices. While this term is formed by combining 'optical' and 'electrode', the operating principles are quite different offering more possibilities relative to electrodes on the one hand, but at the same time being subject to limitations and problems that are not experienced by electrodes. Attractive features of optical sensors relative to electrodes include the following: 1) the signal is optical and not subject to electrical interference; 2) no reference electrode is required; 3) the reagent phase does not have to physically contact the fiber optics and can be in a different environment. It is, therefore, simple to change and in some instances, it will be practical to use a disposable reagent phase. 4) multiple wave lengths can be used and temporal information on chemical reactions (e.g. luminescence) can be obtained. Sensors can be designed that respond simultaneously to two or more analytes distinguished by measurement at two or more wave length combinations. 5) optical sensors can offer cost advantages over electrodes, particularly when a single spectrometer is used for several sensors. Laser illumination may be used for long distance transmission or to get a useful signal from a small amount of reagent.

Optical sensors, however, are also subject to several limitations relative to electrodes: 1) ambient light will interfere with their operation; 2) long term stability may be a problem for some reagent systems; 3) when the amount of reagent phase is small and its detection range is increased by using more intense probe radiation, this will accelerate any photo-degradation process of the reagents. In consequence, in an optical sensor, there may be a trade off between the amount of reagent phase, intensity of probe radiation and stability; and 4) optical sensors may have limited dynamic ranges as compared to electrodes.

The material of the fiber optic determines the usable range of

wave lengths. Silica optics permit measurements in the ultraviolet down
to 220 nm but are relatively expensive. Glass is less expensive and is
suitable for measurements in the visible. Plastic fibers are less
expensive still but are restricted to wave lengths above 450 nm. The
devices may use either bifurcated or single fiber optic bundles.

Because the response of an optrode depends on the equilibrium
constant, optical sensors will measure only the concentration of
analyte in the form available to interact with the reagent phase. For
example, an optical metal ion sensor based on an immobilized ligand
will measure free metal rather than total metal (just like a
potentiometric electrode).

Of interest are the recently developed optical affinity sensors
based on the principle of competitive binding using binding proteins,
antibodies and receptors. As applied to optrodes competitive binding
based sensors make it possible to use analytical reactions that do not
directly produce optical change (79,80).

Fluorescent sensors are particularly well suited for optical
sensing (86). Fluorescence measurement is compatible with a single
strand optic measurement device because the detected radiation can be
distinguished from the probe radiation by wave length. Fluorescence is
a sensitive technique capable of measuring low analyte concentrations.
Non-fluorescent ligands that form fluorescent complexes with metal ions
have been used to prepare sensors for magnesium, zinc, cadmium and
aluminum.

Two wave length fluorescence measurements can be used. The
parameter measured in these sensors is the ratio of fluorescence
intensity admitted at one wave length and excited at another. The ratio
measurement is insensitive to current fluctuations, temperature
quenching, ionic strength and slow loss of reagents, all of which can
affect the single intensity measurement.

Optical sensors can also be based on fluorescence quenching, namely, a
decrease in reagent phase fluorescence upon association with analyte.
Although this approach is inherently less desirable than systems involving
increases in intensity with analyte concentration, it allows access to
analytes that could not otherwise be sensed by fluorescence. A pertinent
example of a sensor based on quenching is the oxygen probe developed by
Peterson et al (87).

A fluorescence-based competitive binding optrode sensor for
glucose has been described by Schultz et al, 1982 (79,80). In this
device, a specific glucose binding reagent, concanavalin-A, is
immobilized on cepharose on the walls of the fiber and, thus, out of
the reagent volume illuminated through the fiber optic. The competing
ligand is dextran, labeled with fluorescein. Increasing glucose
concentration displaces the labeled dextran from the binding sites on
concanavalin-A causing it to be free to diffuse into the illuminated
solution volume. This in turn, leads to an increase in fluorescein,
which is related to glucose concentration. The molecular weight cut off
of the dialysis fiber is low enough to completely retain the 70,000 mw
dextran within the fiber lumen while glucose can freely pass through
the dialysis membrane. The sensor is completed by inserting a single
optical fiber in the lumen of the dialysis fiber, thus allowing
measurement of the unbound dextran.

Future progress in this field will depend on the development of
appropriate reagent phases for a great variety of determinations. A
wide range of approaches and systems are possible.

The application of optical sensors to the gastrointestinal tract is discussed in detail by Dr. Kirt Vener in this volume.

(9) <u>Glucose Sensors</u>:

Glucose sensors are at this time probably the sensing device most widely used for practical application in patients. The clinical need lead to the development of a large number of devices of different design and operating mode, including electrodes, enzyme thermistors, CHEMFETS, optrodes, and others (88,89).

Glucose sensors can be used in the blood stream, in tear fluid or in the peritoneal cavity. Most glucose sensors follow the electro-enzymatic approach (90) and are usually based on glucose oxidation with the enzyme glucose oxidase which causes a decrease in the partial pressure of oxygen, an increase in pH and the production of hydrogen peroxide. The change in all of these chemical components can be used to determine the concentration of glucose. Also, the direct electrocatalytic oxidation of glucose on a platinum electrode has been successful (91). As mentioned above, an optical approach has been used in the form of a fluorescence based affinity sensor (79,80). This sensor is very simple and can be miniaturized. Also, a combination of the glucose oxidase system with luminescence was described (92).

The measurement of the optical rotation of a polarized beam of light allows measurement of glucose in the aqueous humor of the eye which is proportional to the concentration of glucose in blood. A non-invasive glucose sensor, which can be housed on a scleral contact lens based upon this principle, has been proposed. The optical rotation of the beam directed laterally through the anterior chamber of the eye allows the quantitative measurement of glucose (93,94).

Glucose sensors based on chemically sensitive field effect transistors (CHEMFETS) have also been developed (95). The CHEMFETS or ISFETS being considered for use as glucose sensors are based on pH ISFETS in combination with a selective membrane covering the gate. The membrane contains immobilized glucose dehydrogenase, glucose oxidase or some other enzyme to break down glucose into a product which causes a change in the pH of the solution at the interface. The advantage of this approach is that such semiconductor devices can be miniaturized very easily and can be designed to be autoclaved. The electronic part of the Isfet glucose sensor can produce a fast and stable response with low noise at potentially low cost.

If sensors are to be implanted, it has to be possible to calibrate the sensor in-situ. The major problems with all enzymatic glucose sensors implanted in the body are the instability of the immobilized enzyme which degrades over time and, the deterioration of the membrane surface due to interfering blood substances under physiologic conditions in the body, which are rather harsh for a sensor.

The chemosensors for glucose have found wide applications in diabetes management. Their use has clearly demonstrated the circadian time structure of the carbohydrate metabolism. Observations like the 'morning effect' in glucose tolerance made by the use of monitoring devices are now generally known and have been applied to treatment. In diabetes, the combination of glucose sensors with insulin pumps most recently lead to the development of closed loop systems, which monitor and regulate the carbohydrate metabolism of the diabetic automatically in a periodic fashion, serving as 'artificial pancreas' (96).

IV. SUMMARY AND OUTLOOK

Regularly recurring and thus predictable variations in time are a basic property of living matter and are found at all levels of biologic organization from subcellular organelles to the organism as a whole. The question of when a biologic process occurs has been recognized to be as important as to where it occurs and what it consists of. Thus, chronobiology is an integral part of human physiology and determines our response and adaptation to our surrounding. Temporal alterations appear to be of importance in the pathobiology of risk states for common diseases, and further for the development of pathology and disease. The rapidly developing field of chronopharmacology is adding the time dimension to medical treatment, and in some areas may be essential for achieving a therapeutic success within the range of acceptable undesirable side effects.

The impact of chronobiology to applied physiology, work hygiene, preventive medicine, chronopharmacology and pathology, however, will depend critically upon our capability to obtain adequate time series of biophysical and/or biochemical measurements of physiologic functions and to rapidly accomplish inferential statistical quantitation of the parameters of the rhythms observed within a time for this information to be clinically meaningful.

Dry chemistry techniques with relatively inexpensive instrumentation and great simplicity in the performance of the analyses may expand the scope of ambulatory autorhythmometry, to a large number of chemical determinations in saliva, urine, and if necessary blood. Thus, certain infradian rhythms of potential clinical importance (e.g., in the circaseptan frequency range) may become amenable to study. The drug level determinations available with these techniques may lend themselves for chronopharmacologic applications, and together with the study of appropriate reference rhythms for the guidance of chronotherapy of numerous clinical conditions.

Beyond the opportunities provided by these simple chemical instruments and methods, the fast developing sensor technology promises the capability to obtain series of measurements in frequent intervals, over prolonged time spans. Some of the devices presently available or in development require the patient to be connected to an instrument e.g., to a photometer or a fluorimeter, like in the case of the optrodes. Miniaturization in these areas has not yet proceeded to a state to allow availability of portable instrumentation at an acceptable cost. In many other instances, however, like some of the sensors for glucose, miniaturization has reached a point that self-contained closed-loop systems of sensor and insulin pump have become feasible with implantation of the instruments, and long term accuracy and precision of the measurements. In areas like the management of diabetes, growth regulation, in certain fertility problems and in the chemotherapy of malignant diseases with highly toxic substances, the monitoring of certain body functions by invasive methods like implanted sensors may be justifiable. In most present and potential future applications of chronobiology to clinical medicine, including work hygiene, however, rhythms will have to be studied and used as phase reference which can be measured by non-invasive means like the monitoring of variables in saliva, sweat, tear fluid and urine. To be useful and cost-effective in practice, these measurements must be performed on an ambulatory basis with equipment of a size and weight to be compatible with the normal activity of the patient and the method of study, and the equipment used must be socially acceptable.

In the future, microfabrication techniques of biosensors will offer an enormous range of opportunities for chemical analyses. Mass production of many of these components has become feasible at an acceptable price. In addition, the revolution in microcomputer technology has profoundly changed the way analytical information is processed. This wave of technology will produce a dramatic change in the way analytical information can be obtained, evaluated by quantitative statistical techniques and rapidly made available for practical application in human physiology and medicine. The new technology will allow adequate sampling and inexpensive analysis and □as you go□ quasi current data analysis, which are essential for a timely clinical utilization of chronobiologic information.

It is essential to recognize the need for the study of the time dimension in human physiology and medicine, and for its timely application to individual subjects. We have to be aware of the limitation of our present techniques, and the opportunities provided by the recent dramatic progress in electronics and biotechnology. The application of this new technology to the measurement and the evaluation of biologic parameters as a function of time will require a certain investment in funds and effort. This investment, however, will be small in comparison to the potential gains in human well being, prevention of disease and efficacy of diagnosis and treatment which can be expected as a result of a meaningful biomedical application of chronobiology.

REFERENCES
1. Haus E, Lakatua DJ, Sackett-Lundeen LL, Swoyer J: Chronobiology in laboratory medicine. In: Clinical Aspects of Chronobiology, (ed) WT Reitveld, Baarn:Bakker, 13-82, 1984.
2. Haus E, Lakatua DJ, Swoyer J, Sackett-Lundeen LL: Chronobiology in hematology and immunology. Am J of Anatomy 168:467-517, 1983.
3. Nicolau GY, Haus E, Lakatua DJ, Bogdan C, Popescu M, Petrescu E, Sackett-Lundeen L, Swoyer J, Adderley J: Circadian periodicity of the results of frequently used laboratory tests in elderly subjects. Rev Roum Med-Endocrinol 21:3-21, 1983.
4. Nicolau GY, Haus E, Lakatua D, Bogdan C, Petrescu E, Sackett-Lundeen L, Berg H, Ioanitiu D, Popescu M, Chiopan C, Milcu SM: Endocrine circadian time structure in the aged. Rev Roum Med-Endocrinol 20:165-176, 1982.
5. Nicolau GY, Lakatua DJ, Sackett-Lundeen L, Haus E: Circadian and circannual rhythms of hormonal variables in clinically healthy elderly men and women. Chronobiol Internat 1(4):301-319, 1984.
6. Touitou Y, Touitou C, Bogdan H, Chasselut J, Beck H, Reinberg A: Circadian rhythms in blood variables of elderly subjects. Chronobiologia 5:199-200, 1978.
7. Kanabrocki EL, Scheving LE, Halberg F, Brewer R, Bird T: Circadian variations in presumably healthy men under conditions of peace-time army reserve training. Space Life Sci 4:258-270, 1973.
8. Reinberg A, Schuller E, Delasuiere N, Clench J, Helary M: Rhythmes circadiens et circannuelles des leucocytes proteines totales immunoglobulines A Get M: etude chez 9 adultes jeunes et sains. Nouv Presse Med 6:3819-3823, 1977.

368

9. Casale G, Nicola de P: Circadian rhythms in the aged: A review. Arch Gerontol Geriatr 3:267-284, 1984.
10. Halberg F, Lagoguey M, Reinberg A: Human circannual rhythms over a broad spectrum of physiological processes. Int J Chronobiol 8:225-268, 1983.
11. Scheving LE, Halberg F, Kanabrocki EL: Circadian rhythmometry on 42 variables of thirteen presumably healthy young men. In: Proc XII Internat Conf of the Int Soc Chronobiol, Il Ponte, Milano, 47-71, 1977.
12. Moore-Ede MC, Sulzman FM, Fuller CA (eds): The Clocks That Time Us: Physiology of the Circadian Timing System. Harvard University Press, 448 pp, 1982.
13. Minors DS, Waterhouse JM (eds): Circadian Rhythms and the Human. John Wright & Sons, Ltd, England, 332 pp, 1981.
14. Haus E, Kabat HF (eds): Chronobiology 1982-1983. S. Karger Publishing, 568 pp, 1984.
15. Reinberg A, Smolensky M: Biologic rhythms and medicine. Springer Verlag, New York, NY, 1983.
16. Halberg F: Quo vadis basic and clinical chronobiology: procedures and illustrative examples. Am J Anat 168:543-594, 1983.
17. Bingham C, Arbogast B, Cornelissen-Guillaume G, Lee JK, Halberg F: Inferential statistical methods for estimating and comparing cosinor parameters. Chronobiologia 9:397-439, 1982.
18. Halberg F, Engeli M, Hamburger C, Hillman D: Spectral resolution of low-frequency, small amplitude rhythms in excreted 17-ketosteroids; probable androgen-induced circaseptan desynchronization. Acta Endocr Suppl 103:5-54, 1965.
19. Haus E, Halberg F: The circadian time structure. In: Chronobiology-Principles and applications to shifts and schedules. (eds) Scheving LE and Halberg F, NATO Advanced Study Institute, Series D, Sijthoff, Int Publ, Leiden, Netherlands, 47-94, 1980.
20. Sothern RB, Leach CS, Nelson WL, Halberg F, Rummel JA: Characteristics of urinary circadian rhythms in a young man evaluated on a monthly basis during the course of 21 months. In: Chronobiological aspects of endocrinology. J. Aschoff, F. Ceresa, & F. Halberg (eds), pp 73-81, 1974.
21. Levi F, Halberg F: Circaseptan (about 7-day) bioperiodicity - spontaneous and reactive - and the search for pacemakers. La Ricerca 12:323-370, 1982.
22. Nicolau GY, Lakatua D, Sackett-Lundeen L, Haus E: Circadian and circannual rhythms of hormonal variables in clinically healthy elderly men and women. Chronobiologia 10:144, 1983.
23. Halberg F, Lee J, Nelson WL: Time qualified reference intervals-- chronodesms. Experientia 34:713-716, 1978.
24. Haus E, Cornelissen G, Halberg F: Introduction to chronobiology. In: Chronobiology-Principles and applications to shifts and schedules. (eds) Scheving LE and Halberg F, NATO Advanced Institute, Series D, Sijthoff, Int Publ, Leiden, Netherlands, 1-32, 1980.
25. Haus E, Halberg F: Endocrine rhythms. In: Chronobiology-Principles and applications to shifts and schedules. (eds) Scheving LE and Halberg F, NATO Advanced Institute, Series D, Sijthoff, Int Publ, Leiden, Netherlands, 137-188, 1980.

26. Haus E, Lakatua DJ, Halberg F, Halberg E, Cornelissen G, Sackett LL, Berg HG, Kawasaki T, Ueno M, Uezono K, Matsuoka M, Omae T: Chronobiologic studies of plasma prolactin in women in Kyushu, Japan and Minnesota, USA. J Clin Endocrinol Metab 51:632-640, 1980.

27. Ferrari E, Bossolo PA, Daguati M, Canepari C, Ficara S: Lack of adrenocortical rhythmicity in liver cirrhosis. Internat J. Chronobiol 7:239-, 1981.

28. Reinberg A, Smolensky M, Levi F: Clinical chronopharmacology. In: Clinical aspects of chronobiology, WJ Reitveld (ed). Baarn:Bakker, pp. 127-139, 1984.

29. Walker RF, Read GF, Riad-Fahmy D: Radioimmunoassay of progesterone in saliva: Application to the assessment of ovarian function. Clin Chem 25:2030-2033, 1979.

30. Walker RF, Riad-Fahmy D, Read GF: Adrenal status assessed by direct radioimmunoassay of cortisol in whole saliva or parotid saliva. Clin Chem 24:1460-1463, 1978.

31. Maier H, GeiBler M, Heidland A, Schindler JG, Wigand ME: Beeinflussung speichelchemischer Parameter in Abhangigkeit vom Menstruationszylkus. Laryng Rhinol 58:706-710, 1979.

32. Halberg F, Cornelissen G, Sothern RB, Wallach LA, Halberg E, Ahlgren A, Kuzel M, Radke A, Barbosa J, Goetz F, Buckley J, Mandel J, Schuman L, Haus E, Lakatua D, Sackett L, Berg H, Kawasaki T, Ueno M, Uezono K, Matsuoka M, Omae T, Tarquini B, Cagnoni M, Garcia Sainz M, Perez Vega E, Griffiths K, Wilson D, Donati L, Tatti P, Vasta M, Locatelli I, Camagna A, Lauro R, Tritsch G and Wendt HW: International studies of human host and tumor rhythms with multiple frequencies lead toward cost-effective sampling. In: Neoplasms-Comparative Pathology of Growth in Animals, Plants, and Man. Kaiser HN (ed), Wiley & Sons. New York, pp 553-596, 1981.

33. Free AH, Free HM: Seft testing, an emerging component of clinical chemistry. Clin Chem 30:829-838, 1984.

34. Walter B: Dry reagent chemistries in clinical analysis. Analyt Chem 55:498-514A, 1983.

35. Curme HG, et al: Multilayer film elements for clinical analysis: general concepts. Clin Chem 24:1335-1342, 1978.

36. Hay W Jr, Osberg IM: The 'eyetone' blood glucose reflectance colorimeter evaluated for in-vitro and in-vivo accuracy and clinical efficacy. Clin Chem 29:558-560, 1983.

37. Ohkubo A, et al: Multilayer-film analysis for urea nitrogen in blood, serum, or plasma. Clin Chem 30:1222-1225, 1984.

38. Free AH, Free HM: Dry chemistry reagent systems. Lab Med 15:595-600, 1984.

39. Kortum G: Reflectance spectroscopy: principles, methods, applications. Springer-Verlag, New York, NY, 1969.

40. Pesce AJ, Rosen, CG, Pasby TL: Fluorescence spectroscopy. Marcel Dekker Inc., New York, NY, 1971.

41. Williams FC, Clapper FR: Multiple internal reflections in photographic color prints. J Opt Soc Am 43:595-599, 1953.

42. Kuan JW, Lau HKY, Guilbault GG: Enzymatic determination of serum urea on the surface of silicone-rubber pads. Clin Chem 21:67-70, 1975.

43. Burd JF, Carrico RJ, Fetter MC, Buckler R, Johnson R, Boguslaski R, Chistner J: Specific protein binding reactions monitored by enzymatic hydrolysis of ligand-fluorescent dye conjugates. Anal Biochem 77:56-67, 1977.

44. Cornelissen G, Halberg F, Stebbings J, Halberg E, Carandente F, Hsi B: Chronobiometry with pocket calculators and computer systems. La Ricerca in Clinica e in Laboratorio 10:333-385, 1980.
45. Freiser H (ed): Ion selective electrodes in analytical chemistry. Plenum, New York and London, Vol I, 1978 & Vol II, 1980.
46. Thomas RC (Ed): Ion sensitive intracellular microelectrodes. Academic Press, London, 1978.
47. Kessler M, Harrison DK, Hoper J (eds): Recent advances in the theory and application of ion selective electrodes in physiology and medicine. Springer-Verlag, Berlin, 1984.
48. Seiyama T, Fueki K, Shiokawa J, Suzuki S (eds): Chemical sensors. Analyt Chem Symposia Series, Vol 17, Kodansha Ltd, Tokyo; Elsevier; Amsterdam-Oxfird-New York-Tokyo, 1983.
49. Potrin AR, Neuman MR (eds): Proceedings of the Symposium on Biosensors. IEEE/NSF. IEEE84 CH 2068-5, Piscataway, NJ, 118 pp, 1984.
50. Cremer M: Ueber die Ursache der elektromotorischen Eigenschaften der Gewebe, zugleich ein Beitrag zur Lehre von den polyphasischen Elektrolytketten. Ztschr f Biol 47:562-608, 1906.
51. Buck RP: Ion-selective electrodes. Anal Chem 50:17R-29R, 1978.
52. Severinghaus JW, Bradley AF: Electrodes for blood pO_2 and pCO_2 determination. J Appl Physiol 13:515-520, 1958.
53. Guilbault GG: Ion-selective electrodes applied to enzyme systems. Ion Selective Electrode Rev 4:187-231, 1982.
54. Ammann D, Morf WE, Anker P, Meier PC, Pretsch E, Simon W: Neutral carrier based ion-selective electrodes. Ion Selective Electrode Rev 5:3-92, 1983.
55. Simon W, Pretsch E, Morf WE, Ammann D, Oesch U, Dinten O: Design and application of neutral carrier based ion-selective electrodes. Analyst 109:207-209, 1984.
56. Dutsch S, Jenny HB, Schlatter KJ, Perisset PMJ, Wolff G, Clerc JT, Pretsch E, Simon W: Microprocessor controlled ex-vivo monitoring of sodium and potassium concentrations in undiluted urine with ion selective electrodes. Anal Chem 57:578-580, 1985.
57. Oesch U, Dinten O, Ammann D, Simon W: Life time of neutral carrier based membranes in aqueous systems and blood serum. In: Recent advances in the theory and application of ion selective electrodes in physiology and medicine. (eds) Kessler M, Harrison DK, Hoper J, Springer-Verlag, Berlin, 1984.
58. Simon W, Ammann D, Anker P, Oesch U: Ion-selective electrodes and their clinical application in the continuous ion monitoring. Ann NY Acad Sci 428:279-285, 1984.
59. Meyerhoff ME, Fraticelli YM: Ion-selective electrodes. Anal Chem 54:27R-44R, 1982.
60. Aizawa M: Molecular recognition and chemical amplification of biosensors. In: Chemical sensors. (eds) Seiyama T, Fueki K, Shiokawa J, Suzuki S, Kodansha Ltd, Tokyo; Elsevier; Amsterdam-Oxford-New York-Tokyo, 683-692, 1983.
61. Rechnitz GA: Bioanalysis with potentiometric membrane electrodes. Analyt Chem 54:1194-1200, 1982.
62. Plese C, Fox W, Williams K: Vitamin B_6 measured in plasma with a CO_2 selective electrode. Clin Chem 29:407, 1983.
63. Rechnitz GA, Kobos RK, Riechel SJ, Gebauer CR: A bioselective membrane electrode prepared with living bacterial cells. Anal. Chim Acta 94:357-365, 1977.

64. Rechnitz GA, Arnold MA, Myerhoff MA: Bio-selective membrane electrode using tissue slices. Nature 278:466-467, 1979.
65. Cunningham L, Freiser H: Ion-selective electrodes for basic drugs. Analytica Chim Acta 139:97-103, 1982.
66. Mascini M, Zolesi F, Palleschi G: Development of membrane electrode techniques for the determination of hormone factors using enzyme immunoassay. Anal Lett 15(B2):101-113, 1982.
67. Bergveld P, DeRooij NF, Zemel JN: Physical mechanisms for chemically sensitive semiconductor devices. Nature 273:438-443, 1978.
68. Wohltjen H: Chemical microsensors and microinstrumentation. Analyt Chem 56:87A-103A.
69. Bergveld P: Chemically sensitive field effect transistors (CHEMFETS). Trans Biomed Eng 17:70-71, 1970.
70. Janata J, Huber RJ: In: Ion selective electrodes in analytical chemistry. (ed) Freiser H, Plenum Press: New York, NY, Vol 2, Chap 3, 1980.
71. Mansouri S, Schultz JS: Optical glucose sensor based on reversible competitive binding. In: IEEE Sympos on Biosensors, 84 CH 2068-5, (eds) Potrin AR, Neuman MR, 112-115, 1984.
72. Moss SD, Johnson CC, Janata J: Hydrogen, calcium and potassium ion-sensitive FET transducers: A preliminary report. IEEE Trans on Biomed Engin, Vol BME-25, 1:49-54, 1978.
73. McKinley BA, Saffle J, Jordan WS, Janata J, Moss SD, Westenskov DR: In-vivo continuous monitoring of K$^+$ in animals using ISFET probes. Med Instrument 14:93-97, 1980.
74. Sibbald A, Covington AK, Cooper EA, Carter RF: On-line measurement of potassium in blood by chemical sensitive field effect transistors: A preliminary report. Clin Chem 29:405-406, 1983.
75. Oesch U, Caras S, Janata J: Field effect transistors sensitive to sodium and ammonium ions. Anal Chem 53:1983-1986, 1981.
76. Shimada K, Yano M, Shibatani K, Komoto Y, Esashi M, Matsuo T: Application of cather tip ISFET for continuous in-vivo measurement. Med Biol Eng Comput 18:741-745, 1980.
77. Mattiasson B, Borrebaeck C, Sanfidson B, Mosbach K: Thermometric enzyme linked immunosolvent assay (TELISA) Biochim Biophys Acta 483:221-227, 1977.
78. Ikariyama Y, Aizawa M: Bioaffinity sensors. Proc 2nd Sensor Symp, 97-100, 1982.
79. Schultz JS, Sims G: Affinity sensors for individual metabolites. Biotechnol Bioeng Symp 9:65-71, 1979.
80. Schultz JS, Mansouri S, Goldstein IJ: Affinity sensor: A new technique for developing implantable sensors for glucose and other metabolites. Diabetes Care 5:245-253, 1982.
81. Ikariyama Y, Furuki M, Aizawa M: Sensitive bioaffinity sensor with metastable molecular complex receptor and enzyme amplifier. Anal Chem 57:496-500, 1985.
82. Mosbach K, Danielson B: Thermal bioanalyzers in flow streams. Enzyme thermistor devices. Analyt Chem 53:83A-94A, 1981.
83. Seitz R: Chemical sensors based on fiber optics. Analyt Chem 56:16A-34A, 1984.
84. Peterson JI, Goldstein SR, Fitzgerald RV, Buckhold DK: Fiber optic pH probe for physiological use. Anal Chem 52:864-869, 1980.
85. Kirkbright GF, Narayanaswamy R, Welti NA: Studies with immobilized reagents using a flow-cell for the development of chemically sensitive fiber-optic devices. Analyst 109:15-17, 1984.

86. Saari LA, Seitz WR: pH sensor based on immobilized fluoresceinamine. Anal Chem 54:821-823, 1982.
87. Peterson JI, Fitzgerald RV, Buckhold DK: Fiber-optic probe for in-vivo measurement of oxygen partial pressure. Anal Chem 56:62-67, 1984.
88. Penra RA, Mendelson Y: Blood glucose sensors: An overview. In: Proc Sympos on Biosensors, (eds) Potrin AR, Neuman MR, IEEE, 84 Ch 2068-5, Piscataway, NJ, 63-68, 1984.
89. Mosbach K, Danielson B: Thermal bioanalyzers in flow stream enzyme thermistor devices. Anal Chem 53(1):83A-94A, 1981.
90. Clark LC Jr, Lyons C: Electrode systems for continuous monitoring in cardiovascular surgery. Ann NY Acad Sci 102:29-45, 1962.
91. Lerner H: Measurement of glucose concentration in the presence of coreactants with a platinum electrode. Diabetes Care 5:229-237, 1982.
92. Pilosof D, Nieman T.A.: Microporous membrane flow cell with non-immobilized enzyme for chemiluminescent determination of glucose. Anal Chem 54:1698-1701, 1982.
93. Rabinovitch B, March WF, Adams RL: Noninvasive glucose monitoring of the aqueous humor of the eye: Part I: Measurement of very small optic rotations. Diabetes Care 5:254-258, 1982.
94. March WF, Rabinovitch B, Adams RL: Noninvasive glucose monitoring of the aqueous humor of the eye: Part II: Animal studies and the scleral lens. Diabetes Care 5:259-265, 1982.
95. Janata J: Chemically sensitive field effect transistor as a potential transplantable glucose sensor. Diabetes Care 5:271, 1982.
96. Soeldner JS: Treatment of diabetes mellitus by devices. Am J Med 70:183-194, 1981.

CHEMILUMINESCENCE IMMUNOASSAY: A NEW DIAGNOSTIC TECHNOLOGY

Ian Weeks and J. Stuart Woodhead

Dept. of Medical Biochemistry, University of Wales, College of Medicine, Cardiff CF4 4XN, U.K.

Introduction

During recent years immunological techniques have played an increasingly important role in the diagnosis and monitoring of disease. Of these techniques, radioimmunoassay and its related procedures have been extremely successful in providing sensitive and specific tests for a wide range of molecules of biological importance. However, the rapid developments in immunoassay technology which have accompanied the increases in application have revealed important limitations in methods relying on the use of radioisotope labels. Thus, in addition to legislative problems relating to the handling and disposal of radioactive materials, severe restrictions are also imposed by the instability of the radioisotope and the molecule to which it is attached as well as by the detection limit of the radioisotope itself.

Until recently the success of non-isotopic immunoassay systems has been limited. The fact that much therapeutic drug monitoring is carried out by immunoassays based on enzyme or fluorescent labels is due to two major factors. Firstly, there is no requirement for high sensitivity so that samples can be diluted considerably before measurement, thus eliminating much of the potential non-specific interference. Secondly, the modification of the signal by antigen-antibody interaction has precluded the requirement of separation of bound from free label prior to quantitation with the result that many convenient "homogeneous" assay procedures are now in use.

Such procedures are not, however, universally applicable particularly when high sensitivity measurements are required. The detection of enzyme labels can be improved by the use of amplifying, cycling reactions (1). Such procedures are cumbersome and because of their biological nature subject to environmental interference so that automation becomes a key factor in providing reliability. The major drawback·with fluorescence has been the problem of background originating either from the sample or the instrument itself. This has been overcome to some extent by the development of sophisticated instrumentation for the quantitation of rare earth chelates using time-resolved fluorimetry (2).

In contrast to these systems, chemiluminescence provides a relatively simple alternative. Highly Chemiluminescent molecules do not occur naturally so there are fewer problems of background interference. Secondly, the light emission derives from simple chemical reactions which do not require the precise control of temperature and pH such as is necessary with enzymes. Finally, these molecules can be detected with a sensitivity equal to or better than that of ^{125}I using simple photon counting equipment. In this paper we describe the development of immunoassays based on the use of chemiluminescent acridinium esters as labels which demonstrate superior performance compared with methods using radioisotopes.

Chemiluminescence

Chemiluminescence occurs when the excited product of an exoergic chemical reaction reverts to its ground state with the emission of photons. This contrasts with fluorescence where the excitation energy derives from prior irradiation of a ground state molecule. The photoefficiency of the reaction, that is the number of photons emitted per mole of reactant, is referred to as the quantum yield. In chemiluminescent systems studied this rarely exceeds 0.2. The chemical reactions required to generate luminescence are invariably oxidative, two examples being illustrated in figure 1. While both luminol (5-amino-2,3-dihydrophthalazine-1,4-dione) and aryl acridinium esters undergo oxidation under alkaline conditions, the reaction involving luminol is dependent on a catalyst which may be a simple transition metal cation or complex macromolecules such as horseradish peroxidase or cytochromes (3).

There are two fundamental advantages of the reaction of acridinium salts as shown in figure 1 over that involving luminol and its derivatives. Firstly, since there is no requirement for a catalyst the acridinium ester reaction is less likely to be influenced by catalytic factors present in biological samples. The second advantage relates to the relationship between the chemiluminescent molecule and the antigen or antibody to which it is attached. In the case of luminol and its derivatives, considerable quenching of luminescence can be induced by the proximity of protein (4) which may lead to a requirement for chemical modification of the immune complex prior to initiation of the chemiluminescent reaction (5). In contrast, the excited product molecule resulting from acridinium ester oxidation (N-methyl acridone) is dissociated from the remainder of the molecule prior to photonic emission, thus making this process relatively independent of microenvironmental interference.

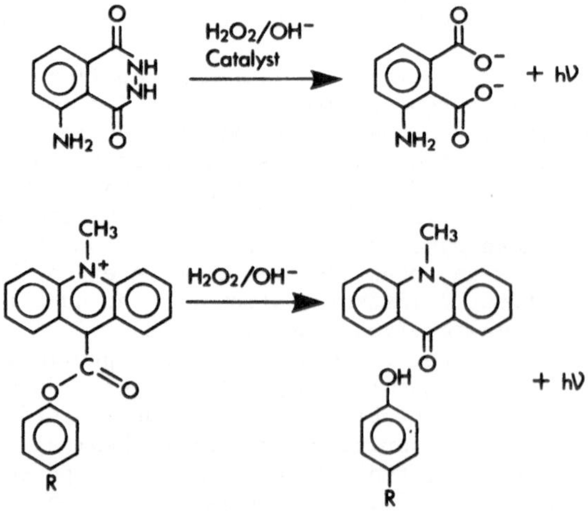

Fig.1. Chemiluminescent reactions of luminol and an acridinium ester.

The preparation of a hydroxysuccinimide derivative of the acridinium ester has enabled us to label a variety of antibodies under mild aqueous conditions to provide stable preparations which show no loss in quantum yield of the product compared with the ester itself (6).

Luminometry

The theoretical problems of measurement of low intensities of emitted light in this context are similar to those encountered in β-counting. Visible radiation and reactions producing it are more naturally abundant than γ-radiation for example, so that care is needed to eliminate non-specific luminescence from the analytical system. Recent interest in luminometry as an analytical tool has prompted the development of several commercially manufactured luminometers, though as yet none has been specifically built for immunoassay quantitation.

The most advanced system currently available is the LB950 Automatic Luminescence Analyzer supplied by Laboratorium Berthold (D7547 Wildbad, FRG), which combines a high sensitivity detector with a transportation device based on a flexible interlocking plastic belt. Tubes carried in the belt are introduced into the measuring chamber by an elevator mechanism and injection of the excitation reagents is automatic. The operating system including injection is controlled by an Apple II Processor utilizing the manufacturer's software. The system is capable of operating a range of luminometric techniques including immunoassays and carries the appropriate data reduction facilities. The throughput is approximately 250 sample tubes per hour.

Chemiluminescence Assay of Polypeptides

While this article is concerned primarily with the development of novel labelling systems, it is important to appreciate that the success of an immunodiagnostic procedure relies as heavily on the design of the immunochemistry as on the choice of label. It has been argued for many years that reagent excess assays using labelled antibodies offer distinct advantages over conventional competitive systems for the measurement of polypeptides in terms of speed, specificity and sensitivity (7,8,9). More recently it has been argued on theoretical grounds that reagent excess systems would profit most from the use of high specific activity labels in terms of overall detection limits provided background noise remains low (10,). This has been impossible to demonstrate using ^{125}I since attempts to increase the incorporation of the radioisotope into the antibody molecule result in progressive losses in immunoreactivity (11). In contrast we have been able to demonstrate a five fold increase in sensitivity in an immunochemiluminometric assay (ICMA) of α_1-fetoprotein (AFP) as a result of increasing the molar incorporation of acridinium ester into monoclonal antibody from 0.3 to 3.0 (12).

The most successful achievement obtained so far with this approach has been the development of an ICMA for human thyrotrophin (13) in which a high specific activity labelled monoclonal antibody is reacted first with the hormone followed by a second reaction with cellulose-linked polyclonal antibody. Following centrifugation, the complex is washed and quantified luminometrically. A dose-response curve for this assay is shown in figure 2. The assay has a sensitivity of detection of 0.003 mU/1, an improvement of at least a factor of ten over a corresponding system using ^{125}I as the label. The clinical usefulness of this assay is illustrated in figure 3 which compares serum thyrotrophin (TSH) results in normal subjects with those obtained in 90 patients with thyrotoxicosis. This ability to discriminate totally the thyrotoxic subjects from normal is important not

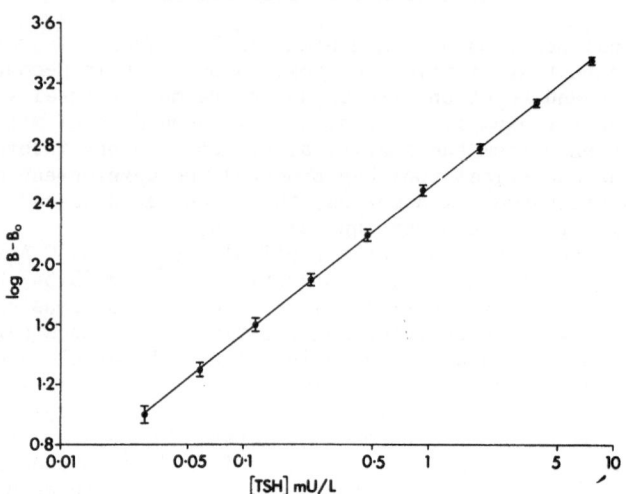

Fig.2.   Dose-response curve for the TSH ICMA.

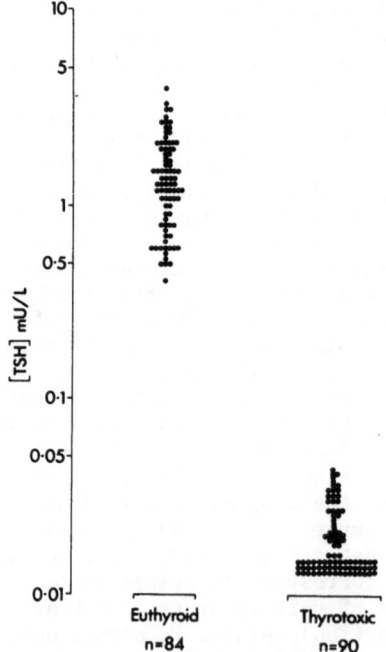

Fig.3.   Circulating TSH in normal subjects and hyperthyroid patients.

only in initial diagnosis but also in the monitoring of treated patients, particularly those having thyroid hormone replacement therapy. This method represents a major breakthrough in providing a rapid and accurate firstline test of thyroid status.

An important aspect of this approach is that it provides a uniform framework for polypeptide assays. A range of monoclonal antibodies have now been labelled by the same procedure and in addition to the tests for AFP and TSH, assays using common methodology have been established for prolactin, chorionic gonadotrophin and ferritin. An important feature of these assays is that the dose-response relationship is linear over a wide range of analyte concentrations, thus simplifying data reduction. Moreover, the reproducibility of this relationship from day to day suggests that simplified calibration may replace the currently obligatory full dose response curves.

Chemiluminescence Assay of Haptens

Most immunoassay laboratories, particularly those concerned with endocrine diagnosis and management, are required to measure analytes which are widely different, not only in their range of concentrations, but also in their molecular size and chemical properties. Thus any new assay technology must have the versatility to embrace this range of analyte measurements. To date a number of chemiluminescent hapten immunoassays have been described, mainly in the field of steroid endocrinology. Initially these procedures were homogeneous, based on changes in the kinetics of lumininescent reactions when luminol labelled haptens were bound to antibody (14). Such phenomena, however, are antibody dependent and are unpredictable, so that more recently a number of heterogeneous steroid assays have been developed using luminol derivatives (5). Such systems still suffer the problem of luminescence quenching when the labelled hapten is associated with antibody so that immune complex dissociation is necessary prior to luminometry.

Our own approach has been to pursue the possibility of using a labelled antibody system for haptens as well as for peptides. In this approach labelled antibody is reacted with a mixture of sample containing the analyte and a solid-phase derivative of the analyte. These latter two compete for antibody binding so that the label bound to the solid-phase varies inversely with the sample analyte concentration. An important feature of this approach is that it can be used to assess the free analyte concentration in a situation where the hapten is associated with endogenous binding proteins. Provided that the solid-phase hapten itself does not interact with binding proteins, the inhibition of labelled antibody uptake on to the solid-phase yields a measure of the free hapten concentration.

Figure 4 shows a standard curve for free T4 obtained with this procedure using acridinium ester labelled antibodies. The total reaction time is 40 minutes and the assay is sufficiently precise to discriminate hyper- and hypothyroid patients from euthyroid subjects.

Conclusions

Chemiluminescent molecules satisfy the requirements of non-isotopic labels for immunoassay in that they are stable and can be detected with high sensitivity using simple equipment. Acridinium esters in particular can be coupled to antibodies to yield high specific activities without compromising either the immunoreactivity of the antibody or the chemiluminescent light emission. Assays based on simple immunochemistry utilising these labels have shown considerably improved performance compared with techniques relying on radioisotope labels. The versatility

378

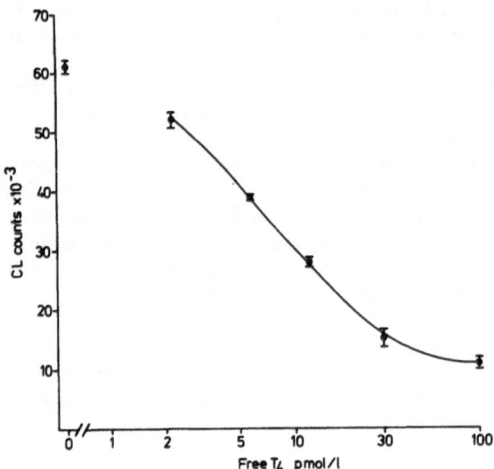

Fig.4. Chemiluminescent labelled antibody assay of free T4.

and performance of chemiluminescent labels makes them a logical
alternative to radioactive compounds.

Acknowledgments

The studies reported in this article were carried out in collaboration
with Maria Sturgess, Kenneth Siddle, Ian Laing, M. Keston Jones and Peter
Evans. The work was supported by Bioanalysis Ltd., Cardiff.

REFERENCES
1. Roddis MJ, Burrin JM, Johannssen A etal: Serum thyrotropin: a first
   line test of thyroid function. Lancet i: 277-278, 1985.
2. Pattersson K, Siitari H, Hemmila I etal: Time-resolved
   fluorimmunoassay of human chorionic gonadotrophin. Clin. Chem. 29: 60-
   64, 1983.
3. Schroeder HR & Yeager FM: Chemiluminescence yields and detection
   limits of some isoluminol derivatives in various oxidation systems.
   Anal. Biochem. 50: 1114-1120, 1978.
4. Schroeder HR, Hines CM, Osborn DD etal: Immunochemiluminometric assay
   for hepatitis B surface antigen. Clin. Chem. 27: 1378-1384, 1981.
5. Collins WP, Barnard GJ, Kim JB etal: Chemiluminescence immunoassays
   for plasma steroids and urinary steroid metabolites, in Hunter WM &
   Corrie JET (eds): Immunoassays for Clinical Chemistry, Churchill
   Livingstone, pp 373-397, 1983.
6. Weeks I, Beheshti I, McCapra F etal: Acridinium esters as high
   specific activity labels in immunoassay. Clin. Chem. 29: 1474-1479,
   1983.
7. Miles LEM & Hales CN: Labelled antibodies and immunological assay
   systems. Nature (Lond) 219: 186-189, 1968.
8. Woodhead JS, Addison GM & Hales CN: The immunoradiometric assay and
   related procedures. Brit. Med. Bull. 30: 44-49, 1974.
9. Hales CN & Woodhead JS: Labeled antibodies and their use in the
   immunoradiometric assay, in Van Vanukis M & Langone JJ (eds): Methods

in Enzymology vol 70, Academic Press, New York, pp 334–355, 1980.

10. Jackson TM, Marshall NJ & Ekins RP: Optimisation of immunoradiometric (labelled antibody) assays, in Hunter WM & Corrie JET (eds): Immunoassays for Clinical Chemistry, Churchill Livingstone, Edinburgh; pp 557–575, 1983.

11. Kemp HA, John R & Woodhead JS: Labeled antibody immunoassays. Ligand Quarterly 5: 27–34, 1982.

12. Weeks I, Campbell AK & Woodhead JS: Two-site immunochemiluminometric assay for human α_1-fetoprotein. Clin. Chem. 29: 1480–1483, 1983.

13. Weeks I, Sturgess M, Siddle K etal: A high sensitivity immunochemiluminometric assay for human thyrotrophin. Clin. Endocrinol. 20:489–495, 1984.

14. Kohen F, Pazzagli M, Kim JB etal: An assay procedure for plasma progesterone based on antibody enhanced chemiluminescence. FEBS Lett 104: 201–205, 1979.

THE APPLICATION OF CHRONOBIOLOGIC TECHNIQUES TO STUDIES IN THE DIGESTIVE SYSTEM†

KIRT J. VENER, National Institute of Arthritis, Diabetes, and Digestive and kidney Diseases, NIH, Bethesda, MD

1. INTRODUCTION

The application of chronobiologic techniques to studies of the digestive system offers many opportunites for basic and clinical investigators interested in gastrointestinal physiology and pathophysiology.

A recent report published by the Department of Health and Human Services, Research Advances, Opportunities, and Needs in Digestive Diseases, (1) reviews the state of the art and the research in 14 areas of gastroenterology research. Among those 14, a number contained research needs which would lend themselves nicely to acquisition of chronobiologic data and analysis, if appropriate technology existed for collection of continuous data. These opportunities and several others will be described below.

2. RESEARCH NEEDS IN THE DIGESTIVE SYSTEM

2.1 Gastrointestinal Motility (2)

The motility in the alimentary canal is a highly complex integrated phenomena which is beginning to be more clearly understood. It is evident that the simplistic approaches which had been taken to explain the integrative nature of motility in the alimentary canal are no longer valid. Important strides have been made in our understanding of the cellular physiology of gut smooth muscle, its nervous control, and the importance of neurohumoral transmitters in the regulation of activity through the myenteric plexus.

Dysrhythmias in motility are among the altered states of bowel function in many persons. The so-called functional digestive disorders, an apparently acquired symptom complex which appears to be psychogenically induced, are believed to afflict between 8 and 22 percent of the American population in any year. Although only a small proportion of individuals with these symptoms seek medical attention, fully half of all referrals to gastroenterologists are patients with these disorders (3). Methods need to be developed for better recording of the slow waves from the gut so that the motility abnormalities associated with clinical conditions, such as the functional digestive disorders, can be better characterized. Existing methods for in vivo measurement suffer from poor signal-to-noise ratios and other difficul-

† The author would like to thank Dr. Harold Roth, Director, Division of Digestive Diseases and Nutrition, NIADDK and Dr. Van Hubbard, Program Director for Nutrition, NIADDK, for their helpful comments and suggestions. The author would also like to thank Ms. Karen Howard for her assistance in gathering the material cited in this manuscript.

* Digestive Diseases and Nutrition Division, Westwood Building, Room 3A16 National Institute of Arthritis, Diabetes, and Digestive and Kidney Diseases National Institutes of Health, Bethesda, Maryland 20205

ties.
2.2 Liver Detoxification (4)

There is a wealth of data which has been accumulating on the predictable periodic behavior of the liver and its importance in detoxification (Table 1.). The recent development of in vitro technology permitting chronobiologic approaches to tissue culture offers the opportunity to further extend our knowledge in isolated tissue systems (5).

Research opportunities in this subspecialty include:

1. Exploitation of microfluorescent probes to monitor intralobular oxygen consumption and regional drug metabolism;
2. Exploitation of the known inhibitory effect of imidazole ring containing compounds on the microsomal oxidizing system, to synthesize and assess the effects on this system of analogues;
3. Investigation in depth of the mechanism(s) of relative preservation of glucuronidation (vs.) oxidation in the presence of liver injury;
4. Assessment of the biochemical basis of impaired hepatic drug detoxification with aging;
5. investigation of the relative importance of impaired microsomal function of shunting in the impaired drug elimination in cirrhosis;
6. further assessment of the mechanisms of drug hepatotoxicity as they relate to the the formation of toxic metabolites and the possible means of interfering with this effect by the use of inhibitors of drug oxidation (i.e., cimetidine and similar agents);
7. Development of test systems for assessing genetic predisposition to drug hepatotoxicity;

TABLE 1. Periodic liver functions related to detoxification.

Function	Reference
Vitamin D metabolism in alcoholics	17
Alcohol metabolism	18, 19
Alcohol dehydrogenase	20, 21
Choloroform toxicity	22
Lysosomal enzymes:	
acid phosphatase	23
arylsulphatase	24, 25
B-acetylglucosaminidase	24
Cathepsin A, B, D	26
Esterases	27
Folic acid metabolism	28
Hexobarbital metabolism	29
Isoproterenol	30
Tyrosine amino transferase	31, 32

382

8. Design of methods for assessing the pharmacodynamic effects of sedatives on the brain of patients with liver disease;
9. Examination of the role of the regulation of hepatic glutathione in terms of turnover, single or multiple pools, effects of fasting, alcohol etc., on these;

Much of the experimentation done on biological rhythms has been descriptive in nature and as a consequence has been subject to criticism. Dr. Schenker's component of the Digestive Diseases Advisory Board Report (4) on research advances, opportunities and needs in digestive diseases identifies a number of excellent suggestions which would permit chronobiolgic investigators to go beyond the conventional homeostatic approaches. Each of the above listed opportunites can be investigate from a chronobiolgic perspective to allow a more accurate understanding of the integrative nature of hepatic function. Such understanding should permit an exploitation of susceptibility-resistance cycles of medication in order to minimize the toxic effects on the host and optimize the susceptibility of the disease state.

2.3 Gallstone Disease (5)

Bile, a concentrated solution which is formed in the liver, serves as an elimination pathway for hydrophobic wastes which cannot be excreted in the urine. In addtion to the waste products, bilirubin and cholesterol, detergent molecules called bile salts are present which solubilize the insoluble constituents of the bile.

In some persons, the insoluble components separate from solution and forming precipitates or crystals. If there is an aggregation of these precipitates or crystals gallstones may form.

There have been a number of chronobiologic investigations which have examined parameters influencing bile secretion (a few are identified in Table 2), and at least one participant of the National Cooperative Gall-

TABLE 2. Periodic phenomena related to gallstone/gallbladder disease.

Function	Reference
Cholic acid:CoA ligase	33
Glycolithocholate sulfotransferase	33
Cholesterol saturation	34
Cholesterol synthesis	35

stone Study suggests that that study might have been improved if time
dependent variables had been included in the study design (7).

Additional lines of investigation dealing with bile and biliary constituents which might benefit if chronobiologic approaches (either in vitro
or in vivo) were used are as follows:

1. Biliary lipid secretion: little is known about the cell biology
   and biophysics of biliary lipid secretion. The control of biliary
   cholesterol secretion is not understood.
2. Biliary calcium secretion: little is known about the mecahnisms,
   characteristics, and regulation of biliary calcium secretion.
3. Chemistry of biliary substituents: structure activity relationships
   of bile acids are poorly understood because the analogues are not
   available. The diglucuronide ester of bilirubin (the major form
   occurring in bile) is not available commercially, precluding its
   study by physical chemists and enzymologists.
4. Enzyme activity in bile: little is known of the factors influencing
   hydrolysis of conjugated bilirubin by beta glucuronidase or hydrolysis of lecithin to lysolecithin in bile.

2.4 Mucosal Blood Flow (8, 9)

The endoscope, a fiber optic device which can be used for direct visual-
ization of the inner surface of the alimentary canal, provides the opportunity for conducting a variety of investigations to answer physiolgic as
well as clinical questions. One opportunity is the improvement of our
understanding of mucosal blood flow.

Oishi and colleagues (10) in Boston have demonstrated that the ulcerogens
cysteamine and acrylonitrile produce more or less severe ulcer lesions
depending on the time of day of administration of the drugs. It has been
further suggested that changes in the blood flow to the susceptible areas
may contribute to or minimize the opportunity for ulcer production (11).
Therefore, if a quantifiable method for the continuous measurement of
mucosal blood flow were developed, such observations could have relevance
to the development and healing of stress ulcer and peptic ulcer. Also, it
may help distinguish between ischemic colitis, ulcerative colitis, antibiotic colitis and Crohn's disease of the colon.

A two-channel endoscope fitted with a hydrogen electrode (to measure
resting blood flow) and a laser-Doppler velocimeter (to measure changes in
blood flow) together could provide a sensitive record of hemodynamics.
Another approach might be to use a magnifying endoscope to visualize the
gastric or duodenal microcirculatory pattern using epi-illumination of
fluorescein in the vasculature. Such techniques could be used to visualize
and study areas of healed or active ulcers in both patients or experimental
animals.

Gastrointestinal surgeons tell us that the implantation of fiber-optic
bundles in experimental animals for the purpose of the continuous data collection is technically feasible (H. Debas, personal communication).

3.0 STATE OF THE ART FOR CONTINUOUS DATA COLLECTION IN THE DIGESTIVE
SYSTEM

Continuous recording within the alimentary canal is presently available
for pH. Several devices have been developed (Biosearch-Sandhill; Velmar
Avionics; Oxford Medalog) and are being used at a number of locations.
These devices appear to be accurate within the approximate range of 0.5 pH
units. Such devices may be of value in some patients in assessing the
contribution of gastric reflux in those who suffer from noncardiac chest
pain. Further, the relationship between gastro-esophageal reflux and
sudden infant death syndrome (SIDS) has neither been confirmed nor denied
and important information may be forthcoming if continuous monitoring

approaches in at risk patients were used. Similarly, a catheter may be placed a short distance up the biliary tree in order to sample biliary secretions.

Clearly, there would be a significant advantage in being able to directly analyze in situ internal secretions for specific constituents without having to first aspirate and then later analyze the material.

4.0 EMERGING TECHNOLOGY FOR CONTINUOUS RECORDING OF DIGESTIVE SYSTEM PARAMETERS

One technology which might provide the accuracy, stability and minimal size requirements to measure constituents of internal secretions is remote spectroscopy using fiber optics. Studies have shown the feasibility of measuring a variety of useful physiologic parameters using a detector placed at the end of a fiberoptic bundle. Investigators at the Oak Ridge Nationl Laboratory have developed remote instrumentation for measuring the concentration of plutonium and uranium in reprocessing solutions (12). Investigators in the Division of Research Services of the National Institutes of Health have prepared a flexible, 0.4mm diameter fiberoptic pH probe which has been used to measure pH in the blood to 0.017 pH units (13, 14). A similar device, the Optrode, has been developed by ST&E Technical Services. The basic operation of these devices in shown in Figure 1.

There seems to be a great potential for the adaptation of this fiberoptic technology for chemical detection. Within the limits of the biocompatibility of the materials to be used in the detector end, it seems feasible that any biological fluid substituent which can induce a color change should be able to be measured using remote spectroscopy. For example, appropriate fiber optic detectors could be developed (technology presently exists but must be adapted to this purpose) and surgically implanted in the

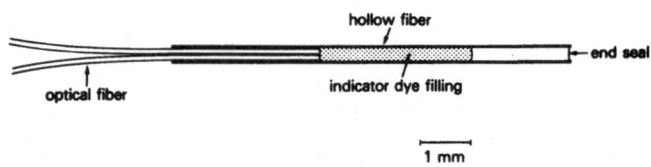

FIGURE 1. pH sensor employs two single strand optic fibers, typically 0.125 mm in diameter, which at the distal (implanted) end are adjacent and parallel and fit inside a Cuprophan dialysis hollow fiber of 0.3-mm diameter. The proximal end of the other fiber is attached to a tungsten light source, fitted with a red and green motor-driven filter wheel, and the proximal end of the other fiber is attached to a photomultiplier tube. The Cuprophan is packed with phenol red dye adjacent to the cut ends of the optic fiber. Hydrogen ions passing through the membrane cause the dye to change its color, and this is quantified by measuring the intensity of green light (550 nm) that is transmitted through the system. The dye is trapped inside the membrane by bonding it to $10-\mu$ polyacrylamide gel microspheres to which $1-\mu$ - diameter, light-scattering microspheres have been added. (Reproduced with permission.) (13)

gall bladder of the prarie dog (a species which spontaneously produces cholesterol gall stones) in order to continously monitor the environment within the gallbladder. The procedures would allow the animal to be free moving in its cage but connected to the activating and recording system by exiting the bundle between the scapulae. Further, it is not outside of the realm of possibility that a package small enough for implantation and telemetry in the dog or larger species could be produced.

For human studies the delivery of a small diameter probe such as the one described above is not difficult if one is simply concerned with sampling in the lumen of the alimentary canal. However, attempting to insert such a device in the biliary tree using a conventional catheter would be very difficult if not impossible. The engineering group that produced the fiber optic pH probe described above has also developed a catheter (the socalled toposcopic catheter or 'topo') which does not need to be pushed into a vessel or duct to be advanced (15, 16). Originally developed for used in the cardiovascular system, it is a continuously everting miniature tube which advances with minimal friction (Figure 2 and Table 3).

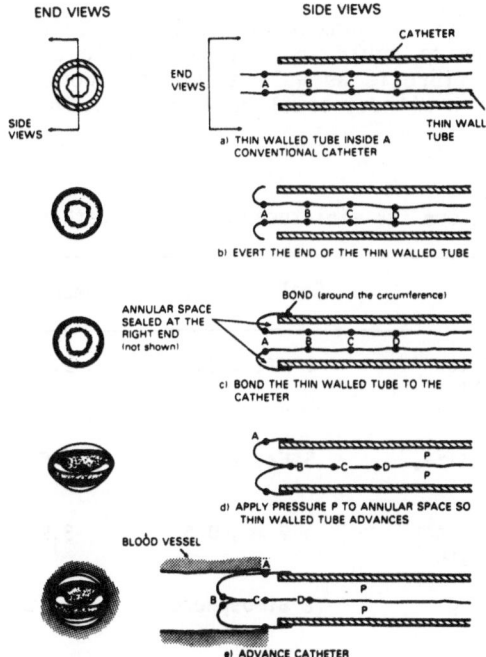

FIGURE 2. Schematic illustration of construction and operation of toposcopic catheter. The rolling action of the everting tube, e.g., point A in parts c, d, and e, has the potential to minimize irritation of the intimal layer as it advances up small diameter tortuous vessels. The conventional catheter is advanced as far as possible, e.g., potentially throught the lumen of an ecdoscope, and the topo element is activated. Retraction in the rolling mode is accomplished by inflating the annulus to a low pressure and pulling on the proximal end of the topo element. (Reproduced with permission) (15).

There are several advantages of the topo over conventional catheters. First, "there is no relative motion and virtually no friction between the topo and the endothelium as it advances and retracts through the blood vessel or biliary duct. This feature minimizes the possibility of damaging the vessel or inducing muscular spasm. Second, there is no need to make the usual design compromise between catheter rigidty (to avoid buckling as it is advanced) and catheter flexibility (to negotiate sharp turns in the vessel)" (16) (Figure 3).

The fiber optic pH probe and the topo have been used in concert with the pH probe traveling through the topo as the topo is everted. One problem which has confronted some GI investigators in trying to continuously monitor gastric pH is the problem of mucus covering the electrode tip so that data become aberrant (V. Hubbard, personal communication). If the pH (or other) probe were held within the confines of the topo and the probe was extruded intermittently, it is likely that the mucus problem would be minimized.

Another possible application of these devices used jointly would be to place fiber optic or other small diameter probes in the biliary tree. Catheter plcacments across the sphincter of Oddi are not uncommon in patients and may be left in place for as long as 72 hours. The possible use of the topo in GI studies is currently being investigated. Preliminary studies with catheterization of the gall bladder in the dog have been performed and prototype topos for use in humans with delivery by the endoscope are being developed. This device could in fact be used to asses the status of patients with cystic fibrosis as well as monitor normal patterns of biliary substituent secretion without bowel content contamination.

TABLE 3. Parameters for miniature toposcopic catheter.

	Small size topo	Medium size topo
Topo element outer diameter, wall thickness	1 mm, 0.06 mm	1.5 mm, 0.1 mm
Outer catheter size, length	5 Fr, 1 m	7 Fr, 1 m
Extension tube outer diameter, length	3.9 mm, 0.6 m	3.9 mm, 0.6 m
Annulus operating pressure	2 atmospheres	2 atmospheres
Flow rate of hypaque contrast media (Na 50%) through lumen for driving pressure of 1.3 atmospheres	5 cc/min	30 cc/min

5.0 SUMMARY
There has been a good deal of additional chronobiologic measurement of GI function but there is great potential for the collection of significant physiologic and pathophysiologic data. The use of fiberoptics may be one promising technology which may enable researchers to generate new chronobiologic insights into many aspects of GI biology.

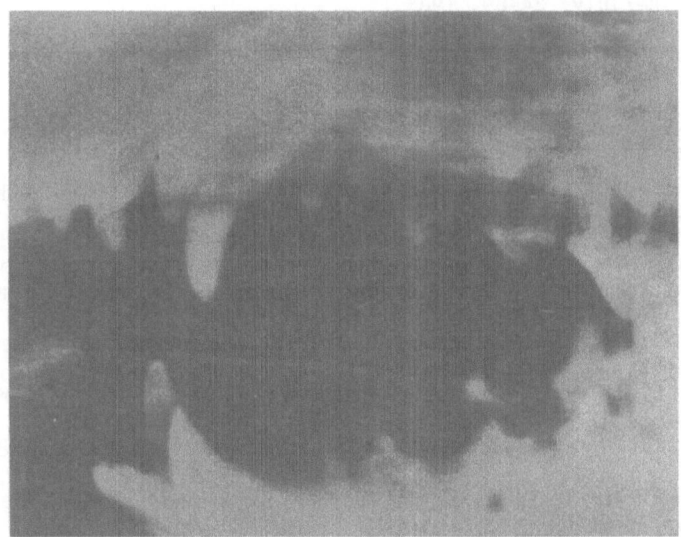

FIGURE 3. Angiogram showing topo catheter at the tip of a canine tongue reached through a branch of the external carotid artery. (Reproduced with permission) (15).

388

REFERENCES

1. McGuigan JE, Trier JS (eds): Research advances, opportunities, and needs in digestive diseases: A report of the National Digestive Diseases Advisory Board. NIH Publication No. 84-2658, 132pp., 1983.
2. Christensen J: Smooth muscle disease and motility, In: Research Advances, Opportunities, and Needs in Digestive Diseases, (eds) J McGuigan and J S Trier. NIH Publication No. 84-2658, 61-67, 1983.
3. Almy TP: Biological adaptation, digestive disorders, and health services. Psychosomatics, 19:200-20, 1978.
4. Schenker S: Liver Detoxification. In: Research Advances, Opportunities, and Needs in Digestive Diseases, (eds) J McGuigan and J S Trier. NIH Publication 84-2658, 105-111, 1983.
5. Gruenberg ML, Walker RD: A new technique for controlled delivery of biochemical regulatory agents to isolated tissue in culture. Biotechniques, June/July: 84-89, 1983.
6. Hofmann, AF: Gallsonte disease. In: Research Advances, opportunities, and Needs in Digestive Diseases, (eds), J McGuigan and J S Trier, NIH Publication 84-2658, 119-122, 1983.
7. Wilson ID: Chronobiology: The gastroenterologist's perspective. In Chronobiology and the Digestive System, (ed) K Vener, NIH Publication No. 84-857, p. 95-99, 1984.
8. Silvis SE: Research opportunities in gastrointestinal endoscopy. In: Research Advances, Opportunities, and Needs in Digestive Diseases, (eds) J McGuigan and J S Trier. NIH Publication 84-2658, 129-132, 1983.
9. Silvis SE, Vener KJ: Report of a seminar on the role of fiberoptic instrumentation in digestive diseases research. Gastrointestinal Endoscopy 29:231-232, 1983.
10. Oishi T, Gallagher GT, Szabo S: Diurnal variation of duodenal ulcer induced by cysteamine. Gastroenterol 82:1139, 1982 (abstract).
11. Szabo S: Biology of disease: Pathogenesis of duodenal ulcer disease. Lab Invest 51:121-147, 1984.
12. Maugh TH: Remote spectrometry with fiberoptics. Science 218:875-876, 1982.
13. Goldstein SR, Peterson JI, Fitzgerald RV: A miniature fiberoptic pH sensor for physiological use. J Biomech Eng 102: 141-146, 1980.
14. Peterson JI, Goldstein SR, Fitzgerald RV, Buckhold DK: Fiberoptic probe for physiological use. Analyt Chem 52:864-869, 1980.
15. Goldstein SR, Jones RE, Sipe JJ, Doppman JL, Boretos JW: A miniature toposcopic catheter for small diameter tortuous blood vessels. J Biomech Eng 102:221-229, 1980.
16. Goldstein SR, Shook DR, Peterson JI, Markle DR, Doppman JL, Patterson RE, Dooley J: The toposcopic catheter and the fiberoptic pH probe - two medical instruments of potential use to gastroenterologists. Gastrointestinal Endoscopy, 29: 236-240, 1983.
17. Lund B, Sørensen OH, hilden M, Lund B: A hepatic conversion of vitamin D in alcoholics with varying degrees of liver affection. Acta Med Scand 202:221224, 1977.
18. Püschel K, Adam G, Agarwal DP, Goedde HW: Circadian aspects of alcohol metabolism in the rat liver. Beitr Gerichtl Med 38:311-316, 1980.
19. Demling MJ, Schnell RC: Circadian rhythms in the biological response and disposition of ethanol in the mouse. J Pharmacol Exp Ther 213:1-8, 1980.
20. Sturtevant RP, Garber SL: Circadian rhythms of alcohol dehydrogenase and meos in the rat. Proc Soc Exp Biol Med 175:299-303, 1984.

21. North C, Feuers RJ, Scheving LE, Pauly JE, Tsai TH, Casciano DA: Circadian organization of thirteen liver and six brain enzymes of the mouse. Am J Anat 162:183-199, 1981.
22. Lavigne JG, Belanger PM, Dore F, Labreque G: Temporal variations in chloroform induced hepatotoxicity in rats. Toxicology 26:267-273, 1983.
23. Twardowski J, Lityńska A, Proniewcz LM, Domoslawski J: Rhythmic changes of some lysosomal hydrolases activity from rat liver. Rhtyhmic changes of acid phosphatase synthesis. Chronobiologia 8:231-242, 1981.
24. Lityńska A: Diurnal rhythm of activity of some lysosomal hydrolases. Folia Biol (Kraków)347-355, 1980.
25. Lityńska A: The effect of adrenalectomy on the diurnal changes of aryl sulphatase activity in mouse liver. Bull Acad Pol Sci 28:399-405, 1980.
26. Obled C, Arnal M, Valin C: Variations through the day of hepatic and muscular cathepsin A (carboxypeptidase A; EC 3.4.12.2), C (dipeptidyl peptidase; EC3.4.14.1) and D (endopeptidase D; EC 3.4.23.5) activities and free amino acids in rats: influence of feeding schedule. J Nutr 44:61-69, 1980.
27. Bhattacharya RD, von Mayersbach H: Circadian variation of liver esterases. Eur J Appl Physiol 46:85-89, 1981.
28. Kretzer G, Hardeland R: Diurnal rhythmicity in folic acid metabolism of rat liver and kidney. Arch Int Physiol Biochem 86:563-567, 1978.
29. Kato H, Saito M: Diurnal variations in response of rat liver tyrosine aminotransferase activity to food intake. Biochim Biophys Acta 627:109-111, 1980.
30. Cahill AL, Ferguson SM, Ehret CF: Chronotypic induction of tyrosine aminotransferase by α-methyl-p-tyrosine. Life Sci 28:1665-1671, 1981.
31. Kirkpatrick RB, Robinson SF, Killenberg PG: Diurnal variation of rat liver enzymes catalyzing bile acid conjugation and sulfation. Biochim Biophys Acta 620:627-630, 1980.
32. Kupfer RM, Northfield TC: Diurnal variation in cholesterol saturation of gall-bladder bile, Gut 24:950-953, 1983.
33. Püschel K, Mätzsch, von Mayersbach H: Chronopharmacologic aspects of hexobarbital oxidation rate in rat. J Toxicol 48:199-204, 1981.
34. Stone JE, Scheving LE, Burns RE, Graham M: Circadian activity of ornithine decarboxylase activity in mouse liver; effect of isoproterenol and Clelland's reagent. In Chronobiology, (eds) L E Scheving, F Halberg, and J E Pauly) Igaku Shoin Ltd., Tokyo, pp. 38-41, 1974.
35. Strandberg TE, Tilvis RS, Miettinen TA: Diurnal variation of plasma methyl sterols and cholesterol in the rat: relation to hepatic cholesterol synthesis. Lipids 19:202-205, 1984.

GASTRIC CONTINUOUS pH MONITORING: A NEW APPARATUS IN CHRONOBIOLOGICAL RESEARCH

*B. Tarquini, P. Lombardi, L.M. Pernice, F. Andreoli
*Istituto di Clinica Medica 2; Istituto di Patologia Chirurgica 1, University of Florence, Italy

1. INTRODUCTION

Among the tools required for a future clinical chronobiology, the instrumentation described here represents only the hardware that has to be complemented with appropriate software for as-one-goes analysis of variables such as gastric acidity. The software is available to determine reference standards against which excess or deficit in gastric acidity or any other pertinent variable can be assessed chronobiologically (Cornélissen et al., 1985; Halberg et al., 1985). This is the more important since several signs and symptoms of diseases related to gastric acid secretory function show prominent circadian, ultradian and infradian variations (Tarquini, 1980). The chronobiological assessment of endoluminal gastric pH, therefore, seems most appropriate to define physiopathological aspects and schedule a proper therapy of these diseases.

Gastric acid secretory function can be detected by an intraluminal pH electrode connected to an external recorder. In order to improve this diagnostic tool, we recently devised a solid-state, battery-operated recorder, capable of collecting data at a high sampling rate.

In this paper, we report correlations between some morphologically well-documented cases of overt gastric disease and of subjects at high risk for peptic ulcer/gastric cancer and their chronobiologically-quantified parameters (temporal morphology) of intragastric pH, determined on the basis of dense data series.

2. MATERIAL AND METHODS

All subjects and patients investigated (table 1) underwent esophageal variable-flux open-tip manometry with multiple remark points of pressure's signal connected to a pressure transducer of

Table 1. 24-h gastric pH rhythm parameters*

Subjects	Diagnosis	N obs	PR	P	M ± SE	A±SE	ø±SE
D.P.	*health*	291	32	.001	1.97 ± .06	1.03 ± .09	-200 ± 5
G.G.	*health*	259	17	.001	1.98 ± .06	.60 ± .09	-228 ± 8
B.V.	*health*	200	41	.001	2.47 ± .12	1.46 ± .19	-232 ± 5
R.V.	*health*	280	35	.001	2.38 ± .06	.95 ± .08	-272 ± 5
B.G.	*health*	280	18	.001	2.72 ± .07	.81 ± .10	-236 ± 7
D.O.	*g.ca.*	263	21	.001	6.49 ± .04	.43 ± .05	-118 ± 7
D.R.	g.ca. h.r.	267	46	.001	5.10 ± .09	1.92 ± .13	-123 ± 4
D.D.C.	*d. ulcer*	285	5	.001	2.05 ± .06	.33 ± .06	-284 ± 15
C.D.	d.ulcer h.r.	308	10	.001	2.26 ± .07	.67 ± .10	-255 ± 9

*h.r.=subjects at high risk for g (gastric), ca (carcinoma) or d (duodenal ulcer); N obs = number of observations considered; PR=percent rhythm; P=P-value in testing the zero-amplitude hypothesis; M=MESOR; A=amplitude; ø=acrophase; SE=standard error; in view of the non-sinusoidality of the data, higher-order harmonics should be considered as well, or methods robust with respect to the exact waveform used.

tensiometric type (Statam P23AA). Records were collected with a Beckman R611 polygraph. This test allowed definition of a correct map of esophageal motility and the dynamics of lower esophageal sphincter (LES). The distance between this structure and the nasal vestibule is very important for the correct position of the endoluminal pH electrode. According to nomenclature, hydrogen-ion concentrations are generally expressed as their logarithms with the sign reversed and indicated by the term pH. Thus, $pH = -log°H+é$ or $°H+é=10^{-pH}$ and an increase in pH indicates a decrease in hydrogen-ion concentration or true gastric acidity.

The 24-hour pH monitoring was implemented, placing, by nose, the electrode (Radiometer) in the patient's stomach, 10 cm under the LES. This position seems to be optimal for two reasons: to prevent the probe from 'fluctuating' in the gastric bubble, and to prevent 'false positives', simulating a duodeno-gastric reflux due to intermittent transit of the electrode in the duodenum. The electrode was then connected with a portable (cm 17 x 9 x 3) solid-state, battery-operated recorder, completely devoid of mechanical parts, of 48 Kbyte capacity (Biocardio Elettronica Mod. G.A.E.P.). This device samples the signal from the endoluminal electrode every 2 seconds, thus collecting about 50,000 data per 24 hours. The recorder is provided with 12 event markers exploring several events during the study: posture (supine, sitting, upright), meals (beginning, end) or the onset of specific symptoms (pain, cough, belch, vomit, regurgitate, etc.). The portable electrode recorder set is checked by buffer with pH 1.4 and 7 before and at the end of each test. The greatest difference allowed between the two measurements is 0.1 UpH.

All subjects and patients admitted to the 24-hour gastric pH monitoring were invited to scrupulously follow a quantitatively-, qualitatively- and temporally-standardized diet at definite hours and to point out, by means of the event markers, all the activities that were carried out and the onset of symptoms during the monitoring span.

At the end of the 24-hour span, the data collected in the memories of the recorder were transferred into a computer (Biocardio Elettronica) for data evaluation by conventional and chronobiological inferential statistical methods (Halberg et al., 1977).

3. RESULTS AND DISCUSSION

Today the diagnosis of gastric diseases has to be morphologically substantiated. The evaluation of acid secretion function is considered accessory or additional. Our results suggest that definite chronobiological features of endoluminal gastric pH correspond to definite morphologic ones.

All dense data series of gastric pH showed statistically significant circadian and ultradian components. In healthy subjects the 24-hour component was prominent over ultradian ones and the circadian amplitude was higher as a group as well as in single series. By contrast, in patients with active duodenal ulcer, but also in a high-risk subject, the extent of circadian rhythmic change in intraluminal pH was small, the acrophase delayed and an 8-hour component was prominent. In the patient with gastric cancer, but also in a high (anamnestically) risk subject, the circadian component remained prominent, the MESOR was high, the amplitude small, and the acrophase occurred earlier than anticipated.

Examination of the 24-h recordings of endoluminal pH reveals an increase in pH around meal times for the healthy subject and for the subject at high risk of developing duodenal ulcer. This observation may prompt the question whether a test procedure should not include a recording under fasting conditions as well, in order to avoid any bias from the effect of food intake. On the other hand, circadian stage dependence of the response to food intake may provide valuable information as well.

In any event, a data base can now be accumulated to determine, under standardized conditions, the pattern of endoluminal pH in healthy subjects for the determination of time-specified reference limits (chronodesms). Circadian recordings of this variable in subjects at risk or in patients with the overt disease could then be compared against such reference limits to detect any excess (or deficit) of gastric acidity (Cornélissen et al., 1985; Halberg et al., 1985). This approach allows not only the detection of an elevation in overall mean gastric acidity, but also the assessment of the timing of any undue excess and thus the correct timing of treatment.

These results await further studies to indicate how this research can be applied to solving clinical problems, to diagnose the disease earlier and to determine what potential benefits subjects with only an increased risk of developing manifest disease could expect.

4. SUMMARY

The reflux both of gastric juice in the esophagus and of biliopancreatic juice into the stomach produces sharp and great changes in luminal pH. These changes are superimposed on circadian, infradian and ultradian variations and can be detected by means of an intraluminal pH electrode connected to an external recorder. This method was used in the past to detect reflux esophagitis. In order to improve this diagnostic tool, we recently devised a solid-state battery-operated recorder, which is capable of collecting about 50,000 data per day. Data are easily transferred into a personal computer with dedicated software. On the portable recorder, 12 event markers are available to the patient. This personal device appears to be useful for a chronobiologic approach with respect to overt disease and, perhaps, in the assessment of increased risk of developing diseases of the upper digestive tract.

REFERENCES

1. Cornélissen G, Sothern RB, Moore JG, Halberg F: Chronobiologic methods for evaluation of gastro-intestinal ulcerogenesis. Abstract, 5th Int. Conf. on Experimental Ulcer. Dig. Dis. Sci. 30: 371, 1985.
2. Halberg F, Carandente F, Cornélissen G, Katinas GS: Glossary of chronobiology. Chronobiologia 4, Suppl. 1, 1977, 189 pp.
3. Halberg F, Moore JG, Cornélissen G: Reference standard for circadian characteristics of human gastric acidity. Abstract, 5th Int. Conf. on Experimental Ulcer. Dig. Dis. Sci. 30: 379, 1985.
4. Tarquini B: Physiopathology of peptic ulcer: a new view. Rass. Med. Sper. 27: 279-302, 1980.

This work has been partially supported by a grant from the Regione Toscana, Italy.
The authors are greatly indebted to Germaine Cornélissen Guillaume and Franz Halberg (both of the Chronobiology Laboratories, University of Minnesota, Minneapolis, MN, USA) for their kind editing of this paper.

Hardware and software needs for the eventually ambulatory clinical chronobiologic laboratory

Norberto Montalbetti* and Franz Halberg**
*Clinical Biochemistry Laboratory, Niguarda-Cà Granda Hospital, Milan, Italy
**Chronobiology Laboratories, University of Minnesota Medical School, Minneapolis, MN, USA

A collection of urine or blood for a span of a day is still practical (1). Prominent circadian rhythms can thus be assessed in a number of variables, as illustrated in Figure 1 (2). There are rhythms with lower frequencies, however, as shown for the urinary excretions of calcium (3,4), illustrated in Figure 2, and of 17-ketosteroids (5), shown in Figure 3. Actually, about-yearly rhythms are not only ubiquitous (6), but they have already been documented for many variables, longitudinally (4). What is particularly noteworthy, circannual rhythms are of very great epidemiologic interest and serve for the prediction of the risk of developing major diseases of our civilization (7). Thus, the need arises for long-term *in vivo* monitoring of variables that are of biomedical interest. It seems reasonable to anticipate that most of the variables determined in the clinical laboratory exhibit a spectrum of rhythms with different frequencies. Their monitoring by *in vivo* probes, placed, e.g., into the circulation or the tissue, can greatly help in continuously or intermittently monitoring biochemical processes, notably when the collection of biological material is not possible (as is the case on too many occasions) for practical or ethical reasons. Thus, there is a need for the following types of devices:

1. Biochemical sensors: specific ion electrodes and sensors coupling the specific action of immobilized enzymes, or receptors, or functional proteins or cells with an electrochemical detection system, implanted in tissues or veins (8-13).
2. Non-invasive methods: already-existing for pO_2, pCO_2, bilirubin and chloride, based on spectrophotometry or conductivity (14,15).

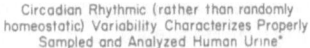

3. Nuclear magnetic resonance: non-invasive, can monitor some biochemical processes in a given region of the body. The specificity is to be increased (16-18).
4. Monitoring of $^{14}CO_2$ or ^{3}H in expired air after administration of tracer substances along with biochemical loads.

It is also desirable to develop simple, portable sampling devices for the collection of blood, urine and other biological fluids (saliva, tears, bronchial or vaginal mucus, intestinal fluids, etc.); these should also include apparatus for the preservation of the samples and their identification.

The collection of samples of biological fluids deriving from a single organ or functional area would allow assessment and monitoring of localized and relatively short-lived, possibly ultradian periodic chemical processes of biological importance.

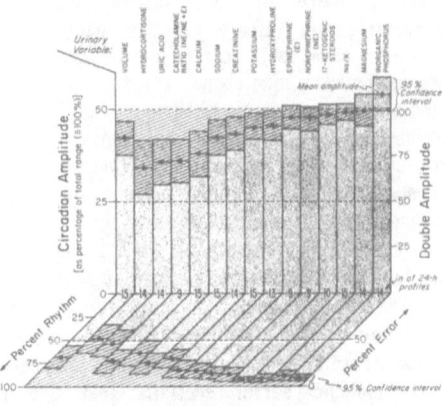

Figure 1 (right).

394

Figures 2 (top) and 3 (bottom).

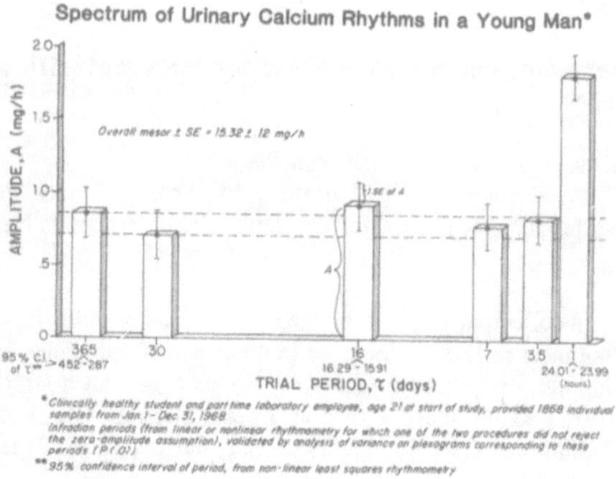

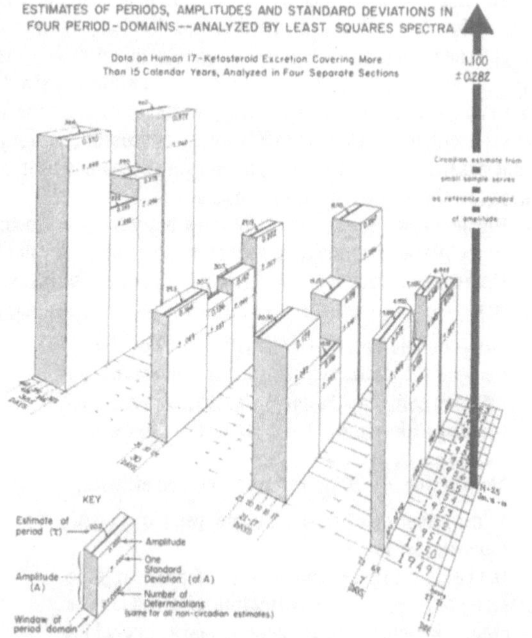

Thompson (19) has proposed *in vivo* bioprobes that not only incorporate a selective receiving site for molecular or ionic recognition, and a transducer which is capable of translating a perturbation of physical chemistry of the determinant-site reaction (interaction) into a useable signal, but he also listed as performance criteria selectivity, sensitivity, fast response, small size, ruggedness, low cost, biocompatibility, calibratability and facile use by means of telemetry. He recognizes that such demands create enormous challenges to the specialist in sensors. Thompson envisions implants for general hospital use, transient probes to replace classical blood tests, short-term implantable probes and the most important ones of interest to the chronobiologist, long-term bioprobes. He amplifies that with respect to biocompatibility, the sensor must not be involved in infection, clot formation or antigenic response. Thompson indicates that protein adsorption or other factors that can affect the sensor's response should be avoided; even if they are, calibration and recalibration, that is the check on drifts, remain major problems. Finally, there is the matter of preventing any tumors. While many implants have been carried by human beings for very long spans, without any obvious harm, it seems to be important, at least in intraperitoneal implantation, to prevent the fixation and fibrotic encapsulation of the implant, perhaps by means of regular mobilization and, for

Spectrum of Urinary Calcium Rhythms in a Young Man*

ESTIMATES OF PERIODS, AMPLITUDES AND STANDARD DEVIATIONS IN FOUR PERIOD-DOMAINS--ANALYZED BY LEAST SQUARES SPECTRA

this reason as well as others, to keep any *in vivo* probes at the smallest possible size. Moreover, implant surfaces may be roughened by sandpaper or coating to reduce fibrosis.

The signals coming from automatic portable devices (see points 1 and 2) should be recorded in a computer-compatible support system and possibly analyzed as-one-goes [at intervals corresponding to the circadian or other period(s) of interest] if not on line. Such analysis can be carried out with chronobiologic serial sections that are relatively simple and readily implemented by microcomputers as illustrated for a biophysical variable, blood pressure (20) in Figure 4. Results thus obtained are equally pertinent for the assessment of biochemical status. For instance, one can assess the statistical significance of a biochemical rhythm, e.g., in blood, as in row 2 of Figure 4, even in data that are irregularly sampled, as shown on top of Figure 4. Such studies could be carried out before and after the change from a drug to a placebo or vice versa, and could examine changes in

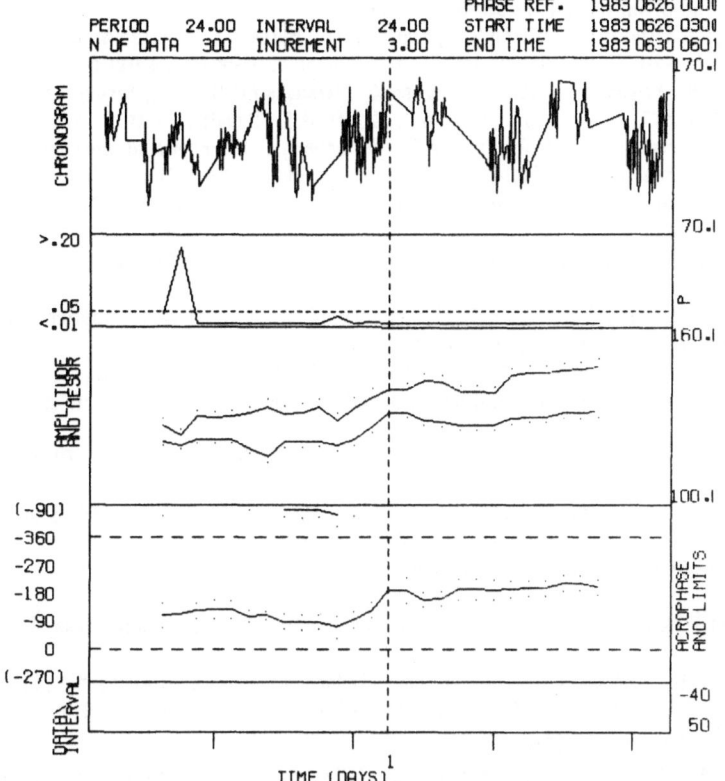

PERIOD 24.00 INTERVAL 24.00 PHASE REF. 1983 0626 0000
N OF DATA 300 INCREMENT 3.00 START TIME 1983 0626 0300
                                 END TIME   1983 0630 0600

TIME (DAYS)

POST-ISOLATION : 62.5Y-OLD "HYPERTENSIVE" MAN(LS):SYSTOLIC BP(MMHG)
(VERTICAL LINE=STOP DRUG. START PLACEBO DAILY AT 0530)

Figure 4.

biochemical rhythm characteristics such as the change in amplitude (distance between lower and upper curves, row 3, Figure 4), in the timing of overall high values shown in row 4, and the changes in MESOR (rhythm-adjusted mean) (the lower curve in row 3, Figure 4).

References

1. Kanabrocki E.L., Scheving L.E., Halberg F., Brewer R.L., Bird T.J.: Circadian variations in presumably healthy men under conditions of peace-time army reserve unit training. Space Life Sci. 1973; 4: 258-270.
2. Halberg F.: Quo vadis basic and clinical chronobiology: promise for health maintenance. Am. J. Anat. 1983; 168: 543-594.
3. Sothern R.B., Leach C., Nelson W.L., Halberg F., Rummel J.A.: Characteristics of urinary circadian rhythms in a young man evaluated on a monthly basis during the course of 21 months. Chronobiologia 1974; 1 (Suppl. 1): 73-82.
4. Sothern R.B., Halberg F.: The spectrum of urinary calcium rhythms in a healthy young man. Chronobiologia 1981; 8: 180.
5. Halberg F., Engeli M., Hamburger C., Hillman D.: Spectral resolution of low-frequency, small-amplitude rhythms in excreted 17-ketosteroid; probable androgen-induced circaseptan desynchronization. Acta endocr. (Kbh.) 1965; Suppl. 103: 5-54.
6. Halberg F., Lagoguey J.M., Reinberg A.: Human circannual rhythms in a broad spectral

structure. Int. J. Chronobiol. 1983; 8: 225-268.

7. Halberg F., Cornélissen G., Sothern R.B., Wallach L.A., Halberg E., Ahlgren A., Kuzel M., Radke A., Barbosa J., Goetz F., Buckley J., Mandel J., Schuman L., Haus E., Lakatua D., Sackett L., Berg H., Wendt H.W., Kawasaki T., Ueno M., Uezono K., Matsuoka M., Omae T., Tarquini B., Cagnoni M., Garcia Sainz M., Perez Vega E., Wilson D., Griffiths K., Donati L., Tatti P., Vasta M., Locatelli I., Camagna A., Lauro R., Tritsch G., Wetterberg L.: International geographic studies of oncological interest on chronobiological variables. In: Neoplasms--Comparative Pathology of Growth in Animals, Plants and Man, H. Kaiser, ed., Williams and Wilkins, Baltimore, 1981, pp. 553-596.

8. Covington A.K.: Ion selective electrode methodology. Boca Raton, Florida: CRC Press, 1980, 272 pp.

9. Mascini M.: Elettrodi ad enzimi, a batteri, ad anticorpi ed a tessuti viventi: applicazioni per la chimica clinica e la biologia. Biochim. Clin. 1984; 8: 1193-1195.

10. McKinley B.D., Hautcheces B.A., Janata J.: In vivo application of ISFETs: summary of current laboratory research and probable future clinical detectors. Ion-Selective Electrode Rev. 1984; 6: 173-208.

11. Mosca A., Carpinelli A.: Sensori elettrochimici di interesse biochimico clinico. Biochim. Clin. 1985; 9: 621-628.

12. Seitz W.R.: Chemical sensors based on fiber optics. Anal. Chem. 1984; 56: 16A-34A.

13. Sibbald A., Covington A.K., Carter R.F.: Simultaneous on-line measurements of blood K^+, Ca^{2+} and pH with a Four-Function ChemFET integrated circuit sensor. Clin. Chem. 1985; 30: 135-137.

14. Rolfe P. (ed.): Non-invasive physiological measurements, vol. 2. Academic Press, 1984, 400 pp.

15. Wimberley P.D., Pedersen K.G., Thode J., Fogh-Andersen N., Møller-Sørensen A., Siggaard-Andersen O.: Transcutaneous and capillary pCO_2 and pO_2 measurements in healthy adults. Clin. Chem. 1983; 29: 1471-1473.

16. Bales J.R., Howe D.P., Harve I., Nicholson J.K., Sadler P.J.: Use of high-resolution proton nuclear magnetic resonance spectroscopy for rapid multicomponent analysis of urine. Clin. Chem. 1984; 30: 426-432.

17. Brown C.E., Battocletti J.H., Johnson L.F.: Nuclear magnetic resonance (NMR) in clinical pathology: current trends. Clin. Chem. 1984; 30: 606-618.

18. Andrew E.R. (ed.): Magnetic Resonance in Medicine (journal). Vols. 1 and 2, 1984 and 1985, Academic Press.

19. Thompson M.: In vivo probes: problems and perspectives. In: Proc. Int. Symp. Laboratory Medicine for the Next Decade: Issues for the 80's and 90's, Hamilton, Ont., Oct. 2-3, 1985, p. 8.

20. Halberg F., Scheving L.E, Lucas E., Cornélissen G., Sothern R.B., Halberg E., Halberg J., Halberg Francine, Carter J., Straub K.D., Redmond D.P.: Chronobiology of human blood pressure in the light of static (room-restricted) automatic monitoring. Chronobiologia 1984; 11: 217-247.

MULTIPARAMETER DATA ACQUISITION SYSTEMS FOR STUDIES OF CIRCADIAN RHYTHMS.

KENNETH R. GROH, CHARLES F. EHRET, WILLIAM J. EISLER, JR., and DONALD A. LeBUIS
Division of Biological and Medical Research, Argonne National Laboratory,
9700 South Cass Avenue, Argonne, Illinois 60439.

INTRODUCTION

Circadian studies require facilities in which many animals can be exposed simultaneously to multiple environmental and biochemical time cues (zeitgebers) and in which their response(s) can be monitored in a noninvasive manner for long periods of time (4,11). Facilities that monitor and record circadian and ultradian metabolic and behavioral responses provide the most sensitive measures that can be obtained of environmental perturbations of the central and autonomic nervous system.

In our laboratory, where we have developed such facilities, we have shown that when low concentrations of phenobarbital are fed ad libitum to rats, circadian rhythms tend to disappear, and the rats become "dyschronic" (5). Also, when dopamine (L-DOPA) is presented before the thermal acrophase (peak) in body temperature, dyschronism occurs, but when L-DOPA is given after the thermal acrophase no alteration of the circadian rhythm in body temperature occurs (3). Long-term, simultaneous monitoring of multiple metabolic circadian cycles such as energy metabolism, animal activity, and body temperature have revealed ultradian (less than 24 hour) rhythms that depend on circadian phase and the perturbations of environmental influences (12). Correlations have been drawn between circadian rhythms of body temperature and the circadian chronotype of the rat. The rat chronotype includes the phase-shifting effects of theophylline and of pentobarbital. The strength of their effect depends on when (at what "phase") in the circadian cycle they are administered (2). The method and timing of zeitgeber administration are also important.

Because of the variation between individual animals, it is beneficial in such experiments as these to have large sample sizes for each experimental condition, and as many experimental conditions as possible. To this end, during the past ten years we have designed, constructed, and used four microcomputer-controlled data-acquisition systems that collect circadian data from organisms that range from populations of eukaryotic cells to individually housed small mammals (rats and mice) (1,4,6,7,10,11). These systems are described further below.

THE DATA ACQUISITION SYSTEMS

Although the computer hardware and software programs that service each facility are strikingly similar, the specific data collected varies among data acquisition systems as dictated by the requirements of the particular experiment and experimental animal. For the mammal, the most common measurements that are collected simultaneously are deep body temperature, animal weight, animal activity, food consumption, oxygen consumption, and carbon dioxide production. Each facility is located in one or more rooms with controlled temperature and humidity and programmable lighting to provide entrainment cycles of light and darkness (LD). A representative circadian facility for mammals is the RATDAS (RAT Data Acquisition System) (Fig. 1). For each individually housed animal, the RATDAS system collects data on body temperature, animal weight, animal activity, and food consumption. Thirty-six rats can be housed in each of

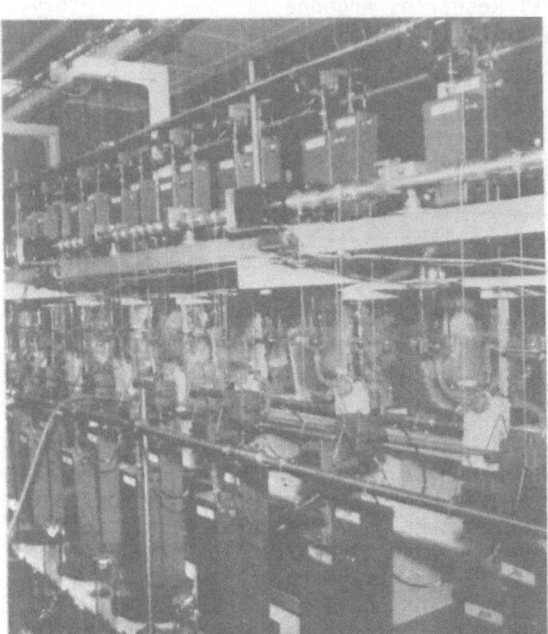

Fig. 1. Battery of cages, showing paired food hoppers supported by force transducers and suspension string; the strings are coiled around horizontal motor-driven rods to raise and lower the hoppers on schedule.

Fig. 2. Cage and food hopper assembly, showing watering device, antenna, and radio-frequency copper-mesh shield. The gridwork cage bottom is supported by a load beam (not shown).

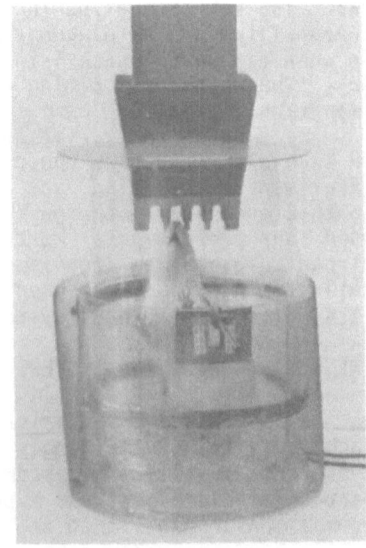

two separate rooms, permitting two different temperature and LD regimens. The animals are individually housed in cylindrical cages (5 inches in diameter x 10 inches in height) (Fig. 2). Each cage is supported by a load-beam transducer, which allows collection of weight and activity data for each animal. Above the cage two food hoppers ("breakfast", "supper") are individually suspended from weight transducers. These hoppers are raised and lowered automatically under programmable control. This feature allows the presentation of different feed-starvation (FS) cycles, during which the content of the diet with or without zeitgebers (i.e., drugs or other diet alterations) and meal timing can be controlled. The food hoppers are continually sampled for weight (i.e., to determine food and/or "zeitgeber" consumed).

Each cage has water available under programmable solenoid control to allow delivery of two different water sources that can contain additional zeitgebers, which can be administered at predetermined phases of the circadian cycle.

Wastes pass through the glass grid-meshwork cage bottom and can be collected for further analysis. "White noise" is also provided to the environmental rooms via continuous-loop audio cassette. This noise desensitizes the rats to sound cues that might be received from most daily building activities. The sounds presented include normal building noise, sounds of animals feeding, sounds of food hopper movement, and other normal room noises.

Body temperature is measured by a miniature temperature radio-telemeter, which is 2.2 x 1.5 cm and weigh 5 g, including the battery (Temp-Tel Engr., Mokena, IL) (Fig. 3, left) and is similar in design to those described by Mackay (8). The telemeter is surgically implanted in the peritoneal cavity and functions for approximately 6 months before requiring battery replacement. These data are generated by a temperature-dependent pulse-modulated transmitter, which has a 1600-1800 kHz carrier frequency. The telemeter (Fig. 3, left) has an effective transmission

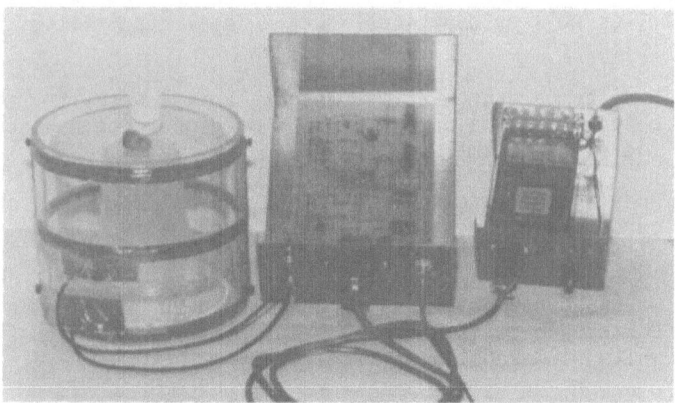

Fig. 3. Telemetry systems for core temperature measurement. Left: Implantable telemeter and antenna; middle: preamplifier; and right: power supply.

range of 30 cm and will transmit temperature measurements between 5 and 40°C ± 0.1°C. The pulse-modulated radio-frequency (RF) signal is collected by a two-plane antenna (horizontal and vertically polarized) fixed to a plastic cylindrical support that loosely fits around the animal cage. Each antenna is tuned (grid-dipped) to a center frequency of approximately 1700 kHz. A RF-shield consisting of fine mesh copper screening (Fig. 2) surrounds each antenna to prevent "cross-talk" between adjacent animals and interference from stray 60 Hz noise. As an additional precaution, each antenna coil is covered with 1-inch-wide, Scotch® RF shielding tape (No. 1245). Each antenna winding is connected to a two-channel preamplifier (Fig. 3, middle), which drives a Teledyne-Philbrick, Model 4702 frequency-to-voltage (F-V) converter, which is trimmed by an offset potentiometer to allow each telemetry-receiver channel to be adjusted to respond identically.

Individual animal weight and animal gross activity information is collected by a load beam transducer that supports the cage bottom (Fig. 2) (Alpha, Model 50N, BLH Electronics, Waltham, MA). The weight-activity signal generated by the animal is amplified (Sensotec, Model SA-10, Columbus, OH), and then a conditioning circuit separates the ac and dc components. The dc signal variations (animal weight) are time-damped and recorded. The ac component (animal activity) is amplified, squared, and integrated.

Data on each animal's circadian consumption of two different food diets are collected by periodically sampling the electric signal of the calibrated load transducer (Unimeasure, Model 60, Konigsberg Instr., Pasadena, CA) from which each food hopper is suspended (Fig. 1). Before each sampling, any food hopper that is being used for feeding during the "F" portion of a FS cycle is raised on computer command, sampled for the weight of food remaining, and then lowered to the animal cage. Water levels remaining can be recorded manually at frequent intervals.

The account given above specifically describes only one of our functional circadian data acquisition systems, RATDAS, which records body temperature, animal weight, animal activity, and food consumed for two different diets. Three other systems; ELFRAT, ELFMAT, and RESPIR collect these same data, as well as additional data. Their capabilities are summarized as follows:

ELFRAT   Body temperature, animal weight, animal activity, and behavior in the presence of 60 Hz high-voltage electric fields (20 animals);

ELFMAT   Body temperature, animal weight, animal activity, oxygen consumption, and carbon dioxide production, in the presence of 60 Hz high-voltage electric fields (8 animals);

RESPIR   Oxygen consumption and carbon dioxide production in eukaryotic cells grown in Petri plates (4 environmental units, 180 Petri plates/unit).

Each data-acquisition system uses a Digital Equipment Corp. (DEC, Maynard, MA) LSI-11 microcomputer to control the system and acquire data. Data I/O requirements have been standardized in each system as much as possible so that the same (or very similar) hardware is used; and computer boards are likewise duplicated in the systems. This feature enables a spare parts inventory to be maintained at minimal cost and avoids costly "downtime" due to breakdown. Malfunctions can be quickly diagnosed and failed components replaced; repair takes place at a noncritical time.

Computer control by the LSI-11 is accomplished by a machine-language program that was designed while the four circadian data-acquisition systems were under development. From a central core of subroutines that are shared by all systems, such as the clock, I/O routines, data formatting for storage, etc., each software program is individualized for the specific data-acquisition system in which it is used. This sharing minimizes the amount of memory occupied by the data-acquisition system program and maximizes the speed at which the program runs. New sampling parameters (animals to be sampled, sampling rate, etc.) can be stored in memory while data is simultaneously collected.

Input and output operations to the system are done by a Teletype 43 terminal (Teletype Corp., Skokie, IL) and a Tandberg TDC 3000 1/4-inch magnetic tape cartridge read-write drive (Innovative Data Technology, San Diego, CA), which include data acquisition program loading and modification, data collection, printing, and storage. Preliminary data processing takes place on a DEC LSI-11 micro- and 11/44 minicomputer; the transformed data is then transferred to and stored in the Argonne Laboratory main computer system (IBM 3330).

After the data have been collected, software packages specifically designed and written for our circadian, long-term data and commercial statistical packages (SAS, BMDP) allow the data to be visualized graphically and to be analyzed statistically. (SAS: SAS Institute, Cary, NC; BMDP: University of California, Berkeley, CA).

RESULTS AND DISCUSSION

The multiparameter, long-term data-collection capabilities of the RATDAS, ELFRAT, ELFMAT, and RESPIR data-collection facilities at Argonne have made possible a diverse spectrum of circadian studies. An example of typical data that are collected in these automated facilities can be seen in Fig. 4. In a group of 10 animals (one animal is represented here), during entrainment by multiple environmental zeitgebers (14 days, days 12-14 shown, 4/20-4/22/85), a strong circadian rhythm is established in body temperature and activity, with maximal temperature and activity occurring at 1200, which is well correlated with the LD: 16:8, L:1600-0800, inactive-active cycle that was established. The FS cycle was coordinated with the LD cycle to reinforce entrainment, FS: 8:16, F:0800-1600.

During entrainment, circadian change in body weight responded to the entrainment cycles, with maximal weight gain approximately 4 hours later than the peak seen in activity and body temperature. While there was a circadian periodicity in weight change during entrainment (periodic gain and loss), a net increase in body weight also occurred.

Later on the last day of entrainment, 4/22/85, the animals in this study were exposed to an electric field (100 kv/m, 60 Hz, 8 h duration, 2000-0400, mid-inactive phase) for 4 days. The rats responded to this circadian perturbation by becoming progressively more dyschronic during and following exposure to the electric field. There was a broadening of the peak (acrophase) in both body temperature and activity and a reduction in the amplitude of body temperature and animal weight (although these

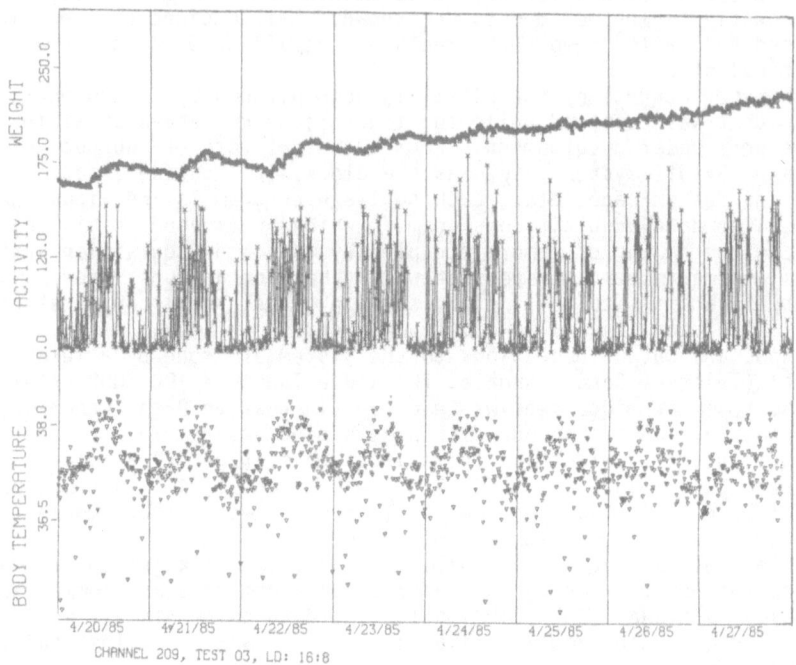

CHANNEL 209, TEST 03, LD: 16:8

Fig. 4. Computer-generated graph of animal core temperature, activity and weight (bottom to top).

peaks were still present). The electric field had a significant effect on the physiological parameters that were monitored. After the 4 days of exposure to the electric field, the animals were subjected to "free-run" conditions of food ad libitum and continual darkness (FF,DD) for 10 additional days. The animals continued to gain weight and ultimately exhibited a phase delay in both activity and body temperature (not shown).

In another representative study, which investigated the effect of low doses of phenobarbital (0.25%) present in food available continuously during FF (9), maximum food consumption occurred during the middle of the "active" phase (D) of the LD cycle (Fig. 5). When the daily results of individuals were combined (Fig. 6), a statistically significant effect of chronic phenobarbital administration was seen on circadian food consumption. In the animals exposed to phenobarbital, only 1 feeding time was seen in the middle of the active (dark) phase. In the control population, a second feeding period occurred, which anticipated the light, and peaked during the beginning of the inactive (light) phase. This difference in feeding answered the earlier presumption that chronic exposure to phenobarbital reduced the amount of food consumed and therefore explained the decrease in weight gained and circadian somnolence in organisms ingesting phenobarbital (9). These results showed no significant difference in the amount of food consumed by the animals: control, 23.0 ± 0.8 g/day vs. phenobarbital, 23.5 ± 0.7 g/day (Fig. 6), but the animals did display a marked reorganization of feeding behavior.

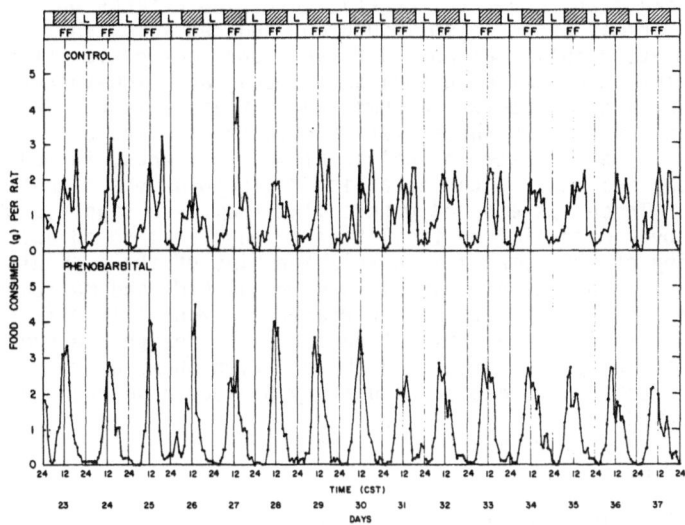

Fig. 5.   Transformation of food consumption data shows bimodal bouts of
food consumption during dark phases in control animals.
From reference (9).

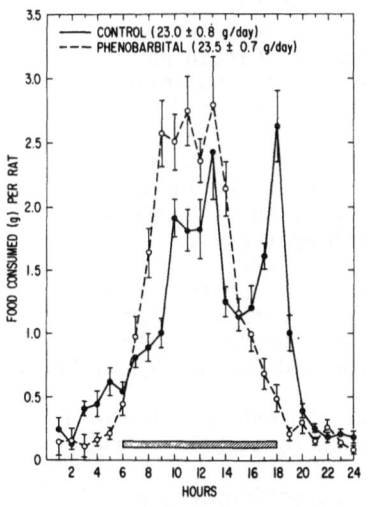

Fig. 6.   Fifteen day summary of food data for
rats (8/group, mean ± SE) shows
bimodal distribution of feeding
bouts in control animals. From
reference (9).

    The advantages of continuous data collection over long time intervals
with many experimental subjects have permitted a diverse catalog of
chronobiologic experimental studies using small mammals (several with
species of rodents), single-celled eukaryotic protozoa, and tissue culture
cells (e.g., rat primary hepatocytes). Circadian studies have been
conducted in the areas of entrainment conditions (LD, FS), phase-shift

inducers, (drugs and other zeitgeber), nutrition effects on established circadian rhythms, dyschronism inducement and recovery, shift-work schedule rotation optimization, "Jet-Lag," corticosteroid effects, catecholeamine-indoleamine metabolism effects, and high-voltage electric-field influence on circadian rhythms and risk assessment. The large sample sizes possible in these systems have exposed and documented the often large variation between individual test subjects, in addition to the average group response to the established circadian experimental conditions. These systems and others like them have significant advantages over more-limited facilities to enable us to advance our understanding of the complex interrelationships of the mechanisms through which circadian rhythms are established, regulated, and maintained.

The need to investigate many circadian phemonena in different species of organisms provided the stimulation for us to design the above automated data acquisition systems described above. With them, a broad spectrum of basic experiments in circadian regulatory biology have been and continue to be conducted.

ACKNOWLEDGEMENTS

We gratefully acknowledge the skillful assistance of Frank Williamson, George Svihla, John C. Meinert, Gordon Holmblad, Carol Fox, and Jeanne Blomquist.

REFERENCES

1. Cahill, A. L. and C. F. Ehret: α-Methyl-p-tyrosine Shifts Circadian Temperature Rhythms. Am. J. Physiol. 243: R218-R222, 1982.
2. Ehret, C. F. and K. W. Dobra: The Oncogenic Implications of Chronobiotics in the Synchronization of Mammalian Circadian Rhythms: Barbiturates and Methylated Xanthines, In The Third International Symposium on the Detection and Prevention of Cancer, H. E. Niebergs (Ed.). New York: Marcel Dekker, pp. 1101-1114, 1977.
3. Ehret, C. F., J. C. Meinert, K. R. Groh, K. W. Dobra and G. A. Antipa: Circadian Regulation: Growth Kinetics of the Infradian Cell, In Growth Kinetics and Biochemical Regulation of Normal and Malignant Cells. B. Derwinko and R. M. Humphrey (Eds.). Baltimore: Williams and Wilkins Co., pp. 49-76, 1977.
4. Ehret, C. F., G. A. Sacher, A. Langsdorf and R. N. Lewis: Exposure and Data Collection Facilities for Circadian Studies of Electric Field Effects Upon Behavior, Thermoregulation, and Metabolism in Small Rodents, In Proceedings of the 18th Hanford Biology Symposium, pp. 198-224, 1979.
5. Ehret, C. F., Van R. Potter and K. W. Dobra: Chronotypic Action of Theophylline and of Pentobarbital as Circadian Zeitgebers in the Rat. Science 188: 1212-1215, 1975.
6. Horseman, N. D. and C. F. Ehret (1982). Glucocorticosteroid Injection is a Circadian Zeitgeber in the Laboratory Rat. Am. J. Physiol. 243: R373-R378, 1982.
7. Jaroslow, B. and W. Eisler: Telemetry of Hibernation. Argonne National Laboratory Report (Publ. 7525), pp. 103-105, 1968.
8. Mackay, R. S.: Bio-Medical Telemetry. John Wiley and Sons, NY, 1968.

9. Peraino, C., C. F. Ehret, K. R. Groh, J. C. Meinert and G. D'Arcy-Gomez: Phenobarbital Effects on Weight Gain and Circadian Cycling of Food Intake and Body Temperature. Proc. Soc. Exp. Biol. Med. 165: 473-479, 1980.
10. Rosenberg, R. S., P. H. Duffy, G. A. Sacher and C. F. Ehret: Relationship Between Field Strength and Arousal Response in Mice Exposed to 60-Hz Electric Fields. Bioelectromag. 4: 181-191, 1983.
11. Runge, W., K. Lange, and F. Halberg: Some Instruments for Chronobiologists Developed or Used in Systems at The University of Minnesota. Inter. J. Chronobiol. 2: 327-341, 1974.
12. Sacher, G. A. and P. H. Duffy: Age Changes in the Rhythms of Energy Metabolism, Activity, and Body Temperature in Mus and Peromyscus. Adv. Exp. Med. Biol. 108: 105-124, 1978.

A CAGE DESIGNED TO IMPROVE COHERENCE OF DATA FROM MEAL-FED
GROUPS OF LABORATORY RODENTS

KAREL M, H, PHILIPPENS Department of Anatomy, Medizinische Hochschule
Hannover, D-3000 Hannover 61, West Germany

INTRODUCTION
In laboratory studies on the phase-responsiveness of rhythmic
functions to food uptake, time-restricted feeding (meal-feeding)
is the method of choice to set the reference event to the animal's circadian system (7). As is rather the rule in studies on
metabolic in- and output, investigations of the effects of meal-
feeding are frequently performed on singly housed animals. In
addition to multiple metabolic analyses this has the advantage
of simultaneously allowing the monitoring of several physiologic
variables in the individual. Elegant technical approaches to
this have been demonstrated in other presentations in this panel.
Short- or long-term isolation of, e. g., the socially organized
rat and mouse, however, may cause profound changes in the animal's physiologic condition and, hence, alter its response to
loads of different kind. Increase of locomotor activity as well
as of sensitivity to d-amphetamine in mice (1), early death of
young mice maintained on a meal-feeding regime (6) are examples
of this. In the isolated rat the adrenocortical response to certain stimuli is prolonged as compared to that observed in grouped animals (5, 8). Although some reports in the literature are
diverging as to certain effects of isolated or grouped housing,
the latter seems to be preferential and, most of all, the more
"natural" way of preparing rats and mice for rhythm studies.

Rank order, on the other hand, may diminish coherence between
group members. Such can be caused by the different impact of
stress due to, e. g., competition for food. When available only
in restricted amounts and during short time spans, the time of
food uptake, the amounts eaten as well as stress by fight-for-
food may differ considerably between different members. Data
collected from animals maintained under such experimental conditions will eventually complicate interpretation.

We constructed a cage equipped for automatic clock-controlled
feeding of rats or mice living in groups. This cage presents a
technical approach to overcome the afore-mentioned undesirable
effects of grouped housing, as its design serves to allow all
group members to take food simultaneously.

Supported by grants from Deutsche Forschungsgemeinschaft/SFB 146
and VW-Stiftung, Hannover AZ 11.2000.

DESCRIPTION
The cage consists of three mutually detachable subunits: the main body, the feeding-compartment, and the food dispenser (FIGS. 1 and 2, A, BC, and D, respectively). Each subunit is constructed of blueishly coloured PVC Transparent plastic plates (Trovidur, Dynamit Nobel, W.-Germany), which are 5 mm thick and form-stable at temperatures below 70°C. The material is resistent to (non-)decomposed excrements.
The main body is 22 cm high and has a floor space of 55 x 34 cm. Through a window in the front-side a PVC Transparent receptacle filled with sawdust and, on top of it, a grid (V-steel rods, 4mm

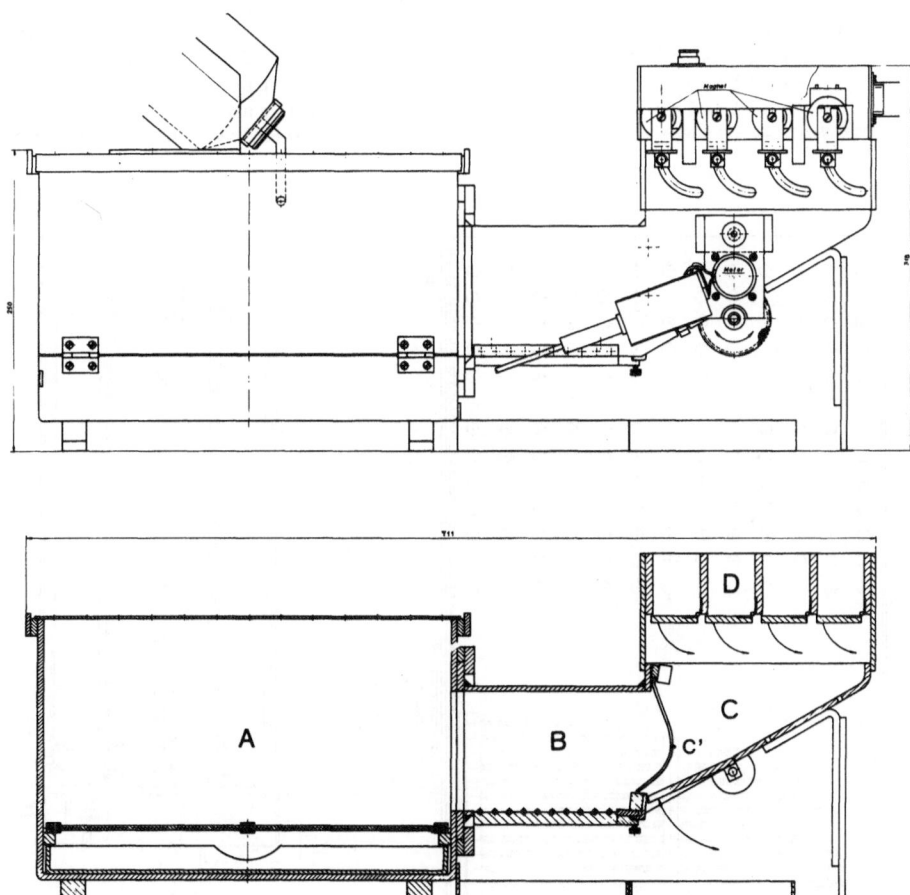

FIG. 1. (Above) Front view of cage. Overall measures: width = 711 mm, height = 330 mm. – (Below) Cross-section (at level of arrows in FIG. 2). A = main body; BC = feeding-compartment (B accessible to animals; C = rack, bottom window closed; c' = wire-grid); D = food dispenser (bottoms of four containers closed). For further explanations, see text.

in diameter) can be put into the bottom part. A V-steel plate
(1 mm thick and with 10 mm-wide perforations) is used as cover
(FIG. 2); one half of the cover is not perforated so as to provide shadow during light spans. The cover also serves to receive
the bottle holder. Animals can enter the feeding-compartment
through a window in the right side-wall of the main body.
The feeding-compartment consists of two halves. The half entered
by the animals is 10 cm high and has a floor space of 16 x 41 cm
(FIG. 1, B). Its bottom consists of a V-steel grid (diameter of
rods = 4 mm). By insertion of plastic plates this half can be
subdivided into several feeding-boxes. The size of these boxes
can be adapted to the animals under study by changing the number
and/or position of the plates. Opposite the entrance of the boxes is the wire-grid (FIG. 1, c') of the rack, which is the other
of the two halves of the feeding-compartment. The shape of the
grid and the slope of the bottom of the rack provide optimal access of the animals to pelleted food. At the end of the feeding-
span, a motor-driven valve serves to open a window in the bottom

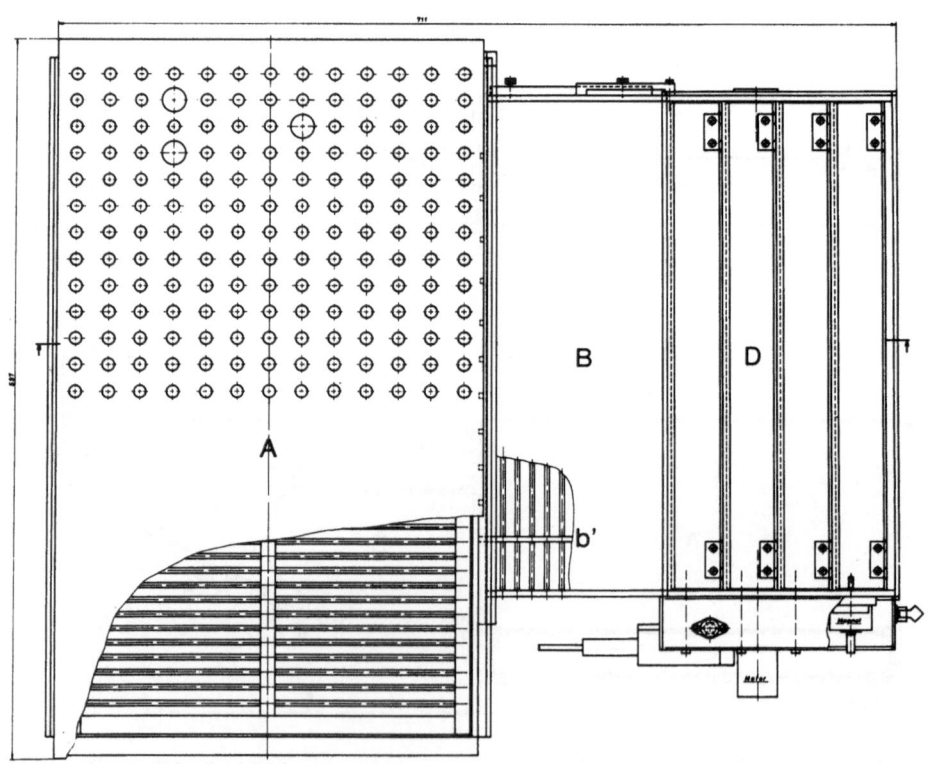

FIG. 2. Cage viewed from above. A, B and D as explained in FIG.
1. Bottom grids in A and B partially visible. b' examplifies
partitioning-plate inserted at one of several possible positions.
Bottoms of containers in D are shown in 'closed'-position.

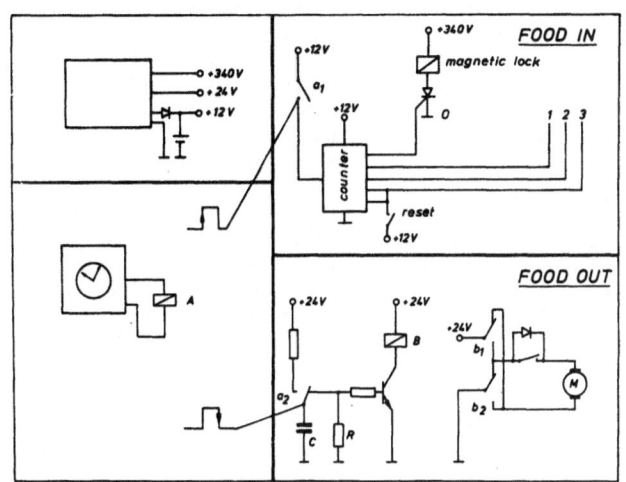

of the rack. Outside the cage, two separate receptacles (PVC Transparent) below the feeding-compartment serve to collect excrements and pellet wastes, respectively.

The food dispenser (FIG. 1, D) is placed on top of the rack. This subunit is 9.7 cm high and measures 18.7 x 41 cm. It is subdivided in four equally spaced pellet containers, each of which can take a maximal load of 600 grams. Pellets are dropped into the rack by unlocking the bottoms. The magnetic

FIG. 3. Circuitry operating the food dispenser (upper right) and the motor for the bottom valve of the rack (lower right).

force of each lock is nullified by a clock-pulsed thyristor (FIG. 3, upper right). After opening the fourth container, the counter in the circuit is reset; however, the magnets have to be put back in their locked position by hand. At the end of the feeding-span, fully opening and then closing the bottom of the rack by the motor (FIG. 3, lower right, M) is completed within 20 seconds. When locking-in back to its resting position (bottom closed), the motor stops operating by putting off a microswitch.

OPERATIONAL CONDITIONS

Up to six adult rats can be housed in the cage. Using a one-meal-per-day schedule allows replenishment of the food dispenser only every fourth day. If desired, the number of feeding-cycles between replenishments can be doubled by mounting a second dispenser above the one of the construction presented here. Other aspects of the design (large size of the main body, easy exchange of receptacles) basically serve to prolong time intervals between changing cages and, thereby, ro reduce disturbation of animals by routine maintenance.

The cage can be equipped for the purpose of automatic monitoring group behaviour, e. g., times and duration of food consumption and locomotor activity.

GENERAL REMARKS

In a preliminary study, ad lib.-fed male rats (Wistar AF/Han) were housed singly each in a standard Makrolon III cage (Altromin, Lage/Lippe, W.-Germany) and subsequently also in the cage presented here. Telemetrical monitoring of the intra-abdominal temperature of the animals during two weeks in each of both environments did not reveal any remarkable change with respect to the rhythmic pattern of the records obtained (not illustrated).

During this study, food consumption of the same animals was determined by daily weighings of the difference between the amount
given and that recovered, respectively. In the average, the consumption did not change (not illustrated), thus providing a further indication for the basic suitability of the new cage as an
environmental unit in the animal quarter. Until now, however, we
did not investigate grouped animals under the same comparative
conditions.
In addition to the advantage of reducing per-animal expenditures
for equipment and routine maintenance, grouped housing, for obvious reasons, is the better condition for the well-being of socially organized rodents (2, 3). However, in rhythm studies on
grouped rats or mice, the application of meal-feeding protocols
has the built-in risk of inducing considerable experimental
noise. On the one hand, rats and mice tend to over-eat so as to
compensate for long time-spans of starvation between meals (7).
As a result of this, the pulse of food uptake and digestion is
obscured as its release from the stomach is prolonged over time
(4). On the other hand, reduction of the amount of food given
during the meals is likely to evoke fighting (9) and cause ine-
qual food consumption by differences in individual competitive
strength. As shown in this contribution, one way of attempting
to prevent such undesirable effects is, to facilitate equal access to food by enabling group members to segregate during the
feeding-span.

REFERENCES

1. Del Pozo F, DeFeudis FV, Jimenez JM: Motilities of Isolated
   and Aggregated Mice; A Difference in Ultradian Rhythmicity.
   Experientia 34, 1302-1304, 1978.
2. Gärtner K: Zur Soziologie der Laboratoriumsratten, physiolo-
   gische Psychologie der Gruppen- und Einzelhaltung. Dtsch.
   Tierärztl. Wschr. 75, 45-48, 1968.
3. Gärtner K: Zur Soziologie der Laboratoriumsratten, physiolo-
   gische Psychologie der Gruppen- und Einzelhaltung. Dtsch.
   Tierärztl. Wschr. 75, 97-100, 1968.
4. Gärtner K, Pfaff J: The Forestomach in Rats and Mice, a Food
   Store without Bacterial Protein Digestion. Zbl. Vet. Med. A,
   26, 530-541, 1979.
5. Moore KE: Studies with Chronically Isolated Rats. Tissue Levels and Urinary Excretion of Catecholamines and Plasma Levels of Corticosterone. Canad. J. Physiol. Pharmacol. 46, 553-
   558, 1968.
6. Nelson W, Cadotte L, Halberg F: Circadian Timing of Single
   Daily Meal Affects Survival of Mice. Proc. Soc. Exp. Biol.
   Med. 144, 766-769, 1973.
7. Philippens KMH: Synchronization of Rhythms to Meal-Timing. In:
   Scheving LE, Halberg F (eds): Chronobiology: Principles and
   Applications to Shifts and Schedules. Nato Advanced Study Institutes Series. Alphen aan den Rijn: Sijthoff & Noordhoff,
   The Netherlands, 1980, pp. 403-416.
8. Plaut SM, Grota LJ: Effects of Differential Housing on Adrenocortical Reactivity. Neuroendocrinol. 7, 348-360, 1971.
9. Volicer L, West C, Greene L: Effect of Dietary Restriction

and Stress on Body Temperature in Rats. J. Gerontol. 39, 178–182, 1984.

ACKNOWLEDGEMENTS
The technical advice and skilful assistance of Mr. R. Albrecht, Mr. R. von der Fecht, and Mr. D. Grunzke is gratefully acknowledged.

LONG TERM RECORDING OF ANIMAL BEHAVIOUR AS A TOOL IN CIRCADIAN
RHYTHM RESEARCH.

W.J. RIETVELD AND A.WIRZ JUSTICE[*]
Department of Physiology, Div. of Medical Chronobiology, Un-
iversity of Leiden, The Netherlands and Psychiatry University
Clinic, Basel, Switzerland.

When studying the biological basis of circadian rhythms, the
investigator is often restricted to the use of animal experimental models since with humans the invasive,rigorous techniques of physiology and anatomy are obviously prohibitive. In
mammalian chronobiology, rodents and lower primates have
proved most suitable for the study of the structural and functional characteristics of the circadian system.
Mammalian circadian rhythms have two oustanding properties.
Firstly under constant environmental conditions they exhibit
free running rhythms with a period somewhat deviating from 24
hours. This observation implies the existence of one or more
physiological mechanisms that are capable of generating a
self-sustaining circadian oscillation. Secondly, when the animal is exposed to light-dark cycles with a period sufficiently
close to 24 hours, its circadian rhythm establishes a constant
phase relationship with the environmental regimen resulting in
an entrainment of organism and environment.
During the last decade the experimental approach to analyse
structure of the circadian system has been focussed on the
search for the central pacemaker as well as on the localisa-
tion of the pathways mediating the signals for entrainment.
A host of recent experiments involving mainly rats and ham-
sters have led to the recognition of the suprachiasmatic nuclei (SCN) of the hypothalamus as the regulator of circadian
rhythmicity. In these experiments neuroanatomical, neurophysiological as well as neuropharmacological techniques have been
used.
In the late sixties it was established that a retinal projection to the hypothalamus existed in lower vertebrates. Using
the autoradiographic tracing method Moore (1973) demonstrated
this pathway in the rat forming a direct connection between
the retina and the SCN, the retino-hypothalamic projection.
In addition to this anatomical finding there is other empirical support for the assumption that the SCN are a major pacemaker. Many behavioural circadian rhythms are abolished by
complete bilateral SCN lesions or surgical isolation (Rusak
and Zucker, 1979).
Electrical stimulation of the SCN alters the phase of circadian rhythms in locomotor activity in rodents (Rusak and Groos,
1982). With the aid of the 2 DG-method, Schwartz et al. (1980)
demonstrated a circadian rhythm in metabolic activity in the
SCN, glucose utilization being high during the light period.
No other brain area exhibit a similar rhythm. In accordance
with this are electrophysiological studies (Inouye and Nawamu-

ra, 1979) showing that in vivo and in vitro the multiunit activity within the SCN is high during the light period, low
during darkness.
From the anatomical point of view the SCN are two small nuclei
lying immediately above the optic chiasm. Each nucleus contains about 10.000 neurones.
Using classical neuroanatomical techniques van den Poll (1980)
described that SCN neurones have relatively simple dendritic
arbors. He identified simple bipolar, curly bipolar, radial,
monopolar and spinous multipolar cells. His findings are recently confirmed by Rietveld et al. (1985), using liposome entrapped lucifer yellow as a specific fluorescent dye for neurones. In addition a large number of peptides is found in
cells and terminals, (Moore,1982).
One fundamental question is in how far the presence of these
specific peptides is genetically predetermined. Cell cultures
of isolated SCN taken shortly after birth will give an answer
to this question. Recent experiments by Marani and Rietveld
(1985), proved the existence of functional neurones in cultures taken from 22 days old rat SCN. Cell homogenates or mi-
cropunches of SCN tissue are placed in a culture medium. Neurones are determined by application of lucifer yellow as well
as by neurofilament antibody labelling. Dual labelling experiments in which antibodies against the various neuropeptides in
the SCN are applied on the cultured cells are done to correlate form, content and development.
An important question to ask is how the SCN is able to generate a periodic 24 hour frequency signal. According to Moore
(1982) the SCN neurones are initially produced as a set of
genetically determined, independent oscillators that become
interconnected during development so that individual neuronal
function now becomes a network function.
To analyse the generation of the time keeping signal within
the SCN different approaches can be followed. Physiologists
use lesion techniques or analyse neuronal firing patterns.
Electrolytic lesions of the rostral part of both SCN in blinded rats alter the period of their freerunning behaviour. After
such partial lesions the rhythms in locomotor activity, food
and water intake, in bodytemperature as well as in urine corticosterone return within a period of 30-60 days but now with
a shorter freerunning period than before the lesion, (Rietveld,1984). Complete lesions of the whole SCN as well as lesions of the caudal part completely disrupt all circadian
rhythmicity, suggesting a dual oscillator system.
Pharmacologists study the effect of drugs on the circadian
pattern of behaviour.

To study circadian rhythms in overt motivational behaviour of
rodents like the rat, a highly versatile system was developed
to monitor food and water intake as well as wheel running activity. Deep body temperature was monitored by a long lasting
miniature telemetry system.
To improve universal use and flexibility a sensor system was
selected in which activation of an approach detector (Pepperl
and Fuchs, Mannheim, FRG) was achieved by food hoppers, drink-

ing bottles or activity wheels. In this way continous monitoring of food approach, licking activity or wheel turning is
possible. The output of the approach detectors is fed into a
DEC PDP 11/03 configuration for temporary storage. A total
number of 128 input lines are available. Temporary storage of
all data is possible up to a period of 72 hours at maximum. In
addition to the approach detector activity, general information (number of the animal, light or dark period, humidity of
the room) is stored simultaneously. By means of asynchronous
communication each half hour the data are automatically
transmitted to a PDP 11/70 computer (operating system RSX
11M+) for further analysis and final storage on disk and magnetic tape, see figure 1.

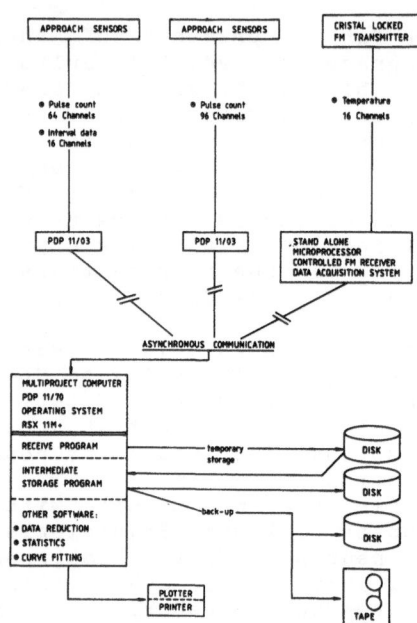

Figure 1. Diagramme of the
connections of the various
sensors to the computer configuration.

Food consists of commercially available pellets with an average weight of 0.124+0.024 g. The drinking bottles are filled
with tap-water. Actual food and water consumption are measured
over a period of 0.5-6.0 days by weighing food and water reservoir at begin and end of each period. For each animal, food
and water consumption are compared to the total number of approaches totalled over the same period of time. Correlation
coefficients between actual and estimated food and water consumption range from 0.90 to 0.99. The slope of the regression
line may range between 1.00 and 6.00. For each rat, however,
this slope is remarkably reproducible. Slope values are fed
into the computer to convert the data into values of actual
food and water intake. The animals are individually housed in
cages each provided with a food hopper, a drinking bottle and
a running wheel. The cages are placed in light, temperature
and humidity controlled rooms.

The door of the food hopper can be closed by an electromagnetic lock to induce meal timing. Similar valves are present in the drinking tubes. A timing programme in the main computer enables indivual blocking of both food and water availability for each individual rat. Anticipation to the meal timing can be recorded by an extra door in front of the actual flap that gives access to the food compartment.

The transmitter used in the temperature measurements is small (size 20x12 mm, weight incl. battery 6.25 g). To reduce battery current (average current 12 micro-Amp, life time more than 12 months) the HF-transmitter stage is periodically switched-off by a low frequency multivibrator. The repetition rate of this multivibrator is temperature dependent (80 msec at 30°C); switch-on time is fixed at 1.2 msec. To obtain the temperature of a transmitter the repetition rate is measured by the decoder. Transmitting frequencies are in the 88-108 Mc FM range. A stable transmitting frequency is achieved by the use of christal locking. Due to this fact a commercially available FM-receiver can be used to receive the transmitted signals. Up to 16 simultaneously recorded channels are scanned and detected by a micro-processor. Transmitter monitor time is 4 sec/90 sec. The number of measurements before averaging is 16x200. Averaging time: 5 minutes. Back-up memory capacity of 24 Kbyte enables a temporary storage of 72 hours of data. The data are automatically transmitted to a PDP 11/70 computer for final storage and analysing. A monitor system enables on-line, video inspection of data simultaneously over all 16 channels over 1 hour or of one channel over 24 hours. Transmitters are made by thick film technique. They have an accuracy of 0.2°C and a resolution of 0.05°C.

In some experiments the animals are placed in metabolic cages with simultanous measurements of food and water intake as well as of body temperature. Urine samples are taken by means of a fraction collector connected to the bottom of the cage to determine urine hormone levels.

For most of the neuropeptides present in these SCN cells it is unknown whether they are involved in circadian timekeeping. The serotonin (5-HT) in the SCN is located in terminals, the perikarya of which are located in the midbrain raphe nuclei. 5-HT may act as a transmitter between these nuclei and the SCN. Electrophysiological studies reveal a response of SCN neurons to iontophoretical application of serotonin (5-HT), and clorgyline a MAO inhibitor. In spite of this there is no effect on free running period after local application of 5-HT into the SCN. However, in case of local implantation of clorgyline near the SCN there is some evidence of an increase in period length. Applying clorgyline through mini osmopumps does not affect free running rhythms in food intake of rats, (Rietveld and Groos, non published observation). Local injection of alpha-bungarotoxin, an irreversible cholinergic antagonist, into the SCN does not affect circadian rhythmicity in pineal activity (Zatz and Brownstein, 1981). Brattleboro rats that lack vasopressin in the SCN show undisturbed circadian rhythms. Injection of vasopressin in the rat SCN does not

416

change the period of freerunning activity rhythms.
Experiments in which the anti-epileptic drug sodium-valproate
is added to the drinking water reveal a reversible shortening
of the period of all kinds of behaviour. After withdrawal of
the drug, the period returns to pre-drug values within a couple of days, see figure 2.

Figure 2, left:double plot of food intake of a rat before,
during and after application of sodium valproate to the drinking water, (arrows mark begin and end of application). Note
the reversible shift in period.

Figure 3, right:double plot of the drinking activity of a rat
before and during application of methamphetamine to the drinking water (arrow).

Although it is an attractive proposition to attribute these
effects to an influence on the pacemaker itself, also more
peripheral effects have to take into account too. Adding methamphetamine to the drinking water results in an internal dissociation of food and water intake as well as in wheel running, see figure 3. In addition so callled circabidian days
(persisting activity during 24 hours, followed by 24 hours of
inactivity) occur. It is not at all evident that this is an
effect on the pacemaker itself. A recent modell proposed by
Daan, Beersma and Borbely (1984), originally designed to describe the timing of human sleep, is based on a sleep (or behaviour) regulating variable (possibly, but not necessarily associated with a neurochemical substance) which increases and

decreases during different states of activity. The onset of behaviour is triggered when the variable approaches an upper threshold; Inactivity occurs when the variable reaches a lower threshold. The thresholds show a circadian rhythm controlled by a single pacemaker for example the SCN. Internal desynchronisation and circabidian days can be simulated by this model in three ways. First by lengthening the period of the pacemaker itself, but also by decreasing the amplitude of the circadian oscillation and by increasing the threshold for initiation of behaviour. The latter case implies an effect on a more peripheral level than that of the SCN. Experimental manipulation of parameters given by the model will exclude some of these possibilities.

Circadian information is conveyed from the SCN towards other hypothalamic area.
However, what do we know about the circadian structure, about the presence of secundary or slaved oscillators.
If secundary synchronizing stimuli, (others than the light-dark alternation), are able to induce rhythms that are not abolished by SCN lesions and if these stimuli entrain those rhythms, it could indicate that other area of the brain contain endogenous oscillators or secundary pacemakers.
Meal timing in the intact, blinded rat is able to synchronize freerunning rhythms in adrenal corticosterone secretion, temperature and brain monoamines. However, in all these experiments a masking effect is more likely to occur than real entrainment, as after the meal timing all rhythms immediately shift back towards a position assuming a free running pacemaker
On the other hand there is experimental evidence that in animals with a bilateral SCN lesion meal timing induces an activity rhythm that shows anticipatory activity before the time of feeding, whereas the rhythm persists for a short time following reinstitution of ad libitum feeding. Ablation of the ventromedial hypothalamic nucleus abolishes these rhythms suggesting a role of a, weak, oscillator in this nucleus, (Krieger, 1980). Recent experiments by Ruis and Rietveld (1985) show that this is also the case in DMH-lesioned animals with an intact VMH.

So although the suprachiasmatic nuclei have been definitively established as the main driving oscillators for a large number of circadian rhythms, several functions still remain to be elucidated. By what mechanisms the endogenous circadian activity is generated, how entrainment is achieved as well as the existence and location of secundary oscillators.
In conclusion development and application of chronopharmacological techniques using programmed application of drugs, either systematically or locally, will be necessary to gain more insight into the role of neuropeptides in the time keeping mechanism as well as in the way this mechanism is entrained to signals from the outside world.

REFERENCES

Daan,S., Beersma,D.G.M. and Borbely, A.A. (1984). Timing of human sleep: recovery process gated by a circadian pacemaker. Am.J.Physiol.,246,R161-R178.

Inouye, S.I. and Kawamura, H. (1979). Persistence of circadian rhythmicity in a mammalian hypothalamic "island" containing the suprachiasmatic nucleus. Proc. Natl. Acad. Sci. USA,76, 5962-5966.

Krieger, D.T. (1980). Ventromedial hypothalamic nucleus lesions abolish food-shifted circadian adrenal and temperature rhythmicity. Endocrinology, 106,649-654.

Marani,E and Rietveld,W.J. (1985). Properties of cultured suprachiasmatic nucleus cells. Neurosc. Lett. Suppl., in press.

Moore, R.Y. (1973). Retino-hypothalamic projection in mammals. a comparative study. Brain Res. 49,403-409.

Moore,R.Y. (1982). The suprachiasmatic nucleus and the organization of a circadian system Trends in Neurosciences,5, 404-407.

Poll,A.N.van den, The hypothalamic suprachiasmatic nucleus of rat: intrinsic anatomy. J.Comp.Neurol.,191,661-702.

Rietveld,W.J.(1984). The effect of partial lesions of the hypothalamic suprachiasmatic nucleus on the circadian control of behaviour. In Annual review of chronopharmacology. (eds A.Reinberg, M.Smolensky and G.Labreque). Pergamon Press, Oxford.

Rietveld,W.J., Marani,E. and Thunnissen,I.E. (1985). Cell composition of the hypothalamic suprachiasmatic nucleus. Proceedings of the 26th Dutch Federation Meeting, 32-33.

Ruis,J . and Rietveld,W.J. (1985). Effects of meal timing in rats with a lesion of the dorsomedial hypothalamic nucleus. Neurosc. Lett. Suppl., in press.

Rusak, B. and Groos, G.A. (1982). Suprachiasmatic stimulation phase shifts rodent circadian rhythms. Science,215, 1407-1409.

Rusak, B. and Zucker, I. (1979). Neural regulation of circadian rhythms. Physiol. Rev.,59, 449-526.

Schwartz, W.J., Davidsen, L.C. and Smith, C.B. (1980). In vivo metabolic activity of a putative circadian oscillator, the rat suprachiasmatic nucleus. J. Comp. Neurol.,189, 157-167.

Zatz, M. and Brownstein, M.J. (1981). Injection of alpha-bungarotoxine near the suprachiasmatic nucleus blocks the effects of light on nocturnal pineal enzym activity. Brain Res.,213, 438-442.

MEASUREMENT OF BRAIN INDOLEAMINE RELEASE IN VIVO: APPLICATION TO
CHRONOBIOLOGY

K.F. MARTIN AND C.A. MARSDEN, Department of Physiology and Pharmacology,
Medical School, Queen's Medical Centre, Clifton Boulevard, Nottingham NG7
2UH, U.K.

1. INTRODUCTION

In the study of circadian rhythms many approaches are available to the
chronobiologist. These range from the relatively simple measurement of
gross locomotor activity (Pittendrigh & Daan, 1976) to the sophisticated
assessment of neuronal activity from multiunit recordings (Borsook et al,
1984). Electrophysiological techniques have been used for a number of
years in order to study neuronal activity. An alternative approach to the
study of this process is to look at neurotransmitter release and
metabolism. In this chapter we shall describe the use of two techniques,
in vivo voltammetry and intracerebral dialysis, used routinely in our
laboratory to study the release and metabolism of 5-hydroxytryptamine
(5HT) in vivo. Both of these techniques can be used in freely moving
animals and are therefore ideally suited to the requirements of the
chronobiologist. The two techniques will be dealt with separately and
then followed by some general remarks.

2. IN VIVO VOLTAMMETRY

At present this technique can only be used to monitor changes in the
extracellular concentrations of 5-hydroxyindole acetic acid (5HIAA) which
is the metabolite of 5HT. It is therefore limited to the measurement of
5HT metabolism in vivo. The principles of in vivo voltammetry have been
presented in detail elsewhere (Adams & Marsden, 1982), and therefore will
only be dealt with briefly here.

2.1. Electrochemical principles. In vivo voltammetry makes use of a
well-known problem for those working with catechol- and indoleamines -
their ease of oxidation (Figure 1). This reaction takes place on the
surface of a carbon electrode which acts as the oxidising agent. Most
neuroscientists are now familiar with the first practical application of
electrochemistry, namely the use of an electrochemical detector combined
with high performance liquid chromatography. Essentially, the in vivo
technique involves the implantation of a miniaturised version of the
electrochemical detector into the brain. However, in vivo there is no
chromatographic separation of the compounds in the extracellular fluid,
therefore one has to rely upon the ability of the voltammetric techniques
to distinguish between the various compounds on the basis of the different
potentials at which these compounds oxidise (Figure 1).

These oxidative reactions occur at the surface of the working electrode
and the electrons generated are proportional to the number of molecules
oxidised. There is no voltage or current flow across the brain at the
potentials used in vivo since the electrons generated are unable to move
distances greater than a few molecular diameters. This means that the

420

electrodes used only detect extracellular compounds in its immediate
vicinity (Cheng et al, 1979).

   The form of the electrochemical signal monitored depends upon the
measurement technique employed and the nature of the working electrode.

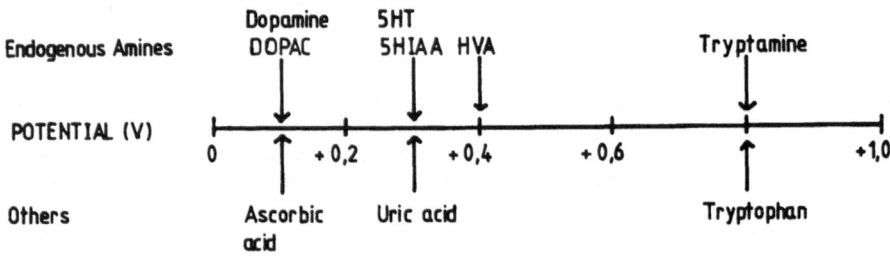

FIGURE 1. (Top) Oxidation of indoleamines to form an orthoquinone and
(bottom) a diagram to indicate the appproximate oxidation potentials of
some of the compounds found in the extracellular space.

2.2. Measurement techniques. Essentially there are two approaches. In
the first method, known as chronoamperometry, a square wave potential is
applied to the working electrode for a fixed time (e.g. +0.5 V for 1 s)
and the current generated during the last 10% of the fixed time measured,
thus avoiding the inclusion of the capacitance current in the measurement.
All compounds which oxidise at or below the applied potential are oxidised
and therefore this technique provides quantitative but not qualitative
information. Its main advantage is the speed at which measurements can be
made.

   The second method is to apply a steadily increasing ramp potential, of
a pre-determined range, to the working electrode. At the oxidation
potential of a compound there will be a peak in the current recorded and
providing there is a reasonable difference between the oxidation
potentials of two or more compounds (e.g. 150 mV) they will produce
separate oxidation peaks. Therefore qualitative as well as quantitative
data can be obtained. Peak resolution can be improved by using
modifications of the basic linear ramp technique, for example, by super-
imposing regular step potentials (of e.g. 30 ms duration, 50 mV amplitude,
2 Hz) on the basic linear ramp. This technique is known as differential
pulse voltammetry (DPV) and is the one used routinely in our laboratory.

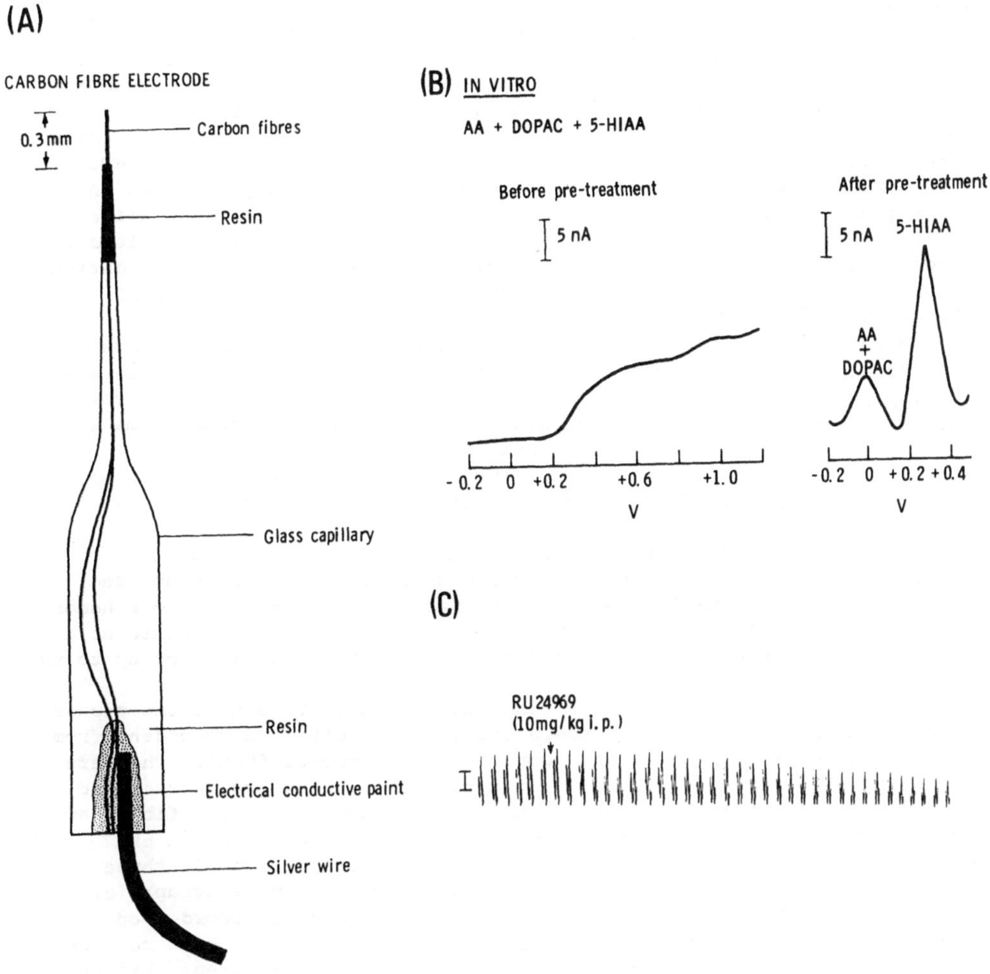

(A)

CARBON FIBRE ELECTRODE

0.3 mm

— Carbon fibres

— Resin

— Glass capillary

— Resin

— Electrical conductive paint

— Silver wire

(B) IN VITRO

AA + DOPAC + 5-HIAA

Before pre-treatment

5 nA

-0.2   0   +0.2   +0.6   +1.0
V

After pre-treatment

5 nA   5-HIAA

AA
+
DOPAC

-0.2   0   +0.2 +0.4
V

(C)

RU 24969
(10mg/kg i.p.)

FIGURE 2. A) The carbon fibre in vivo electrode. B) Typical in vitro voltammograms obtained from a mixture of ascorbic acid (AA), DOPAC and 5HIAA in phosphate buffered saline pH 7.4 before and after an electrical pretreatment consisting of three 20 sec applications of a 70 Hz triangular waveform of 0-3 V, 0-2 V and 0-1 V. C) Typical voltammograms obtained from the SCN in an experiment to study the effect of i.p. administration of the $5HT_1$ receptor agonist RU 24969 (10 mg/kg). The vertical bar represents 1 nA.

2.3. Working electrode. Because the electrochemical signals recorded in vivo are in the nano-amp range the working electrode needs to be made of material with a very low residual current. This has therefore limited electrode construction to carbon based materials. In addition, the working electrode must be able to distinguish between compounds with similar oxidation potentials which are found in the extracellular fluid. For example, a considerable problem was posed by the high levels of

ascorbic acid in the brain (Mefford et al, 1981) which oxidises at a
similar potential to that of dopamine and its metabolite DOPAC. In
addition the indoleamines oxidise at a similar potential to uric acid,
which is also found in high concentrations in the brain (Zetterstrom et
al, 1983). Finally, since ultimately we are interested in
neurotransmitter release, we would also like an electrode to distinguish
between the acid metabolites and the parent amines, dopamine and 5HT.
This latter problem has some way to go before it is fully resolved and is
in part due to the very low extracellular concentrations of the amines
(5×10^{-8}M) compared to the metabolites (5×10^{-6}M). The former problems with
ascorbic acid have been largely overcome (Gonon et al, 1984). Oxidation
of 5HIAA can also be separated from that of ascorbic acid and DOPAC
(Cespuglio et al, 1984).

The working electrodes used in our laboratory (see Figure 2A) are made
from three pyrolytic carbon fibres (each 8 μm diameter) inserted into a
glass pipette pulled to a fine tip. The tip is sealed and the fibres
trimmed to 300 μm length. Electrical contact with the fibres is made
using electrical conductive paint and silver wire and the joint
strengthened with polyester resin. These working electrodes are used with
a silver/silver chloride reference electrode and a silver auxiliary
electrode.

Electrochemical separation between compounds is obtained by
electrically pre-treating these electrodes prior to implantation (see
Figure 2B). Full details are given in Sharp et al (1984). In our hands
these electrodes have remained stable for up to 10 h and Cespuglio et al
(1984) have reported their use in chronically set-up animals for up to two
days.

These carbon fibre electrodes also have the advantage that the tip is
only 20 μm in diameter and is therefore ideally suited to recording from
small brain regions such as the suprachiasmatic nuclei (SCN). They are
implanted into the brain region of interest using standard stereotaxic
procedures. Considerable care is required to ensure that the fibres are
not broken while penetrating the dura. The reference and auxiliary
electrodes are placed in contact with the dura surface and all three
electrodes cemented into place before connection to a polarograph (e.g.
Princeton, Brucker, Metrohm or Tacussel) and the output recorded on a
flat-bed recorder. With freely moving animals a permanent head connector
and electrically 'noise-free' swivel system are also required. Figure 2C
shows a typical recording from the SCN before and after i.p. injection of
the 5HT$_1$ receptor agonist RU 24969 and typical results from
pharmacological interventions are shown in Figure 3.

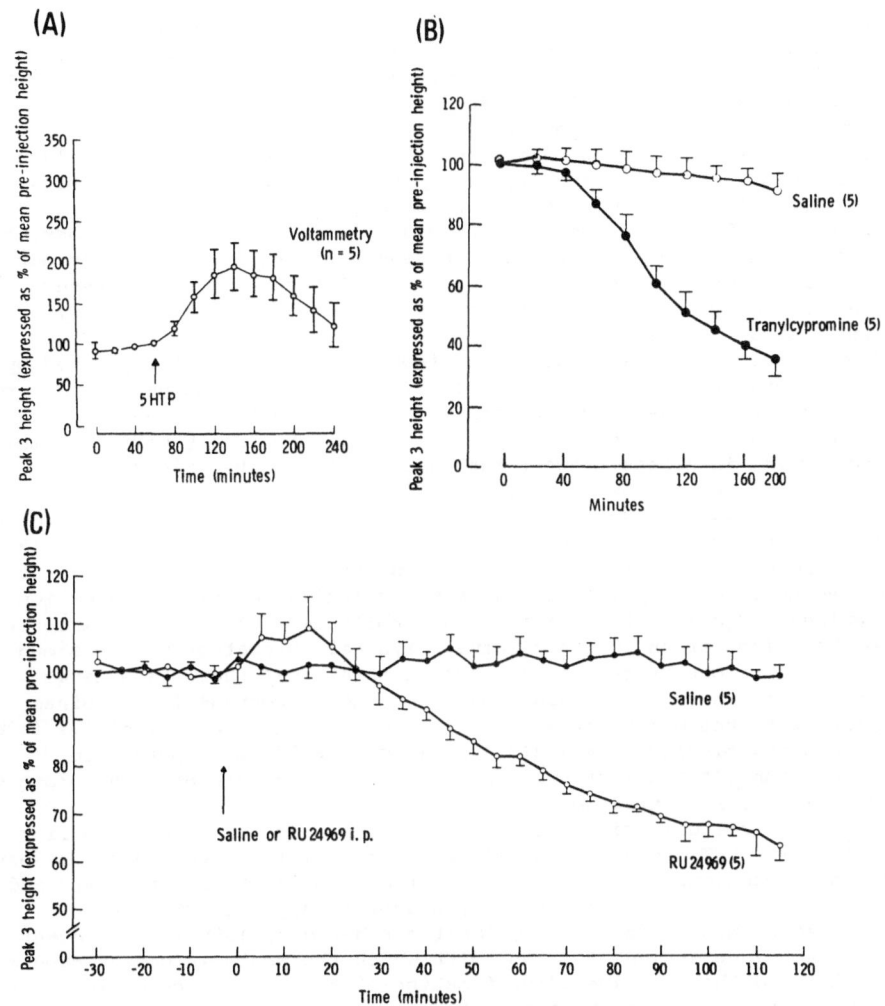

FIGURE 3. Graph showing the effect of A) 5-hydroxytryptophan (25 mg/kg i.p.) and B) tranylcypromine (10 mg/kg i.p.) on extracellular levels of 5HIAA in the striatum of chloral hydrate anaesthetised rats. C) The effect of RU 29496 (10 mg/kg i.p.) on 5HIAA levels in the SCN of anaesthetised rats.

3. INTRACEREBRAL DIALYSIS

This technique is one of several that have been devised to sample the extracellular fluid in the brain. It involves the implantation of a small dialysis tube into the particular brain region of interest. The tube is

then perfused with a physiological salt solution, solutes in the
extracellular fluid will diffuse down a concentration gradient, through
the semi-permeable membrane of the tube into the perfusion medium and be
transported away. The perfusate is collected and assayed in the
appropriate manner for the substances of interest. The range of
substances collected by the dialysis tube is dependent upon the molecular
weight cut-off of the tubing (typically 5,000 Daltons). Thus amines,
their metabolites and amino acids are readily collected and measured
(Ungerstedt, 1984). In addition, providing sensitive radioimmunoassays
are available, extracellular pepetide levels can be estimated. In our
laboratory we measure the indoles in the perfusate with high pressure
liquid chromatography coupled to an electrochemical detector (LCEC)
(Brazell et al, 1985).

The dialysis probe is constructed from a dialysis fibre supported by
two stainless steel cannulae (Figure 4A) and is implanted using standard
stereotaxic techniques. During perfusion one cannula is connected to a
microinfusion pump by polyethylene tubing. In the freely moving animal a
liquid swivel is placed between the pump and the probe (Figure 4B).
Physiological saline (Na^+ 147 mmol, Ca^{2+} 2.3 mmol, K^+ 4 mmol, Cl^-
156 mmol, pH 7.4) is perfused through the probe at a rate of 1 or 2 μl per
minute. The perfusate is collected into an everted eppendorf tube placed
on the end of the other cannula. The eppendorf tube contains 10 μl of
0.1 M Perchloric acid/0.02% sodium metabisulphite to prevent oxidation of
the amines. Usually 20 min samples are collected and injected directly
onto the column of an LCEC apparatus. Typical chromatograms are shown in
Figure 4C. It can be seen from these examples that there is a large
difference in the extracellular levels of the neurotransmitter amines
compared with the metabolites. For instance, Marsden and Routledge (1984)
have reported finding only 1.2±0.1 pmol 5HT per 50 μl of perfusate
compared with 27±2 pmol of 5HIAA per 50 μl of perfusate when the probe was
located in the rat striatum.

Intracerebral dialysis, then, provides a simple method of measuring
extracellular 5HT and 5HIAA as well as extracellular tryptophan. We have
used this technique to study diurnal variations in these parameters and
found that they are all consistently higher at night in the rat
hypothalamus than during the day (Martin & Marsden, 1985). The advantages
of the technique include the ease with which the probe is constructed and
implanted and the positive identification of the substances collected by
the LCEC assay. The major disadvantages of the technique are the
relatively large size of the probe and the long sample collection times
required.

4. CONCLUSIONS

There are now several techniques available for measuring whole and
regional brain 5HT turnover and release. In addition to those described
here there are several others and the reader is directed to Marsden (1984)
for more detailed information on these techniques. Considerable effort
has been put into establishing and validating them and it now seems the
appropriate time for the chronobiologist to take them in hand to increase
our understanding of the role and control of circadian rhythms.

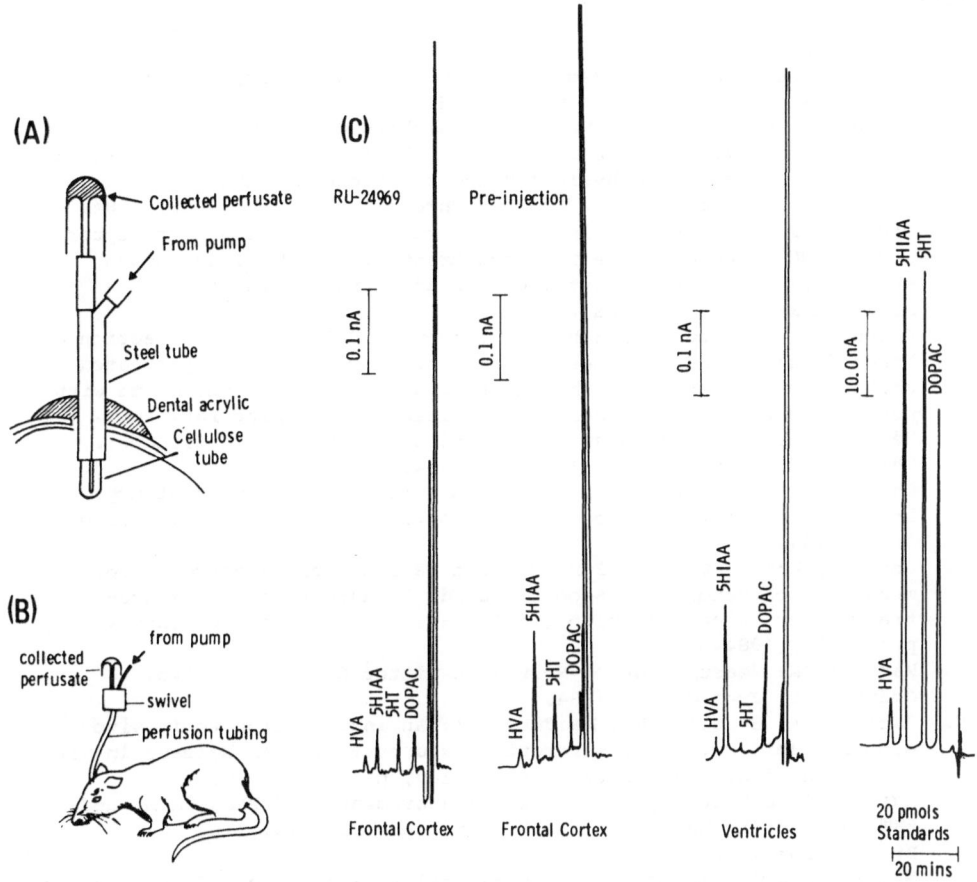

FIGURE 4. A) Diagram of the intracerebral dialysis probe and B) connected to a liquid swivel for collection of perfusate from a freely-moving animal. C. Typical reverse phase LCEC chromatographs of perfusates from rat frontal cortex and striatum. The pre-injection frontal cortex trace was obtained from a sample collected just prior to injection of RU 24969 (10 mg/kg, i.p.). The trace annotated RU 24969 was obtained from a sample collected from 60 to 80 minutes after the injection of RU 24969. Note the decrease in the height of the 5HT and 5HIAA peaks.

ACKNOWLEDGEMENTS
    We thank the Wellcome Trust and M.R.C. for financial support. We would like to thank M P Brazell, N T Maidment and C Routledge for the use of their data in this chapter.

REFERENCES

1. Adams RN & Marsden CA: Electrochemical detection methods for monoamine measurements in vitro and in vivo. In Handbook of Psychopharmacology (Eds LL Iversen, SD Iversen & SH Snyder), Vol 15,
p 1-74. New York: Academic Press, 1982.

2. Borsook D, Moore-Ede MC, Hedberg T, Richardson G & Brennan MJW:
Gamma-aminobutyric acid and the neural basis of circadian timekeeping:
implications for pathophysiology and psychopharmacotherapy of
circadian based disorders. Ann.Rev.Chronopharmac. 1, 53-56, 1984.

3. Brazell MP, Marsden CA, Nisbet AP & Routledge C: The $5HT_1$ receptor
agonist RU 24969 decrease 5-hydroxytryptamine (5HT) release and
metabolism in the rat frontal cortex in vitro and in vivo.
Br.J.Pharmacol. (in press).

4. Cespuglio R, Faradji H, Hahn Z & Jouvet M: Voltammetric detection of
brain 5-hudroxyindoleamines by means of electrochemically treated
carbon fibre electrodes: Chronic recording for up to one month with
movable cerebral electrodes in the sleeping or waking rat. In
Measurement of Neurotransmitter Release in vivo (Ed CA Marsden).
Chichester: John Wiley, p 173-191, 1984.

5. Cheng H-Y, Shenk J, Huff R & Adams RN. In vivo electrochemistry:
behaviour of microelectrodes in brain tissue. J.Electroanalyt.Chem.
100, 23-31, 1979.

6. Gonon F, Buda M & Pujol J-F: Treated carbon fibre electrodes for
measuring catechols and ascorbic acid. In Measurement of Neurotransmitter Release in vivo (Ed CA Marsden). Chichester: John Wiley,
p 153-171, 1984.

7. Marsden CA: Measurement of Neurotransmitter Release in vivo.
Chichester: John Wiley, 1984.

8. Marsden CA, Brazell MP & Maidment NT: An introduction to in vivo
electrochemistry. In Measurement of Neurotransmitter Release in vivo
(Ed CA Marsden). Chichester: John Wiley, p 127-151, 1984.

9. Marsden CA & Routledge C: In vivo measurement of DOPAC, 5HIAA and
5HT in specific brain regions by intracerebral dialysis.
Br.J.Pharmac. 82, 1984.

10. Martin KF & Marsden CA: In vivo diurnal variations of 5HT release in
hypothalamic nuclei. In Circadian Rhythms in the CNS (Eds Redfern PH,
Davis JA, Campbell IC & Martin KF), Macmillan, in press, 1985.

11. Mefford IN, Oke AF & Adams RN: Regional distribution of ascorbate
in human brain. Brain Res. 212, 223-226, 1981.

12. Pittendrigh LS & Daan S: A functional analysis of circadian pacemakers
in nocturnal rodents. V. Pacemaker structure: A clock for all seasons.
J.Comp.Physiol., 106, 333-335, 1976.

13. Sharp T, Maidment NT, Brazell MP, Zetterstrom T, Ungerstedt U,
Bennett GW & Marsden CA: Changes in monoamine metabolites measured
by simultaneous in vivo differential pulse voltammetry and intracerebral dialysis. Neuroscience 12, 1213-1221, 1984.

14. Ungerstedt U: Measurement of neurotransmitter release by intracranial
dialysis. In Measurement of Neurotransmitter Release in vivo
(Ed CA Marsden). Chichester: John Wiley, p 81-105, 1984.

15. Zetterstrom T, Sharp T, Marsden CA & Ungerstedt U: In vivo measurement
of dopamine and its metabolites by intracerebral dialysis: changes
after d-amphetamine. J.Neurochem. 41, 1769-1773, 1983.

AUTOMATIC MONITORING OF OXYGEN UTILIZATION IN INSECTS

D.K. HAYES. Livestock Insects Laboratory, AEQI, Agricultural Research
Service, USDA, Beltsville, MD 20705

1. INTRODUCTION

Insects have long been a favorite model for chronobiologists because of
the relative ease of obtaining specimens and the clear responses by some
of their rhythms to synchronization. However, methodologies for measuring
responses of rhythms to the environmental synchronization and of
perturbations of these rhythms are depending on instruments; insects are
not amenable to self-measurement techniques. This report summarizes
methodology dependent upon determination of oxygen uptake which we used to
follow insect rhythms during the pupal or adult portion of the life cycle,
or after an environmental insult.

2. MATERIALS AND METHODS

Oxygen uptake was determined using a Beckman Oxygen Analyzer Model 777
with additional circuitry consisting of a buck-out circuit which
effectively increased sensitivity of the determination from 2 to 50 fold
(Hayes et al. 1968). Oxygen concentration was assessed by means of a
polarographic electrode; because agitation such as occurs in a Warburg-type
respirometer apparently increases oxygen consumption, the chamber was not
agitated (Hayes et al. 1972). The device was equipped initially with a
recorder, points were selected and slopes were manually computed to
determine rate of oxygen utilization. However, it soon became apparent
that automation of data recording and processing was necessary. With the
Data Systems Division in USDA a simple system was devised for automatically
collecting data from the electrodes using a retransmitting slide wire.
Data were initially collected by a device at the site of oxygen measurement
and transmitted to a PDP 1000 central computer.

A program was developed to compute the rate of oxygen uptake per hour at
2 minute intervals and to plot the chronogram with oxygen uptake per hour
plotted as a fraction of time. The original data and the computations were
stored on a disc.

Technology progressed toward self-contained, computerized laboratory
equipment. A second device which was designed by Ralph Curtis, ARS,
transmitted data obtained in real time to a tape recorder and stored the
data for transmission to a central processing unit for analysis. This is
the system we are using today.

The polarographic electrode can be inserted into a sealed compartment
varying in size from 15 to 1000 ml so that oxygen uptake rates can be
monitored in single insects weighing from 10 mg to 10 g. It is possible to
manipulate humidity, absorb carbon dioxide, supply food and water and
insert other materials when the insect is placed in the chamber.

3. RESULTS AND DISCUSSION

Automatic oxygen uptake rates have been determined on a number of

insects. These studies have either been for the purpose of determining
long-term properties of the rhythms of oxygen uptake or for examination of
effects of manipulation on ultradian rhythms (Hayes 1979).

Rhythms in oxygen utilization have been observed during starvation in the
large Madagascar cockroach, <u>Gromphadorhina portentosa</u> Schaum, in moribund
adults of the face fly, <u>Musca autumnalis</u> DeGeer, and in insects standardized in various photoperiodic regimens. During the course of the observations, some changes in rhythms which could be observed macroscopically,
such as a decrease in amplitude, could be observed (Hayes et al. 1968,
1979). We also have examined the putative ultradian rhythms in the codling
moth and the face fly after treatment with ultraviolet light for 1 hour in
the "B" region of the UV spectrum, i.e. 285-320 nm. This exposure was at
the level that would occur if the ozone layer in the high atmosphere were
reduced by about 15%. After UV-B treatment examination of the macroscopic
longitudinal plot indicates that absolute rate of oxygen uptake is
increased. The apparent ultradian rhythms are no longer visible macroscopically as they are in the insects not exposed to UV-B. I believe that
being able to monitor this immediate effect on the ultradian rhythms
provided a sensitive and partially specific method to evaluate quickly the
effects of an environmental insult on an insect and possibly on other small
organisms as well. Medical applications are beyond the scope of this
paper, but a similar occurrence, that of an increase in respiration which
obscures ultradian phenomena, may also occur in mammals.

4. CONCLUSION

Rhythms in oxygen uptake can be demonstrated effectively and simply by
means of macroscopic and microscopic examination of data obtained using an
automated data collection and computation apparatus. Such data can provide
a means for non-destructive evaluation of effects of treatments or aging on
an experimental subject to predict future responses (e.g., death) and
measure a positive or negative effect resulting from a treatment. Such
evaluations are not possible by simple examination of the specimen, or by
biochemical determination alone. Generally serial sampling of body fluids
in a single insect is impossible. Therefore this type of non-destructive
testing, which affords multiple data points necessary for chronobiological
studies, is especially important.

REFERENCES

1. Hayes, D.K.: Oxygen uptake in selected insects. Chronobiologia VI:109,
   1979.
2. Hayes, D.K., J. Horton, M.S. Schechter and F. Halberg: Rhythm of oxygen
   uptake at several temperatures of codling moth larvae in diapause. Ann.
   Entomol. Soc. Amer. 65:93-96, 1972.
3. Hayes, D.K., M.S. Schechter, E. Mensing and J. Horton: Oxygen uptake of
   single insects determined with a polarographis electrode. Anal.
   Biochem. 26:51-60, 1968.

DISCLAIMER
Mention of a commercial product does not imply endorsement by the USDA.

CONTROLLED RELEASE DEVICES

D.K. HAYES, R.W. MILLER, AND H. JAFFE. Livestock Insects Laboratory, AEQI,
Agricultural Research Service, USDA, Beltsville, MD 20705

   Several types of devices are under study in the Livestock Insects
Laboratory, one of the Agricultural Research Service Laboratories whose
research program is oriented toward the management of populations of animal
ectoparasites. These include devices familiar and unfamiliar to the
participants of this conference and are as follows:
   (1) Boluses for inclusion in the 2nd stomach (reticulum) of cattle, to
release material for control of filth breeding flies and for which timed
release can be manipulated (Miller et al. 1979, Miller and Miller 1985,
Miller and Miller 1978).
   (2) Ear tags - which release material over a 3 month time span.
   (3) Implantable biodegradable devices which can be implanted and which
release one or more materials at a time (Feldmesser et al. 1981, Jaffe et
al. 1977, 1983, 1984).
   (4) Microcapsules administered in various ways (Jaffe 1985).

   A brief summary of each device follows:
   The bolus. This device can be administered to cattle with a balling gun.
although for research purposes it may be placed directly into the reticulum
of fistulated dairy or beef cattle. It lodges in the reticulum and
releases its contents into the digestive tract over a time span from 2
weeks to 6 months. Theoretically release occurs at a steady rate; however,
this device may actually release active contents in a cyclical manner
depending upon the cycles in the gastric portion of the bovine digestive
system. Degradation rates can be measured by studying the changes in the
bolus placed in the reticulum of fistulated animals.
   Release of substances into the digestive tract acts to control ecto- and
endoparasites through either (1) entry of the substance into the blood
stream for various parasitic helminths or (2) entry of a larvicide into
feces to control breeding of filth flies such as the face fly, Musca
autumnalis and the horn fly, Haematobia irritans.
   We have not determined that there are rhythms of the release of the
active ingredient from the bolus. It is clear, however, that by using
several fistulated cows, it would be possible to obtain both an estimate of
possible rhythms as well as to obtain serially independent samples over a
24 hour span to measure degradation. It may be environmentally desirable
to minimize the amount of substances released to the environment. This
could be done by timing of release from the bolus by either multiple
layering as has been done in other devices discussed at this meeting or by
selecting the waxes and other components of the bolus so that the release
can be regulated by the changes in the composition of the reticulum (as may
already occur).
   Eartags. Eartags are devices which contain a pesticide and are clipped
to the ears of cattle. This pesticide becomes distributed on the surface

of the animal in sufficient concentration to kill most insects lighting upon it; the mechanism of coverage of the animal is not entirely understood. A problem encountered with the device has been development of resistance to the insecticide by the target organism.

Implantable tube. This device is a small, porous tube ranging from 0.5-4 cm in length (Jaffe et al. 1983) in which the dimensions are carefully controlled. This tube is usually injected using the same type of device employed to implant hormones in cattle, such as a Synovex® implanter. A liquid solution or a concentrated liquid material placed in the tube moves from the tube at a rate determined by kinetics of diffusion from the tube.

We have shown that synthetic hormone analogues released from this device will interfere - as do antifertility drugs - with the hormonal rhythms of ticks (Jaffe et al. 1984). We know very little about how to vary release rates from these devices over a 24 hour span. Pumps are not practical for use with most farm animals or for many pets, although for truly expensive companion animals such as champion race horse stallions, or for some cattle and sheep pumps could be practical for administration of control chemicals for external or internal pest control.

Microcapsules. The microcapsule is a spherical body in which a pesticide or other active material is surrounded by a substance such as a polymer which regulates the release rate. Typical capsules can be 3-100 μ in diameter with the actual size tailored to the application. Such devices could represent an approach to the beginning of experimental chronotreatment for insects; microcapsules containing hormones can either be injected into insects or into an animal host on which they feed. This is an especially exciting prospect for insect studies because implantation surgery, even in very large insects that can approach the size of a small mouse, presents problems somewhat more complicated in my opinion than surgery in mammals (Redfern 1984).

For the future, we need to continue to develop systems for release of materials in a fashion consistent with the concepts already outlined for chronotherapy in medicine by Halberg et al. (1981), Scheving et al. (1977) and other chronobiologists. Specific modifications and refinements will depend on the application of the technique.

REFERENCES

1. Halberg, F., D.K. Hayes, E.W. Powell and L.E. Scheving: Preface in XIII Intl. Conf. Proc., Halberg, Scheving, Powell and Hayes (eds). The Publ. House Il Ponte, Milan, Italy, 1981.
2. Feldmesser, J., H. Jaffe, P.A. Giang and G. Wolfhard: Experimental controlled-release formulations of a nematicidal amine. Proc. 8th Intl. Symp. on Controlled Release of Bioactive Materials, Ft. Lauderdale, Florida, 1981.
3. Jaffe, H.. D.K. Hayes, D.E. Sonenshine, W.H. Dees and M.J. Thompson: Controlled release reservoir systems for the delivery of insect steroid analogues against ticks. Proc. 10th Intl. Symp. on Controlled Release of Bioactive Materials, San Francisco, California, 1983.
4. Jaffe, H., D.K. Hayes, P.A. Giang, R.O. Drummond and T.M. Whetstone: Injectable formulations for the controlled release of pesticides against ticks on cattle. Proc. 1977 Controlled Release Symposium, Corvallis, Oregon, 1977.
5. Jaffe, H., D.E. Sonenshine, D.K. Hayes, W.H. Dees, M. Beveridge and M.J. Thompson: Effects of the controlled release of ecdysteroids on the development and sex pheromone activity in ticks. Proc. 11th Intl. Symp.

on Controlled Release of Bioactive Materials, Ft. Lauderdale, Florida, 1984.
6. Miller, J.A., F.W. Knapp, R.W. Miller and C.W. Pitts: Sustained-release boluses containing methoprene for control of the horn fly and face fly. The Southwest. Entomol. 4:195-200, 1979.
7. Miller, J.A. and R.W. Miller: Sustained-release bolus formulations containing insect growth regulators for control of livestock pests. Proc. 1978 Controlled Release of Bioactive Materials Symposium, Gaithersburg, Maryland, 1978.
8. Miller, R.W. and J.A. Miller: Feed-through chemicals for insect control in animals. Proc. Agricultural Chemicals of the Future BARC Symp. No. 8, 1983, J.A. Hilton (ed). Rowman and Allanheld, Pubs., Chap. 27, pp. 355-363, 1985.
9. Redfern, R.E., D.K. Hayes, J.D. Warthen, Jr., A.B. DeMilo and T.P. McGovern: Responses of nymphs of the large milkweed bug and pupae of the yellow mealworm to three compounds affecting insect growth. Annual Review of Chronopharmacology, Vol. 1, pp. 239-242, Pergamon Press, 1984.
10. Scheving, L.E., E.R. Burns, J.E. Pauly, F. Halberg and E. Haus: Survival and cure of leukemic mice after optimization of cancer treatment with cyclophosphamide and arabinosyl cytosine. Cancer Res. 37:3648-3655, 1977.

DISCLAIMER
Mention of a commercial product does not imply endorsement by the USDA.

ELECTROPHYSIOLOGICAL RECORDINGS FROM CILIATES

L. JONSSON AND O. SAND, Department of Physiology, University of Iceland, Grensasvegur 12, Reykjavik, Iceland

Several species of ciliates have been extensively used as model systems for studying a variety of physiological and biochemical phenomena (1). Many of these phenomena have electrophysiological correlates, like for instance control of ciliary movements, mechanoreception, chemokinetic behavior and morphological transformation (2,3,4,5,6). It may therefore be of interest to record electrophysiological parameters in chronobiological studies. On this background we will describe a simple method for intracellular recordings from ciliates.

Two different methods have mainly been used for immobilization of the animal before microelectrode impalement of ciliates. The animals may be confined to a small volume of medium, causing the swimming speed to be retarded due to compression by the surface film of the drop. A selected animal is then penetrated by a microelectrode, and possibly by an additional microneedle to keep the animal in position. Normal conditions are then restored by adding medium to the drop. This method was first developed for Paramecium using a hanging drop, making it possible to employ an ordinary microscope (7). However, the technique is simpler using an inverted microscope (4).

In addition to movement by cilia, ciliates contain contractile filaments and are able to alter their body shape (8). This ability is particularly pronounced in some species, like for instance Tetrahymena, which makes it difficult to keep the animals on the microelectrode. This problem is solved using a suction pipette to catch and hold the animal (9). This is easily performed by using an inverted microscope and suitable micromanipulators. The animals may be caught under normal conditions, without retarding the swimming speed. This method may of course also be beneficial for animals with a more rigid body structure, like for instance Paramecium.

Figure 1 presents the technique we are using to record from Tetrahymena. The suction pipette has a tip diameter of about 10 μm, and is connected to either ambient-, subatmospheric- or superatmospheric pressures via a solenoid valve (Mecman, 4431). The subatmospheric pressure is obtained using an air-jet vacuum pump. The suction pipette, which is filled with medium, is positioned centrally in the field of view at a sutable distance above the bottom of the recording chamber. An animal is then brought in position using the controls of the microscope stage. During this procedure the pipette is connected to ambient pressure. When the animal path is

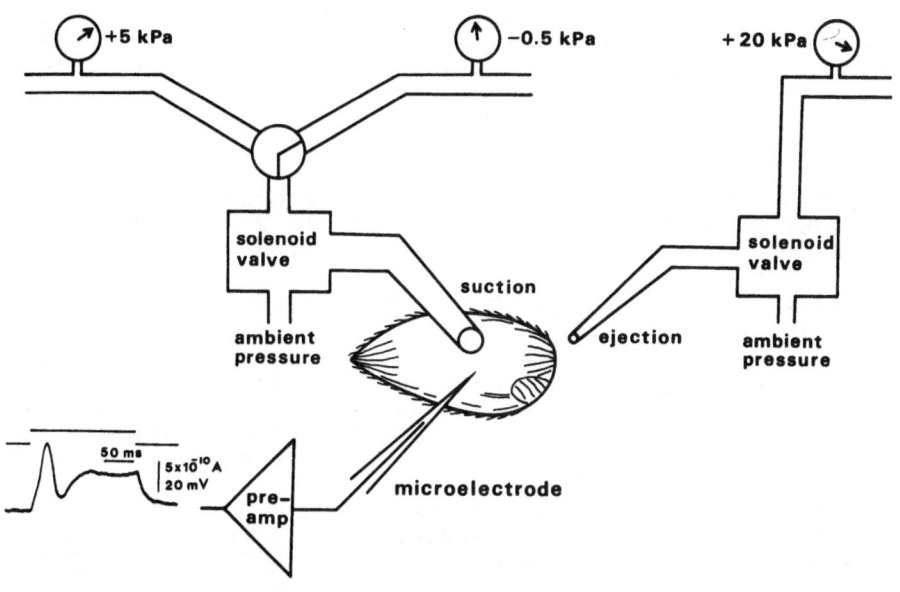

FIGURE 1. Sketch of the experimental set-up. See text for details.

crossing right underneath the tip of the pipette, the solenoid valve is activated using a manual trigger. The animal is then instantly sucked on to the tip of the pipette. The subatmospheric catching pressure is -1 to -1.5 kPa, whereas the holding pressure during the recordings is reduced to -0.5 kPa. The animals are coated with a gel-like material, which easily clogs the pipette. Between each catch the pipette is therefore cleaned by a short flush of medium through the tip. This is obtained by connecting the pipette to a pressure of about +5 kPa.

For chemical stimulation, a similar system may be used for ejecting different solutions on to the surface of the animal (10). To minimize leakage of solution from the ejection pipette between stimulations, the tip diameter should not exceed 5 μm.

The microelectrodes we usually employ for cell penetrations are filled from behind with 4M potassium-acetate adjusted to pH 7.2 by acetic acid. An electrode resistance between 40 and 60 MΩ is suitable for recordings from ciliates. To facilitate the impalement of the cell the electrode holder is attached to a piezoelectric stepper (Physik Instrumente, P-2020). The electrode is connected to standard recording equipment, including a high impedance preamplifier with a bridge circuit for current injection through the recording electrode. The insert in Figure 1 shows an example of the action potential-like on responses to depolarizing current injections in the microstome form of Tetrahymena vorax.

REFERENCES

1. Levandowsky M and S H Hutner(eds): Biochemistry and Physiology of Protozoa. New York: Academic Press Inc, 1979.
2. Eckert R : Bioelectric control of cilia. Science 176, 473-481, 1972.
3. Naitoh Y : Bioelectric basis of behavior in protozoa. Am. Zoologist 14, 883-893, 1974.
4. Van Houten J : Membrane Potential Changes During Chemokinesis in Paramecium, Science, 204, 1979.
5. Machemer, H and S Machemer-Röhnish: Mechanical and electrical correlates of mechanoreceptor activation of the ciliated tail in Paramecium. J. Comp. Physiol.154 A, 273-278. 1984.
6. Jonsson, L, O Sand, T Ö Jonassen and E M Grelland : Microstome-macrostome transformation in Tetrahymena vorax is associated with altered electrical membrane properties. Acta Physiologica Scandinavica, 123, 28A, 1985.
7. Naitoh Y and R Eckert: Electrical properties of Paramecium caudatum: modification by bound and free cations. Z. Vergl. Physiol., 61, 427-452. 1968.
8. Huang B and D Mazia: Microtubules and filaments in ciliate contractility. In Molecules and Cell Movement. (Eds: S Inoué and R E Stephans) 389-409. New York: Raven Press. 1975.
9. Connolly J G and G A Kerkut: The membrane potentials of Tetrahymena vorax. Comp. Biochem. Physiol., 69 C, 265-273, 1981.
10. McCaman R E, D G McKenna and J K Ono : A pressure system for intracellular and extracellular ejections of picoliter volumes. Brain Res., 136, 141-147, 1977.

SUBJECT INDEX

438

AUTHOR INDEX

442

450

LIST OF PARTICIPANTS

Dr. David R. Armstrong, Dir.
Reynolds Medical Ltd.
Cawthorne House
51, St. Andrew St.
Hertford, SG14 1HZ, UK

Dr. Ivan Bourgeois, Dir. of
Research & Support Ctr., EAME
MEDTRONIC BV
Wenckebachstraat 10 6466 NC
Kerkrade-W
THE NETHERLANDS

Asst. Prof. Marco Cavallini
Staff Surgeon
1 Istituto Di Clinica
Chirurgica, Policlinico Umberto I
00161 Rome, ITALY

Dr. Robin G. Clugston
Infusion Pump Coor.
Eli Lilly
Kingsclere Rd., Basingstoke
HAMPSHIRE, RG21 2XA, UK

Dr. Germaine Cornelissen
Research Associate
Univ. of Minnesota, Chrono. Labs.
5-187 Lyon Laboratories
420 Washington AV. S.E.
Minneapolis, MN 55455, USA

Dr. Pietro Cugini, Assoc. Prof. of
Endocrinol./Pathophysiol.
II Clinica Medica, Univ. of Rome
Policlinico Umberto I
00161, Rome
ITALY

Professor Esref Deniz
Head of Med. Biol. Dept.
Faculty of Medicine
University of Ankara
Sihhiye, Ankara, TURKEY

Professor Jean De Prins
Universite Libre de Bruxelles
Stanley 7
B1980 Tervuren
BELGIUM

Dr. Philip De Quae
Universiteit Antwerpen
Unwersiteitsplein 1B-2610
Wilrijh, BELGIUM

Dr. Charles F. Ehret
Senior Scientist
Division of Biol & Med. Res.
Argonne Natl. Laboratory
Argonne, IL 60439, USA

Dr. Dorothy M. Ehret
General Chronobionics
Administrative Asst.
453 South Madison St.
Hinsdale, IL 60521, USA

Dr. Robert E. Fischell
Chief of Technology Transfer
Johns Hopkins University
Applied Physics Laboratory
Laurel, MD 20901, USA

Dr. Simon Folkard
MRC Perceptual & Cognitive
Performance Unit,
Laboratory of Experimental Psychology
Univ. of Sussex Falmer,
Brighton, BN1 9QG,UK

Dr. Robert M. Goodman, Asst. Prof.
Dept. of Physiol. & Biophy.
Hahnemann Univ.
Broad & Vine Sts.
Philadelphia, PA 19102, USA

Mr. Kerry Gordon. Res. Asst.
Dept. of Mathematics
Univ. of Nottingham
University Park
Nottingham, UK

Ms. Carolyn Gorman
Research Assistant
Johns Hopkins Univ.
601 N. Broadway St.
Baltimore, MD 21205   U.S.A.

Professor Keith Griffiths, Dir.
Tenovus Inst. for Cancer Res.
Univ. of Wales, Coll. of Med.
Cardiff CF4 4XX, UK

Dr. Pierre Guiot
Clinical Eval. Eng.
Medtronic BV
1- Wenckebacjstraat 6466
NC Kerkrade
THE NETHERLANDS

Erna Halberg
Chronobiology Laboratories
University of Minnesota
5-187 Lyon Laboratories
Minneapolis, MN 55455,USA

Professor Franz Halberg
Director, Chronobiol. Labs
University of Minnesota
5-187 Lyon Laboratories
Minneapolis, MN 55455, USA

Professor Erhard Haus
Department of Anatomic &
Clinical Pathology
St Paul-Ramsey Hosp. & Med. Ctr.
St. Paul, MN 55101, USA

Dora K. Hayes, Chief
Livestock Insects Lab.
Room 120, Bldg. 307
BARC - East
Beltsville, MD 20705,USA

Professor Martin Healey
Dept. of Microprocessor Eng.
University College
Newport Rd.
Cardiff, CF2 1TA, UK

Ramon C. Hermida , Res. Fellow
Univ. of Minnesota
5-187 Lyon Labs.
420 Washington AV, S.E.
Minneapolis, MN 55455, USA

Dr. Guy Hoffman Service
Psychiatric de 1' hopital
Service Brugmann
Rue van Obbergehen 58
1140 Brussels, BELGIUM

Dr. William Hrushesky, Asst. Prof.
Box 414, Mayo Memorial Bldg.
Univ. of Minnesota
Minneapolis, MN 55455, USA

Mr. Frank Johnson, Technical Mgr.
Oxford Medical Systems Ltd.
1, Kimber Rd., Abingdon
Oxon. OX14 1BZ
UK

Dr. Logi Jonsson, Asst. Prof.
Dept. of Physiology
Univ. of Iceland
Grensasvegur 12
Reykjavik, ICELAND

Martin S. Knapp, Professor
Unit of Medical Inform. Tech.
Univ. Hospital
Queens Medical Centre
Nottingham, NG7 2UH, UK

Priv-Doz. Dr. Peter Knauth
Institut fur Arbeitsphysiol.
an der Universitat Dortmund
Ardeystrasse 67
D-4600 Dortmund 1
WEST GERMANY

Periklis Y. Ktonas, Assoc Prof.
Electrical Engineering Dept.
Univ. of Houston, Univ. Park
Houston, TX 77004
USA

Dr. David V. Land
Natural Philosophy Dept.
University of Glasgow
Glasgow G 12 8 QQ

Dr. Charles N. Leach, Jr.
Director Cardiology
New Britain General Hospital
New Britain, CT 06050 USA

Michele Lucente, Asst. Prof.
Dept. of Cardiology
Catholic Univ
Largo Agostino Gemilli 8
00168 Rome, ITALY

452

Charles A. Marsden, Reader
Dept. of Physiol. & Pharmacol.
Nottingham Univ. Med. School
Nottingham, NG7 2UH
UK

Verlin R. McCall
Mgr. of Product Applications Res.
Del Mar Avionics
1601 Alton Ave. at Red Hill
Irvine, CA 92714, USA

Paul Meis, Assoc. Professor
Dept. of OB/GYN
Bowman Gray School of Medicine
300 So. Hawthorn Rd.
Winston-Salem, NC 27103
USA

Jacques Mirouze, Prof. of Med.
Hospital Lapeyronie
F34059 Montpellier Cedex
FRANCE

Rudolf Moog, Wissen-Angst
Institut fur Arbeitsphysiol.
forschung der Universitat,
Robert-Koch-Strasse 7a
D-3550 Marburg Lahn, W. GERMANY

David R. Owens, Honor. Lect.
Dept. of Medicine
Univ. of Wales Coll. of Med.
Heath Park, Cardiff, CF2 ITA
UK

Professor John E. Pauly
Vice Chan. for Acad. Affairs
Univ. of Arkansas for Med. Sci.
4301 W. Markham St.
Little Rock, AR 72205, USA

Professor Olga Petre-Quadens
Dept. of Med.
Univesitaire instelling antiwerpen
Universiteitsplein 1B-2610 Wilrijk
BELGIUM

Karel Philippens, Senior Lecturer
Dept. of Anatomy, Div. 1
Medizinische Hochschule Hannover
Konstanty-Gutschow-Strasse 8
D-3000 Hannover 61, WEST GERMANY

Antonio G. Rebuzzi, Researcher
Catholic University
Largo Argostino Gemilli 8
00168 Rome, ITALY

Dr. Daniel P. Redmond, Chief
Dept. of Behavioural Biology
Walter Reed Army Inst. of Research
Washington, DC 20307
USA

Dr. Alain Reinberg
Director of Research, CNRS
Fondation A. de Rothschild
29 Rue Manin
75940 Paris Cedex 19, FRANCE

Professor Wop J. Rietveld
Department Head, Physiology
Wassenaarseweg 62
2333 Al Leiden
THE NETHERLANDS

Dr. Salvatore Romano
Assoc. Prof. of Medical Physics
Institute of Medical Physics
Univ. of Florence, Viale Morgogni 85,
50134 Florence, ITALY

Paolo Scarpelli, Director
Postgrad. Med. Sch., Nephrology
Institute of Clinica Medica II
University of Florence
Viale Pieraccini 18
50100 Florence, ITALY

Dr. Lawrence E. Scheving
Rebsamen Prof., Anatomical Sci.
Univ. of Ark. for Medical Sci.
4301 W. Markham St.
Little Rock, AR 72205 USA

Hugh Simpson
Pathology
Royal Infirmiry
Glasgow, GF4 0SF,
UK

Michael H. Smolensky, Assoc. Prof.
Environmental Physiology
University of Texas
Health Science Ctr. @ Houston
Houston, TX 77225, USA

Felix Theeuwes
Vice President of Research
Alza Corporation
950 Page Mill Rd.
Palo Alto, CA 94303 USA

Dr. Peter L. Truran
Salivary Steroid Lab.
Tenovus Int. for Cancer Res.
University of Wales, Coll. of Med.
Heath Park, Cardiff, CF4 4XX UK

Dr. Kirt Vener, Health Sci. Admin.
NIADDK, Westwood Bldg., Rm. 3A16
Natl. Institutes of Health
Bethesda, MD 20205, USA

Richard F. Walker
Steroid Assay Res. Lab.,
Tenovus Inst Cancer Research
Univ. of Wales, Coll. of Medicine
Cardiff, CF 4XX
UK

Michael Weber
Hypertension Ctr. (W130)
V.A. Medical Ctr.
5901 E. 7th Street
Long Beach, CA 90822 USA

Jeffrey M. Williams
Drug Admin. Devices & Systems
Medtronic, Inc.
6972 Old Central Ave. N.E.
Minneapolis, MN 55432, USA

Douglas W. Wilson
Head of Chronobiology
Tenovus Institue for Cancer Res.
Univ. of Wales College of Med.
Cardiff, CF4 4XX, UK

Dr. J. Stuart Woodhead
Reader in Endorcine Biochem.
Univ. of Wales College of Med.
Cardiff, CF4 4XN, UK

Anthony F. Yapel, Jr., Tech. Mgr.
Biomaterials Research
Biosciences Lab. Bldg. 270-2A-08
3M Company, 3M Center
St. Paul, MN 55144 USA

P. Schoenfeld
Erasmus Hospital
Boulevard des Invalides 109
1160 Brussels
Belgium